TOUGH CALLS
— *in* —
Interventional Cardiology

An Instructional Atlas

Edited by

Robert D. Safian, M.D.
Director, Interventional Cardiology
William Beaumont Hospital
Royal Oak, Michigan

Mark Freed, M.D.
Interventional Cardiologist
William Beaumont Hospital
Royal Oak, Michigan

— 1997 —

PHYSICIANS' PRESS

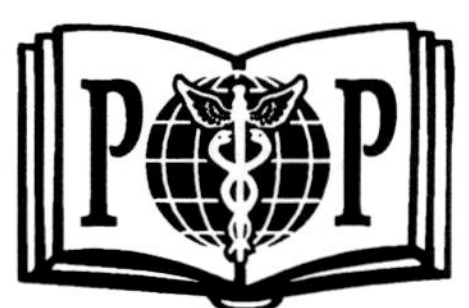

BIRMINGHAM, MICHIGAN

About Physicians' Press

Physicians' Press is a unique entry into the medical publishing industry. Owned and operated by physicians, Physicians' Press specializes in innovative and user-friendly manuals, textbooks, and newsletters in the fields of Interventional Cardiology, Clinical Cardiology, and Internal Medicine. Physicians' Press stands apart from all other medical publishers in being able to produce completely current publications, with literature references ***less than 1 week old*** at the time of book release, compared to 18 months old for most other texts! We frequently receive comments such as "I am astounded at how current your information is," and, "The only books I bother reading are yours, the rest are outdated." Physicians' Press is committed to providing its readers with the most current, practical, and user-friendly information, as we continue to distinguish ourselves as the new gold-standard in medical publishing.

Comments and suggestions should be referred to:

Physicians' Press
555 South Woodward Ave., Suite 1409
Birmingham, Michigan 48009
Tel: (810) 645-6443
Fax: (810) 642-4949

Printed in the United States of America ISBN 0-9633886-6-5

Dedication

To my family (my wife Maureen and my sons Luke and Ryan), my friends, and my interventional colleagues, who provided encouragement, support, and advice.

– Rob Safian

To my family with love, for believing in me when no one else would listen to me, for loving me when no one else would tolerate me, and for reminding me to relax (at least one hour a week).

– Mark Freed

List of Contributors

Donald Baim, MD
Professor of Medicine
Harvard Medical School
Chief, Interventional Cardiology Section
Beth Israel Hospital
Boston, MA

John Bittl, MD
Associate Professor of Medicine, Harvard Medical School; Director, Interventional Cardiology, Brigham & Women's Hospital, Boston, MA

Antonio Colombo, MD
Director, Cardiac Catheterization Laboratory, Columbus Hospital Milan, Italy; Director, Investigational Angioplasty, Lenox Hill Hospital, New York, NY

Michael Cowley, MD
Professor of Medicine, Medical College of Virginia, Richmond, VA

John Douglas Jr., MD
Associate Professor of Medicine/ Cardiology; Co-Director, Cardiac Catheterization Laboratory, Emory University Hospital, Atlanta, GA

Raimund Erbel, MD
Professor of Internal Medicine/Cardiology; Director, Department of Cardiology, University-GHS-Essen, Germany

David Faxon, MD
Professor of Medicine; Chief, Division of Cardiology, University of Southern California School of Medicine, Los Angeles, CA

David Foley, MD
Director, Cardiac Catheterization Laboratory, Erasmus University, Rotterdam, Netherlands

Barry George, MD
Associate Professor of Medicine, Ohio State University, Columbus, OH

Cindy Grines, MD
Director, Cardiac Catheterization Laboratory, William Beaumont Hospital, Royal Oak, MI

Richard Heuser, MD
Director, Interventional Cardiology; Director, Research and Education, Arizona Heart Institute and Foundation, Phoenix, AZ

David Holmes, MD
Director, Adult Cardiac Catheterization Laboratory, Mayo Clinic, Rochester, MN

Dean Kereiakes, MD
Director, The Carl & Edyth Lindner Center for Clinical Cardiovascular Research; Professor of Medicine, The University of Cincinnati College of Medicine, Cincinnati, OH

Morton Kern, MD
Professor of Internal Medicine;
Director, J.G. Mudd Cardiac
Catheterization Laboratory,
St. Louis University Health Sciences
Center, St. Louis, MO

Ferdinand Kiemeneij, MD
Amsterdam Hospital, Department of
Interventional Cardiology,
The Netherlands

Takeshi Kimura, MD
Department of Cardiology, Kokura
Memorial Hospital, Kitakyushu, Japan

Spencer King III, MD
Professor of Medicine/Cardiology;
Director, Interventional Cardiology,
Emory University Hospital,
Atlanta, GA

Martin Leon, MD
Director, Cardiovascular Research,
Washington Hospital Center,
Washington, DC

Frank Litvack, MD
Co-Director, Cardiovascular Intervention
Center, Cedars-Sinai Medical Center,
Los Angeles, CA

Bernhard Meier, MD
Professor and Head of Cardiology,
University Hospital, Geneva, Switzerland

Michael Mooney, MD
Director, Interventional Cardiology,
Minneapolis Heart Institute,
Minneapolis, MN

Marie-Claude Morice, MD
ICPS L'Angio, Centre Cardiologique du
Nord, Saint-Denis, France

Richard Myler, MD
Clinical Professor of Medicine,
University of California; Medical Director,
San Francisco Heart Institute,
Daly City, CA

Masakiyo Nobuyoshi, MD
Vice Medical Director; Chairman of Heart
Center; Director, Department of
Cardiology, Kitakyushu, Japan

William O'Neill, MD
Chief, Division of Cardiology, William
Beaumont Hospital, Royal Oak, MI

Ian Penn, MD
Director, Interventional Cardiology,
Vancouver General Hospital, Vancouver,
British Columbia, Canada

Nicolaus Reifart, MD
Professor of Medicine, Red Cross Hospital
& Heart Center, Frankfurt, Germany

Gary Roubin, PhD, MD
Professor of Medicine, Radiology;
Director, Interventional Cardiology and
Cath Laboratory, University of Alabama-
Birmingham, Birmingham, AL

Timothy Sanborn, MD
Professor of Medicine; Director, Cardiac
Catheterization Laboratory, New York
Hospital-Cornell Medical Center,
New York, NY

Richard Schatz, MD
Research Director, Cardiovascular
Intervention, Scripps Clinic & Research
Foundation, LaJolla, CA

Patrick Serruys, PhD, MD
Professor, Interventional Cardiology,
Erasmus University, Rotterdam,
The Netherlands

Ulrich Sigwart, MD
Director, Department of Invasive Cardiology, Royal Brompton Hospital, London, England

Paul Teirstein, MD
Director, Interventional Cardiology, Scripps Clinic & Research Foundation, LaJolla, CA

Eric Topol, MD
Chairman & Professor, Department of Cardiology; Director, Joseph J. Jacobs Center for Thrombosis and Vascular Biology, The Cleveland Clinic Foundation, Cleveland, OH

Patrick Whitlow, MD
Director, Interventional Cardiology, The Cleveland Clinic Foundation, Cleveland, OH

David Williams, MD
Director, Cardiovascular Laboratory and Interventional Cardiology, The Rhode Island Hospital, Providence, RI

Preface

The explosive growth of interventional hardware has made it extremely difficult to stay abreast of all the latest techniques and strategies. Journal articles and textbooks are helpful, but the information is often outdated by the time of publication. Interventional conferences are also of value, but it is impossible to keep track of "who said what," given the more than 500,000 possible combinations of lesion type, device type and technique, and adjunctive imaging and pharmacotherapy. While a few studies exist to help guide therapy, the interventional clinician's best friends remain experience, judgement, and intuition.

In planning **TOUGH CALLS in Interventional Cardiology**, we hoped to develop an instructional atlas that would be interesting, informative, easy-to-read, and uniquely practical. We did not intend to develop an encyclopedia of information, but rather a grass-roots, nitty-gritty approach to common (and some uncommon) problems that interventional clinicians face on a daily basis.

If we had all the right answers, we would gladly offer them to you. Unfortunately, we do not. We can, however, offer the insights of 35 renowned interventional cardiologists, who have graciously provided their experienced opinions and recommendations to more than 200 challenging cases. Rather than simply present a "show-and-tell" of pretty pictures before and after intervention, we asked our contributors to "think-out-loud," and to express their cognitive decision-making as if a referring physician was asking their opinion. **TOUGH CALLS** allows you to appreciate areas of 'Consensus & Controversy' among this expert staff of high-volume interventionalists, with regard to patient triage, device selection and technique, hemodynamic support, adjunctive imaging and drug therapy, and clinical follow-up. In addition to extensive discussions about newer interventional devices, our contributors offer specific recommendations for interventionalists who perform only conventional balloon angioplasty, thus providing something for everyone.

TOUGH CALLS is divided into 6 sections: In Section 1 (Lesion-Specific Intervention) and Section 2 (Device-Specific Techniques), our contributors detail their interventional strategy and device technique to a wide range of challenging cases. Section 3 (Ischemic Syndromes) and Section 4 (High-Risk Patients) deal with specific clinical syndromes (e.g., acute MI, LV dysfunction, single patent vessel), with emphasis on device selection, hemodynamic support, and patient triage to surgery vs. medical therapy vs. percutaneous intervention. Section 5 (Suboptimal Results) and Section 6 (Miscellaneous) cover a variety of technical problems (e.g., undilatable lesion), complications (e.g., dissection, acute closure, perforation), and mishaps (e.g., stent embolization), representing many of the "Tough Calls" we face every day in the cath lab. The angiographic images are real and mostly represent our own cases; some cases were provided by friends at other institutions, who are acknowledged throughout the atlas. The clinical histories are essentially true, although some of the details have been modified to emphasize certain teaching points, inject a little humor, and break-up the monotony of viewing multiple angiograms. Each case is followed by a brief editorial perspective, which includes pertinent results of a recent survey we performed on the practice patterns of many of the contributors in the atlas.

TOUGH CALLS in Interventional Cardiology represents the latest entry into the Physicians' Press Interventional Library, which includes **The New Manual of Interventional Cardiology**, **The New Manual of Interventional Cardiology Slide Series**, and **The Device Guide**. These complementary publications have been developed to provide the latest information, step-by-step instruction, and insight into advanced clinical decision making.

We hope you enjoy reading **TOUGH CALLS in Interventional Cardiology**, and find it a practical resource for patient care.

Robert D. Safian, MD
Mark Freed, MD

Acknowledgments

"Tough Calls!" would not have been possible without the enormous contribution of the 35 interventional cardiologists from around the world who participated in this atlas. We are deeply indebted to these individuals, who took time from their busy practices to offer their treatment recommendations. We would also like to thank Dianna Frye, who painstakingly collated all of the recommendations for each case, typed the entire text, and formatted all of the pages. Finally, an atlas is only as good is its image quality; we thank Steven Kronenberg at Imprint Graphic Design and the Photography Staff of William Beaumont Hospital and for their time and expertise in preparing the angiographic images.

Notice

The explosive growth of new equipment and drug therapy has resulted in the rapid evolution and acceptance of practice patterns often based on retrospective nonrandomized data and personal experience. Their ultimate role will require close inspection of prospective randomized trials. The clinical recommendations set forth in this book are those of the authors; they are offered as *general guidelines only and are not to be construed as absolute indications*. In addition, not all medications have been accepted by the U.S. Food and Drug Administration (USFDA) for usages described in this manual. The use of any drug should be preceded by a careful review of the package insert, which provides indications and dosages as approved by the USFDA. The reader is advised to consult the package insert before using any therapeutic agent. The authors and publisher disclaim responsibility for adverse effects resulting from omissions or undetected errors.

Table of Contents

SECTION 1: LESION-SPECIFIC INTERVENTION

SECTION 2: DEVICE-SPECIFIC TECHNIQUES

Directional Atherectomy Techniques

Rotablator Techniques

ELCA Techniques

SECTION 3: ISCHEMIC SYNDROMES

SECTION 4: HIGH RISK PATIENTS

SECTION 5: SUBOPTIMAL RESULTS

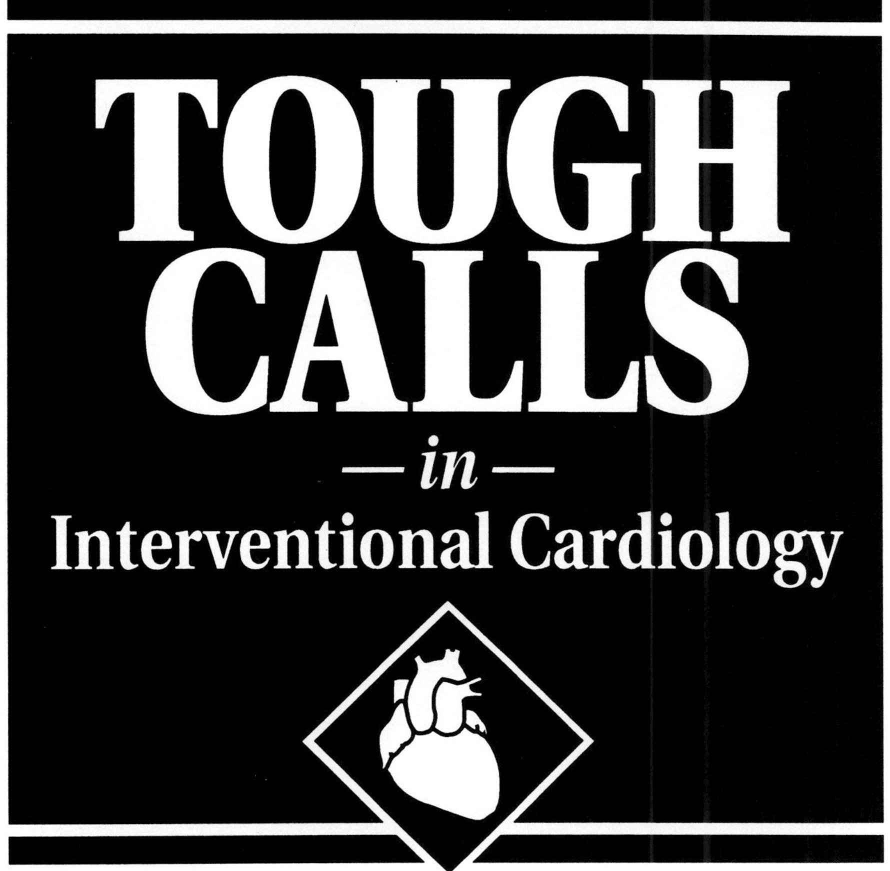

An Instructional Atlas

— Section 1 —

Lesion-Specific Intervention

ECCENTRIC LESION

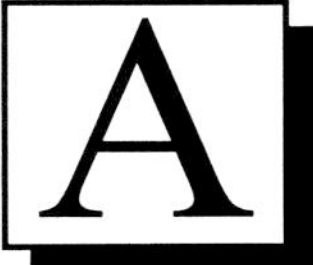

A 55-year-old college professor develops progressive unstable angina after learning that his daughter is president of the Howard Stern fan club. Angiography reveals an eccentric lesion in the mid-LAD (reference diameter = 3.8 mm). Other coronary arteries and left ventricular function are normal.

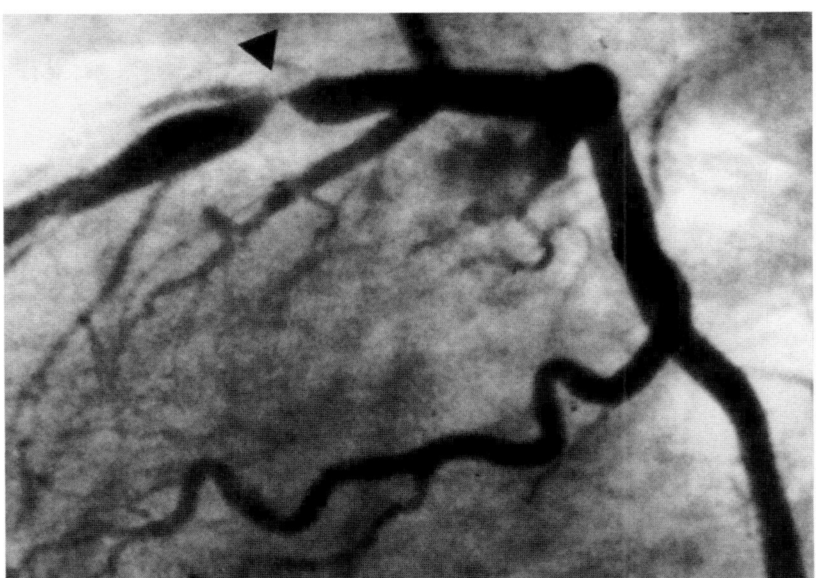

What device would you select to revascularize this patient?

Donald Baim, MD, USA: This patient has unstable angina due to a focal but markedly eccentric lesion in the mid-LAD. Such lesions do poorly with conventional PTCA (in terms of both the acute results and subsequent restenosis), but are very favorably treated by either coronary stenting or directional atherectomy. Assuming that there is no fluoroscopic calcium in this lesion, I favor directional atherectomy as a lower cost procedure with next day discharge.

Marie-Claude Morice, MD, France: This patient has an eccentric lesion in the mid-LAD. Although he has unstable angina, the lesion is smooth and there is no visible thrombus. I prefer stenting this lesion with a Palmaz-Schatz stent or a Nir stent because there are no branches emerging from the lesion, and also to prevent restenosis.

David Faxon, MD, USA: This middle-aged man with unstable angina and clinical indications for revascularization has an eccentric lesion in a large LAD. The lesion is classified by the ACC/AHA Classification as Type B1. While in the past this may have been considered a higher risk lesion, any type of interventional therapy should be successful. However, given the extreme eccentricity, either directional atherectomy or primary stenting is preferable. Since primary stenting is more reliable and more likely to result in a large final lumen, I favor stenting over directional atherectomy. Given the eccentric nature of the lesion, other devices such as TEC, Rotablator, and ELCA are not indicated.

Describe your stent technique and adjunctive medical regimen

Marie-Claude Morice, MD, France: I would perform PTCA with a 0.014-inch Extra-Support guidewire and a 3.5 x 2.0 mm balloon, followed by placement of a Palmaz-Schatz 84 stent crimped on the same balloon, or by a 9 mm Nir stent. This short lesion would be well covered by these short stents. I would use a noncompliant 4.0 x 9-10 mm balloon inflated at 16 ATM to optimize deployment. The procedure would be performed by the femoral approach with a 6F guiding catheter. As with all stents, the patient would receive ticlopidine (250 mg QD) and aspirin (100 mg QD) for one month.

David Faxon, MD, USA: I would use a large-lumen 8F guide and a 0.014-inch x 300 cm Platinum-Plus guidewire. I would predilate with a 3.0 mm balloon followed by implantation of a 4.0 mm Palmaz-Schatz stent, being careful to place the stent just distal to the first septal and diagonal. One concern is that there may be another diagonal emanating from the stenosis, but it is unclear whether or not this would be a technical problem. Following delivery of the stent, I would postdilate with a 4.25 x 10 mm high-pressure balloon and evaluate the results with intravascular ultrasound. If the results are excellent and ultrasound shows good deployment, the medical regimen would be aspirin (325 mg QD) and ticlopidine (250 mg BID). I start antiplatelet therapy several days in advance, so heparinization would be less than 24 hours and the patient would be discharged within 2 days.

Describe your atherectomy technique for this lesion.

Donald Baim, MD, USA: I would position a DVI 10F JL4 guiding catheter and cross the lesion with an ACS 0.014-inch Extra-Support guidewire. Over this wire, I would advance a DVI 7F GTO atherectomy cutter, working in an angiographic view that showed the eccentricity of this lesion to its greatest extent. I would perform initial cuts directed towards the site of maximum eccentric plaque accumulation, beginning at 10-20 PSI and working up to 20-30 PSI depending on tissue retrieval and residual stenosis. If the lumen is anything less than perfect after these atherectomy cuts, I would postdilate using a full-size (balloon/artery ratio = 1) balloon, inflated to 4 ATM. After overnight bedrest, the patient would be discharged the following day on aspirin and a calcium-channel blocker. I do not recommend ReoPro.

David Faxon, MD, USA: One approach is to use a DVI 10F guiding catheter and a 7F Graft AtheroCath, concentrating the cuts on the eccentric portion of the lesion to obtain a residual stenosis < 10%. Directional atherectomy might be preferable to stenting if there is a large diagonal emanating from the lesion. Care needs to be taken so the distal nosecone is in a large and straight portion of the LAD.

What do you recommend for operators who perform only PTCA?

David Faxon, MD, USA: If stenting and directional atherectomy are not options, then PTCA is a reasonable choice. I would start with a slightly undersize balloon (e.g., 3.75 mm) to avoid major dissection, only going to a 4.0 mm balloon if lumen enlargement is suboptimal and a major dissection has not occurred. A perfusion balloon in this setting might be worthwhile if the LAD is large, wraps around the apex, or supplies a large amount of myocardium. In addition, a perfusion balloon would be easy to deliver, might prevent hemodynamic problems during balloon inflation, and would reduce the chance of dissection. Although the EPILOG trial demonstrated efficacy of ReoPro for this type of lesion, my preference is to reserve ReoPro for a suboptimal result ("rescue" ReoPro).

Editors' Perspective: The prevalence of "eccentric" coronary artery stenoses is unknown, and is confounded by varying definitions of "eccentricity" and the fact that more than 60% of lesions appearing concentric by angiography are actually eccentric when examined by intravascular ultrasound. Although most interventionalists would agree that this lesion in the mid-LAD is highly eccentric, there are relatively few data to guide decision-making about proper device selection. Published reports (Table 1) suggest that virtually all devices can be used for eccentric lesions with procedural success rates exceeding 90%. However, since most of these studies failed to differentiate between degrees of eccentricity, it is not certain that equally high success rates could be achieved in highly eccentric lesions such as this one. In fact, the clinical experience (as opposed to published data) of high-volume interventional cardiologists suggests that highly eccentric lesions in large vessels are best approached with directional atherectomy or stenting: In our 1996 survey, nearly 50% of experienced operators would stent such a lesion, and 30% would perform directional atherectomy; the remaining 20% were equally divided between PTCA alone and Rotablator. Dr. Baim raises an important consideration about cost. However, it is likely that in-hospital costs for stenting and directional atherectomy would be similar, provided that adjunctive PTCA was used after atherectomy, and antiplatelet therapy without Coumadin was prescribed after stenting. This patient was treated with directional atherectomy by Dr. Gregory Robertson, and an excellent angiographic result was achieved without adjunctive PTCA (below).

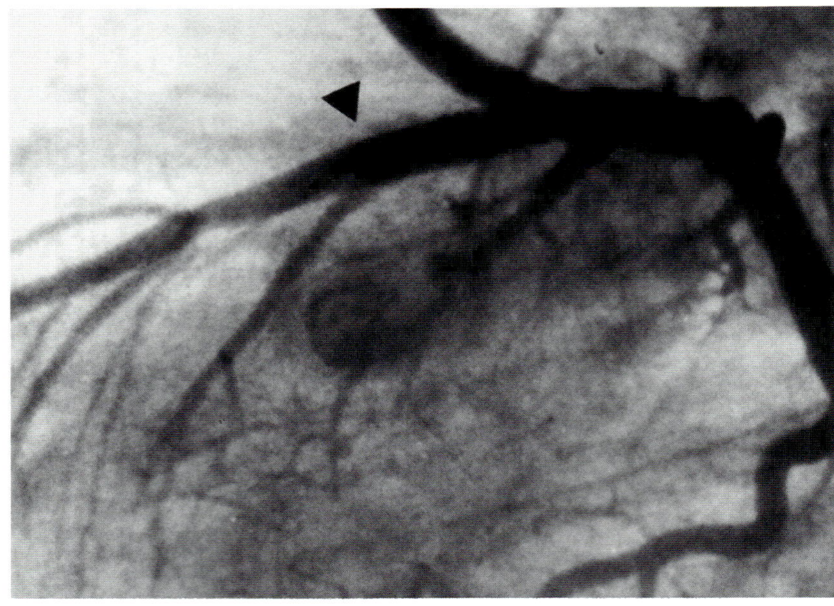

Table 1. Percutaneous Revascularization of Eccentric Stenoses

Series	Modality	Morphology	N	Success+ (%)	Complications* (%)
Tan[824]	PTCA	Concentric	491	93	AC: 2.6
		Eccentric	666	92	3.8
Myler[825]	PTCA	Concentric	304	92	2.6
		Eccentric	475	96	1.1
Popma[833]	DCA	Concentric	71	96	-
		Eccentric	235	94	-
Hinohara[834]	DCA	Concentric	116	92	CABG: 1.7
		Eccentric (mild-mod)	122	86	3.3
		Eccentric (extreme)	85	95	2.4
Warth[835]	Rotablator	Concentric	141	98	0
		Eccentric	205	93	4.4
IVT Registry[836]	TEC	Concentric	207	96	-
		Eccentric	316	92	-
AIS[837] Database	ELCA	Concentric	135	92	-
		Eccentric	174	89	-
Leon[838]	DELCA	Concentric	22	90% overall	Death: 0.9
		Eccentric	110		Q-MI: 0.9
					CABG: 3.8
					AC: 3.8
Ghazzal[839]	DELCA	Extreme eccentricity	62	91%	-

Abbreviations: DCA = Directional Coronary Atherectomy; TEC = Transluminal Extraction Atherectomy; ELCA = Excimer Laser Coronary Angioplasty; DELCA = Direction ELCA; EFS = event-free survival; Q-MI = Q-wave myocardial infarction; CABG = emergency coronary artery bypass grafting; AC = abrupt closure; - = not reported

\+ < 50% residual stenosis after device (and adjunctive PTCA) without death, MI, or emergency CABG

* Single value represents combined incidence of in-hospital death, Q-MI, or emergency CABG, unless otherwise stated

*****

ULCERATED LESION

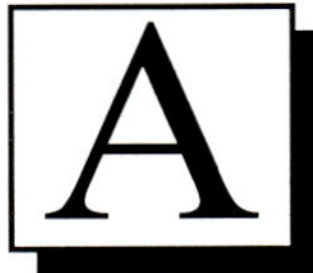

A 58-year-old attorney develops effort angina while running to the courthouse. Angiography reveals a severely ulcerated stenosis in the mid-LAD; moderate proximal and distal lesions are also evident (reference diameter = 3.6 mm). Other coronary arteries and left ventricular function are normal.

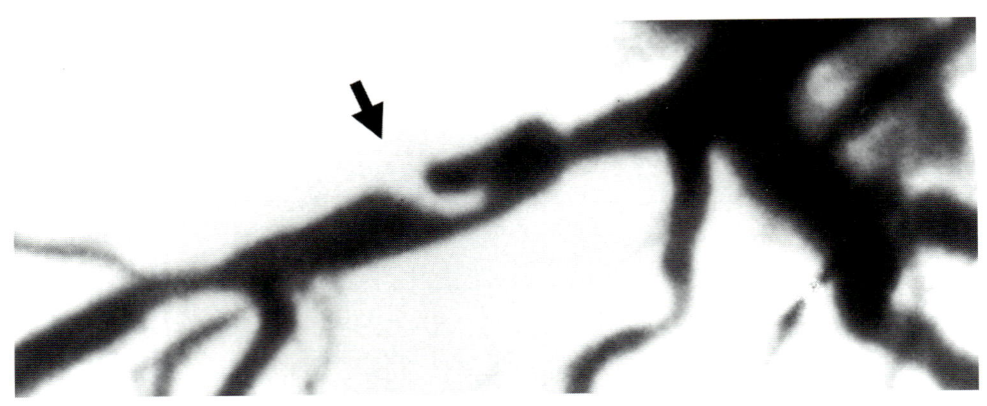

What device would you recommend for this lesion?

Antonio Colombo, MD, Italy: Due to the ulcerated nature of this lesion, I think stent implantation is the best strategy. The ulcerated lesion and the lesion distal to it should both be treated.

Masakiyo Nobuyoshi, MD, Japan: The angiogram shows an ulcerated lesion in a large proximal LAD between the left main trunk and the takeoff of the diagonal branch. Ulcerated lesions adversely affect procedural outcome because of the increased risk of abrupt closure; I recommend stenting. I find that stenting provides excellent angiographic results with very low rates of abrupt closure and restenosis.

John Bittl, MD, USA: The patient has an eccentric lesion in the proximal LAD. As assessed from the angiographic "luminogram," the lesion probably arose from plaque rupture and consists of a flap of intimal tissue or fibrous plaque protruding into the lumen. Conventional PTCA alone is inadequate for this type of lesion because the protruding tissue invariably persists after balloon deflation, leaving a residual stenosis > 50% and a hazy appearance. I recommend primary stenting.

Describe your stent technique and adjunctive medical regimen

Antonio Colombo, MD, Italy: Following placement of a 0.014-inch x 300 cm Extra-Support wire, I would predilate both lesions with a 3.5 mm noncompliant balloon. Two 3.5 mm Palmaz-Schatz stents may be necessary to cover both lesions, but I would deploy the distal stent first. After delivering the second (proximal) stent, an 18 ATM balloon inflation should be performed. It is important to make sure the distal stent completely covers the distal lesion; if more than two stents are needed, stent overlap or a short stent can be considered to avoid covering the proximal diagonal branch. (If the vessel is not tortuous, an alternative approach is to stent from proximal to distal. Using a delivery system, it is usually possible to cross a previously deployed stent, unless it has not been fully deployed). In my experience, inflation at 18 ATM is better than 12 ATM. After a good final result is obtained, the arterial introducer can be removed when the ACT is ≤ 150 seconds. The patient would be treated with long-term aspirin (300 mg QD) and calcium-channel blockers (for 1-2 months); ticlopidine (250 mg BID for 2 weeks) is optional.

Masakiyo Nobuyoshi, MD, Japan: I would perform PTCA with a flexible 0.014-inch x 300 cm guidewire a 3.5 x 20 mm balloon, and place a 3.5 x 15 mm Palmaz-Schatz stent expanded with a 4.0 x 20 mm noncompliant balloon at ≥ 15 ATM. The LAD diameter just proximal to the ulceration is about 3.0 mm, and therefore the initial balloon should be 3.0-3.5 mm. Since the distance from the left main trunk to the second diagonal branch is about 13-15 mm, I would use a 3.5 mm Palmaz-Schatz stent and a 4.0 x 20 mm high-pressure balloon for adjunctive PTCA. After stent deployment, I recommend heparin (10,000-15,000 units/day for 3-5 days), ticlopidine (250 mg BID for 1-3 months), and aspirin (81 mg TID).

John Bittl, MD, USA: I would implant a 3.5 mm Palmaz-Schatz coronary stent using a Cordis 8F 0.086-inch Judkins left short tip guide catheter, an ACS 0.014-inch Hi-torque floppy guidewire, and a 3.5 mm noncompliant balloon inflated at 4 ATM (the same balloon can be used for adjunctive PTCA after stent deployment). The stent should be deployed at 5 ATM, and positioned so the articulation does not "catch" the protruding tissue. After deployment, high-pressure inflation with the 3.5 mm noncompliant balloon should be performed at 18 ATM.

Adjunctive pharmacotherapy should include noncoated aspirin (325 mg QD), ticlopidine (250 mg BID starting at least 48 hours before the procedure), and heparin (12,500 units IV) at the start of the procedure to achieve an ACT > 300 seconds. The sheath should be removed after the procedure when the ACT is < 180 sec. Heparin should be restarted 6 hours after sheath removal, and continued for 36-48 hours if ticlopidine was not started before the procedure.

Would you recommend IVUS?

Antonio Colombo, MD, Italy: If a good angiographic result is obtained (residual stenosis < 10% by visual assessment), an IVUS evaluation should be performed. The smallest cross sectional area inside the stent should be greater than or equal to the cross sectional area of the vessel immediately distal to the stent. I also try to achieve a stent cross sectional area at least 70% of the cross sectional area of a 3.5 mm balloon (the area of a 3.5 mm balloon is 9.6 mm^2; 70% is 6.7 mm^2). If these objectives are not reached, another higher pressure inflation (20-22 ATM) or a bigger (0.25 or 0.5 mm larger) balloon should be used. The decision to use a bigger balloon or higher pressure should be based on the vessel size by IVUS (media to media). The vessel size by IVUS should be used as a reference: Always stay 0.25-0.5 mm below the IVUS reference level when selecting a larger balloon.

Masakiyo Nobuyoshi, MD, Japan: After placing the stent, I recommend ultrasound to corroborate its full expansion. Additional inflations are not necessary unless there is persistent stenosis, in which case high-pressure expansion with a noncompliant balloon is necessary.

Are you concerned about the large diagonal branch?

Antonio Colombo, MD, Italy: The second diagonal branch may be covered by the distal stent; this problem is usually well tolerated. If necessary, a fixed wire system such as a 2.5 mm ACE can be used to dilate the diagonal through the stents struts, and the same balloon can be used to dilate the first diagonal or intermediate branches, if indicated.

Masakiyo Nobuyoshi, MD, Japan: A large second diagonal branch takes off just distal to the ulcerated lesion. Care must be taken so the stent does not obstruct this second diagonal artery, by placing the distal end of the stent just proximal to the origin of the second diagonal artery.

Editors' Perspective: **There are virtually no data to guide therapy for lesions with marked ulceration and abnormal contour, but the consensus appears to strongly favor stenting: In our survey, more than 60% of high-volume interventionalists recommended stenting, 20% recommended PTCA alone, and the remaining 20% were equally divided between directional atherectomy, Rotablator, and TEC. Dr. Richard Schatz often states that when stenting, lesion morphology is a relatively unimportant consideration compared to vessel caliber, inflow, and runoff. We were somewhat surprised that more operators did not select directional atherectomy for this lesion, but suspect that the moderate lesions proximal and distal to the ulcerated target lesion dissuaded many operators from performing atherectomy. In addition, stenting is probably easier than directional atherectomy. PTCA was performed on this lesion in 1989 (before the availability of stents and atherectomy devices) but did not enlarge lumen dimensions (below, middle panel), as predicted by Dr. Bittl, so the patient was treated with laser balloon angioplasty, with an excellent angiographic result (below, right panel). Eight months later, restenosis was treated with directional atherectomy. In contemporary practice, we favor stenting such lesions. For operators who perform PTCA or directional atherectomy, this is the kind of angiographic and clinical scenario in which the use of ReoPro is likely to be beneficial.**

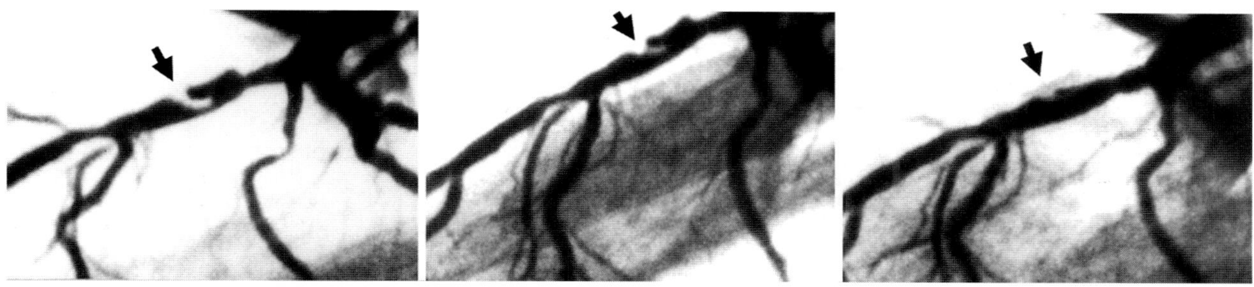

*****

INTRALUMINAL HAZINESS

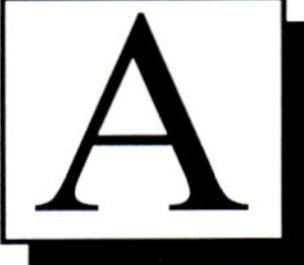

A 65-year-old women suffers a recent non-Q-wave myocardial infarction. A low-level stress test reveals anterior ischemia. Cardiac catheterization demonstrates a significant stenosis in the mid-LAD (reference diameter = 2.9 mm) with intraluminal haziness. Other vessels are normal and left ventricular ejection fraction = 45%.

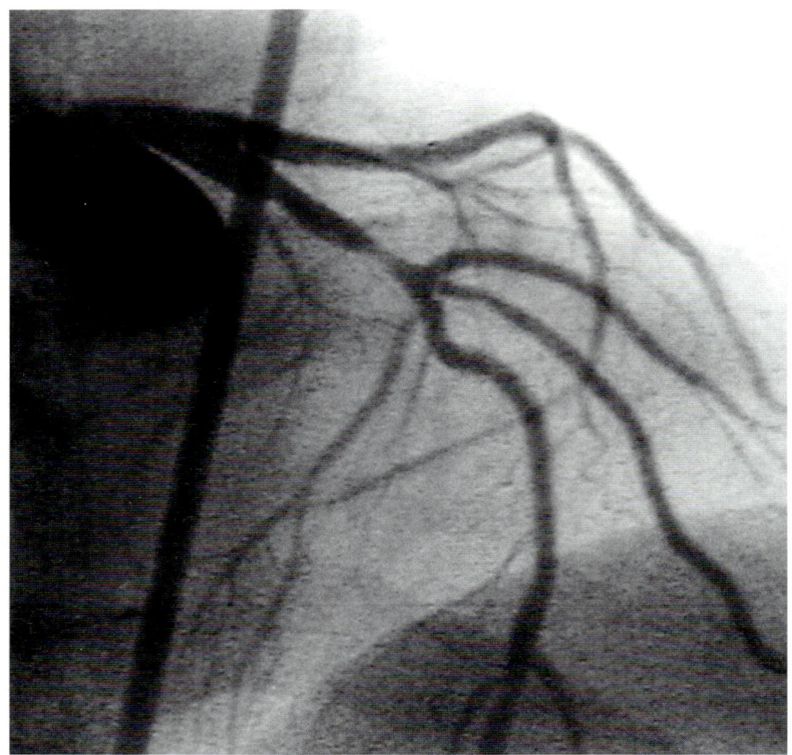

Describe your impression about the intraluminal haziness.

John Douglas Jr., MD, USA: The patient has a severe stenosis; percutaneous revascularization is indicated. It is unclear whether there is intraluminal thrombus; a similar angiographic appearance can be produced by a very eccentric atherosclerotic plaque which becomes evident when the lesion is analyzed in multiple views (in this case a cranial LAO projection would be helpful). If intraluminal haziness is present in other views, thrombus is likely and this factor increases the risk of abrupt closure. I would treat with aspirin and heparin for 3-4 days before intervention, to accelerate thrombolysis and reduce complications.

Ian Penn, MD, Canada: This patient has a hazy stenosis of indeterminate severity at the trifurcation into a septal and diagonal branch. The plaque begins 3 cm from the origin of the LAD. Lesion length is a major predictor of restenosis, especially in the proximal LAD. Intraluminal haziness and lesion at a trifurcation are predictors of abrupt closure, and the myocardial territory at risk is significant.

Michael Cowley, MD, USA: The angiogram shows a high-grade stenosis in the mid-LAD with intraluminal haziness, and there are several large diagonal branches just beyond the lesion, as well as distal tortuosity. The lesion has irregular margins consistent with recent instability, plaque disruption, and residual platelet-fibrin thrombus. This clinical picture and lesion morphology are associated with a higher incidence of acute closure, dissection, distal embolization, and no-reflow.

What device would you recommend?

John Douglas Jr., MD, USA: The trifurcation just beyond the lesion and the smaller, tortuous distal vessel increases the risk of dissection with balloons and other devices. I recommend PTCA with a perfusion balloon, which is simple and cost-effective. In my experience, prolonged inflations are frequently more effective than short inflations in lesions with thrombus.

Ian Penn, MD, Canada: Lesion length, indeterminate stenosis severity, trifurcation lesion, and recent non-Q-wave myocardial infarction should warn the interventionalist that PTCA may cause abrupt closure; I recommend stenting.

Michael Cowley, MD, USA: I recommend directional coronary atherectomy. My results with directional atherectomy for these complex thrombus-containing lesion have been excellent with high success and low complication rates, in contrast to results with PTCA for such lesions.

Describe your technical approach.

John Douglas Jr., MD, USA: I would use a 3.0 x 20 mm Lifestream, positioning the distal end of the balloon proximal to the large septal branch. Because of LAD tortuosity at the tip of the perfusion balloon, I would not withdraw the 0.010-inch guidewire. I would perform a 15 minute inflation, and then observe the vessel for another 15 minutes.

Ian Penn, MD, Canada: The major decision here is which stent to use and how to manage the trifurcation area. A coil stent would provide a margin of error so that inadvertent distal placement would preserve access to the diagonal branches. Alternatively, precise placement of a rigid stent with a double marker balloon would be suitable. I would use a JL4 guide, a 0.014-inch Hi-torque floppy wire, and no wire to protect the diagonal branches. I prefer a double marker balloon to allow precise placement. The lesion length can be measured during predilation. I would deliver the stent so that the distal end is at the trifurcation; it is important to use the same angiographic projection to minimize error. Adjunctive PTCA at 18-20 ATM (balloon/artery ratio ~ 1.15) would be my intended technique.

Michael Cowley, MD, USA: I recommend a 6F GTO AtheroCath and a 0.014-inch Extra-Support wire. I would perform circumferential cuts, starting at 10 PSI and gradually increasing to 30 PSI. I would aim for a final stenosis < 10%, using adjunctive PTCA if needed for residual narrowing or luminal irregularity at the target lesion, with a slightly oversized balloon at 3 ATM.

Are any adjunctive imaging devices useful for this lesion?

Ian Penn, MD, Canada: I use intravascular ultrasound to ensure adequate stent expansion, since underdilation in this location contributes to early and late closure. I do not perform angioscopy routinely after stent placement even in hazy stenoses, but use ultrasound to ensure adequate stent placement, aiming for a minimum stent/artery cross-sectional area ratio of 0.9.

Do you recommend any other adjunctive medical therapies?

John Douglas Jr., MD, USA: If thrombus reforms and does not respond to 3 or 4 prolonged inflations, I would position a 3.0 mm Dispatch catheter at the lesion and infuse urokinase (10,000 units/ml at 0.5 ml/minute for 30 minutes) and repeat the perfusion balloon inflation if needed. If there is definite thrombus during the PTCA, I would use ReoPro (0.25 mg/kg bolus and 0.125 mcg/kg/min for 12 hours). This approach will result in procedural success in 95-98%; no other device or strategy has better initial or long-term results in this setting.

Ian Penn, MD, Canada: Although the presence of thrombus may be a predictor of subacute stent thrombosis, Coumadin has not been shown to be beneficial. I therefore use aspirin alone or aspirin plus ticlopidine, and concentrate on achieving good stent apposition. In this patient, I would use aspirin alone if I obtained a good ultrasound and angiographic result, and I would add ticlopidine if there were any suboptimal findings. The role of ReoPro for suboptimal stent results is unproven.

Michael Cowley, MD, USA: If there was residual thrombus after directional atherectomy, I would give local intracoronary thrombolytic therapy with a 3.0 mm SciMed Dispatch catheter and infuse urokinase (150,000 units over 15 minutes). If distal embolization occurred, selective infusion of urokinase would be given through the balloon, assisted by mechanical fragmentation of the thrombus. If thrombus was confirmed in the lesion by the presence of clot within the excised tissue or evidence of embolization, I would then infuse IV heparin for 24-48 hours; ReoPro would also be desirable to lower the risk of vessel closure.

Editors' Perspective: This case is a difficult one because of the uncertainties associated with intraluminal "haziness." As mentioned by Dr. Douglas, such a finding is nonspecific and may be associated with thrombus or atherosclerotic plaque. Different approaches to this patient reflect different interpretations of intraluminal haziness and its impact on procedural outcome. Although angioscopy can readily differentiate plaque from thrombus, none of the above experts recommended its use. Our impression is that although angioscopy can be useful, it's use is not mandatory, since intraluminal haziness itself is not a compelling angiographic finding. Among the interventionalists surveyed, recommendations included stenting in 50%, PTCA in 36%, and directional atherectomy in 14%. For this particular patient, intravenous ReoPro is certainly reasonable if the patient is treated with PTCA or directional atherectomy; its use as an adjunct to stenting and other devices awaits testing.

*****

THROMBUS

A 65-year-old woman suffers an inferior Q-wave myocardial infarction and 2 episodes of post-infarction angina on day 5, despite continuous IV heparin. The patient never received thrombolytic therapy. Cardiac catheterization demonstrates a subtotal stenosis in the mid-RCA (reference vessel = 3.2 mm) with a moderate intraluminal filling defect. Other vessels are normal and left ventricular ejection fraction = 45% with severe posterobasal hypokinesis.

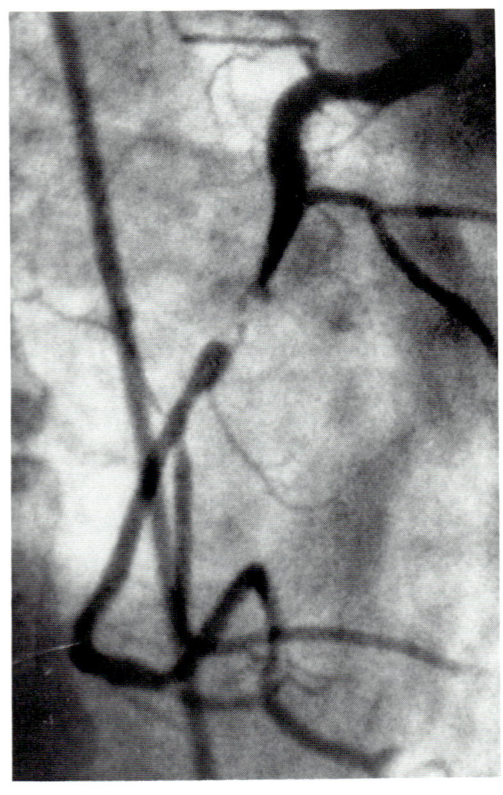

What do you think about the intraluminal filling defect, and what impact does it have?

David Faxon, MD, USA: This case illustrates the dilemma of managing residual thrombus in a patient with recent Q-wave myocardial infarction who continues to have post-infarction angina on IV heparin. The angiographic appearance suggests recanalization of an acute thrombus. The major concern for PTCA alone is that thrombus significantly increases the risk of acute complications. However, studies have shown that even with visible thrombus, PTCA is not associated with increased risk if the patient is pretreated with heparin for at least 3 days. Since this patient has been on heparin for 5 days, I would proceed immediately with PTCA using a 3.5 mm balloon. I would avoid directional atherectomy, laser, or stenting in this setting. However, TEC and the newer thrombectomy catheters may be options for those who have access to these devices.

Gary Roubin, MD, PhD, USA: I would use a Lumax 8F right Judkins guiding catheter, a 0.014-inch Traverse guidewire, and a 3.0 mm semicompliant balloon. I would perform a 3-5 minute inflation at 12-16 ATM. If the lesion looks reasonable after PTCA (residual stenosis < 30% and stable appearance for 5 minutes), I would terminate the case, remove the sheaths the same day, and discharge the patient the next day on aspirin.

Raimund Erbel, MD, Germany: This patient has a complex ulcerated lesion in the RCA. The severe luminal narrowing and distal filling defect suggest that thrombus is present. A higher risk of acute closure, distal embolization, and no re-flow has to be anticipated. I recommend PTCA with a 3.0 x 20 mm Europass.

Do you recommend other adjunctive imaging techniques?

David Faxon, MD, USA: Since the angiographic appearance is quite typical of thrombus, imaging techniques such as angioscopy or intravascular ultrasound are not necessary.

Raimund Erbel, MD, Germany: Intravascular ultrasound should be performed to assess the lesion characteristics and calcification, and guide selection of the appropriate balloon size.

What adjunctive medical therapies would you recommend?

David Faxon, MD, USA: Another adjunct is placement of a Roubin Infusion Catheter, and infusion of urokinase (250,000-500,000 units over 1 hour). Even if significant resolution of the thrombus does not occur, I would proceed with PTCA. ReoPro would also be useful instead of thrombolysis, using a bolus and infusion before PTCA. I would continue the ReoPro infusion for 12 hours and remove the sheaths immediately after the procedure. Ionic contrast affords a little more protection in the presence of significant thrombus, but bradycardia would be significant. Following successful PTCA, at least 24 hours of heparin is important.

Raimund Erbel, MD, Germany: I recommend heparin (15,000 units IV and 3,000 units IC), nitroglycerin (3 mg/hr IV), and intracoronary nitroglycerin. Adjunctive ReoPro should be considered since this is a high-risk lesion.

If a suboptimal result is obtained, is stenting an option?

Gary Roubin, MD, PhD, USA: If the result is suboptimal, I would advance the balloon catheter distal to the lesion, replace the wire with an extra-support guidewire, and implant a 3.5 mm Gianturco-Roubin stent. Adjunctive ReoPro is reasonable. I would postdilate with a 3.5 mm balloon at 14-16 ATM. I would stop heparin, remove the sheaths the same day, and discharge the patient on aspirin (325 mg BID), ticlopidine (250 mg BID), and subcutaneous low molecular weight heparin (30 mg BID for 10 days). I recommend followup angiography within 6 months, and repeat PTCA, if necessary.

Raimund Erbel, MD, Germany: Adjunctive stenting is recommended with a heparin-coated Palmaz-Schatz stent. Apart from aspirin and ticlopidine, no other therapy is prescribed. I recommend IVUS to assess stent alignment with the vessel wall and to identify flaps protruding into the lumen.

If the patient has a recent history of peptic ulcer disease, what approach would you recommend?

David Faxon, MD, USA: If the patient has contraindications to thrombolytics such as active peptic ulcer disease, I would use TEC or PTCA alone, since I anticipate reasonable success.

Gary Roubin, MD, PhD, USA: If the patient has a history of peptic ulcer disease, I would have a higher threshold for placing a stent. If there is a residual stenosis < 50% and TIMI 3 flow, I would depend on PTCA alone (and discharge the patient on enteric-coated aspirin). If the lesion shows marked recoil or threatened closure, I would place a stent but be prepared to stop low molecular weight heparin and ticlopidine if the patient has gastrointestinal bleeding.

Editors' Perspective: Although angiography is relatively insensitive for detecting thrombus, most interventionalists agree that definite globular intraluminal filling defects, especially when identified in multiple projections, are the angiographic hallmarks of thrombus. Over the last several years, a variety of pharmacological and mechanical strategies have been employed, but the optimal therapy for patients with intracoronary thrombus is unknown. PTCA (Table 2) and virtually all atherectomy, laser and stent devices (Table 3) have been associated with greater risk of abrupt closure, no-reflow, and distal embolization in this setting. There seems to be general agreement that the risk of intraprocedural complications can be reduced by treating intracoronary thrombus prior to percutaneous intervention, but there is little agreement on how this should be accomplished. Potential strategies include prolonged pretreatment with aspirin and intravenous heparin; intracoronary or intravenous infusion of thrombolytic drugs (urokinase is usually employed, but tPA has also been used); local delivery of thrombolytic agents; and extraction of thrombus by mechanical devices such as TEC, the AngioJet, or the Hydrolyzer.

As described by Dr. Faxon, the risk of PTCA in thrombus-containing lesions can be reduced by intravenous heparin infusion for 2-14 days followed by inflations with slightly oversized balloons. Intracoronary heparin has also been used, but should be diluted and infused slowly to prevent arrhythmia. Although local delivery of heparin has been shown to decrease platelet deposition in the arterial wall after experimental PTCA, further clinical studies are needed. The ideal duration of heparin infusion after intervention is a matter of debate. Since rebound hypercoagulation after abrupt discontinuation of heparin has been reported, it may be prudent to slowly taper the heparin infusion over 24-72 hours.

Table 2. Impact of Pre-Procedural Thrombus On PTCA Outcome

Series	N (Patients)	Description	Results
White[607]	74	Angioscopic thrombus in 61%	Thrombus group with more in-hospital ischemia (16% vs 10%; p=0.03) and major cardiac events (14% vs 2%, p=0.03).
Mehran[626]	245	Randomized trial of IC urokinase vs. placebo	UK group with more abrupt closure (15% vs. 5.9%; p=0.03) and major cardiac events (17.3% vs. 6.8%; p=0.02).
Hillegass[608]	238	Unstable angina with thrombus	Decreased success (80%); Increased abrupt closure (11%) and CABG (9%).
	1476	Unstable angina without thrombus	PTCA outcome similar to stable angina.
	450	Stable angina	
Tan[609]	46	Thrombus in 3.6% of 1248 lesions	Thrombus group with more abrupt closure (8.7% vs 3.1%; p=0.04).
Violaris[610]	159	Thrombus in 4.5% of 3529 lesions	Thrombus group with more late reocclusion (13.8 vs 5.3%, p<0.001).
Tenaglia[611]	93	Thrombus in 12% of 779 lesions	Thrombus group with more abrupt closure (6.1 fold).
Myler[612]	82	Thrombus in 10.5% of 779 lesions	Thrombus group with more major cardiac events (7.3% vs 1%, p>0.003).
Pavlides[627]	30	IC urokinase: 250,000-500,000 over 20 min; IV urokinase: 250,000-3MU over 30-60 min	Urokinase did not improve PTCA success, but did improve cardiac event rate (19% vs 3%) if thrombus was present.
	27	No urokinase	
Chapekis[628]	21	Continuous IC urokinase (120,000 U bolus, 120,000 U/hr x 24 hrs). IV Heparin: 1000 U/hr.	Distal embolization in 5%. No acute closures.
Kiesz[629]	29	IC urokinase (250,000 U bolus every 5 min, up to 1.5 MU or until thrombus resolves)	Complete resolutions of IC thrombus in 83%; PTCA success in 93%.
Mooney[595]	112	Aspirin, dipyridamole, nifedipine; intraprocedural heparin (IV: 10,000 and IC: 3000U). Balloon: artery ratio = 1.2	Acute closure (7%); nonobstructive residual thrombus (24%); emergency or elective CABG (7%).
Laskey[630]	35	Aspirin, heparin pre-PTCA	PTCA success (94%); acute occlusion (6%)
	18	Aspirin, no heparin pre-PTCA	PTCA success (61%); acute occlusion (33%).

Abbreviations: IC = intracoronary; IV = intravenous; CABG = coronary artery bypass surgery; MU = million units

Table 3. Impact of Thrombus On New Devices

Series	N	Device	Outcome
Grinstead[663]	109	GRS	Angiographic success (84%); post-stent thrombus (27%).
Meany[647]	183	TEC (SVG)	Angiographic success not affected by thrombus.
Dooris[650]	59	TEC (SVG)	Thrombus group with lower clinical success (69% vs. 88%) and more angiographic and clinical complications (no-reflow and Q-wave MI).
Al-Shaibi[646]	124	TEC (SVG)	Less CK elevation compared to PTCA.
Moses[644]	59	TEC	Thrombus a predictor of distal embolization after TEC.
Baumbach[659]		ELCA	Thrombus group with 6.4-fold decrease in procedural success.
Agrawal[664]	77	GRS	Pre-stent filling defect not predictive of stent thrombosis.
O'Neill[631]	345	All devices	Thrombus group with lower angiographic success (85% vs. 93%), increased embolization (6% vs. 0.6%) and more cardiac events (9% vs. 3%).
Emmi[634]	58	DCA	Thrombus: More ischemic complications (15.5% vs. 7.9%) and CABG (10.3% vs. 3.9%).
Estella[658]	12	ELCA	Thrombus: Decreased clinical success (58% vs. 95%).

Abbreviations: GRS = Gianturco-Roubin stent; TEC = transluminal extraction catheter; SVG = saphenous vein graft; ELCA = excimer laser coronary angioplasty; DCA = directional coronary atherectomy; MI = myocardial infarction; CK = creatine kinase; CABG = emergency coronary artery bypass surgery

Several observational studies have reported efficacy for thrombolytic agents before and after PTCA (Tables 2,4). However, the majority of randomized trials have failed to demonstrate clinical benefit for routine administration of thrombolytics during PTCA for unstable angina, and the TAUSA trial actually demonstrated an increased risk of acute MI. (A possible explanation for this apparent discrepancy is that many of the observational studies reported results in cases with "definite" thrombus, whereas the TAUSA trial reported results in clinical syndromes where "thrombus was *likely* to be present.") Taken together, these studies suggest that thrombolytic therapy should not be used indiscriminately, but should be reserved (if at all) for situations in which definite thrombus is present. Although not specifically tested in thrombus-containing lesions, ReoPro has been shown to decrease the incidence of ischemic complications and clinical restenosis in high-risk patients undergoing PTCA or directional atherectomy. Small reports suggest that "rescue ReoPro" may be useful for thrombus after PTCA (using the regimen in the EPIC trial or an intracoronary bolus of 20 mg), but further studies are needed.

Table 4. PTCA Outcome: Impact of Post-Procedural Thrombus

Series	N	Adjunctive Therapy	Results
Muhlestein[700]	16	Rescue ReoPro	Reduced thrombus score and improved TIMI flow; procedural success (100%).
Grines[705]	34	IC lytics during primary PTCA	Post-PTCA thrombus not predictive of ischemic events; more ischemia after lytics (18.4 vs 10.6%; p = 0.10).
Lincoff[707]	43	IC UK or tPA for abrupt closure	PTCA success (44%) not related to lytics.
Chapekis[628]	12	IC UK (120,000 U bolus, 120,000 U/hr x 24 hrs). Heparin IV: 1000 U/hr.	Acute closure (8%).
Pavlides[706]	256	UK	Major cardiac events increased (21% vs 9%, p=0.1) after UK for abrupt closure.
deFeyter[708]	34	IC UK	Success (65%)
Schieman[596]	48	IC UK 100,000-250,000 units over 20-65 minutes. Heparin infusion and aspirin x 5 days	No re-PTCA, MI, or in-hospital death.
Haft[709]	36	IC UK or tPA	Success (72%).
Gulba[710]	27	IC and IV tPA	Initial success (82%); reocclusion within 36 hrs (55%).

Abbreviations: IC = intracoronary; IV = intravenous; tPA = tissue plasminogen activator; CABG = emergency coronary artery bypass surgery; N = number of patients; UK = urokinase

The ideal mechanical treatment for thrombus is unknown. TEC is very efficient at removing fresh globular thrombus, but the risk of adverse events is increased. However, preliminary data from the TOPIT trial suggest that compared to PTCA, there is a lower incidence of non-Q-wave myocardial infarction after TEC. In the VEGAS-2 trial, the Possis AngioJet will be compared to intracoronary urokinase for lesions with thrombus. Finally, studies of therapeutic ultrasound for dissolution of thrombus are in progress. In our interventional survey, the device of choice for thrombotic lesions was PTCA, which was recommended by 41% of operators. Other devices included TEC in 29%, stents in 11%, and directional atherectomy in 18%. This patient was treated with TEC by Dr. Barry Kramer, resulting in significant clot extraction. Residual intraluminal filling defects, thought to represent dissection, were treated effectively with adjunctive PTCA (next page).

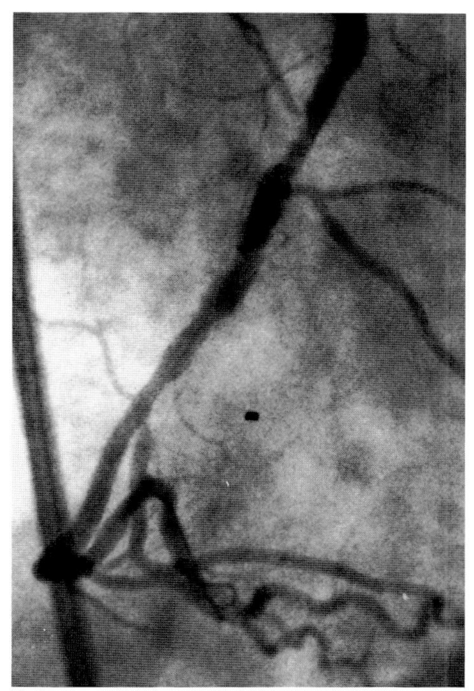

*****

TOTAL OCCLUSION: LAD

A 63-year-old physician presents to your office with a 4-month history of progressive angina. Myocardial perfusion imaging reveals ischemia at a low workload. Cardiac catheterization reveals total occlusion of the proximal LAD (reference vessel = 3.2 mm) and right-to-left collaterals. Other vessels and left ventricular function are normal.

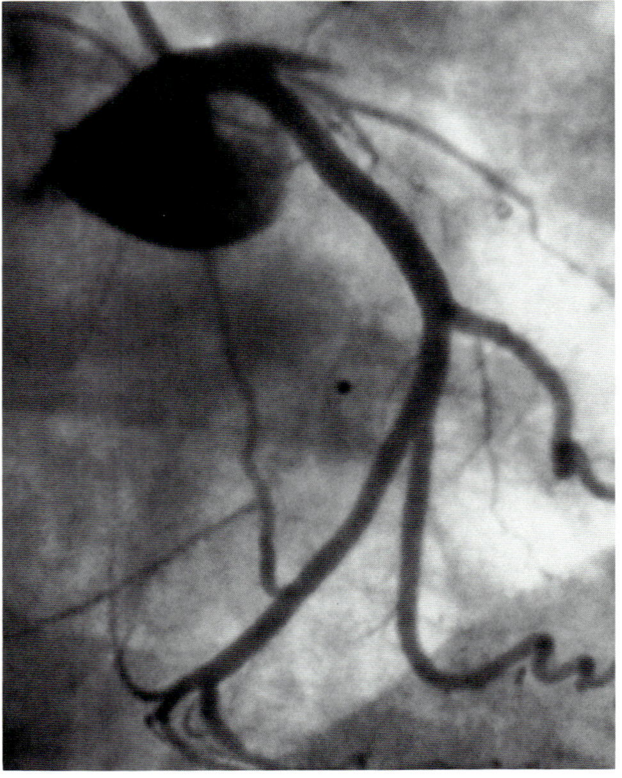

What features favor successful revascularization?

Dean Kereiakes, MD, USA: This patient has a proximal, tapered total occlusion of the LAD without bridging collaterals. Although the length of the occluded segment is unknown, the patient has a "clinical" duration of occlusion of less than 4 months. The easy access, tapered morphology and known duration of occlusion favor successful percutaneous revascularization.

Bernhard Meier, MD, Switzerland: The chronic total occlusion can be assumed to be 4 months old. On the basis of documented ischemia and the lack of previous infarction, a recanalization attempt is indicated. The nicely tapered stump and the right-to-left collaterals promise a fairly high technical success rate.

John Douglas Jr., MD, USA: This patient has total occlusion of the proximal LAD, probably of 3-4 months duration. He is an excellent candidate for percutaneous revascularization. I recommend conventional PTCA. The tapered contour of the occlusion usually funnels the guidewire to the proper site, heightening the probability of success. However, we don't know the length of the occluded segment or the size or complexity of the distal vessel, all of which influence equipment selection, early success, and long-term outcome.

Describe your technical approach.

Dean Kereiakes, MD, USA: I would initiate PTCA with an 8F JL4 short tip guiding catheter (High-Flow Cordis Bright-Tip), a 2.0 mm low-profile balloon, and a 0.014-inch Traverse guidewire. After initially probing the occlusion with the Traverse wire, I would bring the 2.0 mm balloon into the proximal LAD and exchange for a 0.014-inch floppy guidewire. After predilating with a 2.0 mm balloon and intracoronary nitroglycerin administration, the length of the target lesion and caliber of the occluded vessel could be better assessed.

Bernhard Meier, MD, Switzerland: I would insert a 7F JL4 guiding catheter and use a 0.021-inch Magnum wire (1 mm ball tip). First I would insert the ball tip into the stump and probe it until the wire buckles; passage with the wire alone is virtually impossible in chronic occlusions. Then I would back it up with a 3.5 mm Magnarail balloon and advance the balloon all the way to the ball tip where it will stop. Pushing the wire a few millimeters and following with the balloon to back it up or pushing the two as a unit is frequently successful. When reaching the distal vessel, the wire will move freely. At this time I would pass the balloon over the sturdy guidewire. Balloon inflations over the entire occluded segment can be carried out for several minutes (no ischemia is expected).

John Douglas Jr., MD, USA: The key to success in total occlusion angioplasty is atraumatic penetration of the lesion. I would approach this one very gently with a soft, 0.010-inch Approach wire, or a 0.014-inch Choice wire. It is surprising how often persistence with a soft wire will lead to success. I would use a 0.018-inch compatible balloon of appropriate diameter based on visual estimates of the diameter of the distal vessel and length of the occluded segment (using 30 mm or longer lengths to span the entire occlusion). If there is uncertainty about vessel diameter or distal branching, I would start with a 2.0 x 20 mm balloon and make a decision regarding the definitive balloon after the vessel is partially dilated and treated with intracoronary nitroglycerin. A 10-minute inflation is usually well-tolerated and enhances the angiographic appearance of the treated segment.

What would you recommend if your approach fails?

Dean Kereiakes, MD, USA: If attempts to recanalize the occlusion with a 0.014-inch Traverse guidewire are unsuccessful, I would exchange for a standard wire (with a 2 mm hockey stick bend) and then a Magnum wire system to probe the occlusion. A laser tip guidewire could be used in this situation.

Bernhard Meier, MD, Switzerland: The Magnum wire will not fail to cross the occlusion but it may fail to reenter the true lumen. If this occurs, the procedure will have to be abandoned since other wires will invariably follow the subintimal path created by the Magnum wire. A further attempt a few weeks later, however, is possible.

John Douglas Jr., MD, USA: If the initially chosen wires fail, it is likely that an incremental strategy will succeed (0.018-inch Gold Tip Glide wire, 0.014-inch Hi-torque intermediate, 0.014-inch Hi-torque standard, or 0.018-inch Hi-torque standard). If it is not possible to cross the lesion, I would recommend a medical trial (beta blocker, nitrates, calcium channel blocker) before considering surgical therapy. If the patient was anxious for a percutaneous success and the distal features were particularly encouraging (short segment occlusion, single vessel disease, large caliber vessel), I would discuss other possible strategies such as selective administration of thrombolytic drugs for several hours, repeat PTCA, or laser wire recanalization.

Describe your adjunctive medical regimen.

Dean Kereiakes, MD, USA: As some element of intracoronary thrombus is no doubt present (particularly occlusions of shorter duration), I recommend weight-adjusted ReoPro bolus and 12-hour infusion. Our standard protocol for post-procedural heparin and vascular access hemostasis is as follows: Heparin is administered during the procedure to achieve an ACT of 250-300 seconds (Hemochron). Femoral vascular access lines are removed when the ACT is ≤ 170 seconds and manual compression is applied for ≥ 1 hour. Following 1 hour of manual compression, the femstop device is applied for 4-12 hours (applied pressure is 20 mmHg less than systolic blood pressure for 30 minutes, 40 mmHg less than systolic blood pressure for 30 minutes, then ½ systolic pressure. Every 4 hours the pressure is reduced to 40 mmHg for 15 minutes). When the femstop has been removed, a standard pressure dressing is applied for 8-12 hours. Most often, heparin is not restarted and Coumadin is not necessary.

Bernhard Meier, MD, Switzerland: No heparin is necessary after the intervention and the patient can be treated with aspirin alone (whether a stent has been placed or not). The patient can be discharged the next day.

John Douglas Jr., MD, USA: Following successful PTCA, heparin should be continued for 18-24 hours; I would not use ReoPro.

Does stent implantation have a role?

Dean Kereiakes, MD, USA: If the vessel caliber is ≥ 3.0 mm as suspected in this case, I would place a 3.5 mm Palmaz-Schatz stent and postdilate with a 3.5 x 9 mm Titan balloon at ≥ 16 ATM. Intravascular ultrasound would be performed to assure optimal stent deployment. I believe that stents can reduce restenosis and reocclusion following PTCA of chronic total occlusions.

Bernhard Meier, MD, Switzerland: Stent insertion is only necessary if the angiographic result is not satisfactory. A Palmaz-Schatz stent can be crimped on the Magnarail balloon and implanted using an implantation pressure of 16 ATM. No additional balloon is necessary.

John Douglas Jr., MD, USA: Preliminary data regarding Palmaz-Schatz stenting in total occlusions is encouraging; I therefore have a low threshold for stenting single, short segments that have suboptimal angiographic appearance after several prolonged inflations.

Editors' Perspective: The LAD occlusion was treated by conventional PTCA without difficulty (below) (see p. 34 for additional comments).

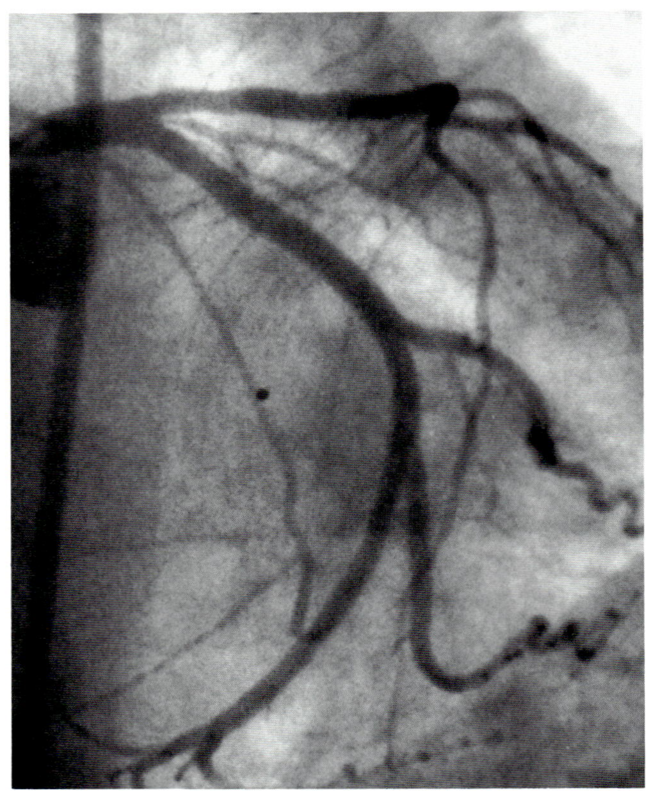

*****

TOTAL OCCLUSION: RCA

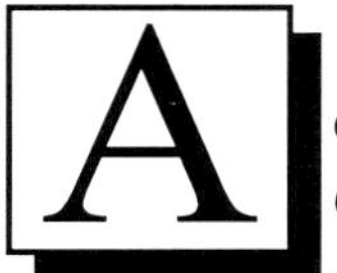

A 55-year-old engineer presents to your office with a 4-month history of decreased exercise capacity. Myocardial perfusion imaging reveals ischemia at low workload. Cardiac catheterization reveals total occlusion of the RCA (reference vessel = 4.5 mm). Other vessels and left ventricular function are normal.

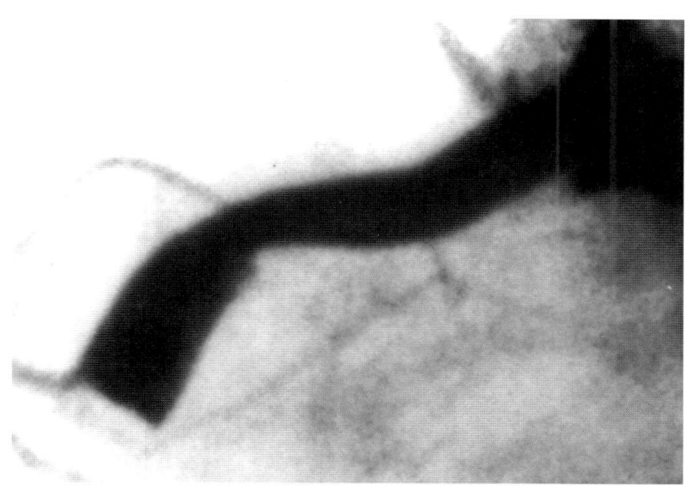

What features favor successful revascularization?

Dean Kereiakes, MD, USA: This patient has an abrupt, non-tapered total occlusion of a large dominant RCA without bridging collaterals. The length of the occluded segment is unknown, but the age of the occlusion (4 months) suggests that PTCA is feasible.

Bernhard Meier, MD, Switzerland: This chronic total occlusion of the RCA has to be assumed to be < 4 months old according to the patient's clinical symptoms. Unfortunately, the stump is not tapered and it is difficult to select a starting place to probe the occlusion. The outside corner must be avoided to prevent the wire from entering the small branch which originates from the occlusion.

John Douglas Jr., MD, USA: This is a total occlusion with retrograde thrombosis, producing a blunt, non-tapered occlusion. The length of the thrombosed segment is uncertain and nothing is known about the distal vessel. Success depends on the ability to wire the lesion and on the extent of thrombosis; I estimate success at 50-75%.

Describe your technical approach.

Dean Kereiakes, MD, USA: The slight downsloping takeoff of the RCA lends itself to engagement with an Amplatz guiding catheter, to maximize back-up. I would use an 8F AL1 or 2 guide catheter, a 4.0 mm low profile balloon, and a 0.014-inch Traverse guidewire.

Bernhard Meier, MD, Switzerland: I would use a 7F JR4 guiding catheter, a 0.021-inch Magnum wire, and a 4.0 mm Magnarail balloon which can be overdilated to 4.5 mm. With a sharp J-tip on the Magnum wire immediately behind the ball tip, the best entry site of the occlusion can be probed. Once the occlusion has been entered, it will be easy to work down the artery.

John Douglas Jr., MD, USA: I recommend a 0.014-inch Hi-torque floppy wire and a 0.018-inch compatible 4.0 x 30-40 mm balloon at low pressure, for 10-15 minutes.

What do you recommend if your approach fails?

Dean Kereiakes, MD, USA: If attempts to cross the occlusion are unsuccessful, I would change to a 0.014-inch standard guidewire and then a Magnum wire, positioning the balloon in the proximal RCA to maximize support. In my experience, total occlusions with an abrupt and smooth cut-off usually have a significant thrombus burden; I would position a Tracker catheter at the occlusion for a continuous infusion of urokinase (240,000 units/hour). I would perform repeat angiography and a second attempt at recanalization in 12-24 hours.

Bernhard Meier, MD, Switzerland: If all attempts fail to find the true lumen, another guidewire is not recommended since it will enter the false channel. If the ball tip fails to cross the occlusion or passes into the small sidebranch, a 0.014-inch Magnum wire can be used. If it meets the same fate, a conventional guidewire can be used. With this approach, it is virtually always possible to enter the occluded segment, but subintimal passage is more common than with the Magnum wire. If the occlusion is short, this case is a good one for the excimer laser wire.

John Douglas Jr., MD, USA: If necessary, a 0.018-inch Gold Tip Glidewire can be used, followed by gentle probing with intermediate and then standard 0.014-inch wires. If the lesion cannot be crossed with a wire and there are additional favorable features (such as a large distal vessel), I recommend selective intracoronary urokinase infusion (50,000 units/hour for 8 hours) and repeat angiography the following day, hoping for some recanalization.

Describe your adjunctive medical regimen.

Dean Kereiakes, MD, USA: I recommend intravenous ReoPro, as described previously; Coumadin is not needed. If the occlusion can be crossed with a guidewire, I would dilate this artery with a 4.0 mm low-profile balloon and place a 4.0 mm Palmaz-Schatz stent. Intravascular ultrasound would be performed to size the vessel and select a proper high-pressure balloon; it is likely that a 4.5 mm or 5.0 mm Sub-4 peripheral balloon will be required.

Bernhard Meier, MD, Switzerland: No heparin is necessary after intervention; aspirin alone is indicated. The patient can be discharged the next day. ReoPro is indicated only if visible thrombus persists after recanalization. If there is a suboptimal result due to dissection or recoil, a Wallstent or GR-II stent would be ideal.

John Douglas Jr., MD, USA: Intracoronary urokinase (500,000-1,000,000 units over 2-4 hours) would be administered only for persistent thrombus and compromised lumen after multiple, prolonged inflations. If considerable thrombus is present, ReoPro will be administered.

Editors' Perspective: The RCA occlusion in this case was refractory to conventional PTCA techniques. Prolonged urokinase infusion resulted in partial recanalization, followed by successful TEC atherectomy and adjunctive PTCA by Dr. William O'Neill (see p. 34 for additional comments).

*****

TOTAL OCCLUSION: BRIDGING COLLATERALS

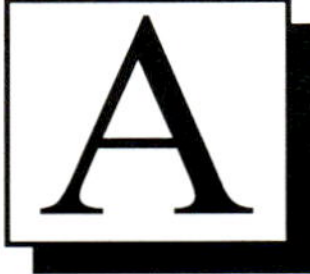

A 55-year-old female presents to your office with a 4-month history of progressive angina. Myocardial perfusion imaging reveals ischemia at low workload. Cardiac catheterization reveals total occlusion of the RCA (reference vessel = 4.5 mm) with faint left-to-right collaterals. Other vessels and left ventricular function are normal.

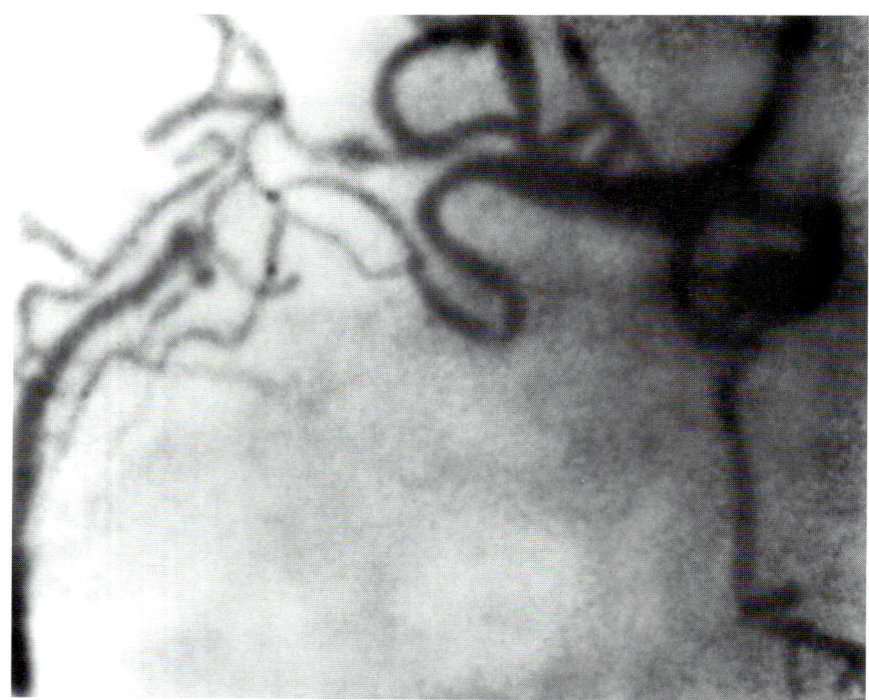

What features favor successful revascularization?

Dean Kereiakes, MD, USA: This case illustrates a difficult anatomic situation. The patient has a 10-15 mm long occlusion and bridging collaterals. The RCA is a large vessel and has a slightly upward takeoff. The length of the occluded segment and the presence of bridging collaterals are associated with reduced primary success.

Bernhard Meier, MD, Switzerland: The angiogram reveals a very old chronic occlusion of the RCA (rich in collaterals). On the other hand, the occlusion is very short (about 1cm), there is a nice stump, and symptoms only date back 4 months.

John Douglas Jr., MD, USA: This is a long total occlusion of the RCA with bridging collaterals. The presence of an extensive network of bridging collaterals suggests an old occlusion; successful PTCA is less likely. Careful analysis of the angiogram suggests that there is a tapered proximal segment. These angiographic features coupled with a 4 month history of angina indicate a PTCA success rate of 50% and a restenosis rate of at least 50%.

Describe your technical approach.

Dean Kereiakes, MD, USA: I would approach this case with an 8F AL1 or 2 guiding catheter depending on the size of the aorta, to maximize guide catheter back up. I would use a 2.0 mm low-profile balloon over a 0.014-inch standard guidewire with a short (≤ 2.0 mm) hockey stick bend.

Bernhard Meier, MD, Switzerland: Since the takeoff of the RCA is less favorable than in the previous case, I would select a 7F AL2 guiding catheter, a 0.021-inch Magnum guidewire, and a 3.0 mm Magnarail balloon. The difficulty in this case is avoiding the bridging collaterals at the tip of the stump.

John Douglas Jr., MD, USA: I would start with a 1.5 x 20 mm balloon (0.018-inch compatible), a 0.010-inch Approach wire, and an incremental wire strategy as in the previous case.

What do you recommend if your approach fails?

Dean Kereiakes, MD, USA: If attempts to cross this occlusion are unsuccessful, I would use the Magnum wire system. The laser tip guidewire could be very useful in this case because of the ability to coaxially align it with the occluded segment in an orthogonal view.

Bernhard Meier, MD, Switzerland: An attempt a few weeks later is always possible. A 0.014-inch Magnum wire with a smaller ball tip should be tried first and then a conventional 0.014-inch guidewire stiffened by the Magnarail balloon. If this fails, the case has to be given up, since a laser wire will probably perforate the sidebranch. The chance of success in this scenario is the lowest of the three chronic total occlusions.

John Douglas Jr., MD, USA: I recommend medical therapy.

Editors' Perspective: Chronic total occlusions account for 10-20% of coronary interventional procedures, and inability to revascularize these lesions is the most common reason for referring patients for CABG. The most common causes of failed intervention include the inability to cross the occlusion with a guidewire (80%), failure to cross the occlusion with a balloon (15%), and inability to dilate the stenosis (5%). Unfortunately, none of the currently available interventional devices are useful if the occlusion cannot be crossed with a guidewire. Compared to nontotal occlusions, where PTCA success exceeds 90%, successful PTCA is achieved in only 47-81% of total occlusions (Tables 5, 6). Several factors influence case selection and predict PTCA success (Table 7), including the type of occlusion (complete vs. functional total occlusion; Tables 5, 8), the length and duration of occlusion (Tables 8, 9), and the presence of sidebranches (Table 8), a tapered stump (Table 8), and bridging collaterals (Table 7). After assessment of these clinical and morphological factors, equipment selection and technique are extremely important. To minimize the increased procedural time, cost, frustration, and radiation exposure (Table 10) associated with PTCA of chronic total occlusions, it is best to anticipate problems and optimize the technical strategy at the beginning of the procedure. It is crucial to select a guiding catheter that will provide coaxial alignment and maximal backup support for guidewire and balloon advancement. In general, the best "power" guides for the left coronary artery include the left Voda (which derives its support from the opposite wall of the aorta) and the left Amplatz (which derives its support from the left Sinus of Valsalva). Voda-like guides, such as the XB and geometric left, are also excellent choices. For the right coronary artery, a left Amplatz or right Voda will provide maximal support for most vessel configurations. A double-loop Arani also provides excellent support but is difficult to manipulate and engage the ostium. Multipurpose catheters are especially useful for vessels with vertical downward takeoffs.

Table 5. PTCA of Nontotal vs. Chronic Total Coronary Occlusion: Acute Outcome

Series	Group	N	Success (%)	Complications (%)* D / MI / CABG	Acute Closure (%)
Berger[955]	Nontotal	1295	-	0 / 1.4 / 0	
	Total	139	-	0 / 1.5 / 0.3	
Favereau[927]	Nontotal	2065	96	1.4	1.8
	Total	292	67	1.7	8
Tan[928]	Nontotal	1157	93	0.4 / 0.7 / 2.1	3.3
	Total	91	66	0 / 0 / 0	0
Ruocco[929]	Nontotal	1429	82	0.7 / 4.8 / 3.5	1.5
	Total	271	59	1.8 / 3.6 / 3.3	4.1
Myler[930]	Nontotal	779	94	1.7	-
	Total	122	76	1.6	-
Plante[931]	Nontotal				
	Stable Angina	637	-	4	-
	Unstable Angina	442	-	8	-
	Total				
	Stable Angina	44	48	2.5	-
	Unstable Angina	46	65	2.0	-
Stone[932]	Nontotal	6950	96	0.9 / 1.5 / 1.7	-
	Total	905	72	0.8 / 0.6 / 0.8	-
Safian[933]	Nontotal	711	90	0.4 / 3 / 2	-
	Functional	102	78	1 / 3 / 3	-
	Total	169	63	0 / 0 / 2	-

Abbreviations: D = in-hospital death, MI = in-hospital myocardial infarction, CABG = emergency coronary artery bypass grafting; - = not reported

Definitions: Nontotal occlusion = 51-99% stenosis (TIMI flow ≥ 2); Functional total occlusion = 99% stenosis (TIMI flow = 1); Total occlusion = 100% stenosis (TIMI flow = 0)

* Single number represents overall complication rate

Table 6. PTCA of Chronic Total Coronary Occlusion: Acute Outcome

Series	N	Success (%)	Complications* (%) D / Q-MI / CABG	Other
Berger[955]	139	-	0 / 1.4 / 2.9	
Favereau[927]	367	67	1.7	
Kinoshita[934]	433	81	0.3 / 0 / 0	Cardiac tamponade (1%)
Tan[928]	91	66	0 / 0 / 0	Acute closure (0%)
Ishizaku[935]	111	62	0 / 1.6 / 0	Non-Q-MI (5%)
Tan[936]	312	61	0.3 / - / 1.6	
Shimizu[937]	468	75	- / - / -	
Stewart[938]	100	47	1 / 0 / -	Non-Q-MI (5%)
Maiello[939]	365	64	0 / 0.6 / 0.3	Perforation (0.6%)
Myler[930]	122	76	1.6	
Ivanhoe[940]	480	66	1 / 2 / -	
Ruocco[929]	271	59	2 / 1 / 2	Acute closure (4%)
Bell[941]	354	66	0.3 / 1.7 / 2.5	
Stone[932]	971	72	0.8 / 0.6 / 0.8	

Abbreviations: D = death; Q-MI = Q-wave myocardial infarction; CABG = emergency coronary artery bypass grafting; - = not reported

* Single number represents overall complication rate

After selection of an ideal guiding catheter, the choice of guidewires is largely at the discretion of the operator (Table 11). The most popular approach is sequential use of floppy, intermediate, and standard guidewires, which can successfully traverse 50-70% of chronic total occlusions. The Choice PT guidewire is an excellent wire for crossing chronic total occlusions. For refractory total occlusions (Tables 11-13), alternative approaches include the Glidewire, the Magnum wire, the laserwire, vibrational angioplasty, rotational angioplasty catheter system (ROTACS), and prolonged infusion of intracoronary thrombolytic agents, which may successfully cross 50% of "refractory" total occlusions.

Once the occlusion is crossed with a guidewire, contemporary studies show no definite advantage of laser or atherectomy over balloon angioplasty. In contrast, preliminary data from Japan suggest that stents offer better immediate and long-term results than PTCA. The practice of interventional cardiology reflect these data: 56% of respondents in our survey recommend PTCA as the primary revascularization

strategy for chronic total occlusions. Other strategies included stents in 28%, Rotablator in 11%, and excimer laser angioplasty in 6%. In our practice, we recommend stenting if the total occlusion can be covered by ≤ 3 stents and the vessel diameter is > 2.5 mm. This RCA occlusion could not be successfully crossed with a guidewire, and the patient was treated medically.

Table 7. Chronic Total Coronary Occlusions: Predictors of PTCA Outcome

Procedural Success	Procedural Failure
Functional occlusion	Total occlusion
Occlusion age < 12 weeks	Occlusion age > 12 weeks
Length < 15 mm	Length > 15 mm
Tapered stump	Abrupt cut-off
No sidebranch at point of occlusion	Sidebranch present
No intracoronary bridging collaterals	Extensive bridging collaterals ("caput medusa")

Table 8. The Impact of Occlusion Characteristics on PTCA Outcome

	Success (%)			
Series	Length Short/Long	Occlusion Type Functional†/ Total††	Tapered Stump Yes / No	Bridging Collaterals Yes / No
Kinoshita[934]	-	-	-	75 / 83
Tan[936]	-	-	69 / 43	70 / 20
Maiello[939]	71 / 60+	68 / 69	83 / 51	67 / 29
Ivanhoe[940]	-	78 / 60	73 / 60	-
Stone[932]	85 / 69++	83 / 74	88 / 59	18 / 85

Abbreviation: - = not reported

† Functional occlusion = faint, late antegrade filling beyond the lesion

†† Total occlusion = absence of antegrade filling beyond the lesion

\+ Short (≤ 15 mm); Long (> 15 mm); ++ Short (≤ 10 mm); Long (> 20 mm)

Table 9. Impact of Occlusion Duration on PTCA Outcome

Series	Occlusion Duration	N	Success (%)
Tan[928]	< 3 mos	42	76
	> 3 mos	49	57
Ishizaka	< 1 mo	11	91
	> 1 mo	100	56
Myler[930]	< 1 week	99	87
	1-12 wks	73	88
	> 3 mos	49	59
Bell[941]	< 1 week	60	74
	1-4 wks	15	93
	1-3 mos	243	67
	> 3 mos	45	64
Maiello[939]	< 1 mo	73	89
	1-3 mos	77	87
	> 3 mos	110	45
Stone[932]	< 12 wks	29	90
	> 12 wks	39	74

Table 10. Chronic Total Coronary Occlusion: Time, Equipment, and Cost

Series	Occlusion Type	Procedure Time (min)	Radiation Time (min)	Equipment Guides/Wires/Balloons	Cost ($)
Stewart[938]	Total	73	30	-	-
	Nontotal	59	18	-	-
Bell[943]	Total	74	31	2.0 / 2.7 / 1.8	1947
	Nontotal	59	18	1.5 / 1.5 / 1.3	1398

Abbreviations: - = not reported

Table 11. Treatment of Occlusions Resistant To Crossing with PTCA Guidwire

Series	N	Device Success (%)*	Final Success (%)**
Glidewire			
Freed[96]	59	54	39
Rees[962]	33	58	52
Hosney[963]	8	-	88
Magnum Wire			
Pande[964]	28	45	39
Haerer[950]	102	32	32
Laserwire			
Serruys[1006]	252	58	-
Vibrational PTCA			
Rees[967]	18	89	78
ROTACS			
Danchin[968]	50	-	66
Kaltenbach[969]	152	-	65

Abbreviations: ROTACS = Rotational Angioplasty Catheter System; - = not reported
*Device success = cross occlusion with device
**Final success = procedural success after adjunctive PTCA

Table 12. Intracoronary Thrombolysis for Occlusions Resistant to Guidewire Crossing

Series	N	Lytic	Results	Other
Ajluni[977]	25	UK (100,000-240,000 U/hour x 8-25 hr) via infusion wire + guide catheter	↑ coronary flow (28%); PTCA success (52%).	MI (8%); significant bleeding (8%); length of stay (5.1 days).
Zidar[972]	60	UK (1.6-3.2 MU x 8 hrs) via infusion wire + guide catheter	PTCA success 52-56% for all doses	More bleeding and vascular complications at higher doses.
Cecena[978]	20	UK bolus (120,000 U IC) + up to 200,000 U/hr x 24 hrs via infusion wire + guide catheter	↑ coronary flow (90%); PTCA success (94%).	No MI or emergent CABG; blood transfusion (10%).
Vaska[979]	11	tPA (5-10 mg/hr x 6 hrs) via infusion wire	↑ coronary flow (91%); PTCA success (82%).	No death, MI, or emergent CABG; acute closure (10%).

Abbreviations: UK = Urokinase; MI = in-hospital Q-wave myocardial infarction; CABG = emergency coronary artery bypass grafting; MU = million units; IC = intracoronary

Table 13. Randomized Trials of Chronic Total Coronary Occlusions

Trial	N	Design	Success (%)*	Comments
Magnum Wire				
Pande[964]	100	Magnum PTCA	45 67	Magnum success after PTCA failure (39%); PTCA success after Magnum failure (12%).
Haerer[950]	102	Magnum PTCA Omniflex	32 68 59	Magnum failures salvaged by other systems (48%).
ELCA				
Appleman[970]	103	ELCA PTCA	65 61	No difference in 6-month clinical endpoints or reocclusion (AMRO Trial).
ROTACS				
Danchin[968]	100	ROTACS PTCA	66 60	
STENTS				
Sato[971]	60	Stent PTCA	100 -	No subacute stent thrombosis; bailout stenting after PTCA (39%).
Lytic Infusion				
Zidar[972]	60	Intracoronary urokinase (0.8 MU, 1.6 MU,3.2 MU)	-	PTCA success after all lytic regimens (52-56%, p = NS). More bleeding and vascular complications at higher doses. Reocclusion (9%); restenosis (59%); target vessel revascularization (36%).

Abbreviations: ELCA = Excimer Laser Coronary Angioplasty; ROTACS = Rotational Angioplasty Catheter System; MU = million units (given over 8 hours); - = not reported

*Success = crossing occlusion with a guidewire

*****

CALCIFIED LESION

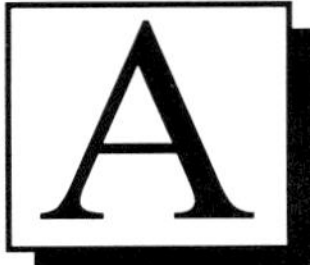

A 70-year-old man develops progressive angina. Angiography reveals a severe, heavily calcified stenosis in the mid-LAD (reference vessel diameter = 2.9 mm; arrows indicate calcification). Other vessels and ventricular function are normal.

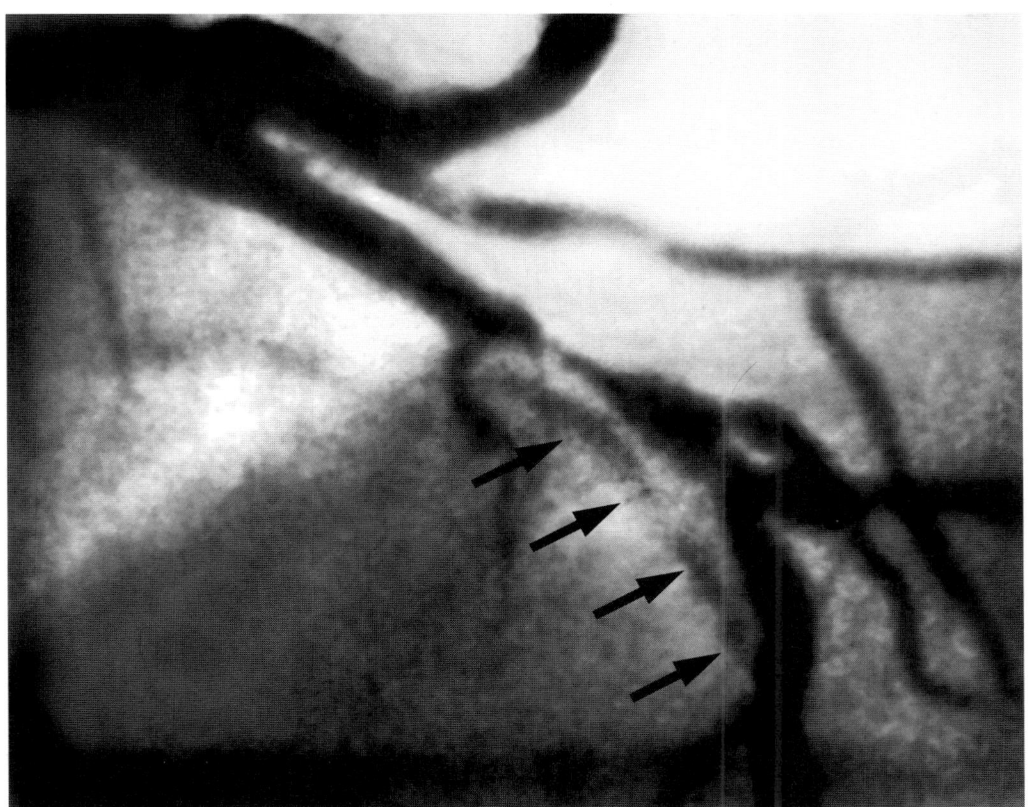

How does this lesion morphology influence your selection of devices for percutaneous revascularization?

John Douglas Jr., MD, USA: This patient has a long, calcified, mid-LAD stenosis. The lesion length, bulk, and degree of calcification increase procedural complications and restenosis. I am concerned about occlusive dissection with conventional PTCA, inability to effectively cut and debulk with directional atherectomy, and somewhat concerned about the large amount of debris that would have to be generated to effectively debulk this lesion with rotational atherectomy. However, I have had good success with rotational atherectomy in similar cases and would favor this approach.

Richard Myler, MD, USA: Since fluoroscopy reveals heavy calcification in the lesion, it must contain an arc of calcium of at least 180° and most likely has (at least) a moderate superficial component. The lesion is 15-20 mm long, though IVUS might indicate a longer segment. A small proximal septal and moderate size diagonal branches do not have significant stenoses, but no doubt their origins will be engaged with any device. The vessel caliber offers several device options, but the presence of abundant calcification is the sine qua non for rotational ablation. At present, no other device (or balloon) is as effective.

Describe your technical approach to this lesion.

John Douglas Jr., MD, USA: I recommend a 10F JL4 guide catheter, a step-burr sequence (1.5 mm, 2.0 mm, 2.25 mm burrs), and adjunctive PTCA with a 3.0 x 30 mm balloon inflated to 3-4 ATM.

Richard Myler, MD, USA: I recommend a sequential Rotablator approach (1.75 mm, 2.0 mm, 2.25 mm burrs). This approach should result in a 20-30% residual stenosis. If the results are excellent (residual stenosis < 20%, smooth contour, no dissection or spasm), I might "stand-alone" with the Rotablator. If not, I recommend low-pressure adjunctive PTCA with a PET balloon at 1-2 ATM for 2 minutes to avoid barotrauma. A 9F JL4 large lumen guide (0.092-inch or larger) will accommodate the 2.25 mm burr. Routine pre-procedure therapy includes aspirin, calcium channel blockers, and heparin to achieve an ACT of 300-350 seconds.

What specific recommendations can you offer to enhance procedural success and safety?

John Douglas Jr., MD, USA: To promote microvascular dilation during rotational atherectomy, I use nitroglycerin (2 mg/L) and verapamil (5 mg/L) in the Rotablator flush solution. Slow passage of the burr is critical to allow transit of atheromatous microparticles through the capillary bed. Following rotational atherectomy and adjunctive PTCA, intravenous heparin (PTT 2-times control) and nitroglycerin (20 mcg/min) would be continued overnight, followed by discharge on the first post-procedure day.

Richard Myler, MD, USA: I would advance the burr very slowly, avoiding any deceleration > 5000 RPM from baseline. Then I would "polish" the lesion with several slow back and forth passes, to avoid heat production, arterial spasm, "slow-flow", or "no-flow." I would retract the burr after 45-60 seconds and allow distal perfusion and clearance of debris. With rotational ablation, "festina lente" — make haste slowly.

Is IVUS useful for this lesion?

John Douglas Jr., MD, USA: Intravascular ultrasound is helpful to assess the degree of superficial calcification and success of atherectomy.

Richard Myler, MD, USA: IVUS will indicate the distribution of mural calcification (superficial vs. deep) and influence device selection. I would perform IVUS during the procedure to select the appropriate device (most likely Rotablator), and to assess the amount and distribution of calcium, lesion length, and true arterial reference diameter. After Rotablator, IVUS may indicate the need for further rotablation, adjunctive PTCA, or stenting. The procedure can be performed successfully without IVUS (as it has been in the past) — but with this wonderful new diagnostic tool, why not use it?

Is conventional PTCA alone an acceptable revascularization strategy?

John Douglas Jr., MD, USA: Prior to the availability of rotational atherectomy, I used conventional PTCA on similar lesions with reasonable success, and this is an option for experienced operators. However, this type of anatomy is not recommended for the novice balloonist. High-pressure PTCA with a 2.5 x 30 mm Bandit or Predator is acceptable.

Richard Myler, MD, USA: This case is much better performed with rotablation, which achieves higher success and lower complications than PTCA for heavily calcified lesions.

Editors' Perspective: In general, fluoroscopy and angiography are insensitive for assessing the degree and distribution of calcium in a lesion, which probably explains the variable success rates reported for PTCA of calcified lesions (Tables 14, 15). Studies using IVUS to accurately identify the length, arc, and depth of calcification, suggest that dissection often develops at the transition between calcified and noncalcified plaque, possibly due to nonuniform shear forces generated during balloon expansion.

Table 14. Influence of Lesion Calcium on Acute Outcome After PTCA

Series	Morphology	N	Success (%)
Tan[781]	Calcified	81	74
	Non-calcified	1076	94
Myler[783]	Calcified	140	92
	Non-calcified	639	95

Table 15. Lesion Calcium and Ischemic Complications After PTCA

Series	Morphology	N	Complications (%)	Comments
Tan[781]	Calcified	81	14	Incidence of abrupt closure.
	Non-calcified	1076	2.5	
			D/MI/CABG	
Danchin[785]	Calcified	285	0.8 / 3.5 / 0	
	Non-calcified	1801	0.7 / 3.0 / 1	
Myler[783]	Calcified	140	3.6	Overall incidence of complications
	Non-Calcified	639	1.3	
Ellis[787]	Calcified	46	-	Relative risk of complications = 1.5

Abbreviations: D = death; Q-MI = in-hospital Q-wave myocardial infarction; CABG = emergency coronary artery bypass grafting; - = not reported

Table 16. New Interventional Devices for Calcified Lesions: Acute Outcome

Series	Device	Morphology	N	Success (%)*	Complications (%)** D / Q-MI / CABG	Other
Dussaillant[820]	ROTA/STENT	Calcified	83	-	0	FDS(%): 12
	ROTA/DCA	(vessel ≥ 3mm)	120	-	-	16
	ROTA/PTCA		235	-	-	24
Warth[792]	ROTA	All lesions	346	95	2.6	
		Calcified	107	97	1.9	
Ellis[793]	ROTA	Calcified	232	91	-	
MacIssac[794]	ROTA	Noncalcified	108	95	0.5 / 0.5 /2.4	RS(%): 50
		Calcified	3	94	1.3 / 0.6 / 2.2	54
			107			
			8			
Altmann[795]	ROTA	No/mild Ca++ Mod.	182	96	0.7 / 0 / 1.4	EFS(%): 67
		Ca++	378	96	0.7 / 0 / 2.1	75
Reisman[796]	ROTA	Undilatable stenoses	67	96	0 / 0 / 1.5	RS(%): 36
Popma[797]	DCA	All lesions	306	95	-	EFS(%): 72
		Mild-mod Ca++	60	94	-	80
Hinohara[798]	DCA	Type A	105	98	0	
		Calcified	70	87	5.7	
TEC[800] database	TEC	Noncalcified	278	96	-	
		Calcified	154	89	-	
Bittl[801]	ELCA	Undilatable stenoses	36	92	-	Non-Q-MI: 6%
Bittl[802]	ELCA	Calcified	170	83	-	RS(%): 43
Levine[804]	ELCA	Calcified	95	96	0 / 2 / 2	
deMarchena[804]	Holmium-laser	All lesions	365	94	2.7	
		Calcified	111	90	4.5	

Abbreviations: DCA = Directional Coronary Atherectomy; TEC = Transluminal Extraction Atherectomy; ELCA = Excimer Laser Coronary Angioplasty; EFS = 1-year event-free survival; AC = Abrupt Closure; RS = Restenosis; FDS = Final Diameter Stenosis; - not reported

* Success = final residual stenosis < 50% (after adjunctive PTCA) without death, Q-wave MI, or emergency CABG

** Single value denotes overall in-hospital complication rate

Potential approaches to calcified lesions (Table 16) include the Rotablator, conventional PTCA with high-pressure noncompliant balloons, "force-focused" angioplasty using high-pressure balloons and a second parallel guidewire next to the balloon, cutting balloon angioplasty, and excimer or infrared laser angioplasty. Rotablator has emerged as the device of choice due to its ability to effectively and preferentially ablate hard calcified plaque; it may also result in fewer dissections compared to PTCA. Eighty-six percent of interventionalists in our survey recommended Rotablator as their device of choice for angiographically-calcified lesions. Although earlier studies of excimer laser angioplasty suggested little benefit compared to PTCA, contemporary use of the saline infusion technique may improve laser results. The need for IVUS is controversial: Although 93% of the high-volume interventionalists in our survey use IVUS in their practice, routine IVUS (defined as IVUS in at least 50% of cases) is used by only 4% of operators. Furthermore, 48% of operators use IVUS in < 10% of their cases! This lesion was treated successfully by Drs. Lowell Satler and Jeffrey Popma, using Rotablator atherectomy, adjunctive PTCA, and IVUS (below).

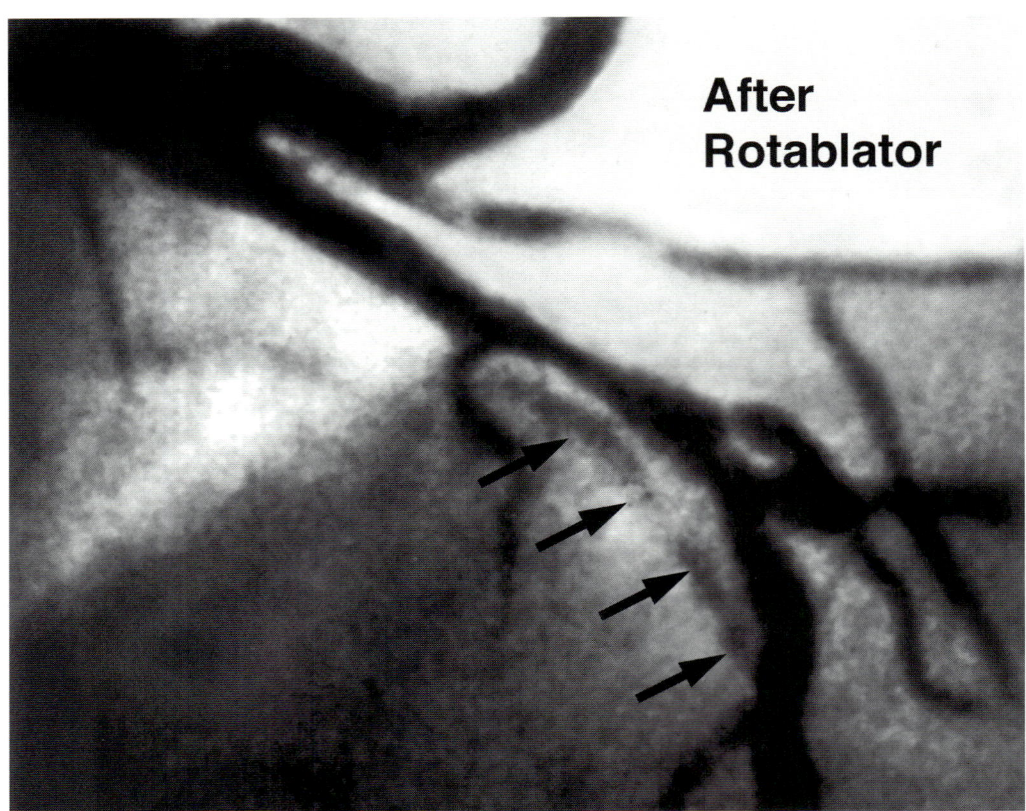

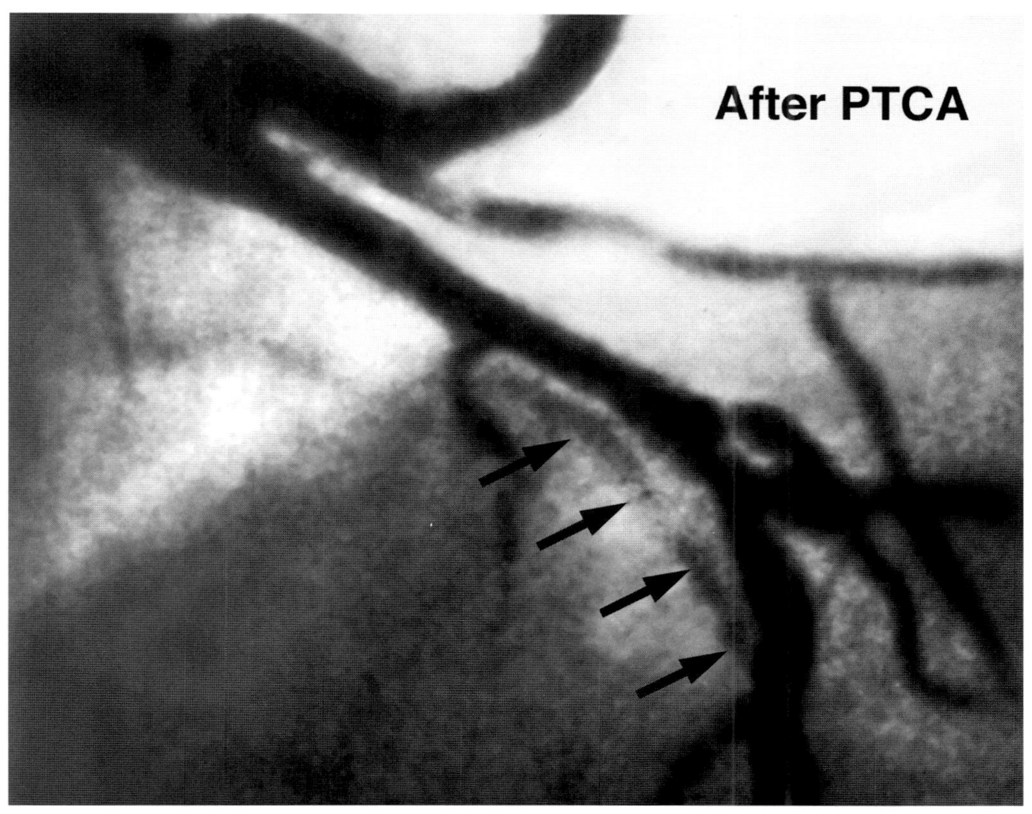
After PTCA

*****

LONG LESION

A 58-year-old medical malpractice attorney with a history of coronary artery bypass surgery 12 years ago presents with unstable angina. Cardiac catheterization reveals a long stenosis in the proximal and mid-LAD (reference vessel = 3.1 mm). The LCX and RCA are occluded, but vein grafts to these vessels are patent. The vein graft to the LAD is occluded at its origin. Left ventricular function is normal.

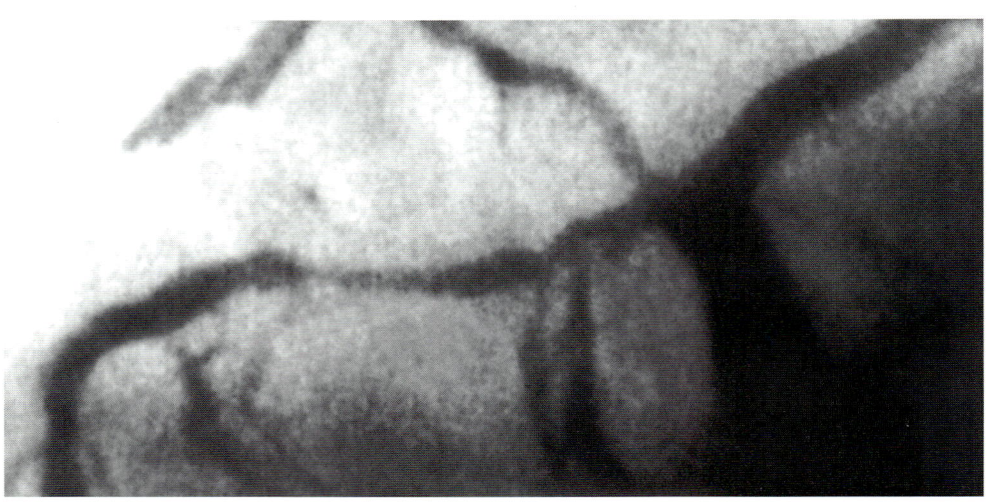

Describe your technical approach to this lesion.

Raimund Erbel, MD, Germany: The patient has a long history of coronary artery disease, recent unstable angina, and a long, irregular type C lesion in the LAD. This type of lesion has high complication and restenosis rates. Hard and inelastic lesions are particularly suitable for the Rotablator. I would use two or three 20-30 second passes with the Rotablator, starting with a 1.25 mm burr, followed by 1.75 mm and 2.15 mm burrs. Definitive lumen enlargement would be achieved by adjunctive PTCA at low pressure. After Rotablator, no-reflow and coronary spasm can occur. Therefore, nitroglycerin (3 mg/hour) and nifedipine (0.5-1.5 mg/hour) are mandatory; nonionic contrast is recommended. To assess the efficacy of the treatment, repeat angiography at 6-12 hours is suggested, to decide whether or not additional PTCA is necessary.

William O'Neill, MD, USA: This patient has patent vein grafts to the RCA and LCX. Therefore, he presents as "single" vessel disease with normal left ventricular function. Some might argue that an initial trial of medical therapy should be initiated. However, the LAD has severe, diffuse disease and I doubt this patient will have adequate relief of symptoms. With access to all interventional devices, I prefer the Rotablator. I would use a 9F guiding catheter with sideholes, and prepare the flush solution with verapamil (10 mg) and nitroglycerin (4 mg) in 1000 cc of heparinized saline. The lesion can be wired easily with a Rotablator-C wire. I would start with a 1.5 mm burr, increase to a 2.0 mm burr (burr/artery ratio ~ 0.6), and complete the procedure with a 3.0 x 40 mm balloon at 2-3 ATM.

Richard Heuser, MD, USA: In this long, straight lesion, I think rotablation is the preferred therapy, particularly because it will decrease the incidence of dissection. I recommend a JL4 guide, a Rotablator-C wire, and a 1.75 mm burr. I would then increase to a 2.0 mm followed by a 2.15 mm burr in a step-wise fashion. Using short runs (< 15 seconds) and urokinase, nitroglycerin, and heparin in the Rotablator flush, no-reflow and spasm are very rare. Short ablation times nearly eliminate the need for temporary pacemakers.

Is conventional PTCA a reasonable approach?

Raimund Erbel, MD, Germany: PTCA alone will lead to significant dissection and potential vessel occlusion, and is not recommended.

William O'Neill, MD, USA: Since this patient presents with unstable angina, cardiologists with only PTCA available should attempt to stabilize this patient for 5-7 days on IV nitroglycerin, aspirin, heparin and ticlopidine. Then PTCA can be attempted with an 8F guiding catheter, a 2.5 x 40 mm balloon (ACS Edge, SciMed Cobra or Cordis Predator), an extra-support wire, and an oscillating inflation technique at 4-6 ATM. If results are suboptimal, I would perform a prolonged inflation (7-10 minutes) with a 3.0 x 40 mm balloon at 2-4 ATM.

Richard Heuser, MD, USA: For interventionalists who only perform PTCA, this patient should be referred to a site where stents are available. Remember, this is a medical malpractice attorney, so we are already dealing with a pain in the rear end.

If the final result is suboptimal, is stenting reasonable?

Raimund Erbel, MD, Germany: Stenting is reasonable, if necessary. I recommend a GR-II or Microstent if the vessel is not calcified, and a Palmaz-Schatz stent if the vessel is calcified.

William O'Neill, MD, USA: I am concerned about using stents in this vessel because three large septal perforators are present. Also, the proximal portion of the stent would have to be placed at the origin of the LAD, which might compromise flow from the left main coronary artery.

Richard Heuser, MD, USA: Although a stent could be placed over the Rotablator-C wire, I would exchange for an Extra-S'port or Platinum-Plus wire. I would use multiple Palmaz-Schatz stents or a 40 mm GR-II stent to cover the stenosis. I would start with the distal lesion and move proximally, making sure all areas are covered. After all stents are deployed, I would postdilate with a 3.5 mm noncompliant balloon. I would image with intravascular ultrasound to ensure ideal apposition, symmetry, and stent diameter. I would prescribe aspirin and ticlopidine, and discharge the patient the following morning.

Are any other adjunctive therapies useful in this setting?

Richard Heuser, MD, USA: I am concerned that this patient might have thrombus in this lesion. With the clinical scenario of unstable angina, this is the type of patient who would benefit from ReoPro (0.25 mg/kg bolus and 10 mcg/min for 12 hours) with a modified dose of heparin (75 units/kg), to reduce complications. I would remove the sheaths after intervention when the ACT is < 180 seconds, and not use any additional heparin.

Editors' Perspective: Percutaneous revascularization of lesions > 20 mm in length is "standard fare" for many interventional cardiologists, and excellent results can be achieved, particularly with long (30-40 mm) and tapered balloons (Table 17). For long lesions, interventionalists in our survey recommended Rotablator in 43%, PTCA in 33%, stents in 14%, and excimer laser angioplasty in 10%. These recommendations reflect currently published data, which do not suggest clear superiority of any single

device for long lesions (Table 18). Furthermore, device choice is heavily influenced by other associated clinical and angiographic characteristics, including left ventricular function, the presence of other coronary artery disease, lesion angulation and calcification, and proximal vessel tortuosity. This particular lesion is well-suited for long-balloon PTCA or the Rotablator. In this case, successful Rotablator atherectomy and adjunctive PTCA were performed by Dr. Michael Cowley (below).

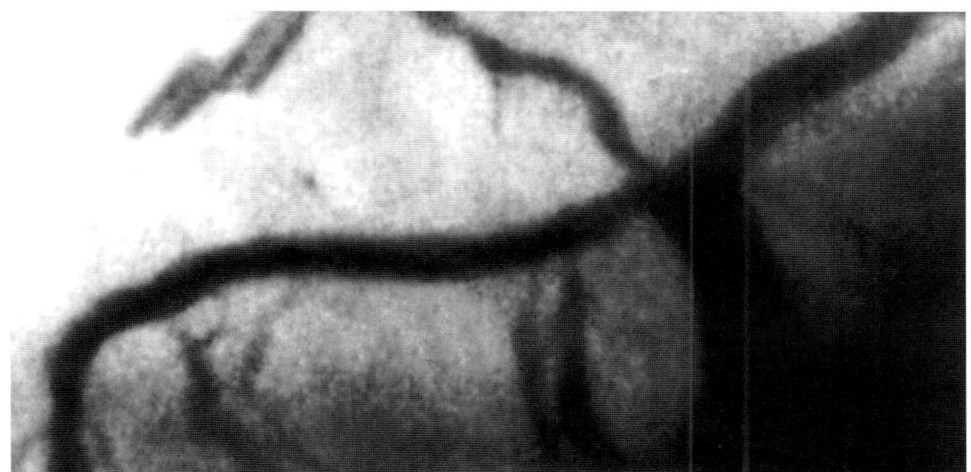

Table 17. Balloon Angioplasty of Long Lesions: Acute Outcome

Series	Balloon Length†	Lesion Length†	N	Success (%)	Complications (%)* D/Q-MI/CABG	DISS (%)	AC (%)
Appelman[884]	-	>10	157	79	0 / 1.3 / 1.9	55	0.6
Tan[876]	20-40	< 10	959	95	-	-	1.5
		10-20	153	85	-	-	11
		> 20	45	74	-	-	16
Kaul[877]	20-40	11-20	112	96	1 / 1 / 1	24	3
		> 20	29	97	0 / 3 / 0	32	3
Cates[878]	80	> 40	54	91	- / - / 4	-	-
Mooney[879]	-	> 10	327	93	0 / 1 / 1.5	29	5
Myler[880]	-	≤ 10	365	95	2.1	-	-
		11-20	278	91	0	-	-
		> 20	136	89	0	-	-
Zidar[881]	20	< 10	579	95	1.2 / - / 4.8	6.6	5.9
	20	> 10	149	90	0.7 / - / 8.1	18.1	14.1
	≥ 30	> 10	90	98	1.1 / - / 3.3	8.9	5.6
Savas[882]	40	> 20	109	90	2	35	7
	40	> 20**	69	88	1	20	7
Goudreau[883]	20	> 20	39	97	2.5	-	-

Abbreviations: AC = acute closure; DISS = dissection; D = in-hospital death; Q-MI = in-hospital Q-wave myocardial infarction; - = not reported; CABG = emergency coronary artery bypass grafting

† Length in millimeters

* Single number denotes overall in-hospital complications rate

** Bend ≥ 45°

Table 18. New Device Angioplasty of Long Lesions

Series	Device	Length (mm)	N	Success (%)	D/Q-MI/CABG (%)*
AMRO Trial[884,906-7]	ELCA	> 10	151	80	0 / 1.3 / 4.5
	PTCA	> 10	157	79	0 / 1.3 / 1.9
Litvack[908]	ELCA	< 10	1832	91	6
		10-19	1042	92	4.6
		20-29	467	89	6.6
		≥ 30	251	87	7.3
Warth[900]	Rotablator	≤ 10	588	-	- / 0.2 / -
		11-25	195		- / 2.1 / -
Ellis[901]	Rotablator	0-4	286	-	4.2
		5-8	69		10.1
		9-12	27		18.5
		13-16	6		50
Reisman[902]	Rotablator	< 10	953	95	0.6 / 0.7 / 2.6
		11-15	180	97	0.6 / 0 / 1.1
		15-25	143	92	2.1 / 2.8 / 1.4
Teirstein[903]	Rotablator	≤ 10	12	92	-
		> 10	30	70	-
Mooney[879]	DCA	> 10	88	97	0 / 1 / 1
Robertson[904]	DCA	< 10	250	93	- / - / 2
		10-19	59	90	- / - / 5
		≥ 20	19	79	- / - / 10
TEC[905] Registry	TEC	< 10	266	93	-
		10-20	220	93	-
		> 20	38	95	-
deMarchena[909]	Holmium laser	≤ 10	123	97	2.7
		11-20	193	94	3.1
		> 20	49	90	0
Maiello[910]	Stent	> 20	108	93	0 / 3 / 3
Shaknovich[922]	≥ 3 PSS	50	54	-	1.8 / 0 / 1.8
Akira[911]	PSS	>20	62	-	-
	GRS		26	-	-
	Wiktor		21	-	-

Abbreviations: D = in-hospital death; Q-MI = in-hospital Q-wave myocardial infarction; CABG = emergency coronary artery bypass grafting; TEC = Transluminal Extraction Catheter; ELCA = Excimer Laser Coronary Angioplasty; GRS = Gianturco-Roubin stent; PSS = Palmaz-Schatz stent; RS = restenosis; - = not reported

* Single number denotes overall in-hospital complication rate

*****

OSTIAL LESION: DIAGONAL BRANCH

A 50-year-old marathon runner develops severe angina at 3 km and while playing tennis. Myocardial perfusion imaging demonstrates ischemia at a moderate workload. Coronary angiography reveals a focal, noncalcified stenosis at the origin of the second diagonal branch (reference vessel = 3.2 mm). Other vessels and LV function are normal.

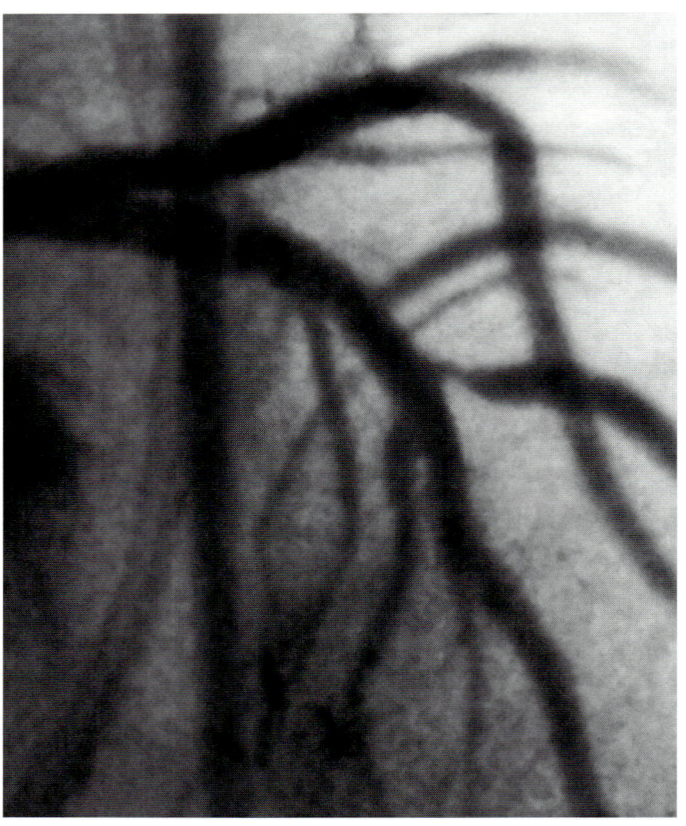

Is PTCA alone suitable for this type of lesion?

John Douglas Jr., MD, USA: This patient has a severe stenosis in a large diagonal artery at its origin. Lesions at vessel origins respond less favorably to conventional PTCA. Vessel recoil, suboptimal lumen enlargement, and dissection of the parent vessel are relatively common. In this patient, disease extends into the LAD, which has mild narrowing proximal to the large septal branch (enhancing the probability of injury to the LAD after PTCA).

Nicolaus Reifart, MD, Germany: The angiogram shows a focal, noncalcified lesion at the origin of the second diagonal branch. These lesions are easy to dilate, but the residual stenosis is usually 40-50% due to recoil and dissection.

Dean Kereiakes, MD, USA: This young patient has a focal, noncalcified stenosis involving the origin of a large diagonal branch. The ostial location is associated with an increased risk of suboptimal results and restenosis after PTCA.

What is your first choice for treating this patient?

John Douglas Jr., MD, USA: There is no angiographically-visible calcification in the lesion and the diagonal is large enough to consider directional atherectomy. In addition, the patient is relatively young and symptoms are of recent onset, both favoring directional atherectomy. I am a little concerned about the ectasia or post-stenotic dilation of the diagonal, which suggests that the lesion is chronic. I would defer my final decision on strategy until the procedure. If there is any calcification in the lesion on fluoroscopy (more sensitive than cine) or if the post-stenotic dilation of the diagonal is confirmed, I would perform intravascular ultrasound. Significant superficial calcification would favor a rotational atherectomy approach; otherwise, I recommend directional atherectomy.

Dean Kereiakes, MD, USA: The best percutaneous therapeutic option for this patient (in the absence of lesion calcification) is directional coronary atherectomy.

Describe your stent approach.

Nicolaus Reifart, MD, Germany: I would perform PTCA with a 0.014-inch Hi-torque floppy guidewire and a 3.0 x 20 mm balloon. If the residual stenosis is > 30% (recoil or dissection), I would place a half Palmaz-Schatz stent. The Palmaz-Schatz stents in Germany can be cut and crimped on the same balloon used for predilation. To place this short stent correctly, high resolution angiographic equipment is needed. Another option is the 8 mm Microstent, which is more radiodense. My specific antiplatelet and anticoagulation regimen is as follows: Aspirin (500 mg IC) before PTCA; heparin (20,000 units IV) during PTCA; heparin (5,000 units IV) after stenting; and ticlopidine (250 mg BID) and aspirin (100 mg BID) for 4 weeks after discharge.

Describe your directional atherectomy approach.

John Douglas Jr., MD, USA: I recommend a 7F GTO AtheroCath over a 0.014-inch Platinum-Plus wire with 8-10 circumferential cuts at 1 ATM. I would repeat atherectomy and perform adjunctive PTCA for residual stenosis > 20%.

Dean Kereiakes, MD, USA: I would use a DVI 10F JL4 guide catheter, a 0.014-inch Extra-Support guidewire, and a 7F EX or GTO atherectomy device. I would perform 6-8 cuts in a circumferential fashion at 15-20 PSI (GTO) or 20-30 PSI (EX). Following atherectomy, I recommend PTCA with a 3.25 mm balloon if necessary, to optimize the result.

Describe your Rotablator approach.

John Douglas Jr., MD, USA: Rotational atherectomy is a third percutaneous option, but will produce less complete debulking in this relatively large vessel. I recommend a 9F guide; sequential 1.5 mm, 2.0 mm, and 2.25 mm burrs; and a 3.25 mm balloon inflated at 3 ATM.

Dean Kereiakes, MD, USA: I favor Rotational atherectomy if significant calcification is present in the target lesion. A very reasonable approach includes a 9F JL4 short-tip guiding catheter, a 0.009-inch Rotablator-C wire, and sequential 1.75 mm and 2.25 mm burrs. The 1.75 mm burr would be operated at 180,000 RPM with a gentle pecking motion, being careful to avoid deceleration ≥ 5,000 RPM. The 2.25 mm burr would be operated at 160,000 RPM with the same technique, and the duration of rotablation would be 30-45 seconds per pass. Following rotablation with a 2.25 mm burr, I would utilize a 3.25 mm balloon at 2 ATM for 2-3 minutes, to optimize the result.

<u>Editors' Perspective</u>: The lesion at the origin of the diagonal branch was treated by directional atherectomy using a 7F EX AtheroCath, followed by adjunctive PTCA (below) (see p. 64 for additional comments).

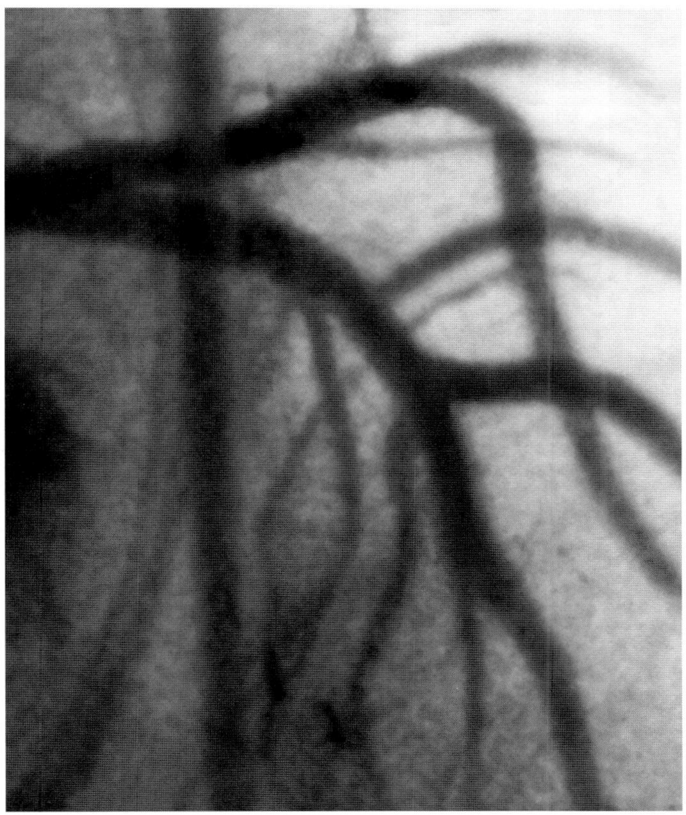

*****

OSTIAL LESION: CALCIFIED RCA

A 50-year-old sheet metal worker develops progressive exertional angina. Myocardial perfusion imaging reveals ischemia out a moderate workload. Coronary angiography reveals a subtotal calcified stenosis of the ostium of the RCA (reference vessel diameter = 2.8 mm; arrows indicate calcification). Other vessels and LV function are normal.

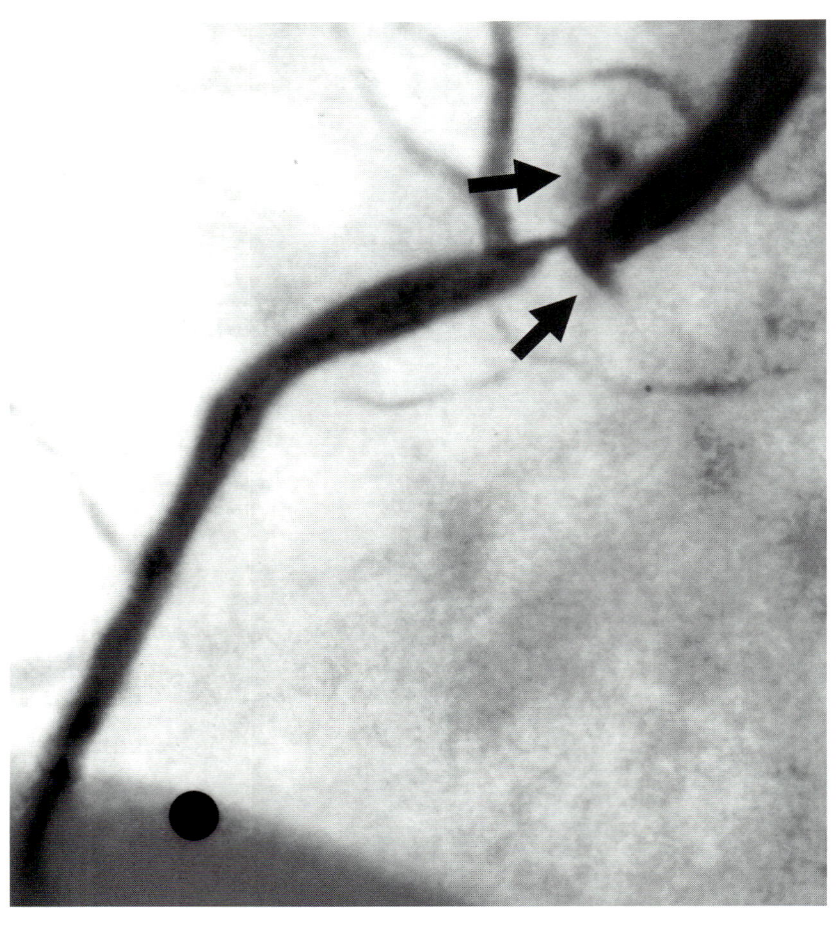

Is PTCA alone suitable for this lesion?

John Douglas Jr., MD, USA: The culprit is a severe lesion at the ostium of a medium-size RCA with angiographic calcification in the aorta, at or near the ostium. Ostial RCA stenoses have an increased incidence of complications and restenosis, regardless of treatment strategy. Lesion calcium further increases the chance of technical difficulty, and precludes effective PTCA, directional atherectomy, and stenting. Given the relatively modest size of the vessel, the extent of diffuse atheromatous disease, and the angiographic calcium, I recommend rotational atherectomy.

Nicolaus Reifart, MD, Germany: This patient has a subtotal calcified stenosis of the ostium of a diffusely diseased RCA. With PTCA, the risk of dissection is high. Even without dissection, the acute results are mediocre because of elastic recoil. Therefore, I recommend Rotablator.

Dean Kereiakes, MD, USA: This angiogram reveals a very focal (5-8 mm) but densely calcified ostial stenosis in a dominant RCA, unsuitable for PTCA. This slightly downsloping takeoff is optimal for rotational atherectomy.

Describe your Rotablator approach.

John Douglas Jr., MD, USA: I would use a 9F JR 3.5 guide with sideholes and sequential 1.5 mm, 2.25 mm, and 2.5 mm burrs. I would insert a prophylactic temporary pacemaker.

Nicolaus Reifart, MD, Germany: I recommend an 8F JR4 guiding catheter (an Amplatz catheter might dissect the vessel). I recommend a Rotablator-C wire and a 1.75 mm burr to debulk the lesion. The platform speed should be 175,000-190,000 RPM and should not decrease more than 5,000 RPM during ablation. To avoid total A-V block, I would administer atropine (1.0 mg) prior to the procedure, limit the ablation sequences to ≤ 10 seconds, and wait 10-20 seconds between runs (to allow flushing of debris and normalization of the heart rate). The Rotablator flush should contain saline, heparin (20,000 units/L), verapamil (10 mg/L) and nitroglycerin (4 mg/L).

Dean Kereiakes, MD, USA: I would approach this case with a 9F JR4 short-tip guiding catheter, a 0.009-inch Rotablator-C wire, and sequential 1.5 mm and 2.0 mm burrs. I would operate these burrs at 180,000 RPM with a gradual pecking motion and ablation duration of 30-60 seconds.

After Rotablator, how would you further enlarge the lumen?

John Douglas Jr., MD, USA: I would perform adjunctive PTCA with a 3.0 mm balloon.

Nicolaus Reifart, MD, Germany: After rotablation, I would use a noncompliant 3.0 x 20 mm balloon at 2 ATM. If the balloon does fully expand at 4 ATM, I would exchange for a 2.0 mm burr to debulk more calcium. With my technique of cautious debulking (burr = 50-60% of reference vessel diameter) followed by PTCA, I achieve very good acute results and very low complication rates. A more aggressive burr strategy may increase major complications and no-reflow, without decreasing restenosis.

Dean Kereiakes, MD, USA: After Rotablator, I would perform PTCA with a 3.0 mm balloon, place a 3.0 mm Palmaz-Schatz stent in the ostium, and then postdilate with a 3.0 x 9 mm Titan at 18 ATM.

Can this lesion be stented?

Dean Kereiakes, MD, USA: Attempts at primary stent placement in this type of lesion are fraught with problems: Significant elastic recoil can significantly obstruct the stent unless tissue ablation or removal is performed prior to stent placement. Because the degree of recoil cannot be ascertained prior to stent placement, I feel it is important to debulk plaque prior to stent deployment. If recoil occurs through the stent, I would place a second overlapping stent of the same diameter, and repeat high-pressure inflations. I find this to be the only effective way to fortify the radial strength of the stent, to counteract elastic recoil.

<u>Editors' Perspective</u>: The calcified lesion at the ostium of the RCA was treated by Rotablator atherectomy and adjunctive PTCA (below) (see p. 64 for additional comments).

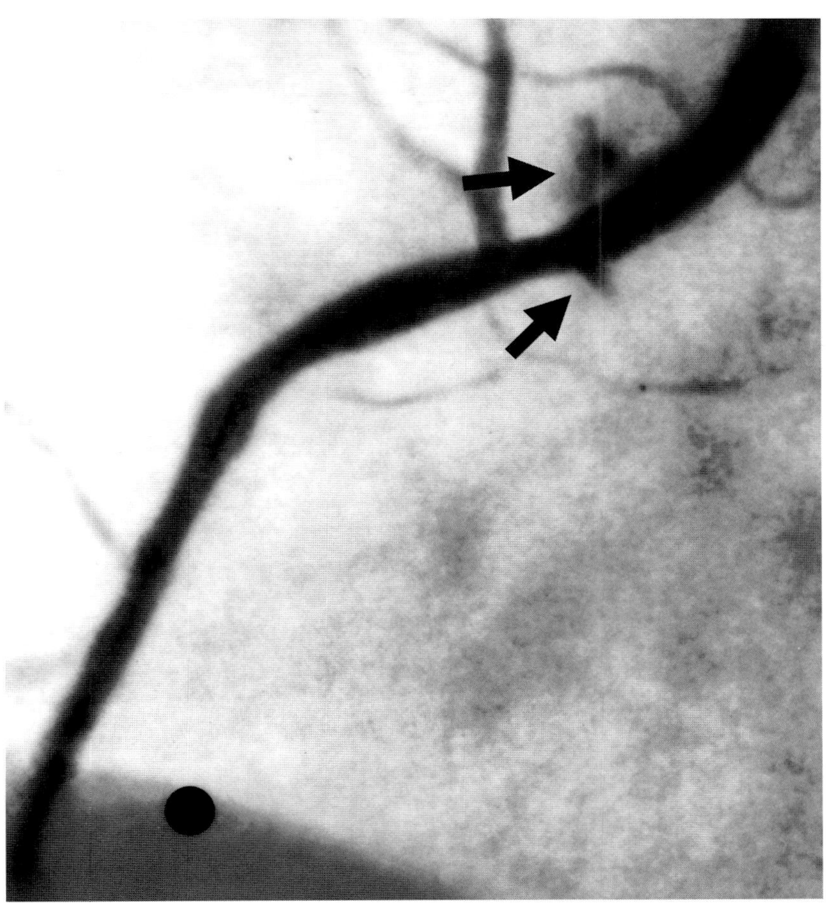

*****

OSTIAL LESION: LAD

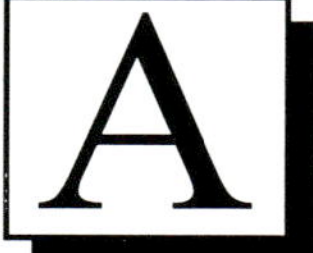

A 64-year-old pilot presents to your office with severe exertional angina. Myocardial perfusion imaging reveals ischemia at low workload. Coronary angiography reveals a severe stenosis at the origin of the LAD (reference vessel diameter = 3.8 mm). Other coronary arteries and left ventricular function are normal.

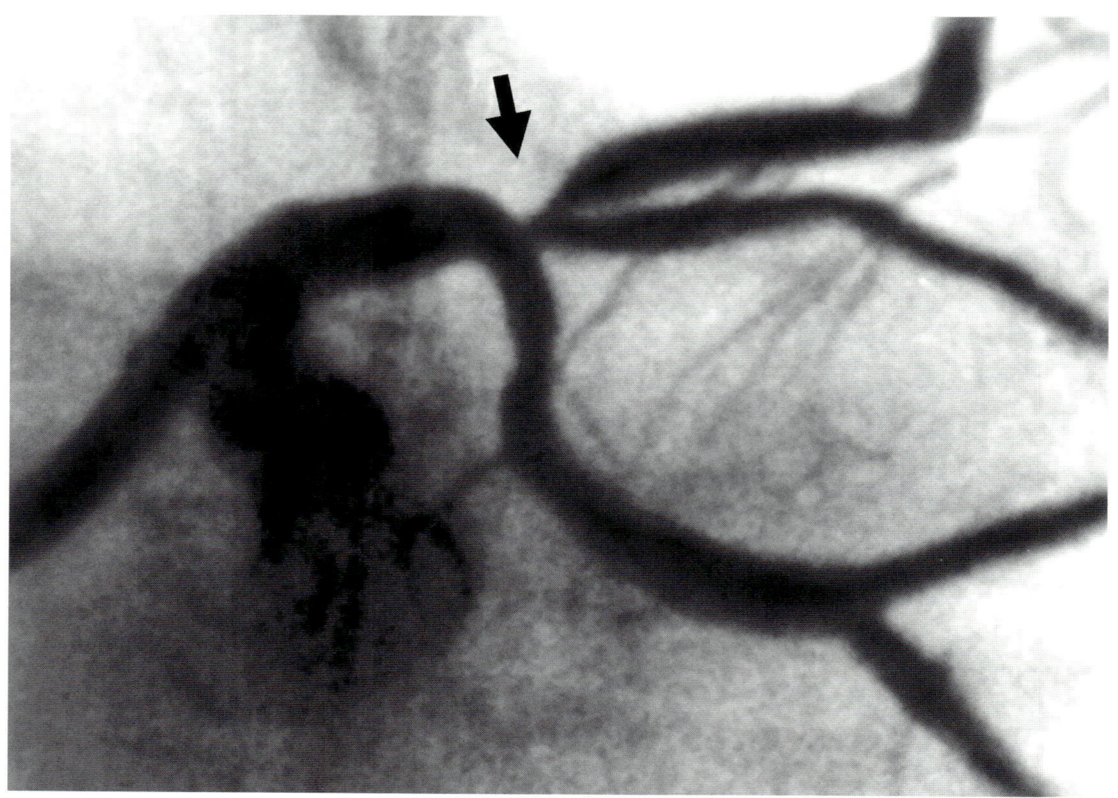

Is this patient suitable for percutaneous revascularization?

John Douglas Jr., MD, USA: This patient has a high-grade stenosis at the origin of a large

LAD, without angiographic calcification. This type of lesion causes apprehension because of the proximal location and extension of the plaque into the left main coronary artery. However, in my experience, acute complications are very rare with PTCA or directional atherectomy; restenosis is common with both. Stenting is not a good option since the stent will have to cover the large ramus and extend into the origin of the LCX.

Nicolaus Reifart, MD, Germany: This patient has a severe stenosis at the origin of the LAD. This type of lesion has prognostic relevance; the percutaneous revascularization technique must be as safe as bypass surgery. Many cardiologists and cardiac surgeons prefer surgery, but randomized comparisons between CABG and PTCA for this type of lesion have not been reported. For PTCA and directional coronary atherectomy, the lesion is not technically challenging. However, the incidence of out-of-lab abrupt closure is 3-5%, which may result in high mortality. Furthermore, the risk of restenosis is 40%. Nevertheless, percutaneous intervention is reasonable; my goal is to achieve a residual stenosis < 20%.

Dean Kereiakes, MD, USA: This patient has a focal, eccentric, noncalcified stenosis at the origin of the LAD. The left main is large and the origin of the LCX and ramus are not involved. Percutaneous revascularization is safe and reasonable.

Describe your preferred approach to this lesion.

John Douglas Jr., MD, USA: I recommend directional atherectomy using a 7F graft AtheroCath and a 0.014-inch Platinum-Plus wire. I would perform 8-10 cuts (avoiding the inferior quadrant) and adjunctive PTCA with a 4.0 mm balloon at 2-3 ATM. If the angiographic result is excellent, the patient will be discharged the following day.

Nicolaus Reifart, MD, Germany: I would perform PTCA with a 0.014-inch Extra-Support wire to facilitate precise stent placement, and a 4.0 x 20 mm perfusion balloon to allow 30-60 second inflations without severe angina or hemodynamic compromise. After full inflation at 6 ATM, the inflation would be repeated twice at 6 ATM and the inflation pressure would be increased only if the residual stenosis exceeds 30%. PTCA would be followed by placement of a Palmaz-Schatz stent; precise placement is crucial and should be verified in at least two views (LAO 40° caudal 25°; and 90° LAO). The stent would be mounted on a 4.0 mm balloon and deployed at 10 ATM, with higher pressure only if on-line QCA reveals a residual stenosis > 0%. The patient would be placed on my routine post-stent treatment (aspirin and ticlopidine for 4 weeks). I recommend a followup angiogram at 4-6 months to ensure a good long-term result.

Dean Kereiakes, MD, USA: I would approach this patient with a DVI 10F JL4 guiding catheter, a 0.014-inch Extra-Support guidewire, and a 7F GTO AtheroCath. I would perform the first atherectomy cut with the window oriented in a superior direction in the RAO projection, since the eccentric plaque is on the roof of the LAD. I would perform circumferential cuts at 30 PSI with the cutter window oriented at 9, 12 and 3 o'clock, and a single pass at 15 PSI with the cutter window directed at 6 o'clock toward the relatively uninvolved LCX. I recommend adjunctive PTCA with a 4.0 mm perfusion balloon to optimize the result, if necessary.

What would you do if the result is "suboptimal"?

John Douglas Jr., MD, USA: If the angiographic result is suboptimal following several adjunctive balloon inflations, I would insert a 4.0 mm perfusion balloon for 10-20 minutes. I would avoid stenting unless needed for bailout, and would use ReoPro to reduce post-procedure ischemic complications.

Editors' Perspective: There is one consistent theme in the percutaneous approach to ostial lesions: PTCA alone does not achieve adequate lumen enlargement, due to lesion rigidity and elastic recoil. None of the interventional cardiologists we surveyed recommend PTCA for ostial lesions. The most favored approach is Rotablator, recommended by 37%, followed by directional atherectomy in 26%, stenting in 21%, and excimer laser angioplasty in 16%. Multi-device therapy (Table 19) based on associated lesion morphology (Table 20) is more often applied to ostial stenoses than any other lesion type.

Table 19. New Device Angioplasty of Ostial Stenoses: Acute Outcome

Series	Device	Lesion	N	Success (%)	D/Q-MI/CABG (%)*
Waksman[858]	All devices	AO native AO SVG	184 122	89 94	3 2
Ellis[859]	ROTA	-	68	91	-
Cowley[860]	ROTA	RCA	109	93	2.8 / 0 / 1.8
Commeau[861]	ROTA	AO BO	32 110	97 94	3 / 3 / 3 0.9 / 0.9 / 0.9
Koller[862]	ROTA TEC	AO, BO AO, BO	29 72	93 90	3 / 3 / 3 1.3 / 0 / 4.1
Stephan[863]	DCA	AO BO	30 73	70 92	0 / 0 / 3 0 / 0 / 0
Boehrer[851] (CAVEAT)	PTCA DCA	LAD LAD	33 41	87 86	0 / 0 / 3 0 / 2 / 5
Popma[864]	DCA	AO, BO	81	98	-
Robertson[865]	DCA	AO BO	41 75	78 92	4.9 0
Litvack[866]	ELCA	-	280	89	7
deMarchena[867]	ILCA	-	23	91	4
Sawada[852]	PTCA ELCA DCA Stent	LAD, LCX	80 24 29 22	90 88 90 100	- - - -
Brogan[869]	ROTA DCA	AO, BO	101 58	97 97	0 / 0 / 2 0 / 0 / 1
Colombo[874]	Stent	AO	35	100	0
DeCesare[875]	Stent	LAD	23	100	0
Rocha-Singh[870]	Stent	AO, BO	41	93	5 / 0 / 0
Teirstein[872]	Stent	AO, BO	28	89	7

Abbreviations: D = death; Q-MI = Q-wave myocardial infarction; CABG = emergency coronary artery bypass grafting; AC = acute closure; AO = aorto-ostial; BO = branch-ostial; DCA = directional coronary atherectomy; ROTA = Rotablator; ELCA = excimer laser coronary angioplasty; ILCA = infrared laser coronary angioplasty; TEC = translumunal extraction catheter; - not reported

* Single number denotes overall in-hospital complication rate

Table 20. Ostial Lesion Morphology and New Interventional Device Selection

Morphology	DCA	TEC	Rotablator	ELCA	Stent
Type A	+	-	+	+	+
Thrombus	+[a]	+	-	+	+[b]
Calcification	±[c]	-	+	±	+[b]
Long	-	-	±	±	±
Eccentric	+	-	+	+[d]	+
Angulation	-	-	-	-	-
Dissection	±	-	-	-	+
Ulcerated	+	-	+	+	+
Restenotic	+	-	+	+	+

Abbreviations: + = Favorable; - = Unfavorable; a = Lesions with a large amount of clot should probably not be attempted; b = May be considered after Rotablator (calcified lesions) or TEC (thrombus-containing lesion); c = New calcium cutter may be useful; may be considered after Rotablator; d = Directional ELCA may have a role

The lesion at the origin of the LAD was treated by directional atherectomy without adjunctive PTCA (below).

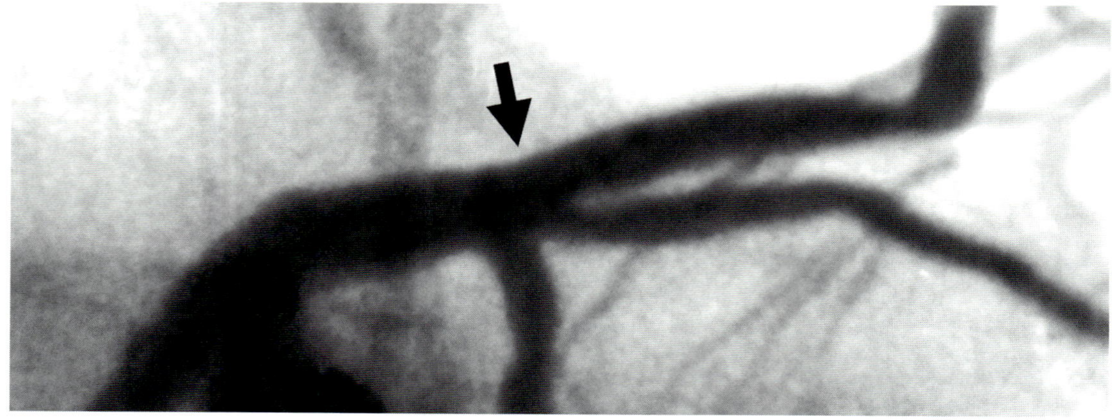

*****

ANGULATED LESION: INNER CURVE

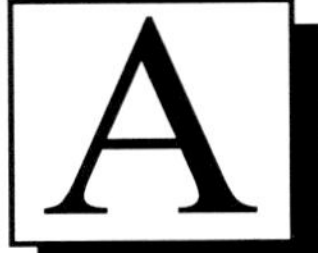

48-year-old firefighter develops angina while exercising on a Nordic track at home. Coronary angiography reveals a severely angulated stenosis in the proximal LAD (reference vessel = 3.4 mm). Other coronary arteries and left ventricular function are normal.

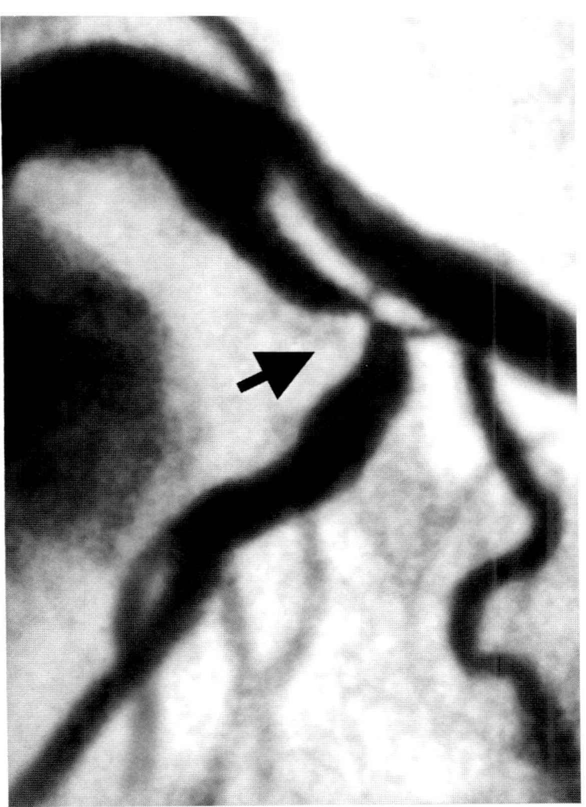

How does this lesion morphology influence your choice of devices for percutaneous intervention?

Spencer King III, MD, USA: This patient has an eccentric stenosis in a large proximal LAD. There is unusual angulation and the bulk of the plaque is located on the inner curve. Angulated lesions have greater propensity for dissection, and eccentric lesions have more recoil. Although PTCA can be performed, I favor directional atherectomy.

David Holmes, MD, USA: This patient has a severely angulated stenosis in a large proximal LAD. Severe angulation increases the potential for dissection with conventional PTCA, perforation with Rotablator, and delivery problems with large devices such as directional atherectomy. The two most reasonable options are stenting or perfusion balloon angioplasty (with conditional stenting, if the result is suboptimal). I favor a primary stent approach.

Are there any devices you would specifically avoid?

Spencer King III, MD, USA: Unless there is heavy calcification, I would not consider Rotablator because of the risk of dissection.

David Holmes, MD, USA: I would specifically avoid the Rotablator in this setting unless the vessel is heavily calcified.

Describe your stent approach.

David Holmes, MD, USA: Because of the angulation, I would choose a guiding catheter that gives optimal support and coaxial alignment, such as an Amplatz guide. The specific guidewire is dependent upon the stent; a GR-II stent and 0.014-inch Extra-Support wire are preferable. If the vessel does not straighten, I would use a 0.018-inch Extra-Support wire. I would predilate with a 3.0 mm balloon to allow passage of the stent. If a Palmaz-Schatz stent is used, I would avoid positioning the articulation at the stenosis. I would postdilate with a 3.75 mm balloon at 16-18 ATM, and perform intravascular ultrasound to document ideal stent apposition. If stent apposition and angiographic appearance are normal, the patient will be given aspirin (325 mg QD) and ticlopidine (250 mg BID) for one month.

Describe your atherectomy approach.

Spencer King III, MD, USA: Directional atherectomy will allow debulking of the lesion along the inner curve; I would not cut on the outer curve. After taking 6-8 cuts on the inner curve with a 7F AtheroCath, I would examine the result: If multiple large tissue samples are retrieved and the residual stenosis is < 25%, I would follow with a 3.5 mm balloon. If I do not retrieve adequate tissue samples, I would reinsert the AtheroCath at 45 PSI. A 300 cm extra-support guidewire is helpful here, and allows easy exchanges. Although the 7F device will probably pass the lesion, this can be aided by gentle device rotation to reduce friction. If the AtheroCath does not pass, I would predilate with a 2.5 mm balloon to facilitate passage.

If the result is suboptimal, what would you do?

Spencer King III, MD, USA: If dissection is observed or the result is unsatisfactory, I would place a 3.5 mm Palmaz-Schatz stent and postdilate with a 3.75 mm balloon at 14-16 ATM.

What would you recommend if new devices are not availabe at your center?

David Holmes, MD, USA: I would treat this lesion with the same guiding catheter, an extra-support wire, and a 3.5 mm perfusion balloon. Prolonged inflation in this setting will result in the best chance for a good initial result, short of stent implantation. ReoPro is useful in high-risk lesions such as this, and I would aim for an ACT < 300 seconds during the procedure, with no further heparin after PTCA.

Spencer King III, MD, USA: This lesion is best managed by operators who are experienced with directional atherectomy and stents; however, PTCA is certainly not contraindicated.

<u>Editors' Perspective</u>: The angulated lesion in the LAD was treated by conventional PTCA with a 3.5 x 40 mm balloon, leaving a mild residual stenosis (below) (see p. 73 for additional comments).

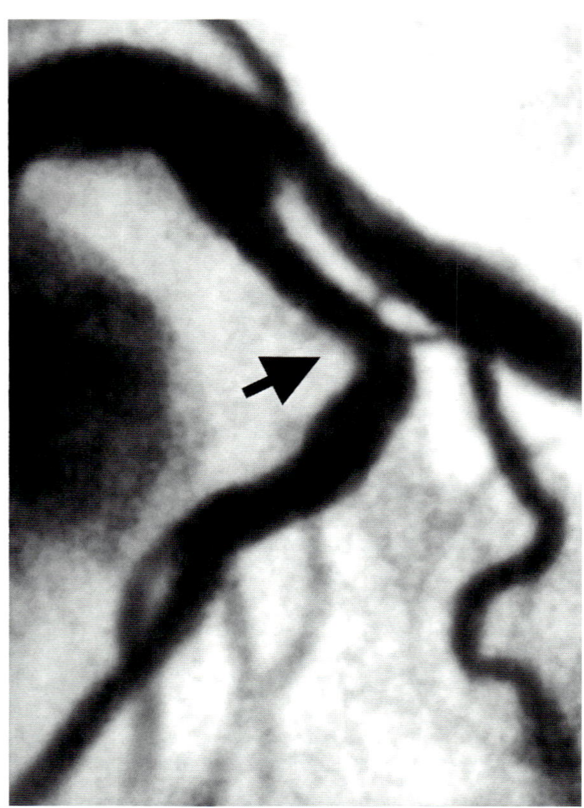

*****

ANGULATED LESION: OUTER CURVE

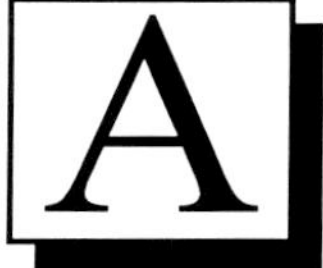
53-year-old firefighter develops angina. Coronary angiography reveals a severe angulated stenosis in the RCA (reference vessel = 3.1 mm). Other coronary arteries and left ventricular function are normal.

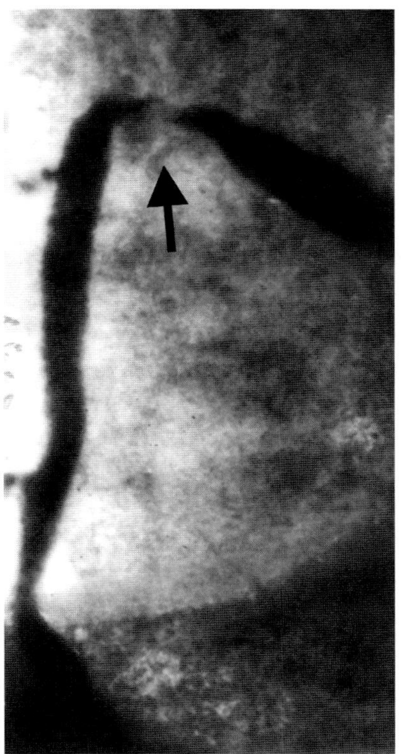

How does this lesion morphology influence your approach?

David Holmes, MD, USA: This patient has a severely angulated, irregular stenosis in the RCA; the lesion is on the outer curve of the bend. This lesion has a substantial down-side to it: Severe angulation impacts device delivery and performance.

Spencer King III, MD, USA: The lesion is complex and has the appearance of possible thrombus. I would first perform PTCA with a 30 mm balloon to minimize straightening of the angulated segment. Pretreatment with ReoPro is useful.

Are any devices not recommended in this setting?

David Holmes, MD, USA: I would avoid Rotablator and laser in this setting because of potential perforation. Directional atherectomy could be used, but it would be difficult to deliver the AtheroCath to the lesion.

Spencer King III, MD, USA: Rotablator is clearly contraindicated here based on lesion angulation and potential thrombus.

Describe your technical approach to this lesion.

David Holmes, MD, USA: Optimal guiding catheter support is important; I recommend a short-tip 8F AL1 with sideholes. Given the excessive tortuosity, I would implant a Gianturco-Roubin stent or a Wallstent (investigational use in the United States). For the Gianturco-Roubin stent, I would use a 0.018-inch Extra-Support wire, a 2.5-3.0 x 30 mm balloon, and a 3.0 mm Gianturco-Roubin stent. The GR-II stent is lower profile and is much better than the original design. I would deploy the stent at 6-7 ATM and then use a 3.5 x 30 mm high-pressure balloon at 16 ATM. If the angiographic result is optimal, I would treat the patient with aspirin and ticlopidine. I do not use IVUS with the Gianturco-Roubin stent because of the potential for snagging the stent coils. If the stent does not look ideal, or if there is plaque protruding through the stent, I would deploy another stent.

Spencer King III, MD, USA: A Judkins-style guide will probably work, although the ostium is slightly upgoing. If the fit is inadequate, I would switch to an AL1 guide for better back-up. I would use a Hi-torque floppy guidewire to maintain the curvature of the artery, and dilate with a 3.0 x 30 mm balloon at 4-6 ATM. If PTCA results in dissection or significant recoil, I would implant a Gianturco-Roubin stent.

What would you recommend for the more distal stenosis?

David Holmes, MD, USA: The distal stenosis may be more severe once the proximal lesion is treated. If it is more than 50%, I would perform PTCA at low pressure to avoid dissection, and implant a stent. Generally, I prefer to stent all dilated segments in the same artery if the vessel is not too small.

Spencer King III, MD, USA: I would utilize the same balloon for the distal stenosis, using low-pressure inflations, if possible.

If new devices are not an option, can this lesion be approached with conventional PTCA?

David Holmes, MD, USA: I would use a 3.25-3.5 x 40 mm balloon at low pressure. I would inflate very slowly and try to maintain pressure for as long as possible to mold the artery. Several series suggest that long balloons result in satisfactory outcome in angulated lesions.

What would you recommend if the result is suboptimal?

Spencer King III, MD, USA: If there is dissection, incomplete expansion, or persistent filling defects, I would place a 3.5 mm Gianturco-Roubin stent because of its flexibility.

Editors' Perspective: Increasing lesion angulation has an adverse impact on PTCA success and complications (Table 21), and severely angulated lesions are problematic for virtually all laser and atherectomy devices due to the risk of dissection and perforation from ablation or plaque removal. Directional atherectomy can be used in some angulated lesions, but the AtheroCath may be difficult to deliver because of rigidity of the housing; when used, undersized and/or short-window devices may facilitate device delivery. In our interventional survey, 65% of operators recommended

conventional PTCA. Long (30-40 mm) balloons may be especially useful in these lesions to enhance conformability and avoid excessive straightening forces. Stents were also recommended by 35% of operators, particularly those from Europe and Asia. The discordance of opinion about stents for angulated lesions may reflect the favorable experience with newer stent designs (such as the GR-II stent, Nir stent, Microstent, MultiLink stent, Palmaz-Schatz stent with spiral articulation, and Wallstent), which are not yet available in the United States. From a technical standpoint, stenting of angulated lesions often requires strong guiding catheter support and coaxial alignment, use of heavy-duty or extra-support guidewires, adequate predilation of the target lesion, and modifications of the delivery system for certain stents. For example, delivery of the articulated Palmaz-Schatz stent may require a "buddy-wire" approach or use of the "stentless delivery balloon" technique. The "buddy-wire" approach requires two extra-support or heavy-duty guidewires to straighten the vessel. Once the stent delivery system is positioned across the lesion, the "buddy-wire" is removed and the stent deployed. The "stentless-delivery balloon" technique involves removing the stent delivery balloon from the delivery sheath, and replacing it with another low-profile balloon. Once the low-profile balloon/delivery sheath is advanced across the lesion, the low-profile balloon is exchanged for the stent delivery balloon; the sheath is then retracted and the stent deployed. If tufts of plaque or dissection flaps protrude through the stent struts or coils, implantation of another overlapping stent is required. In the present case, the angulated lesion in the RCA was treated by PTCA using a 3.0 x 40 mm balloon. Final angiography revealed mild residual stenosis and a small intimal dissection (below).

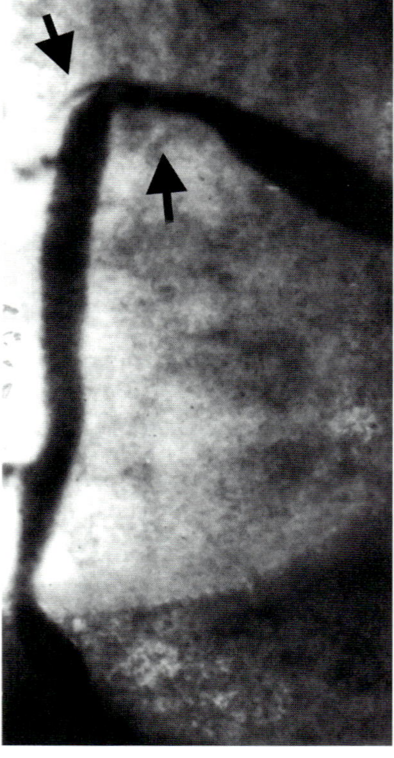

Table 21. Effect of Lesion Angulation on Acute PTCA Outcome

Series	N	Angulation (degrees)	Success (%)	Complications** (%)
Tan[756]	991	< 45	94	2.2†
	136	45-90	88	8.8†
	30	> 90	83	13†
Myler[765]	543	< 45	94	1.3
	158	45-90	95	2.5
	78	≥ 90	94	2.6
Savas[766]	69*	≥ 45	88	1
Ellis[757]	189	Type A	92	2
	144	≥ 45	72	13++
	32	≥ 60	53	-

- = Not Reported
++ Dissection occurred in 46% of angulated lesions compared to 8% of non-angulated lesions
* All lesions ≥ 2 cm in length were treated with long (40 mm) balloons
** In-hospital death, MI, or emergency CABG unless otherwise indicated
† Incidence of acute closure

*****

TORTUOUS RCA

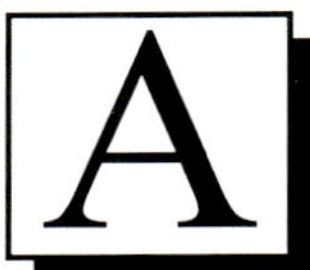

A 58-year-old hospital administrator develops unstable angina. Cardiac catheterization demonstrates a focal 80% stenosis in the proximal RCA (reference vessel = 3.2 mm), which is an extremely tortuous vessel. Other coronary arteries and left ventricular function are normal.

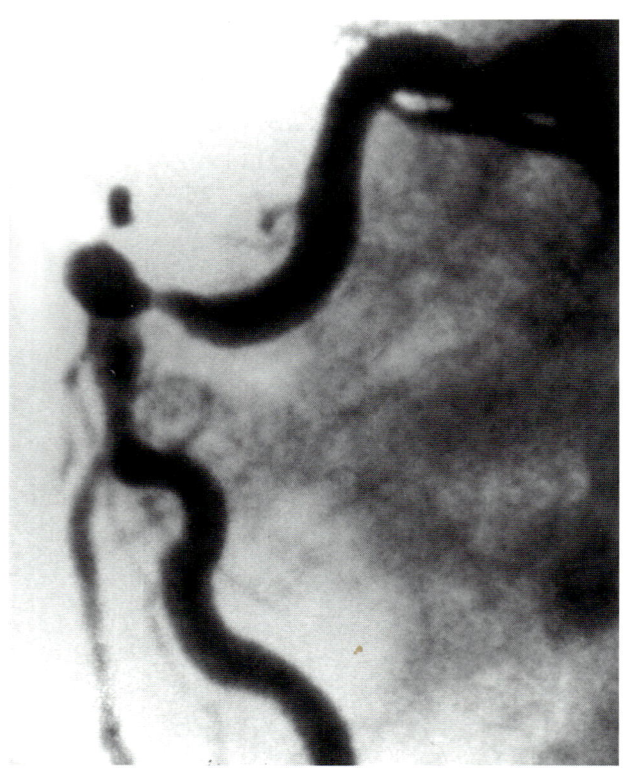

Is this challenging lesion suitable for percutaneous intervention, or is CABG a better choice?

Richard Heuser, MD, USA: This patient has a focal stenosis in a very tortuous RCA. This is definitely a high-risk lesion; if I did not do anything but angioplasty and the patient was unstable, I would send the patient for an internal mammary graft to the distal RCA, or refer the patient to another site where stents and other devices are available.

Richard Schatz, MD, USA: This patient presents with unstable angina and a severe stenosis in the RCA, which is extraordinarily tortuous. This is an excellent example where both clinical presentation and anatomy will conspire against a high success rate after percutaneous intervention. The presence of unstable angina suggests a thrombotic component to the lesion, and is associated with a higher risk of abrupt closure. Likewise, tortuosity increases the risk of dissection and abrupt closure. The combination of adverse clinical and anatomic features suggests that this patient will be at higher risk for procedural complications; this patient should be handled only by someone who is prepared to do immediate bail-out stenting. If the mid-lesion at the takeoff of the marginal branch is critical, this patient is not a great candidate for PTCA or coronary stenting; elective bypass surgery should be considered.

Assuming percutaneous intervention is feasible, what device would you recommend?

Richard Heuser, MD, USA: This clinical scenario could be improved dramatically with administration of ReoPro, no matter which device is selected. I recommend conventional PTCA.

Richard Schatz, MD, USA: Due to the high potential for procedural complications in this particular patient, I would select a device that gives the greatest reliability and predictability during the procedure— the Palmaz-Schatz coronary stent is my first choice. I do not recommend ReoPro, since it is unnecessary with successful stenting. If stent delivery is unsuccessful, ReoPro might increase the risk of bleeding during or after CABG.

Takeshi Kimura, MD, Japan: This patient has a focal, slightly eccentric stenosis involving a tortuous RCA, and a mild distal stenosis. Since the distal vessel is so tortuous making stent implantation extremely difficult, I prefer to treat the proximal "culprit" lesion with PTCA alone.

Describe your PTCA technique.

Richard Heuser, MD, USA: I would use a 0.014-inch x 300 cm Extra-S'port wire and a large lumen (0.086-inch inner diameter) 8F guide. Although the severe lesion is focal, the plaque extends 2-3 cm. I would begin with a 2.5 x 30 mm balloon at low pressure, and a 3.0 mm or 3.5 mm balloon, if necessary. Bolus (0.25 mg/kg) and infusion (10 mcg/min for 12 hours) of ReoPro is strongly recommended.

Takeshi Kimura, MD, Japan: I would perform PTCA with an 8F JR 4.0 guiding catheter, a 0.014-inch guidewire, and a 3.25 x 20 mm semicompliant, over-the-wire balloon. Since I am reluctant to place stents in this lesion, I would perform 2-3 inflations for 2-3 minutes each. Meticulous attention must be paid to proper positioning of the balloon; PTCA in the distal bend might lead to severe dissection.

What would you do if the PTCA result is suboptimal?

Richard Heuser, MD, USA: Because this lesion is so eccentric and the vessel is so tortuous, I would very quickly exchange for a stiffer wire such as a 0.014- or 0.018-inch Platinum-Plus wire (I prefer a 0.018-inch Platinum-Plus wire with a Gianturco-Roubin stent) if the PTCA result is suboptimal. The likelihood of success with the Palmaz-Schatz stent is greater than 90%. I would use a 3.0 mm or 3.5 mm Palmaz-Schatz stent and pull back the sheath a little bit, exposing the tip of the delivery balloon to facilitate tracking. A 3.5 x 40 mm GR-II stent or Wallstent is also an excellent choice, if available. No matter which stent is used, I would postdilate to at least 18 ATM and use intravascular ultrasound to confirm apposition and correct sizing. I would discharge the patient the following morning on aspirin and ticlopidine.

Richard Schatz, MD, USA: One must be prepared to stent any vessel if PTCA is the first line of therapy. If a Judkins guide and a flexible wire are placed and the patient develops abrupt closure, it is very unlikely that an emergency stent could be placed successfully. Trying to change the initial equipment for specialized equipment could prove hazardous, with loss of guidewire position during guiding catheter transfer. Remember that even in experienced hands, rescue for ischemic failure occurs in 10% of patients undergoing routine PTCA.

Takeshi Kimura, MD, Japan: If the final angiographic result is clearly suboptimal despite repeated balloon inflations, I would perform stent implantation. I would exchange the guidewire for a 0.014-inch x 300 cm Extra-Support guidewire, followed by placement of a 3.5 x 10 mm Palmaz-Schatz stent or a 3.5 x 8 mm Microstent. Post-stent dilation must be performed with a 3.5 x 9 mm noncompliant balloon at 15-18 ATM.

Describe your technique for planned stenting.

Richard Schatz, MD, USA: My impression of the tortuous appearance in the LAO projection is that there is also a "switch-back" in the RAO projection, making guiding catheter selection critical. There is no substitute for careful planning for optimal guiding catheter support and a super-stiff guidewire to straighten out the complex target; this case could not be successfully stented with a Judkins guide and a Hi-torque floppy wire. The only guide that will work well here is an AL1 with sideholes; the Cordis guiding catheter is my first choice due to its stiffness. A short-tip guide will decrease the chance of guiding catheter-induced dissection. After passing the "push" test, I would advance a 0.014-inch Cordis Stabilizer wire to the distal vessel, and using the Cordis Titan as a transfer catheter, I would exchange the Stabilizer wire for a 0.014-inch Platinum-Plus wire. Without a doubt, this is the stiffest wire on the market and will straighten the entire vessel. I would cut a Palmaz-Schatz stent in half, remount the 7 mm "half-stent" on the distal marker of the stent delivery balloon to allow precise placement, and leave the greatest length of the balloon proximal to the lesion (where it can do the least damage). There is an obvious balloon-stent mismatch when a half-stent is used, so this must be taken into account when planning stent placement. I would predilate this lesion with a 3.5 x 9 mm Cordis Titan at 1-2 ATM for 10 seconds. Stent deployment and high-pressure balloon inflations should take < 10 seconds; there is no advantage to prolonged inflations. Angioscopy, ultrasound, and Doppler FloWire are not indicated in this case if we assume that the operator completes the final inflation at 20 ATM, and multiple views reveal a "step-up" and "step-down" at either end of the stent. The patient would receive aspirin and ticlopidine and be discharged 6-24 hours after the procedure.

What technical aspects of this procedure are essential to ensure success?

Richard Schatz, MD, USA: The most common mistakes are improper selection of guiding catheters and inappropriate waste of time using standard "non-power" guides and floppy guidewires. Another mistake is failure to recognize that the morphologic appearance of the vessel will change drastically when a super-stiff wire is used, creating pseudolesions due to kinking. One must resist the temptation to "fix" or "repair" these pseudolesions with extra stents, PTCA, or lytic therapy. Another mistake is to use a 15 mm Palmaz-Schatz stent since the extra metal is unnecessary. If the operator places the half-stent on the trailing marker, most of the delivery balloon will be distal to the target lesion during stenosis deployment, exposing the opportunity for distal dissection. If PTCA is the primary therapy, all of the above recommendations (regarding guiding catheter and wire) must be followed.

Editors' Perspective: Rotablator and stents were not available when this procedure was performed. Because of the eccentricity in the RCA lesion, we felt that conventional PTCA would fail; the patient was treated by directional atherectomy using a short-tip 9.5F JR4 guiding catheter, a flexible guidewire, and a 6F short-cut EX device. Two passes and multiple cuts were made, leaving an excellent angiographic result without complication (below) (see p. 86 for additional comments).

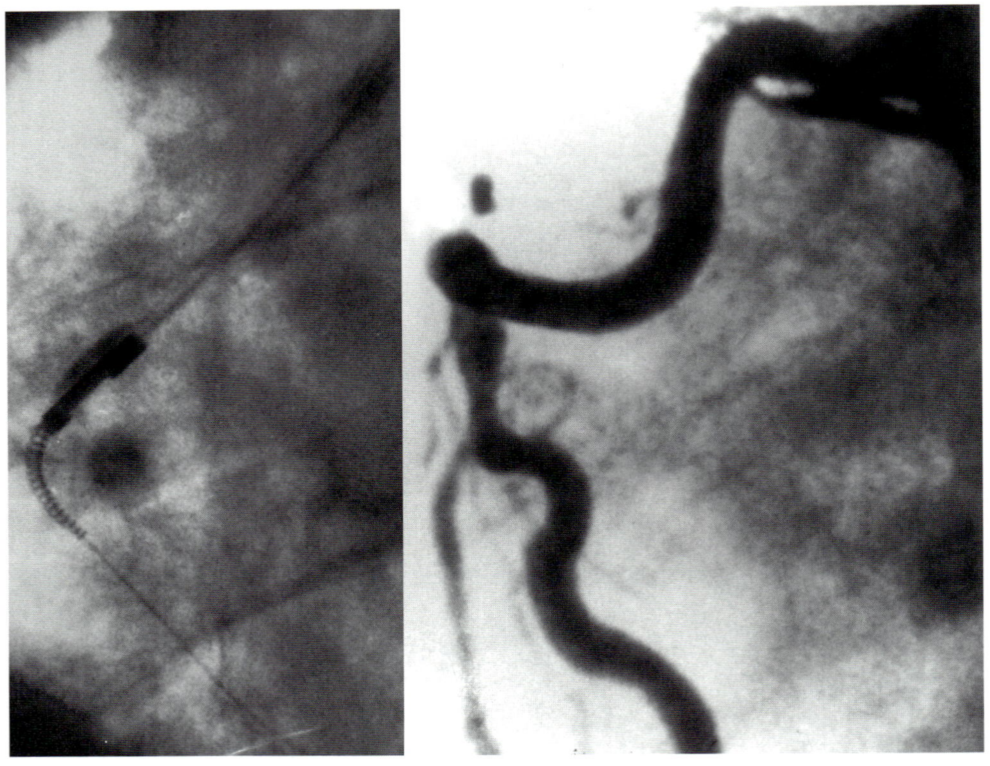

*****

TORTUOUS CIRCUMFLEX

A 63-year-old editor develops unstable angina after learning his name is misspelled on the cover of his book. Cardiac catheterization demonstrates a tubular 80% stenosis in the distal LCX, which is a large dominant vessel (reference diameter = 3.2 mm). The proximal LCX originates at a right angle, and the mid-LCX is tortuous. Other coronary arteries and left ventricular function are normal.

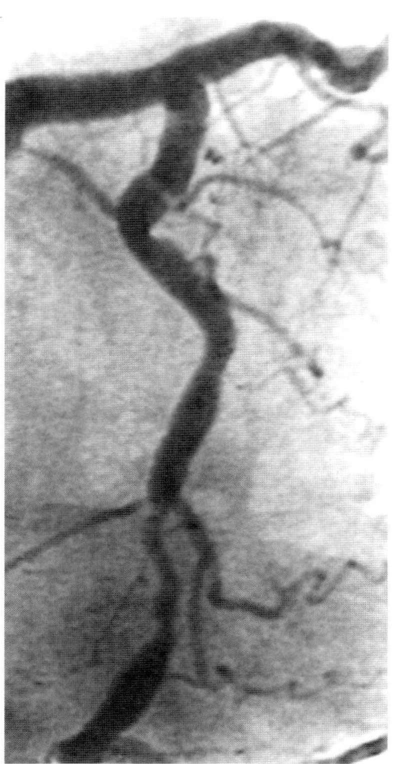

What approach would you recommend?

Richard Heuser, MD, USA: In this patient with unstable angina, I would treat with a bolus and infusion of ReoPro. This is a very complex stenosis in a dominant LCX that is going to be difficult to treat with any device. I would attempt to place a Palmaz-Schatz stent.

Richard Schatz, MD, USA: The angiogram shows an 80% stenosis in the distal LCX, which is a large vessel. The lesion is 12-15 mm in length, and therefore has a higher restenosis risk than a focal lesion. Although it would be easy to get wires and balloons to the target lesion, it would be impossible to deploy any coronary stent due to the right angle takeoff of the LCX. Therefore, this anatomical feature alone has an adverse impact on procedural success. If the operator does not think he can stent this electively, then he certainly would not be able to stent it emergently. In this case, due to the extreme tortuosity of the proximal vessel and its right angle takeoff, I would perform PTCA alone. If PTCA results in dissection, I would add "rescue" ReoPro. If calcification was obvious by fluoroscopy or ultrasound, rotational atherectomy would be a good choice due to its predictability and reduction in acute complications.

Takeshi Kimura, MD, Japan: This patient has a tubular high-grade stenosis involving an extremely tortuous LCX. Due to long lesion length, I expect a suboptimal PTCA result and higher risk of abrupt closure. I would perform elective coronary stenting.

Given the complexity of the anatomy, what do you recommend for operators who only perform PTCA?

Richard Heuser, MD, USA: I would not attempt intervention if stents were not available at my institution. I would refer this patient for stent implantation or CABG.

Richard Schatz, MD, USA: This tortuosity would prevent passage of any stent, so I would not even consider it an option. If the patient develops acute closure unresponsive to a perfusion balloon, the patient should go to emergency surgery. This vessel is a dominant vessel, which means that if it occludes, one should expect significant bradycardia and hypotension. The operator should be prepared for intraaortic balloon pumping and pacing. As long as emergency bypass surgery is available, this patient can be handled by interventionalists who perform only PTCA, since none of the modern bailout devices would be helpful.

Takeshi Kimura, MD, Japan: PTCA was an acceptable option in the pre-stent era. However, considering the expected higher complication rate (especially emergency CABG), I recommend referring the patient to a center in which new trackable stents are available.

Describe your technique for intervention.

Richard Heuser, MD, USA: The question remains: What is the safest way to dilate this vessel? Whether you treat this patient with a balloon, Rotablator, or a stent, guiding catheter and guidewire selection are crucial. A stiffer wire will improve and widen your options. I favor using an 8F AL2 guiding catheter, crossing the stenosis with a 0.014-inch Extra-S'port wire, predilating with a 2.5 mm noncompliant balloon, and inserting a Microstent, GR-II, or Palmaz-Schatz stent. I would postdilate with a 3.5-4.0 mm balloon. I would use intravascular ultrasound to evaluate the result and would discharge the patient the following day on aspirin and ticlopidine.

Richard Schatz, MD, USA: In this case, I suggest a 3.0-3.5 mm extremely low profile balloon with great pushability, flexibility, and trackability, such as the SciMed Bandit. Relatively equivalent choices are be the SciMed Trio, the Medtronic Evergreen, or the Cordis Trakstar. I would not use a monorail balloon in this case since it limits my ability to exchange.

Takeshi Kimura, MD, Japan: Flexible and trackable stents are required to negotiate proximal vessel tortuosity. Since the length of the lesion is greater than 15 mm, I would choose multiple 3.5 x 8.0 mm Microstents or a single 3.5 x 20 mm GR-II stent. I would use an 8F AL2 guiding catheter, a 0.014-inch Hi-torque floppy guidewire, and a 3.0 x 20 mm over-the-wire balloon. I would then exchange for a 0.014-inch x 300 cm Extra-Support guidewire. After stent deployment, I would perform high-pressure inflations at 15-18 ATM with a 3.5 x 20 mm noncompliant balloon. Anticoagulation consists of aspirin and ticlopidine, without Coumadin.

Editors' Perspective: See p. 86 for comments.

*****

TORTUOUS CIRCUMFLEX: ABRUPT CLOSURE

Percutaneous intervention is performed on the distal LCX (see previous case), resulting in abrupt closure. The patient develops bradycardia and hypotension.

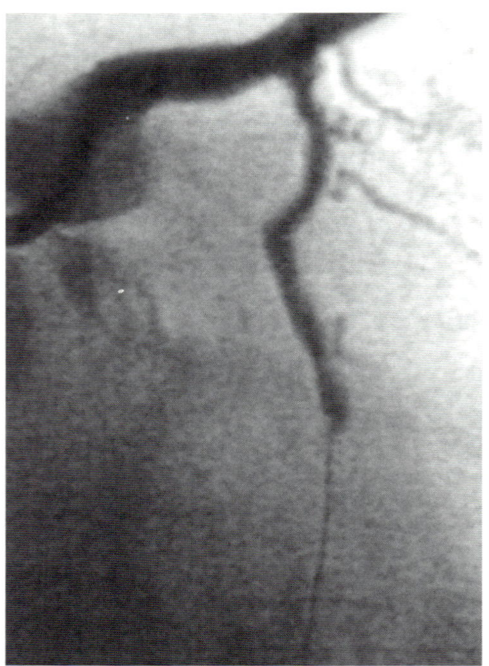

What would you do first to stabilize this patient?

Richard Heuser, MD, USA: I would first place a temporary pacemaker and an intraaortic balloon pump. I would then place a GR-II stent, and postdilate with a high-pressure balloon. If it is not beautiful, I would send the patient to the operating room. If the vessel is beautiful and the patient is doing well, I would wait for at least 15-20 minutes and perform a repeat angiogram.

Richard Schatz, MD, USA: Following percutaneous intervention, the patient develops abrupt closure with bradycardia and hypotension. Unless flow is restored promptly, this patient has a very high risk of acute and chronic complications. We can assume that the culprit is dissection with superimposed spasm and thrombus. Expedience in restoring flow is paramount. I would select the balloon that is already on the table (rather than waste time and expense of another specialized balloon). I would advance the balloon as quickly as possible to the target site and inflate it repeatedly, trying to restore some flow while an intraaortic balloon pump is placed. A pacemaker is required, as well.

Takeshi Kimura, MD, Japan: I would concentrate on reestablishing coronary flow rather than establishing hemodynamic support (such as intraaortic balloon pump or CPS). While injecting noradrenaline and atropine, I would redilate the lesion followed by stent implantation. Reestablishment of flow is very important to assess the length of dissection before stent implantation. Stents should be placed from distal to proximal to cover the entire dissection.

What would you do if the result is suboptimal?

Richard Heuser, MD, USA: It is important to remember that the patient comes first, and if you cannot place a stent and the patient continues to be bradycardic and hypotensive, emergency surgery is indicated. It is certainly better to stabilize the patient with a temporary pacer, an intraaortic balloon pump, and a perfusion balloon, prior to surgery.

Richard Schatz, MD, USA: If there is no flow after repeat PTCA, I would assume that there is significant recoil and I would reach for the SciMed Dispatch balloon. The Dispatch, unfortunately, is somewhat clumsy and may not track. Once in place, I would inflate the Dispatch for 10-20 minutes while balloon pumping and pacing are established. I am taking advantage of the wide central lumen of the Dispatch, not drug delivery. If there is no distal flow with the Dispatch then I would immediately reach for a 3.0-3.5 x 40 mm Lifestream-40. I would inflate this to 6 ATM for as long as tolerated, hoping to establish distal flow. If the perfusion balloon or Dispatch does not pass, I would very quickly try a 0.014-inch Platinum-Plus guidewire. I do not believe that stent delivery would be possible in this case, so as long as bypass surgery is available, I would accept that as the ultimate outcome. I would not use ReoPro, since it will have no impact on the mechanical obstruction due to dissection.

Takeshi Kimura, MD, Japan: If stents are not available, prolonged balloon inflation (10-15 minutes) with a perfusion balloon and prompt institution of balloon pump counterpulsation are recommended. Emergency bypass surgery is required if prolonged inflations fail with a perfusion balloon.

Editors' Perspective: The approach to lesions in tortuous vessels has been simplified by guiding catheters that offer stable coaxial alignment and powerful support, extra-support guidewires, and low-profile balloon catheters for enhanced pushability and trackability. Nevertheless, despite improvements in PTCA hardware, tortuous vessels increase the risk of procedural failure (Table 22) and remain a source of frustration for all interventional cardiologists. Although non-balloon devices have increased the application of percutaneous techniques, with few exceptions, stents, lasers, and atherectomy devices offer little advantage over PTCA. Because of their large caliber and relative inflexibility (particularly devices made of steel), attempts to "force" these devices into tortuous vessels can result in vessel injury. Although the Rotablator burr is rigid, burr rotation reduces friction and facilitates advancement into tortuous vessels. In our interventional survey, 80% of operators rely on conventional PTCA for primary revascularization of tortuous vessels, while 20% prefer stents. Although most operators recommend PTCA, the risk of abrupt closure mandates that operators have experience in stenting tortuous vessels. Considerations are similar to those described for angulated lesions, including use of power guides, extra-support guidewires, and specialized stent techniques such as the "buddy-wire" approach and the "stentless delivery sheath" technique. In situations where failed angioplasty cannot be treated with stents, additional options include perfusion balloons (for prolonged balloon inflations), long balloons (to tack-up dissections at the junction between plaque and normal wall), and emergency CABG.

Table 22. Effect of Proximal Tortuosity on Acute PTCA Outcome

Series	N	Anatomic Subgroup	Success (%)	Other (%)	
Tan[1]	965	No tortuosity	93	Acute closure:	3
	142	Moderate	93		4.2
	50	Severe	84		6
Ellis[2]	189	Type A	92	Acute complications:	2
	65	Proximal tortuosity	72		15
Gossman[3]	53	No Shepherd Crook	98	Difficulty crossing	13
	51	Shepherd Crook	86	lesion:	33

In the present case, the LCX stenosis was treated with a 3.0 x 20 mm balloon, with the hope of revascularizing the tubular stenosis in the distal vessel. After development of a long, spiral, flow-limiting dissection, atropine and neosynephrine were given to support the blood pressure, and a temporary pacemaker was inserted. While the intraaortic balloon pump was being prepared, a 3.0 x 40 mm long balloon was advanced and inflated to 6 ATM (we were reluctant to use a perfusion balloon because of the length of the dissection and concerns about losing guidewire position during passive perfusion). After 2 overlapping 5-minute inflations with the 40 mm balloon, there was no residual stenosis or dissection (below). Hemodynamic performance improved, and the patient was monitored overnight in the intensive care unit without further complication.

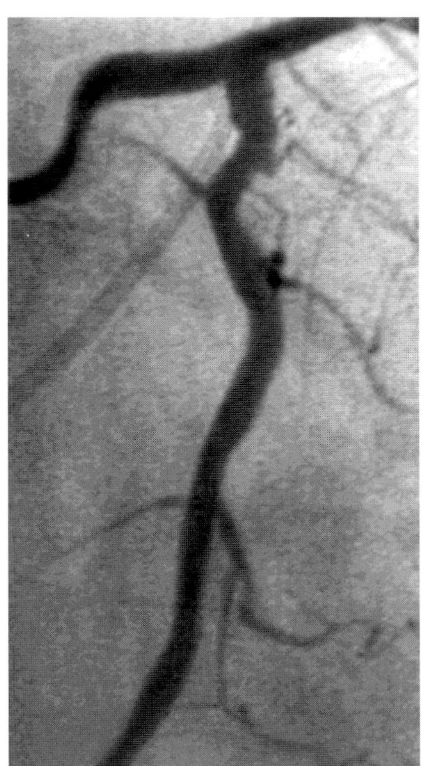

*****

LESION PROXIMAL TO BIFURCATION

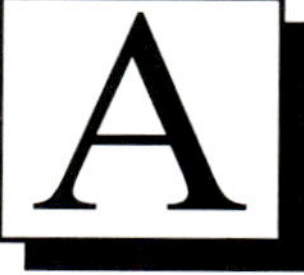

A 45-year-old construction worker presents with progressive exertional angina. Coronary angiography reveals a severe stenosis just prior to the LAD bifurcation (mid-LAD = 3.2 mm, diagonal = 2.8 mm). Other vessels and left ventricular function are normal.

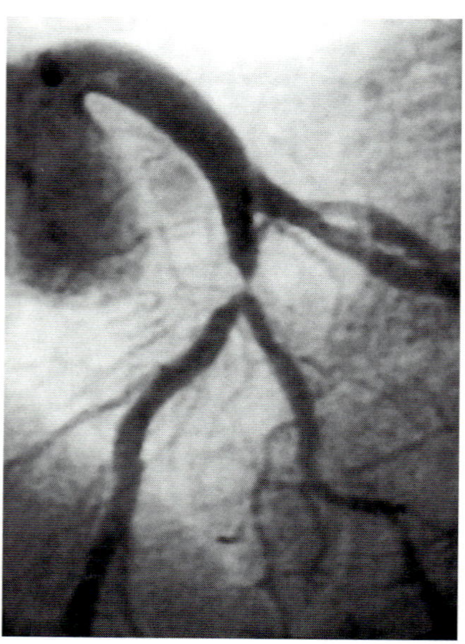

What is the risk of sidebranch occlusion?

Dean Kereiakes, MD, USA: This patient has a focal, concentric, noncalcified stenosis in a large LAD. Although a moderate size first diagonal branch originates from the distal portion of the stenosis, the origin of the diagonal branch is not involved. The risk of sidebranch occlusion is low, and there is no need to protect this vessel with a guidewire.

Ulrich Sigwart, MD, England: This relatively young patient has a true bifurcation stenosis in the LAD at the origin of the first diagonal branch. There is quite a bit of atheroma extending into the main vessel distal to the bifurcation, but the most severe lesion is proximal to the bifurcation.

The risk of branch occlusion is low.

How would you approach this lesion?

Dean Kereiakes, MD, USA: I would use a DVI 10F JL4 guiding catheter, a 0.014-inch Extra-Support wire, and a 7F GTO or EX AtheroCath. I would make atherectomy cuts with the window oriented anteriorly and posteriorly in the LAO cranial view, to excise the bulk of plaque proximal to the diagonal branch. In my opinion, directional atherectomy is less likely than PTCA to cause shifting plaque or compromise the diagonal branch.

Ulrich Sigwart, MD, England: I recommend conventional PTCA, and stent implantation only if necessary. Guidewire selection is not crucial in this case, but I generally use extra-support wires which ease subsequent handling of stents. An 8F guiding catheter (0.086-inch lumen) is the best option in this situation, to accommodate kissing balloons. I would use a 3.0 x 20 mm semicompliant balloon-on-a-wire (because of the lower shaft profile in case kissing balloons are needed).

What would you recommend if there is a suboptimal result?

Dean Kereiakes, MD, USA: If the origin of the diagonal is compromised, I would direct the 0.014-inch guidewire into the diagonal branch and perform directional atherectomy with the 7F AtheroCath at low pressure (≤ 15 PSI).

Ulrich Sigwart, MD, England: I would place a second wire in the diagonal branch and perform kissing balloon inflations with a 3.0 mm balloon in the LAD and a 2.5 mm balloon in the diagonal branch, at low pressure. I would not hesitate to place a Multilink stent across the lesion, to maintain access to the diagonal branch.

LESION DISTAL TO BIFURCATION

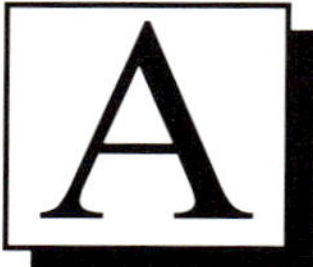

A 49-year-old carpenter presents with progressive exertional angina. Coronary angiography demonstrates a subtotal stenosis in the mid-LAD just after the diagonal branch (mid-LAD = 3.2 mm, diagonal = 2.8 mm). Other vessels and left ventricular function are normal.

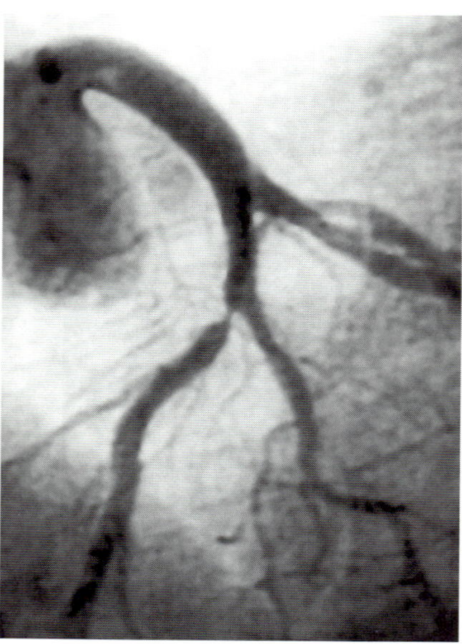

What is the risk of sidebranch occlusion?

Dean Kereiakes, MD, USA: This patient has a focal noncalcified stenosis in a large LAD immediately distal to a moderate size diagonal branch. There is no need for sidebranch protection since the origin of the diagonal branch is not involved, and plaque shift across the diagonal is unlikely.

Ulrich Sigwart, MD, England: This patient has a type A lesion just distal to the bifurcation. I do not foresee any particular problem in performing PTCA. The risk of sidebranch occlusion is minimal.

How would you approach this lesion?

Dean Kereiakes, MD, USA: This type of stenosis will respond very well to conventional PTCA or directional atherectomy. I would use a DVI 10F JL4 guiding catheter, a 0.014-inch Extra-Support guidewire, and a 7F GTO or EX AtheroCath. The EX device allows better visualization of the diagonal origin and potentially better positioning of the cutter window; the GTO device has a larger shaft, allowing less adequate contrast visualization in vessels < 3.5 mm diameter. I would make 6-8 atherectomy cuts in a circumferential fashion. If adjunctive PTCA is required to optimize lumen diameter or smooth intimal irregularities, I would use a 3.25 mm Flowtrack or Lifestream perfusion balloon inflated gradually (1 ATM every 30 seconds to a maximum of 4 ATM). PTCA alone is an acceptable strategy in this case, and could be performed with a 7F or 8F JL4 high-flow guiding catheter, a 0.014-inch Hi-torque floppy guidewire, and a 3.25 mm balloon.

Ulrich Sigwart, MD, England: I recommend PTCA with a 3.0 mm balloon at fairly high pressure.

What would you do if there is a suboptimal result?

Ulrich Sigwart, MD, England: I would implant a MultiLink, Nir, or coil stent to preserve access to the diagonal branch.

BIFURCATION LESION: COMPLEX LAD-DIAGONAL LESION

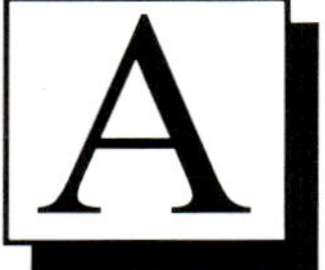

A 48-year-old cabdriver develops angina after learning that his wife is pregnant with triplets. Coronary angiography demonstrates a severe stenosis in the proximal LAD, involving the first diagonal branch (mid-LAD = 3.2 mm; diagonal = 2.8 mm). Other vessels and left ventricular function are normal.

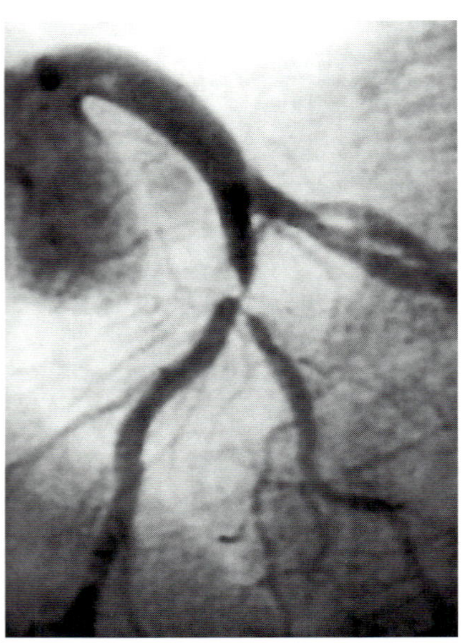

What is the risk of sidebranch occlusion?

Dean Kereiakes, MD, USA: This patient has a complex stenosis with a focal, noncalcified eccentric stenosis in a large LAD and a high grade ostial stenosis in the first diagonal branch. There is a definite risk of sidebranch occlusion.

Ulrich Sigwart, MD, England: This is a difficult case. The risk of sidebranch occlusion is significant.

How would you approach this lesion?

Dean Kereiakes, MD, USA: The diagonal branch originates from the distal border of the LAD stenosis. In this scenario, I believe it is optimal to predilate and/or protect the sidebranch prior to treating the LAD. For this reason, I would begin with a DVI 10F JL4 short-tip guiding catheter, and a large bore Namic dual Y-adapter. I would place a 0.014-inch x 300 cm Traverse wire in the LAD and in the diagonal branch, and predilate the origin of the diagonal branch with a 3.0 mm noncompliant MC Rail. The angle of takeoff of the diagonal is > 90° because of the distortion created by the plaque in the LAD. If the diagonal branch cannot be wired, I would proceed with directional atherectomy of the LAD using a 7F GTO or EX device at relatively low (≤ 20 PSI) pressure, in an attempt to reorient the diagonal origin. This should provide better access to the origin of the diagonal branch. At this time, I would wire the diagonal branch and make circumferential cuts with a 6F GTO AtheroCath at low (20 PSI) pressure. In my experience, tissue ablation and/or removal is clearly the optimal strategy for recanalizing ostial diagonal branches. It is unlikely that simultaneous balloon inflations will be required. Thus, although I would attempt to protect the sidebranch in this case, it may not be possible; I would therefore attempt to reorient the origin of the diagonal branch by performing directional atherectomy on the LAD.

Ulrich Sigwart, MD, England: As the stenosis in the diagonal branch is truly ostial and originates at a right angle to the LAD, it may be difficult to wire this branch. I would not waste too much time trying to wire the first diagonal branch, but go for the LAD first. After a slightly undersized dilation (3.0 mm balloon at low pressures), it is usually much easier to access the diagonal branch. If necessary, the diagonal branch can be wired using an intermediate or standard wire. A kissing balloon technique may be required; an 8F guiding catheter is recommended.

What would you do if there is a suboptimal result?

Ulrich Sigwart, MD, England: If the result is unsatisfactory after sequential high pressure inflations with a 3.0 mm balloon in the LAD and a 2.5 mm balloon in the diagonal branch, I would perform kissing balloon angioplasty at low pressure. Bifurcational stents can be deployed if necessary, but this is technically demanding.

BIFURCATION LESION: MULTIPLE LESIONS

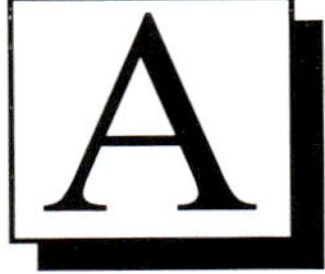

A 61-year-old housewife presents with dyspnea on exertion and myocardial perfusion imaging reveals ischemia at a low workload. Coronary angiography demonstrates a severe stenosis in the mid-LAD and in the diagonal branch (mid-LAD = 3.2 mm, diagonal = 2.8 mm). Other vessels and left ventricular function are normal.

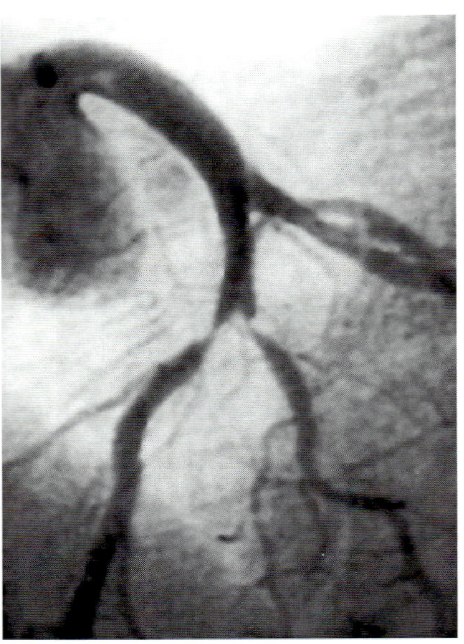

What is the risk of sidebranch occlusion?

Dean Kereiakes, MD, USA: There is a focal, noncalcified, eccentric stenosis in the LAD distal to (not involving) the origin of a large diagonal branch. The proximal (not ostial) diagonal branch also has a high-grade stenosis. Sidebranch protection is not required.

Ulrich Sigwart, MD, England: In contrast to the previous case, this is not a bifurcation stenosis. Each branch is affected separately and the lesion starts 2-3 mm after the bifurcation in the LAD and 2 mm in the diagonal branch. Sidebranch protection is not necessary.

How would you approach this lesion?

Dean Kereiakes, MD, USA: I would perform sequential directional atherectomy on the LAD, and then on the diagonal branch. I would use a DVI 10F JL4 guiding catheter, a 0.014-inch x 300 cm Extra-Support wire, and a 7F EX AtheroCath. After 6-8 atherectomy cuts in a circumferential fashion at 20-30 PSI in the LAD, I would redirect the 0.014-inch guidewire into the diagonal branch and perform directional atherectomy with the 7F EX at low pressure (15-20 PSI). Adjunctive PTCA is recommended to optimize results or smoothe intimal irregularities, using a 3.25 mm balloon in the LAD and a 3.0 mm balloon in the diagonal branch, at 4 ATM.

Ulrich Sigwart, MD, England: I would perform sequential PTCA with a 2.5 mm balloon in the diagonal branch and a 3.0 mm balloon in the LAD.

What would you do if there is a suboptimal result?

Ulrich Sigwart, MD, England: If a major dissection occurs, I would place a stent (in either vessel).

TRUE BIFURCATION LESION

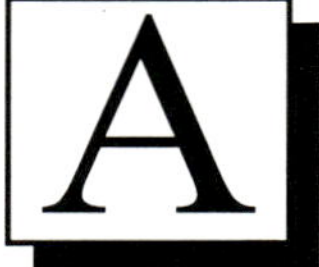

A 52-year-old army sergeant develops angina during his morning exercise routine. Coronary angiography demonstrates a true LAD-diagonal bifurcation lesion (mid-LAD = 3.2 mm; diagonal = 2.8 mm). Other vessels and left ventricular function are normal.

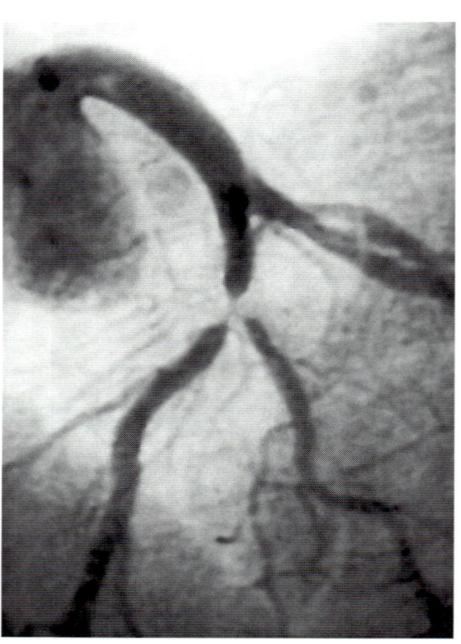

What is the risk of sidebranch occlusion?

Dean Kereiakes, MD, USA: This angiogram demonstrates a true bifurcation lesion involving a large LAD and a moderate diagonal branch. It is optimal to remove plaque to prevent the inevitable plaque shift and sidebranch compromise which occurs after conventional PTCA. The risk of sidebranch occlusion is high.

Ulrich Sigwart, MD, England: This is a bifurcation lesion par excellence; PTCA with a double wire technique is the best approach, since the risk of sidebranch occlusion is high.

How would you approach this lesion?

Dean Kereiakes, MD, USA: I recommend a DVI 10F JL4 guiding catheter, a large bore Namic dual Y-connector, and two 0.014-inch Traverse wires in the LAD and diagonal branch. I recommend predilating the diagonal branch with a noncompliant 3.0 mm balloon. The diagonal dilation system would be removed, followed by directional atherectomy of the LAD with a 7F GTO or EX AtheroCath with 6-8 circumferential cuts at 15-30 PSI. The 0.014-inch guidewire would be placed into the diagonal, followed by circumferential low-pressure (≤ 15 PSI) cuts. If necessary, kissing balloon inflations can be performed with a 3.5 mm balloon in the LAD and a 3.0 mm balloon in the diagonal branch. Simultaneous inflations are usually unnecessary because shifting plaque is uncommon after directional atherectomy.

Ulrich Sigwart, MD, England: I would use 2 extra-support wires in the LAD and diagonal branch, and perform kissing balloon angioplasty; the likelihood of bifurcational stenting is high. Directional atherectomy is also a good choice using a 7F AtheroCath.

> Editors' Perspective: **The majority of bifurcation lesions involve the LAD and diagonal branch. Originally considered a contraindication to PTCA because of the risk of sidebranch occlusion, contemporary interventional practice commonly employs PTCA and other devices for a wide variety of lesions involving vessel bifurcations. The risk of sidebranch occlusion is always a concern and depends on two important factors (Table 23): the proximity of the branch to the parent vessel lesion, and the degree of stenosis of the branch ostium. The need for sidebranch protection (Table 24) depends on the risk of sidebranch occlusion, the anticipated technical difficulty passing a wire into the sidebranch, and the amount of viable myocardium supplied by the branch. Older techniques using double guiding catheters have been virtually abandoned because of the availability of large-lumen guiding catheters, low-profile balloon catheters, and special triadapters able to accommodate two balloons and guidewires without sacrificing guide support or opacification of the target vessel. There are several techniques for bifurcation angioplasty, each with its own advantages and disadvantages (Table 25). Although bifurcation angioplasty can be performed with high success rates, the risk of procedural failure and complications are higher than for PTCA of non-bifurcation lesions (Table 26).**

Table 23. Parent Vessel-Side Branch Relationships[712,714,716,718,719]

Anatomy	Risk of side branch occlusion	Technical difficulty in passing a wire into branch	Protection required
Branch uninvolved by parent vessel lesion but in jeopardy due to transient occlusion during PTCA	Low (< 1%)	Low	No
Branch originates from diseased parent vessel segment; branch is normal	Moderate (1-10%)	Low-Moderate	Probably yes; depends on vessel size
Branch ostial stenosis > 50%	High (14-35%)	High	Yes

To address the problem of shifting plaque, which may lead to suboptimal PTCA results in the branch and/or parent vessel, atherectomy devices and stents have been applied to bifurcation lesions. Directional atherectomy (DCA) can be performed (Table 27) using sequential guidewires and atherectomy, first of the parent vessel, then the branch. This technique may lead to sidebranch occlusion, which must then be retrieved by further directional atherectomy (or PTCA). Another atherectomy technique uses "kissing" guidewires in the parent vessel and branch, followed by sequential atherectomy of each. Although this technique can preserve access to the sidebranch during DCA of the parent vessel, it is more cumbersome and technically challenging than use of sequential wires. Furthermore, Nitinol guidewires must be used to prevent inadvertent damage to the guidewire during atherectomy. In our practice, we find that the sequential guidewire technique is easier than the "kissing" guidewire technique; occlusion of the sidebranch is usually transient, and the branches are usually readily crossed with a guidewire, allowing successful salvage by DCA or PTCA. Rotablator is not generally recommended for bifurcation lesions since sidebranch protection is impossible, although in our experience, occluded sidebranches can usually be crossed with a guidewire and salvaged by Rotablator or PTCA.

Stents can be implanted in the parent vessel and branch, and offer the best opportunity for maximum lumen enlargement by elimination of elastic recoil and shifting plaque. However, these techniques are technically demanding and should not be performed by inexperienced stent operators. Data now suggest that sidebranch occlusion, which occurs in 5-10% of stent procedures (incidence similar to PTCA), can be retrieved through most coil and slotted stents. Several technical points about retrieving sidebranches through stents deserve emphasis: First, the parent vessel stent should be fully expanded with high-pressure balloons. Second, unicore guidewires should be used to cross stent struts to minimize prolapse of the guidewire away from the branch ostium. Third, high-pressure, low-profile balloons or fixed wire-balloon catheters are best used to access the sidebranch through stent coils or struts. Finally,

the proximal end of the balloon is best left across the stent (in the parent vessel) to prevent balloon entrapment after balloon inflation. Among physicians who responded to our interventional survey, 58% recommended directional atherectomy as their primary revascularization strategy, PTCA in 26%, stents in 11%, and Rotablator in 5%.

Table 24. Need for Sidebranch Protection

Sidebranch Protection Recommended	1. **Any sidebranch > 2.0 mm in diameter that has an ostial stenosis ≥ 50% and originates from the parent vessel lesion.** "True" bifurcation lesions are associated with a high incidence of sidebranch occlusion and a low salvage rate when left unprotected.
	2. **Any sidebranch > 2.0 mm in diameter (without ostial stenosis) originates from the parent vessel lesion.** Although it is usually possible to retrieve these occluded sidebranches, their large caliber justifies protection. In such lesions, a double guidewire approach is reasonable; if sidebranch occlusion occurs, sequential PTCA or a kissing balloon technique may be employed.
Protection Probably Not Necessary*	1. **The sidebranch is normal and does not originate from the parent vessel lesion.** Even though the sidebranch may be transiently covered by the inflated balloon in the parent vessel, the risk of occlusion is low.
	2. **The sidebranch is < 1.5 mm in diameter and would not receive a bypass graft during CABG.**
	3. **The sidebranch supplies a small amount of viable myocardium.**
	4. **Isolated stenoses of the origin of the sidebranch usually do not require protection of the parent vessel.**

* If sidebranch occlusion does occur, it can be retrieved by PTCA or not retrieved at all, depending on the clinical situation.

Table 25. Technical Approaches to Bifurcation Angioplasty

Approach	Advantages	Disadvantages
Guiding Catheter Technique		
Two-guide approach	• Large variety of balloon catheters to choose from • Excellent visualization	• Two arterial punctures • More procedural complexity • Potential ostial injury
One-guide approach	• One access site • Less risk of ostial injury • Less time consuming	• Limited choice of balloons, wires • Impaired visualization
Protection Technique		
Double-guidewire	• Access to both vessels • Better visualization • Less expensive if same balloon can be used for both branches	• More wire entanglement
Double balloon-on-the-wire	• Allows immediate salvage PTCA of branch	• More wire entanglement • Cannot upsize or exchange without giving up wire position • Impaired visualization
Double balloon over-the-wire	• Access in the parent vessel to both vessels • Allows salvage PTCA of branch	• More wire entanglement • Impaired visualization
Inflation Technique		
Sequential balloon inflation	• Requires less hardware • Can use same balloon for both vessels	• More wire entanglement • Does not eliminate "snow-plow" • Balloon may not match diameter of parent vessel proximal and distal to branch
Kissing balloon inflations	• Minimizes "snow-plow" • Allows PTCA without overdilating vessel distal to bifurcation	• More complex procedure • More wire entanglement • May overdilate vessel proximal to bifurcation

Table 26. Results of PTCA for Bifurcation Lesions

Series	Sidebranch Protected	N	Success (%)	Complications (%)	Restenosis (%)
Tan[752]	Bifurcation - Yes	135	95	2.2*	-
	Bifurcation - No	52	85	3.8*	-
	Non-bifurcation	970	93	3.4*	-
Lewis[729]	Bifurcation	-	74	3.7	61
	Non-bifurcation	-	86	6.1	52
Myler[715]	Bifurcation - Yes	17	94	0	-
	Bifurcation - No	106	89	3.8	-
	Non-bifurcation	656	95	1.4	-
Ciampricotti[714]	Bifurcation - No	22	95	0	-
Weinstein[718]	Bifurcation - Yes	35	97	0	42
	Bifurcation - No	21	76		16
Renkin[712]	Bifurcation - Yes	34	97	2.9	-
	Bifurcation - No	8	88	12.5	-
Thomas[721]	Bifurcation - Yes	54	87	6.0	30
George[713]	Bifurcation - Yes	52	98	3.8	53

Abbreviations: - = not reported
* = abrupt closure

Table 27. Results of DCA in Bifurcation Lesions

Series	N	Success (%)	MC (%)	SBO (%)
Lewis [729]	-	88	9.5	50
Mansour[727]	8	100	0	0
Hinohara[724]	22	91	4.5	-

Abbreviations: MC = major in-hospital complications (death, Q-wave myocardial infarction, emergency coronary artery bypass grafting); SBO = sidebranch occlusion; - = not reported

*****

PROTECTED LEFT MAIN LESION

A 70-year-old chancellor of a major university with a history of coronary bypass surgery 1 year ago develops progressive angina. Coronary angiography demonstrates a severe stenosis in the left main (reference vessel = 5.1 mm). The vein graft to the OM is occluded, but the LIMA to the LAD and the native RCA are patent. Left ventricular function is normal.

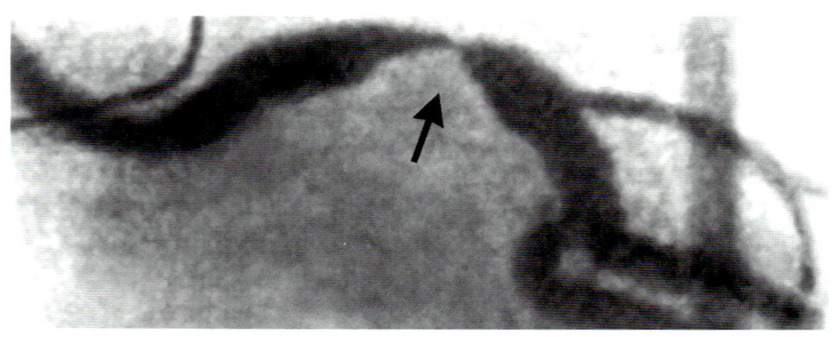

What is your assessment of the risk of intervention?

David Williams, MD, USA: Typically, left main lesions are not considered suitable for percutaneous revascularization because of safety concerns. In this instance, however, myocardium jeopardized by the left main lesion is limited to the distribution of the LCX. Accordingly, the patient can be viewed as having "single" vessel disease, and the risks of intervention are much less.

Timothy Sanborn, MD, USA: This patient has an angulated, eccentric, "protected" left main stenosis. Since reoperation runs the risk of damage to the patent LIMA, I recommend catheter-based intervention.

What is your device of choice for percutaneous intervention?

Takeshi Kimura, MD, Japan: Vessel closure after stenting this large native vessel is extremely unlikely, and late restenosis is lower than after directional atherectomy. A biliary stent will give the best radial support for this artery. Since biliary stents are not available in my laboratory, I would use a Palmaz-Schatz coronary stent.

David Williams, MD, USA: I've had particularly good experience with debulking by rotational atherectomy followed by stenting lesions of this type for two reasons: First, the lesion is at least one year old and has a greater chance of being dense and possibly calcified. Second, the lesion is eccentric, and rotational atherectomy can preferentially ablate eccentric plaque. Since the largest burr (2.5 mm) will not result in adequate lumen enlargement, adjunctive PTCA and stenting are required to avoid restenosis.

Describe your technical approach.

Takeshi Kimura, MD, Japan: I would perform PTCA with an 8F JL4 large lumen (> 0.084-inch) guiding catheter without sideholes, a 0.014-inch x 300 cm Extra-Support guidewire, and a 4.0 x 20 mm balloon. Then, I would place a 4.0 x 20 mm Palmaz-Schatz coronary stent with spiral articulation. After initial stent deployment, postdilation should be performed with a 5.0 x 9 mm noncompliant balloon at 15-18 ATM. The potential problems with coronary stents for this vessel are protrusion of plaque through the expanded stent struts, and stent shortening. When significant protrusion of the plaque is observed, additional stent implantation inside the stent is acceptable, preferably after evaluation by intravascular ultrasound. The anticoagulation regimen consists of aspirin (243 mg QD) and ticlopidine (200 mg QD).

David Williams, MD, USA: I would start with a 1.75 mm burr with progressive increases in burr size by 0.25-0.5 mm increments, up to a final burr of 2.5 mm. The procedure will be completed with a balloon/artery ratio of 1.0-1.1. If the final angiographic outcome is not ideal, I would stent the lesion. A 10F guide with sideholes (ID = 0.108-0.110 inches) is required to accommodate a 2.5 mm burr. After positioning the guide catheter in the left coronary artery, I would advance a Rotablator-C wire into the distal LCX and begin rotablation with a 1.75 mm burr in the nondiseased platform segment. I would then advance the burr across the entire lesion, approaching the LCX. If initial rotablation does not cause sustained ischemia or impaired flow, I would use a 2.0 mm burr. As burr size increases, ischemia is more likely. I would use a 2.25 mm burr followed by a final 2.5 mm burr. I would select a balloon capable of tracking over the Rotablator wire, such as a SciMed Cobra-18 or a Cordis Trakstar, inflating for at least 120 seconds at a pressure adequate to achieve a balloon/artery ratio of 1:1. It is important that the Rotablator flush solution contain verapamil and nitroglycerin. IVUS would be used to optimize stent deployment.

Timothy Sanborn, MD, USA: I would select an 8F large lumen (0.086-inch) SL4 guiding catheter. Once I confirm good backup support, I would cross with a 0.014-inch Extra-Support wire, and dilate with a 4.0 mm balloon, followed by placement of a 4.0 mm Palmaz-Schatz coronary stent. I would place the articulation just distal to the lesion. Maximal stent expansion would be achieved with a 5.0 mm balloon inflated at 14-18 ATM. IVUS is recommended to confirm proper stent expansion, so that anticoagulation will not be needed.

What other devices can be used for this lesion?

Takeshi Kimura, MD, Japan: Directional atherectomy with adjunctive PTCA is acceptable.

David Williams, MD, USA: Alternative treatments include PTCA alone or directional atherectomy. Directional atherectomy is well suited for eccentric lesions, although the angulated nature of this artery makes directional atherectomy less desirable.

Timothy Sanborn, MD, USA: While I generally prefer directional atherectomy for eccentric lesions, there appears to be more angulation and tortuosity distal to the lesion, which could be traumatized by the nosecone of the AtheroCath.

Is conventional PTCA reasonable?

Takeshi Kimura, MD, Japan: PTCA alone is acceptable.

David Williams, MD, USA: It is possible that this lesion could be handled by PTCA alone, although it is likely that the result will be suboptimal due to residual stenosis and dissection.

<u>Editors' Perspective</u>: **In this case, conventional PTCA was attempted, but full balloon expansion could not be achieved because of lesion rigidity (even in the absence of gross calcification by fluoroscopy). At the time this procedure was performed, Rotablator and stents were not available. Because of the eccentric nature of the lesion, excimer laser angioplasty was performed using a 1.8 mm directional laser fiber followed by PTCA. Excimer laser seemed to facilitate subsequent balloon inflation, although there was a moderate persistent residual stenosis (below). Today, we would treat this patient with the Rotablator and a biliary stent (see p. 111 for additional comments).**

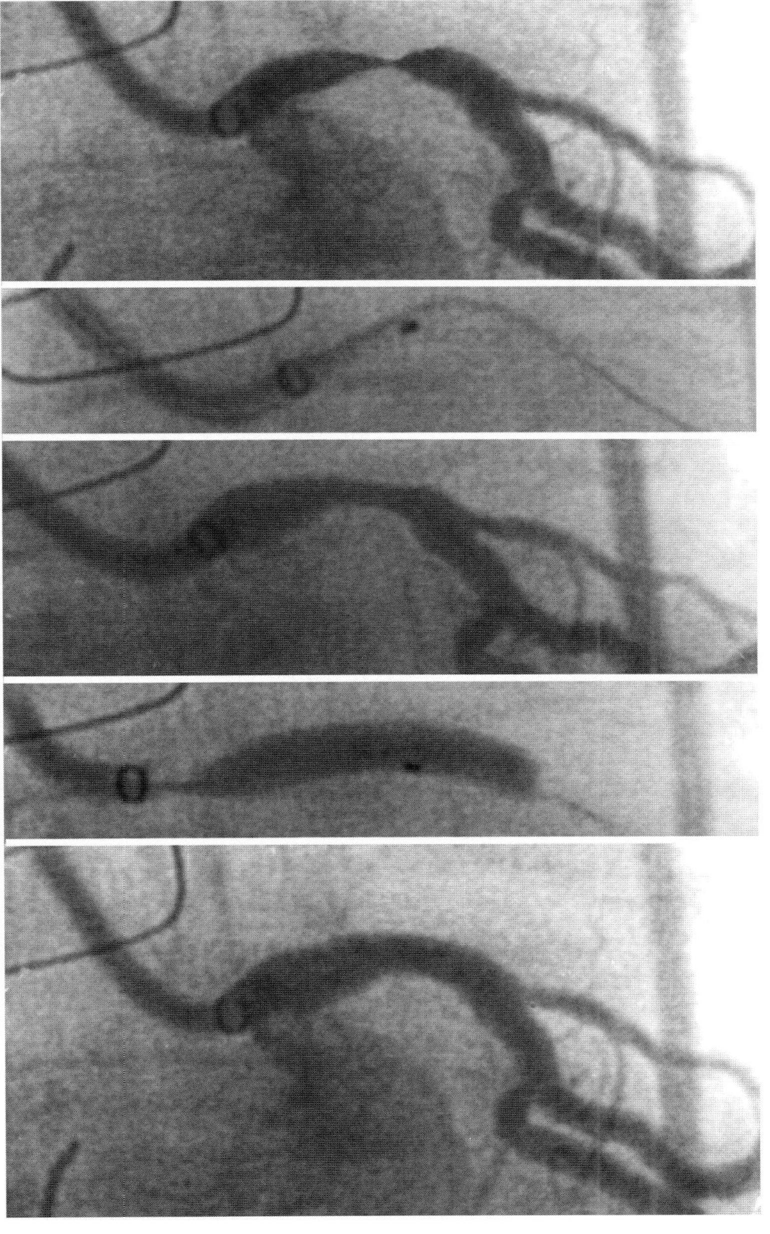

*****

LEFT MAIN BIFURCATION LESION

A 65-year-old politician develops angina after learning that his opponent has just proposed a large tax cut. Coronary angiography demonstrates a severe ulcerated stenosis at the distal left main bifurcation (left main = 4.2 mm, LCX = 3.8 mm). The vein graft to the OM is occluded, but other grafts and left ventricular function are normal.

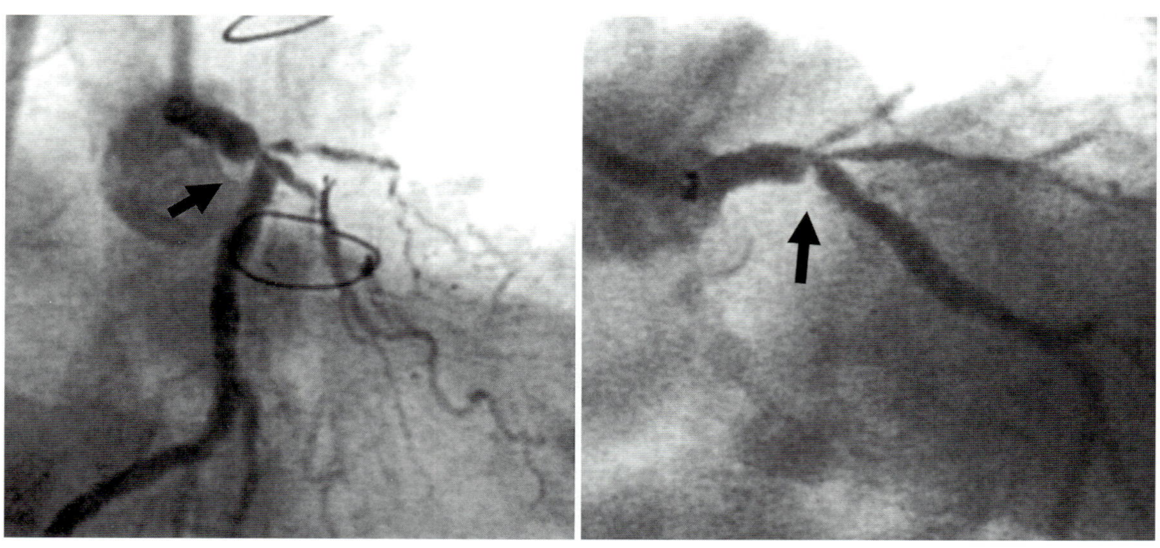

How does this type of lesion morphology influence your choice of devices for revascularization?

Takeshi Kimura, MD, Japan: The angiogram shows a very short slit-like stenosis in a bend in the distal left main. I recommend stent implantation with IVUS guidewire.

David Williams, MD, USA: This individual has a very eccentric lesion in the distal left main coronary artery. The lesion is located on a moderately angulated segment. Unlike the previous patient, this lesion is considerably more complex in that it has an unusual eccentric contour and very short length. I recommend directional atherectomy for this lesion because of marked eccentricity and short length. Furthermore, the left main and circumflex are large and should be able to accommodate the AtheroCath.

Timothy Sanborn, MD, USA: This is a protected left main lesion that I would treat with directional atherectomy (7F Graft device).

Describe your technique for intervention.

Takeshi Kimura, MD, Japan: Intravascular ultrasound is helpful to evaluate the degree of plaque accumulation in the proximal LCX. If IVUS reveals significant plaque accumulation, I would perform PTCA with an 8F AL1 or AL2 large lumen (> 0.084-inch ID) guide without sideholes, a 0.014-inch Extra-Support guidewire, and a 3.5 x 20 mm noncompliant balloon. I would then place a 3.5 x 20 mm Palmaz-Schatz stent with spiral articulation. After initial stent deployment, I would postdilate with a 4.0 x 20 mm noncompliant balloon at 16-18 ATM. Final optimization of stent expansion should be performed with IVUS. Anticoagulation consists of aspirin (243 mg) and ticlopidine (200 mg).

David Williams, MD, USA: I recommend a 7F Graft AtheroCath, a 10F JL4 guide, and a 0.014-inch Hi-torque floppy wire in the LCX. The window should be directed toward the lesion and a series of cuts performed along the inferior aspect of the left main. I would follow atherectomy with a 4.0 mm balloon to obtain the best possible acute outcome. Directional atherectomy is associated with an increased incidence of CK release due to distal embolization. Should embolization occur, intracoronary verapamil or diltiazem may be necessary. If atherectomy fails, I would consider rotational atherectomy or stenting. If the vessel is inflexible, I would perform rotational atherectomy and stent placement (RotaStent).

What techniques should be avoided?

Takeshi Kimura, MD, Japan: Directional atherectomy may be effective, but results are somewhat unpredictable. This kind of slit-like stenosis responds poorly to conventional PTCA. Interventionalists who perform only PTCA should refer the patient to a center experienced with stents.

Editors' Perspective: Directional atherectomy was performed, achieving an excellent angiographic result (below) (see p. 111 for additional comments).

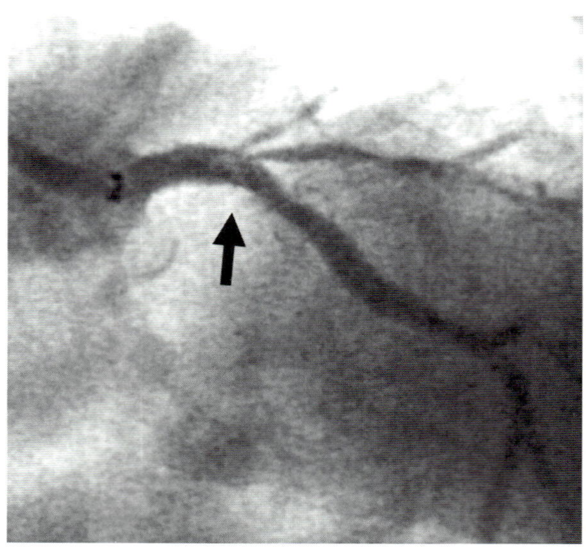

*****

UNPROTECTED LEFT MAIN BIFURCATION LESION

A 64-year-old executive develops angina running to catch a plane. Coronary angiography reveals an eccentric, ulcerated, severe stenosis involving the distal left main bifurcation (left main = 3.6 mm, LAD = 3.4 mm, LCX = 3.1 mm). There is mild tapering of the proximal LCX. All grafts to the left coronary artery are occluded, but the RCA and left ventricular function are normal.

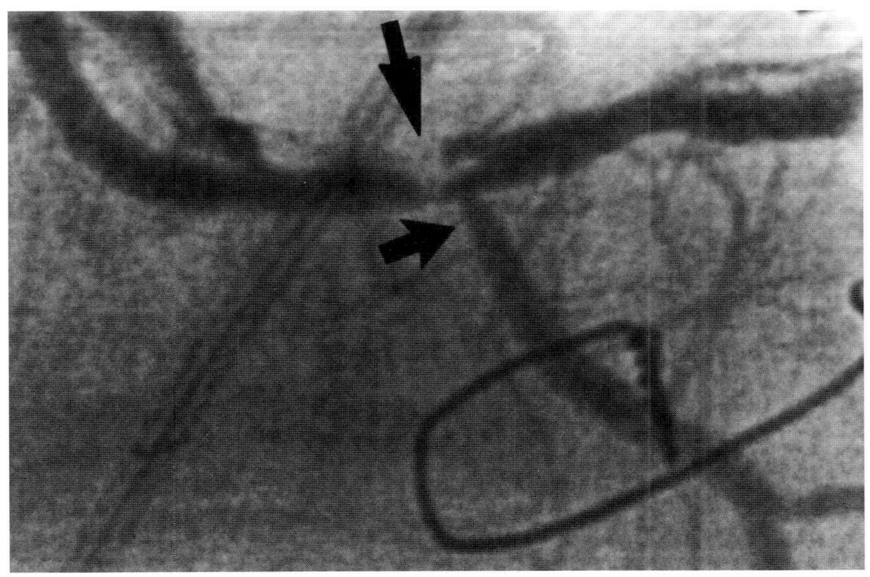

Would you recommend percutaneous intervention or redo CABG for this patient?

Takeshi Kimura, MD, Japan: This patient has a highly eccentric ulcerated lesion involving an unprotected distal left main bifurcation. The most important issue for patient management is the choice of percutaneous intervention or redo coronary bypass surgery. It is difficult to assess relative advantages and disadvantages of the two strategies in terms of mortality, morbidity, and long-term outcome. I have to consider factors such as the availability of internal mammary artery grafts and technical issues during prior surgery. Although lesion morphology is very complex, the lesion is so focal and the reference diameter is so large, I expect excellent results with percutaneous intervention with new devices. Interventionalists who perform only PTCA should refer the patient for redo surgery or to a center experienced in IVUS, atherectomy, and stent implantation.

David Williams, MD, USA: This patient has left main coronary disease characterized by a very bulky, eccentric, irregular and ulcerated lesion in the distal left main, extending into the LAD and LCX. This lesion is extremely complex and friable. The grafts to the LCX and LAD are occluded; acute occlusion will result in extensive left ventricular ischemia and infarction. The most appropriate treatment for this patient is repeat coronary bypass surgery.

Timothy Sanborn, MD, USA: This "unprotected" left main coronary artery lesion is very irregular and may contain fresh thrombus. There is a very high risk of embolization with any intervention. Unless repeat coronary artery bypass surgery (with a LIMA to the LAD and a vein graft to the obtuse marginal) is considered excessively risky, I recommend redo bypass surgery.

If percutaneous intervention is reasonable, what device would you recommend?

Takeshi Kimura, MD, Japan: My approach is to start with IVUS to assess the degree of superficial calcification and to predict hemodynamic changes during intervention. Since the LCX is large, I prefer directional atherectomy rather than stent implantation to preserve access to the LCX. I would begin with a 10F JL4 guiding catheter, a 0.014-inch x 300 cm Extra-Support guidewire, and intravascular ultrasound. If the arc of superficial calcium exceeds 180°, I would pretreat with a 2.0 mm Rotablator burr, followed by a 7F AtheroCath (guidewire in the LAD). Since there is mild tapering of the proximal LCX, I would perform sequential atherectomy in the LCX. If final plaque burden by IVUS exceeds 50-55%, I would perform adjunctive PTCA with a 4.0 mm balloon at 4-6 ATM. If the final diameter stenosis exceeds 20%, I would consider stent implantation.

Timothy Sanborn, MD, USA: There is growing experience in Europe with stenting bifurcation lesions of this type. However, until more experience and long-term follow-up have been achieved, I recommend repeat bypass surgery.

Is hemodynamic support recommended during percutaneous intervention?

Takeshi Kimura, MD, Japan: If blood pressure falls during IVUS, I would use a prophylactic intraaortic balloon pump. If the patient tolerates IVUS, I would not use any prophylactic support device.

Editors' Perspective: Increasing numbers of patients with left main disease are being referred for percutaneous revascularization. The typical patient we see today is elderly, has had CABG 5-10 years ago, and presents with progressive angina and occlusion of vein graft(s) to the LCX, thus creating a situation commonly referred to as a "protected" left main stenosis (e.g., patent LIMA protects the LAD if there is injury to the left main). "Protected" left main lesions, the functional equivalent of LAD or circumflex lesions (depending on which graft is occluded), pose much less risk than "unprotected" left main lesions, and can be treated using conventional equipment and techniques with high success and low complication rates; given the large caliber and proximal location of these vessels, stenting or directional atherectomy (preceded by Rotablator if significant calcium is present) is the percutaneous treatment of choice.

Less commonly, grafts to the LAD and LCX are occluded, and the left main stenosis is "unprotected;" these patients are at much higher risk of severe ischemic complications since the myocardium supplied by the entire left coronary artery is in jeopardy. The most important initial decision is whether patients with unprotected left main lesions are suitable candidates for repeat bypass surgery. This decision is based on multiple factors including left ventricular function; the presence of valvular disease, other coronary arterial lesions, and comorbid medical conditions; and the availability of suitable conduits for bypass. There are now several preliminary studies from Europe describing the favorable results of stenting unprotected left main lesions, and when percutaneous intervention is required, stenting is favored because of the reliable lumen expansion. Significant calcification is common, so Rotablator may be useful for initial lesion modification and debulking. In some cases, prophylactic hemodynamic support may not be necessary, although a temporary pacemaker and access to the contralateral femoral artery (for IABP or CPS) are recommended. The need for supported angioplasty (Table 28) is often guided by consideration of the jeopardy score (Figure 1) and baseline left ventricular function (Figure 2); a variety of systemic and regional support systems may be utilized (Table 29).

Table 28. Potential Candidates for Supported Angioplasty

- Target vessel supplies the majority of viable myocardium.
- Ejection fraction < 20-30%.
- Jeopardy score > 3.
- Cardiogenic shock and multivessel disease.

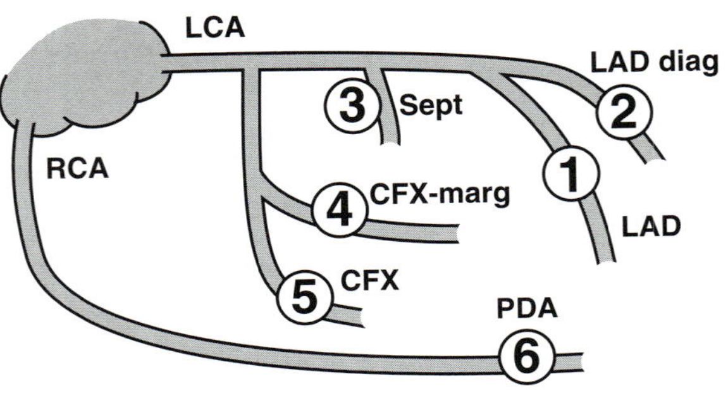

Figure 1. Jeopardy Score

Six arterial segments are used to calculate the jeopardy score, which considers the total region of jeopardized myocardium (supplied by the target vessel and providing collaterals to other regions) and the degree of baseline LV dysfunction. Scoring system:

- 1 point: for each myocardial region supplied by the target lesion.
- 1 point: for each myocardial region supplied by a vessel with diameter stenosis ≥ 70%.
- 0.5 point: for each myocardial region that is hypokinetic at baseline and not supplied by a vessel with significant stenosis.

Table 29. Overview of Supported Angioplasty

I. Systemic Support	
Intra-Aortic Balloon Pump (IABP)	**Advantages**: Extensive clinical experience. Provides afterload reduction. May result in improved outcome for selected high-risk PTCA patients and for those unable to be weaned from CPS. **Disadvantages**: Requires stable cardiac rhythm for optimal function. Probable slight increase in vascular complications.
Percutaneous Cardiopulmonary Bypass Support (CPS)	**Advantages**: Provides systemic support independent of ventricular function or cardiac rhythm. **Disadvantages**: Does not prevent myocardial ischemia during balloon inflation (or during acute closure). Not intended for long term support. Does not unload ventricle.
Ventricular Assist Devices	**Advantages**: Systemic support independent of ventricular function or cardiac rhythm. Long-term support possible. **Disadvantages**: Surgical placement required. Limited clinical experience.
Left Atrial-Femoral Bypass	**Advantages**: Systemic support independent of ventricular function or cardiac rhythm. Able to provide support for longer periods than CPS. **Disadvantages**: Requires transseptal puncture. Limited clinical experience. Limited flow rates.
II. Regional Myocardial Support	
Autoperfusion Catheters	**Advantages**: Allows better tolerance of prolonged balloon inflations. Better outcome for patients with abrupt closure. **Disadvantages**: Large profile limits access to distal lesions or tortuous vessels. Requires mean arterial pressure > 65 mmHg for effective passive perfusion.
Active Hemoperfusion	**Advantages**: Less ischemia during balloon inflations. **Disadvantages**: Limited clinical experience. Potential for hemolysis at high flow rates.
Adjunctive Pharmacotherapy	**Advantages**: Ease of administration. **Disadvantages**: Least effective of all local approaches.

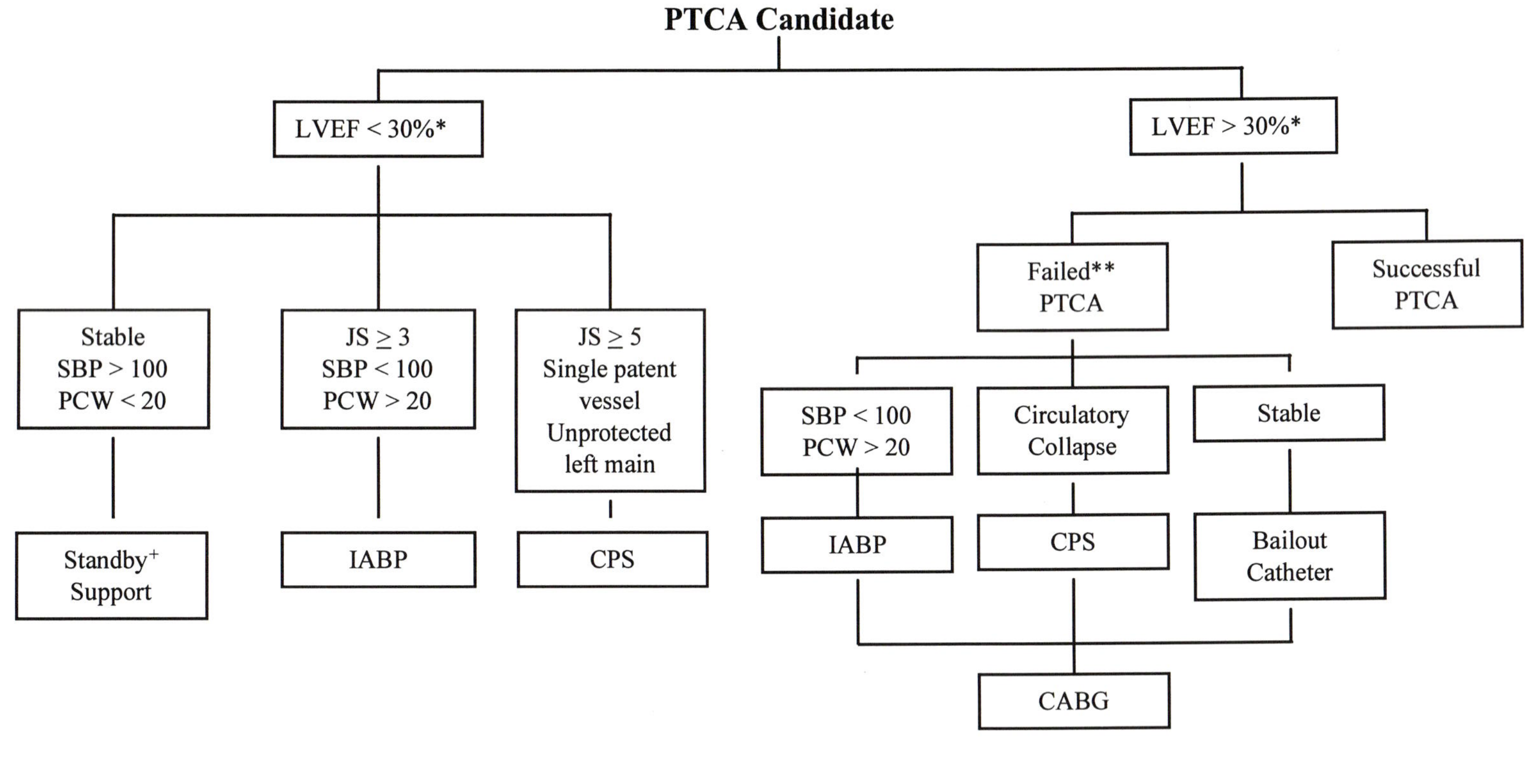

Figure 2. Selection of Patients for Supported Angioplasty

Abbreviations: LVEF = left ventricular ejection fraction; SBP = systolic blood pressure; PCW = pulmonary capillary wedge pressure; JS = jeopardy score; IABP = intra-aortic balloon pump; CPS = percutaneous cardiopulmonary bypass support; CABG = emergency coronary artery bypass grafting

* Autoperfusion balloons may be useful.

** Bailout catheters are recommended if emergency CABG is needed.

\+ Standby implies contralateral femoral vascular access; IABP or CPS ready if needed.

This patient was problematic — redo bypass surgery was recommended, but since there were no suitable venous or arterial conduits, percutaneous intervention was performed. A PS204 biliary stent was implanted using a DVI 10F JL4 guide, a 0.018-inch x 260 cm Platinum-Plus guidewire, and a 4.0 x 20 mm Schwarten delivery balloon. Predilation was performed using a 3.5 x 20 mm Cobra-18, and postdilation was performed with a 4.0 x 10 mm NC Cobra-18 at 16 ATM. Final angiography revealed no residual stenosis or ulceration, and the mild lesion at the origin of the LCX was not changed (below). A prophylactic pacemaker and intraaortic balloon pump were used prior to intervention, and there were no hemodynamic problems or arrhythmias.

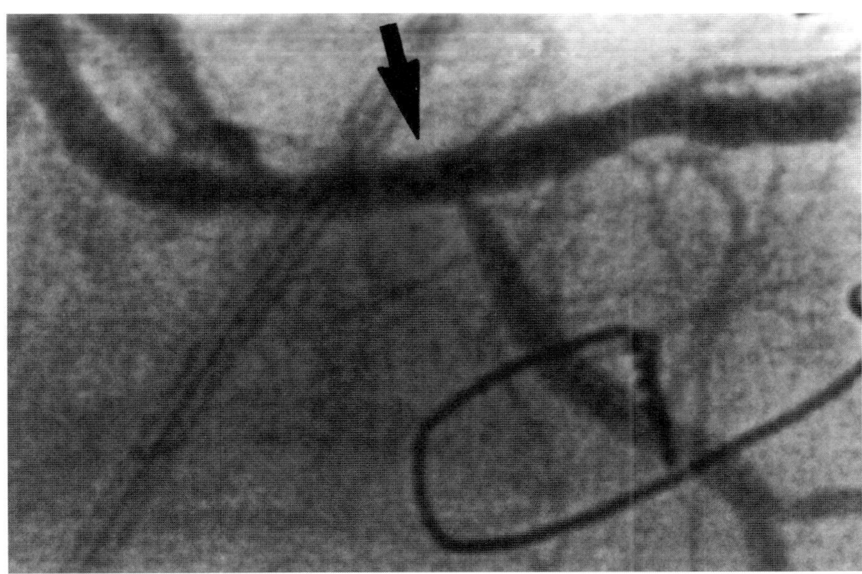

*****

DEGENERATED VEIN GRAFT

A 68-year-old minister with a history of coronary artery bypass surgery 8 years ago develops angina while climbing a ladder to the roof of his church. An exercise test is positive at a low workload. Coronary angiography reveals a patent LIMA to the LAD and a patent vein graft to the obtuse marginal branch. The native RCA is occluded, and the vein graft to the PDA has moderate degeneration in the mid-body of the graft (reference vessel diameter = 3.5 mm). Left ventricular function is normal.

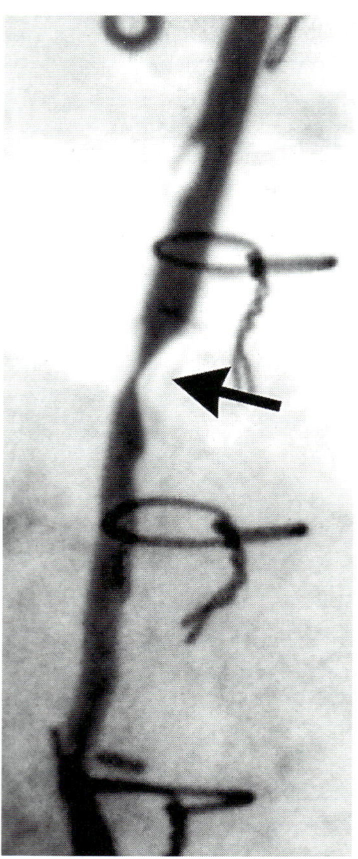

Is percutaneous intervention reasonable for this type of degenerated vein graft?

Patrick Serruys, MD, PhD, The Netherlands: This is a degenerated bypass graft with a severe focal stenosis, and considerable disease extending perhaps 40 mm in length. Nowadays, I consider this type of problem eminently suitable for percutaneous intervention, with the appropriate devices.

Frank Litvack, MD, USA: This patient is quite symptomatic and clearly in need of definitive intervention. The vertically oriented vein graft to the RCA has a tight mid-shaft lesion and diffuse moderate disease in the proximal and distal body of the graft. In a relatively young patient with this anatomy, I would not consider repeat bypass surgery at this time; percutaneous intervention is indicated.

Marty Leon, MD, USA: Based on the clinical syndrome and the anatomic considerations, vein graft intervention is indicated. There is a severe eccentric stenosis in the mid-body of the vein graft, with multiple adjacent stenoses consistent with moderate degeneration, at higher risk for distal embolization and restenosis.

What device would you recommend?

Patrick Serruys, MD, PhD, The Netherlands: The treatment of choice for this type of problem is a Wallstent measuring 1-1.5 mm larger than the maximal vessel diameter (by on-line QCA). I would treat the entire segment of disease, anchoring the Wallstent proximally and distally in what appears to be relatively healthy tissue. The Schneider Hannibal wire provides excellent support; the ACS Extra-Support wire creates some friction in the Wallstent and is not desirable under these circumstances. The constrained Wallstent has a diameter of 1.57 mm; I would choose a 60 mm stent which will shorten to 45-50 mm when dilated to 3.5-4 mm. I can easily position the Wallstent using an 8F giant-lumen El Gamal or multipurpose guiding catheter. With experience, it is possible to reposition or drag the Wallstent proximally as the constraining sheath is retracted, if necessary. The Wallstent is absolutely ideal for covering the entire segment of disease with one stent. Postdilation should follow with a 4.0 mm noncompliant balloon at 14-16 ATM. After successful implantation, my medical therapy is aspirin and ticlopidine. If there is thrombotic material, I recommend a 12-hour infusion of ReoPro.

Frank Litvack, MD, USA: I would perform PTCA and stent placement. Using the equipment available in the United States, I would insert an 8F multipurpose guide and cross the lesion with a 0.014-inch x 300 cm Extra-Support guidewire. I would predilate with a 3.5 mm noncompliant balloon, and place a 3.5 mm Palmaz-Schatz stent in the mid-portion of the graft at the most severe lesion. I would place 1 or 2 more stents in the proximal graft towards the ostium to cover the proximal area of diffuse disease. If the distal graft looks worse, I would not hesitate to place additional stents. I would postdilate all stents at 15-20 ATM. I see no need to debulk this graft prior to stent implantation. I would treat the patient with aspirin and ticlopidine, but I would not use prophylactic ReoPro unless there is visible thrombus.

Marty Leon, MD, USA: Vein graft disease is best managed with endovascular stents. Acute complications, distal embolization, and 6-month restenosis rates are lower with stents compared to PTCA or ablative technologies. I would select a 2.0 mm Spectranetics excimer laser catheter and perform 1-2 passes with the saline infusion technique before stent placement. An alternative is extraction atherectomy with a 7.5F cutter followed by stent placement. In saphenous vein grafts ≥ 4 mm in diameter, I prefer to use biliary stents. Since the target lesion is in a straight portion of the graft with a downward orientation, I would deploy a P154 biliary stent on a 4.5 mm Schwarten peripheral balloon at 6-8 ATM. I recommend a 9F multipurpose guide and a 0.014- or 0.018-inch Extra-Support or Platinum-Plus guidewire. The decision to treat contiguous segments of moderate disease proximal and distal to the target lesion is controversial. At present, I favor treating areas of moderate stenosis if careful ultrasound examination confirms significant plaque mass to justify therapy, using at least 2 additional P154 biliary stents. My preference is to treat with aspirin, ticlopidine (for 2 weeks), ReoPro, and low-dose heparin (for 36 hours). I would discharge the patient on Lovenox (30 mg BID for 2 weeks). At the end of this 2-week period, I would slowly begin oral Coumadin for 3-6 months, and perform repeat angiography in 3-6 months to assess lesion progression and stent patency.

What particular complications do you expect?

Frank Litvack, MD, USA: Any type of intervention on this vein graft is associated with risk of distal embolization. I am not particularly worried about this graft in that the patient's symptoms are stable and it is unlikely that fresh thrombus is present. However, I would be prepared to deal with embolization and no reflow; if these occur, I would use intracoronary nitroglycerin and/or verapamil.

Marty Leon, MD, USA: There is significant likelihood of distal embolization, even after predilation with a balloon catheter. Therefore, I would "pretreat" the severe stenosis with excimer laser angioplasty or extraction atherectomy before stent placement. In working on degenerated saphenous vein grafts, one must accept a "less than perfect" result. I would not be aggressive with pre-stent preparation of the vein graft, and I would be content with a 2 mm channel after excimer laser or TEC. I would implant the stent on a nominal size balloon, and be very careful regarding post-stent dilation. Data suggest that if stent dimensions exceed 4 mm in the body of saphenous vein grafts, restenosis rates are low and there is little to be gained by achieving a residual stenosis closer to 0%. In fact, there is much to lose from the standpoint of distal embolization and plaque herniation through the stent struts: Be careful about aggressive post-stent high pressure dilations in degenerated vein grafts. Although I generally use Hexabrix, conventional ionic contrast is acceptable. In degenerated vein grafts, I am extremely aggressive with adjunctive medical therapy. I would pretreat with verapamil (100-200 mcg IC) via a transport catheter distal to the lesion, prior to laser or TEC. Given the complexity of the vein graft, I would give intravenous ReoPro.

Is this patient suitable for conventional PTCA alone?

Patrick Serruys, MD, PhD, The Netherlands: This type of lesion is extremely unattractive for PTCA, which is associated with a high risk of distal embolization, suboptimal results, and restenosis > 60%.

Frank Litvack, MD, USA: This type of diffuse vein graft disease is associated with prohibitive clinical and angiographic restenosis rates after conventional PTCA. If an interventional cardiologist is not equipped with coronary stents, I do not recommend PTCA, but rather referral of the patient to a center with stent capability.

Marty Leon, MD, USA: Degenerative disease in saphenous vein grafts represents a lesion substrate only suitable for advanced angioplasty techniques. The combination of frequent procedure-related complications and high incidence of late restenosis, makes this lesion unacceptable for conventional PTCA alone. If the procedure is undertaken, it should be performed by skilled interventionalists in a center with access to advanced modalities, including atheroblation, Wallstents, and biliary stents.

Would you use any other alternative imaging approaches?

Patrick Serruys, MD, PhD, The Netherlands: Only angioscopy can clarify the presence of thrombus and atheromatous material. This might change my general approach to the patient, but from a practical point of view, I consider angioscopy to be somewhat academic, and I would proceed without angioscopy. I would perform intravascular ultrasound only if stent underexpansion is suspected.

Frank Litvack, MD, USA: Assuming the angiographic result is excellent, I do not utilize intravascular ultrasound, but rely on high-pressure inflations and the angiographic appearance of the graft.

Marty Leon, MD, USA: I would certainly use intravascular ultrasound to correctly size the vein graft and lesion length, and most important, to determine if the adjacent segments of moderate disease are sufficient to justify additional stents.

Editors' Perspective: The ideal treatment for degenerated vein grafts is unknown. In the setting of other disease requiring revascularization, repeat CABG should be strongly considered. In situations where other grafts are patent and there is significant degeneration of one graft, the choices generally consist of medical therapy (with significant chance of progressive disease, vein graft occlusion, and myocardial infarction) versus percutaneous intervention (with significant chance of distal embolization, no-reflow, restenosis, reocclusion, and myocardial infarction). Clearly, there are no "good" choices.

However, recent experience suggests that percutaneous approaches using multiple devices and adjunctive pharmacotherapy to maximize lumen diameter and reduce complications offer hope. The most important complication to avoid is no-reflow, since it is common (~ 15% of degenerated vein graft interventions), frequently leads to myocardial infarction and/or death, and cannot be treated by mechanical techniques such as stents or bypass surgery. The etiology of no-reflow in uncertain, but is most likely related to distal embolization and microvascular spasm. Angioscopy can reliably identify vein graft characteristics that increase the risk of no-reflow (e.g., thrombus, friability), but passage of the angioscope itself can lead to no-reflow. Fortunately, ~ 65% of no-reflow is reversible by intracoronary administration of calcium channel blockers (although the likelihood of irreversible no-reflow is higher in degenerated vein grafts than in other situations). To minimize the risk of no-reflow, we empirically administer verapamil prior to any intervention in vein grafts and just prior to insertion of each device. Although this approach is not supported by clinical trials, it is virtually never associated with verapamil-induced hypotension or severe bradycardia. We also recommend a prophylactic pacemaker for interventions on degenerated vein grafts to the RCA or a dominant LCX, since no-reflow in this setting is commonly associated with significant bradycardia and hypotension. A pulmonary artery catheter is extremely useful for monitoring left heart filling pressures, especially during prolonged periods of no-reflow and hypotension (several companies manufacture pulmonary artery catheters with pacing capability).

There are no reliable mechanical methods for avoiding no-reflow (except not to

intervene on degenerated vein grafts). Extraction devices (TEC) may cause less embolization than PTCA, but are still associated with a significant risk of no-reflow. Nevertheless, a popular approach in degenerated vein grafts is to perform initial TEC atherectomy followed by a 2-4 week period of oral anticoagulation and subsequent stenting, although 10-20% of such grafts may occlude during the intervening period. Recently, there has been renewed interest in ablative laser technologies. Although preliminary studies in small numbers of patients suggest potential benefit, laser techniques are still limited by small device size (particularly in large caliber vessels) and the universal need for other adjunctive devices, which themselves can lead to no-reflow and a high incidence of restenosis. Thrombectomy devices such as the AngioJet and Hydrolyzer are theoretically attractive, but may be more useful for removal of fresh thrombus rather than organized, adherent, degenerated material. In the United States, the most commonly used stents for vein grafts are the Palmaz-Schatz stent and the Palmaz biliary stent; in Europe, the Wallstent is widely used, and currently offers the largest variety of stent diameters and lengths. Stents covered with synthetic (Gortex, Dacron, PTFE) or natural (autologous vein) surfaces hold future promise for dealing with degenerated vein grafts. In our interventional survey, 71% of respondents recommended stents as their primary approach for degenerated vein grafts, while TEC atherectomy, which is commonly used just prior to stenting, was recommended by 29%. This patient was treated rapidly and effectively with a single 3.5 mm Palmaz-Schatz coronary stent, a 0.014-inch Hi-torque floppy guidewire, and an 8F multipurpose guide (below). IVUS and angioscopy were not employed.

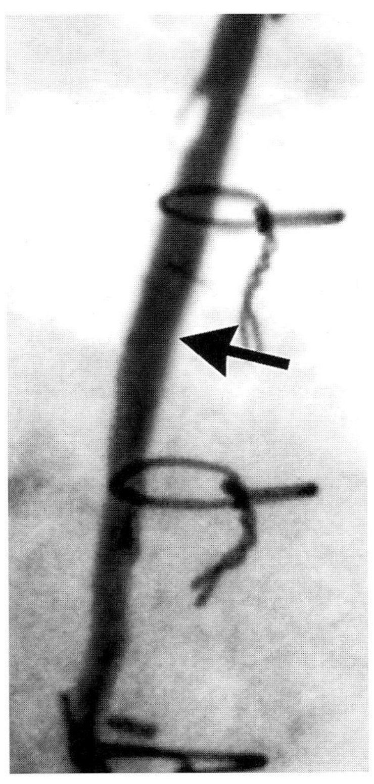

*****

VEIN GRAFT: COMPLEX LESION

A 68-year-old farmer with a history of coronary artery bypass surgery 10 years ago, develops progressive angina while working the fields. Myocardial perfusion imaging reveals ischemia at a low workload. Coronary angiography reveals a complex ulcerated stenosis in the vein graft to the LAD (reference vessel diameter = 4.1 mm). Other grafts and left ventricular function are normal.

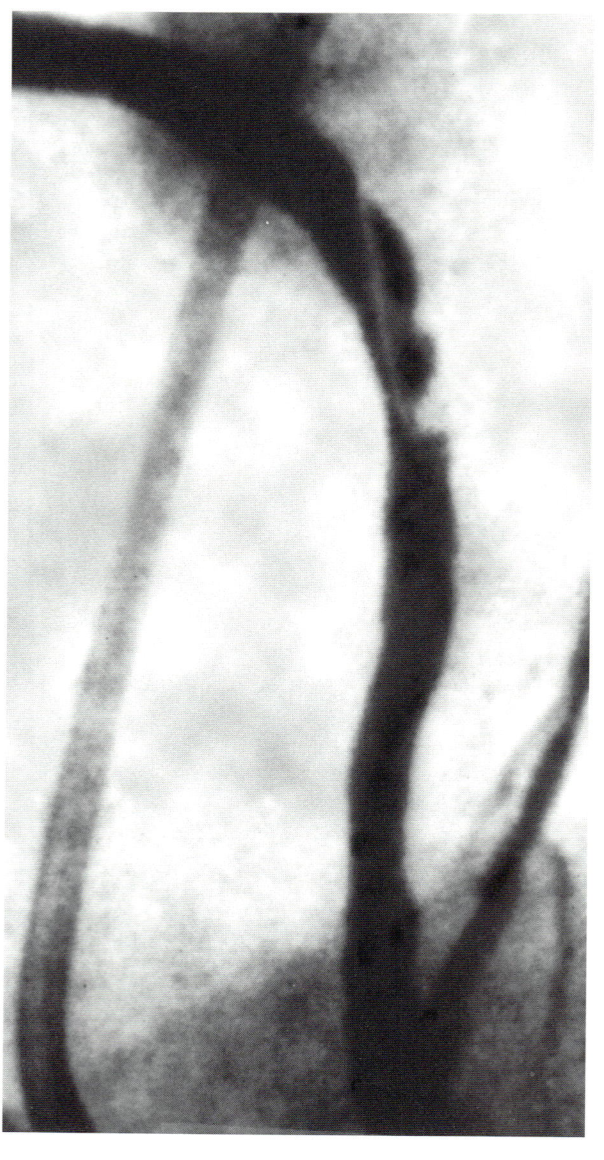

Describe your impression of this complex lesion.

David Holmes, MD, USA: This patient has a complex ulcerated stenosis in the vein graft to the LAD. The pathology of these vein grafts is usually awful; I am concerned that there is thrombus in this lesion. There are multiple approaches, all of which have advantages and disadvantages. Regardless of the approach, I recommend a bolus and infusion of ReoPro, starting before intervention.

Paul Teirstein, MD, USA: This patient has a complex, ulcerated but fairly focal lesion in the body of the saphenous vein graft.

Bernhard Meier, MD, Switzerland: A 10-year-old vein graft to the LAD shows an irregular lesion in its mid-portion. This is the only problem, and certainly responsible for the ischemia.

What device would you recommend?

David Holmes, MD, USA: I would choose a 4.0 mm Dispatch catheter and a 0.014-inch wire. I would infuse heparin and urokinase (500,000 units) into the wall of the vessel. I would then insert an articulated PS204 biliary stent.

Paul Teirstein, MD, USA: I would place one or two Palmaz-Schatz stents into the lesion.

Bernhard Meier, MD, Switzerland: It would be best to implant a stent without predilation to minimize the risk of distal embolization.

Describe your technique.

David Holmes, MD, USA: Multipurpose guiding catheters are excellent in this setting. The goal of initial therapy is to debulk the lesion, prevent embolization, and facilitate stent implantation.

The biliary stent is optimal; I would position the stent to cover the entire lesion. The articulated stent is preferred over the rigid nonarticulated stent. I would deliver the stent on a 4.5 mm Total Cross or Advantage balloon, and postdilate with the same balloon at 12 ATM. I think this would give a superb angiographic result, and I would treat the patient with aspirin and ticlopidine. Another stent which is quite promising in vein grafts is the Wallstent.

Paul Teirstein, MD, USA: I would use an 8F Amplatz or hockey stick guide without sideholes. I would cross the lesion with a 0.014-inch Extra-S'port guidewire, then predilate with a 3.0 mm balloon. I would then use a high-pressure balloon to optimally expand this stent to at least 16 ATM. If the angiographic result is pristine, I would remove the sheaths on the evening of the procedure, and discharge the patient the next day on aspirin and ticlopidine (250 mg BID).

Bernhard Meier, MD, Switzerland: This lesion may be tough to dilate and it is likely that the stent will not pass the lesion without predilation. Since the lesion is short, an 18 mm Palmaz-Schatz stent is a good choice. I would approach this case with a 6F multipurpose or AL3 guiding catheter. I would pass a guidewire into the LAD and predilate the lesion with a 4.5 mm balloon. If distal embolization does not occur, further risk is small. A Palmaz-Schatz stent can be crimped on the balloon and deployed at 14-18 ATM. If a good angiographic result is achieved, no heparin is needed after intervention; aspirin with or without ticlopidine is sufficient. The patient can be discharged the next day.

Are other devices reasonable?

David Holmes, MD, USA: Conventional PTCA is possible, but if distal embolization occurs, the physician will wish PTCA hadn't been performed! Directional atherectomy may give an excellent result. A promising approach is TEC atherectomy followed by stent implantation, to reduce the risk of embolization.

Do you anticipate any particular complications?

David Holmes, MD, USA: The problems with old vein grafts with complex ulcerated stenoses are distal embolization and myocardial infarction. With any approach, the potential for embolization is real and can result in major problems. I recommend adjunctive ReoPro as an important strategy to reduce complications in patients with complex lesions containing thrombus.

Paul Teirstein, MD, USA: The major potential pitfall of this procedure is no-reflow due to distal embolization. If this occurs, I would use a Schneider PMC catheter (monorail with a through-lumen) and inject verapamil into the distal vein graft and native coronary artery. Although some advocate ReoPro to reduce distal embolization in degenerated vein grafts, there are no data to support its use.

Would you recommend any other imaging devices?

David Holmes, MD, USA: I recommend IVUS after stent implantation to document apposition to the vessel wall. Other alternative imaging modalities such as angioscopy might be useful to identify thrombus, but are not required.

Paul Teirstein, MD, USA: Intravascular ultrasound would be used as part of a randomized research trial.

Bernhard Meier, MD, Switzerland: There is no need for intravascular ultrasound.

Editors' Perspective: Focal, complex lesions in nondegenerated vein grafts are usually treated by stenting, and 95% of the interventional cardiologists in our survey confirmed such an approach. Numerous observational studies reported low rates of major ischemic complications and restenosis rates of 20-40% for de novo lesions (which may be as high as 60% for restenotic lesions) (Table 30). For vein grafts, the Palmaz-Schatz stent may soon be approved by the FDA, and a multicenter trial of the Wallstent is in progress in the United States and Canada. Although not commonly used as sole therapy in vein grafts, other techniques have been used, including conventional PTCA (Table 31), TEC (Table 32), directional atherectomy (Table 33, 34), and excimer laser angioplasty (Table 35).

Table 30. Results of Stents in Saphenous Vein Grafts

Series	Stent	Lesions (N)	Succ. (%)	SAT (%)	Complications (%) D/MI/CABG	VSR/XF (%)	RS (%)
Wong[1097]	PSS	624	98.8	1.4	1.7 / 0.3 / 0.9	8.0 / 6.3	30
Rechavia[1098]	PSS,B	29	100	0	0	3.4 / 6.8	-
Wong[1099]	PSS,B	309	95.3	1.7	1.3 / 0.9 / 0.4	8.4 / 25	-
Denardo[1100]	PSS,B	300	93.3	6.7	0	(16.7)	-
Piana[1101]	PSS,B	200	98.5	0.6	- / 0.6 / 0	8.5 / 14.0	17
Eeckhout[1102]	Wall,Wik	58	100	2	0	(14)	33
Keane[1103]	Wall	29	97	3.4	0	3.4 / 6.8	32
Fenton[1104]	PSS	209	98.5	0.5	0.4 / 0 / 0	17.2 /12	34
Leon[1105]	PSS	589	97	1.4	1.7 / 0.3 / 0.9	7.5 / 15.5	30
Fortuna[1106]	Wik	101	95	2	1 / 3 / 1	-	-
Pomerantz[1084]	PSS	84	99	0	0	(5)	25
Bilodeau[1107]	GRS	37	-	-	0	-	35
Strauss[1108]	Wall	145	-	8	- / - / -	-	39
deScheerder[1109]	Wall	95	100	10	1.4 / 4.3 / 2.8	(33)	47
Urban[1110]	Wall	14	100	0	0	7.7 / 7.7	20

Abbreviations: Succ. = procedural success; RS = restenosis; SAT = subacute thrombus; D = death; MI = in-hospital Q-wave myocardial infarction; CABG = emergency coronary artery bypass surgery; VSR/XF = vascular surgery repair/blood transfusion (number in parentheses indicates combined vascular and bleeding complications if not identified separately); Wall = Wallstent; Wik = Wiktor stent; PSS = Palmaz-Schatz stent; B = biliary stent; GRS = Gianturco-Roubin stent; - = not reported

Table 31. Results of PTCA in Saphenous Vein Grafts

Series	N	Graft Age (months)	Success (%)	D/MI/CABG (%)	Restenosis (%)
Tan[1032]	50	50	86	-	39
Morrison[1033]	89	98	93	3 / 3 / 1	51
Unterberg[1034]	55	46	89	-	-
Miranda[1035]	409	> 12	94	-	-
Meester[1036]	59	56	86	1.2 / 8.3 / 2.4	-
Plokker[1037]	454	67	90	0.7 / 2.8 / 1.3	-
Douglas[1038]	672	≤ 120	90	1.2 / 2.3 / 3.5	-
Jost[1039]	49	40	94	0	-
Webb[1040]	168	66	85	0	50
Dorros[1041]	241	-	91	2.3 / 5.2 / 1.4	-
Platko[1042]	107	50	92	2 / 5.9 / 2	61
Pinkerton[1043]	100	60	93	-	-
Cote[1044]	83	51	86	0	23
Ernst[1045]	33	-	97	0	31
Douglas[1046]	235	-	92	0	-
Reeder[1047]	19	38	84	5.3 / 5.3 / 0	73

Abbreviations: D = death; MI = myocardial infarction; CABG = emergency coronary artery bypass surgery; - not reported

Table 32. In-hospital Results of TEC Atherectomy in Saphenous Vein Grafts

	Meany[1068]	Twidale[1069]	Safian[1066]	Popma[1067]
No. lesions	650	88	158	29
Adjunctive PTCA (%)	74	95	91	86
Success (%)	89	86	84	82
Complications (%)				
Myocardial infarction	0.7	3.4	2.0	3.7
Death	3.2	0	2.0	10.3
Acute closure	2.0	5.0	5.0	-
Distal embolization	2.0	4.5	11.9	17
No-reflow	-	-	8.8	-

Abbreviation: - = not reported

Table 33. In-hospital Results of Directional Atherectomy in Saphenous Vein Grafts

Series	No. Lesions	Success (%)	Major Complications (%)*
Holmes[1089]	149	89	4.7
Stephan[1137]	57	86	0
Cowley[1081]	363	85	2.5**
Garratt[1085]	26	96	3.8
Pomerantz[1084]	35	94	0
DiScasio[1083]	96	97	1.4
Ghazzal[1087]	286	87	2.1
Selmon[1086]	87	91	2.6
Kaufmann[1082]	14	93	7

* Major complications = death, myocardial infarction, or emergency coronary artery bypass surgery

** US DCA Registry: Vascular repair (3.5%); non-Q-wave MI (3%); restenosis rate (57%; 38% for de novo lesions, 75% for restenotic lesions)

Table 34. DCA vs. PTCA in Saphenous Vein Grafts (CAVEAT II)[1089]

	DCA No. (%)	PTCA No. (%)
No.	149 (100)	156 (100)
Graft age (years)	9.5	9.9
Lesion location		
Aorto-ostial	22 (14.8)	14 (9.0)
Proximal body	42 (28.2)	57 (36.5)
Mid-body	57 (38.3)	52 (33.3)
Distal body	28 (18.8)	43 (27.6)
Distal anastomosis	8 (5.4)	7 (4.5)
Lesion length (mm)	10.9	11.0
In-hospital results (%)		
Success	89.2	79.0*
Final diameter stenosis	31.5	37.6**
Acute closure	7 (4.7)	4 (2.6)
Distal embolization	20 (13.4)	8 (5.1) +
Perforation	1 (0.7)	0.00
Q-wave-MI	2 (1.3)	3 (1.9)
Non-Q-MI	24 (16.1)	15 (9.6) ++
CABG	1 (0.7)	2 (1.3)
Death	3 (2.0)	3 (1.9)
Composite endpoint	30 (20.1)	19 (12.2) ++
Follow-up results (%)		
Restenosis	47 (45.6)	48 (50.5)
Late cardiac event	(49.3)	(44.3)
Target lesion revascularization	(18.6)	(26.2) ++

Abbreviations: CABG = emergency coronary artery bypass grafting; DCA = directional coronary atherectomy; MI = myocardial infarction

* p <0.05; + p < 0.01; ** p < 0.001; ++ p < 0.10

Table 35. In-hospital Results of ELCA in Saphenous Vein Grafts

Series	No. Lesions	PTCA (%)	Success (%)	Complications (%)*
Strauss[1090]	125	83	89	3.7
DeMarchena[1093]	34	-	100	0
Bittl[1091]	545	91	92	6.1
Litvack[1092]	480	-	92	-

Abbreviations: PTCA = adjunctive balloon angioplasty; - = not reported

* Death, myocardial infarction, or emergency coronary artery bypass surgery

This lesion was readily treated by Dr. Donald Baim using a single Palmaz-Schatz stent with excellent results.

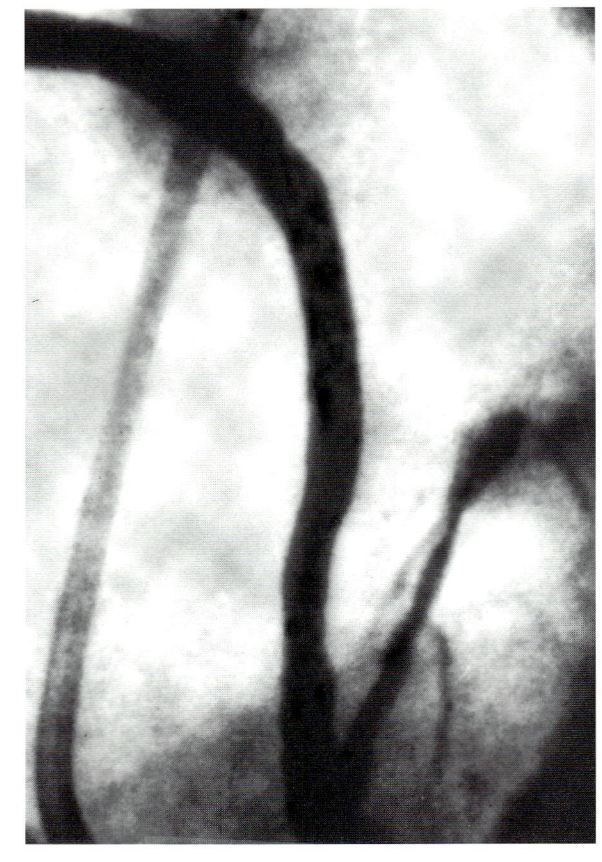

*****

VEIN GRAFT: AORTO-OSTIAL LESION

A 68-year-old senator with previous coronary artery bypass surgery 10 years ago, develops progressive angina during filibuster of the 1996 Tax Reform Bill. Myocardial perfusion imaging reveals ischemia at a low workload. Coronary angiography reveals patent vein grafts to the PDA and obtuse marginal branch and a severe ostial stenosis in the vein graft to the LAD (reference vessel diameter = 4.3 mm). Left ventricular function is normal.

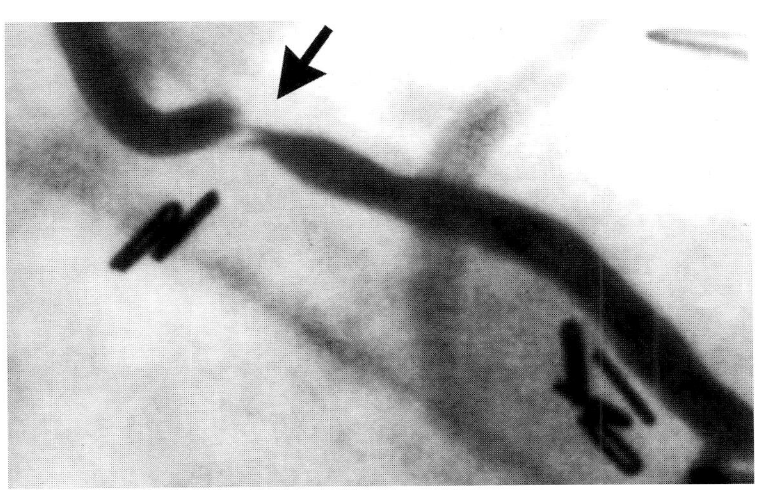

Describe your impression about this lesion.

Morton Kern, MD, USA: This patient has a 10-year-old vein graft to the LAD with an ostial stenosis. This stenosis may also contain thrombus, but after 10 years most likely consists of atherosclerotic plaque. The body of the vein graft is normal.

Patrick Whitlow, MD, USA: The lesion appears eccentric, short, and severe, but without calcification, ulceration, or thrombus. The vein graft is not diffusely degenerated. Therefore, the initial risk of percutaneous intervention is low, and the chance of distal embolization is 3%. Restenosis is a concern, and target vessel revascularization is > 20%, even with new devices.

Marie-Claude Morice, MD, France: The lesion is short and located at the ostium of the graft to the LAD.

What device would you recommend?

Morton Kern, MD, USA: I would perform primary stent placement, to reduce restenosis and achieve a satisfactory angiographic result without dissection or thrombus.

Patrick Whitlow, MD, USA: Since aortoostial lesions are difficult to dilate due to recoil, a stent which resists radial compression will give the best result.

Marie-Claude Morice, MD, France: The lesion is short; however, I would select a 15 mm stent and a 20 mm balloon to stabilize the stent in the ostium, to avoid stent embolization during deployment. Despite stenting, the risk of further evolution of this lesion is high. For restenosis, I propose mammary artery grafting.

What technical "pearls" are essential for successful outcome?

Morton Kern, MD, USA: Guide catheter backup and seating may be difficult. Placement of ostial stents requires precise positioning with retraction of the guide catheter and alignment of the stent just inside the aortic wall. Take enough time to position the stent correctly!

Patrick Whitlow, MD, USA: I would make sure that a balloon fully expands without a waist before placing a stent, because suboptimal stent expansion will lead to restenosis or thrombosis. The Palmaz biliary stent is made of thicker metal and is more radioopaque than the coronary stent, and I particularly like biliary stents for aortoostial lesions. Optimal stent placement requires that 1 mm of stent extends into the aorta to completely cover the aortic anastomosis. Since the stent has to be hand-crimped, it is important to make sure that the stent is firmly crimped on the balloon. Most of the hand crimping should be applied to the middle of the stent and not to the ends, to make sure the balloon material is not damaged. I always inflate the balloon first before mounting the stent, since the winged balloon material tends to hold the crimped stent in position more reliably than an uninflated balloon.

Marie-Claude Morice, MD, France: The difficulty in this case is that the lesion is located at the ostium. Very precise and stable stent implantation is mandatory! I would use a short-tip guide to avoid deep intubation, which can damage the stent struts. To ensure correct positioning of the stent, I would push it a little distal, then pullback slowly on the guiding catheter and the delivery balloon; selective injections confirm adequate positioning. Then I would deploy the stent firmly, holding the guiding catheter and the balloon to avoid any movement.

Describe your interventional approach.

Morton Kern, MD, USA: I would use a 0.086-inch large-lumen right Judkins or Amplatz guiding catheter for support, a 0.014-inch Extra-Support guidewire, predilate with a 3.5-4.0 mm balloon, and implant a P104 Palmaz biliary stent. Alternatively, a 4.0 x 15 mm Palmaz-Schatz stent can be used. After placing the stent, I would use a 4.0 x 10 mm Titan at 15-20 ATM. If the angiographic result is perfect, I would consider the procedure complete. Heparin would be stopped after 4 hours, the sheath pulled, and the patient would be treated with aspirin and ticlopidine.

Patrick Whitlow, MD, USA: I would predilate the lesion using a 4.0 x 20 mm balloon (polyethylene or nylon) to make sure that low-to-moderate pressure resolves any waist, followed by placement of a P154 Palmaz biliary stent using the same balloon. The stent would be postdilated with a 4.5 mm high-pressure balloon. A 9F guiding catheter (JR4 or multipurpose) and a 0.018-inch extra-support wire are recommended. I avoid PET balloons for stent delivery for fear of balloon rupture at low pressure, but PET balloons are excellent for postdilation.

Marie-Claude Morice, MD, France: I would dilate this lesion with a 4.0 mm balloon over a 0.014-inch Extra-Support guidewire, followed by a Palmaz Schatz stent crimped on the same balloon. I would overdilate the stent would a 4.5 mm x 9-10 mm noncompliant high-pressure balloon. As for all our stent patients, this patient would receive aspirin (100 mg QD) and ticlopidine (250-500 mg QD).

Are other devices useful?

Morton Kern, MD, USA: Ostial saphenous vein graft lesions respond poorly to PTCA. Oversize balloons may be an alternative, but cause higher rates of dissection. PTCA of ostial vein graft lesions is associated with elastic recoil and high restenosis rates; atherectomy and/or stents are favored.

Patrick Whitlow, MD, USA: Directional atherectomy can be utilized and may give a good result, but these ostial lesions frequently have very fibrous or calcified plaque which resist balloon expansion and are difficult to completely excise with present AtheroCaths. If predilation fails to resolve a waist in the balloon or the lesion is calcified, I recommend Rotablator prior to stent placement. Aortoostial vein graft lesions should be referred to centers with stents.

Marie-Claude Morice, MD, France: Although I like Wallstents in grafts, it is not my first choice in this case for one reason: If you know the precise distal position of a Wallstent, you never know where the proximal end will be, because of stent shortening.

Would you recommend other imaging modalities?

Morton Kern, MD, USA: If there are irregularities in the stent, I would use intravascular ultrasound to ensure full stent apposition.

Patrick Whitlow, MD, USA: Ultrasound is very useful to determine the composition of plaque before intervention. It is useful in this case to make sure that there is no calcification and to determine if the stent is optimally expanded after deployment. If optimal stent placement and expansion are confirmed by ultrasound, the patient can be treated with aspirin alone, and require only one day in-hospital. The cost savings from decreased length of stay outweigh the cost of the ultrasound catheter.

Marie-Claude Morice, MD, France: I would use IVUS to optimize stent deployment and to ensure ideal positioning of the stent. Failure to properly position the stent will increase the risk of restenosis.

Editors' Perspective: The percutaneous approach to ostial vein graft lesions is complicated by rigidity and elasticity of the aorta. Because of the known limitations of PTCA, other approaches are favored, although no single modality has emerged as the device of choice. Many interventionalists favor stenting such lesions, based on the ability of stents to resist elastic recoil. For many, the issue is not whether to stent, but which stent to use. There are two important technical considerations when stenting ostial vein lesions: First, care must be taken to ensure that rigidity of the wall of the aorta does not preclude full stent expansion. IVUS may be used to identify lesion calcium, which may have an adverse impact on stent expansion. If superficial calcium is identified, Rotablator atherectomy is a useful adjunct (except in lesions in the body of the vein graft), and may facilitate subsequent stent expansion. Second, the technique of stent implantation is challenging, requiring special skill and patience. In order to properly deploy a stent in the ostial location, the stent must protrude 1-2 mm into the aorta; failure to completely cover the aortoostial junction increases the risk of stent thrombosis and vessel occlusion. Since the guiding catheter cannot be positioned inside the ostium, stenting must be accomplished with a "weak" guide position, which reduces guide support and the ability to properly image the ostial lesion. After stent deployment, care must be taken to avoid damaging the stent struts or coils with the guiding catheter tip. IVUS may be useful to assess ideal stent deployment, and to ensure that the lesion is completely covered by the stent. In some cases, overlapping stents may be needed to provide enough radial strength to resist elastic recoil. Although observational studies suggest a high restenosis rate for ostial stenting, we suspect that a large fraction of these cases were due to improper stent position and/or incomplete stent expansion. Directional atherectomy may be useful for ostial vein graft lesions, but is technically challenging for reasons similar to those for stenting. Although excimer laser can also be used, it's use is limited to debulking prior to more definitive lumen enlargement with PTCA, directional atherectomy, or stents. This particular lesion was successfully treated by Drs. Lowell Satler and Jeffrey Popma using a 7F Graft AtheroCath and adjunctive PTCA, with excellent results (below).

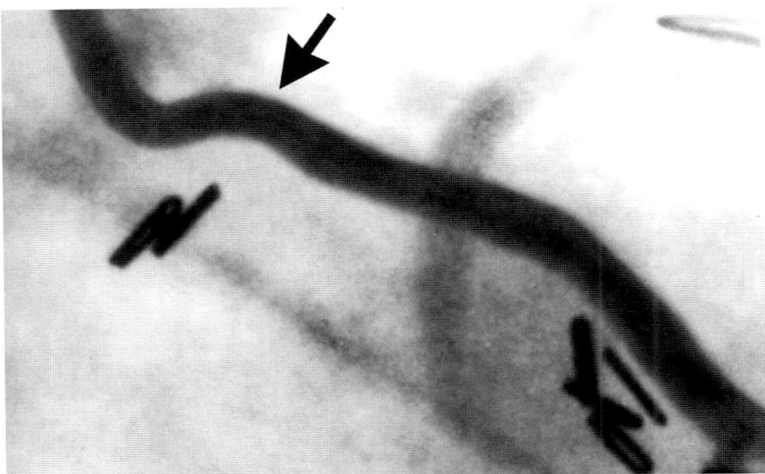

*****

VEIN GRAFT: DISTAL ANASTOMOSIS

A 60-year-old executive vice president of a bank, with a history of coronary artery bypass surgery 10 years ago, presents with progressive angina. Myocardial perfusion imaging reveals ischemia at a low workload. Coronary angiography demonstrates patent vein grafts to the PDA and obtuse marginal branch. Left ventricular function is normal. The vein graft to the LAD has a severe diaphragm-like stenosis at the distal anastomosis (vein graft = 4.1 mm, native LAD = 3.0 mm).

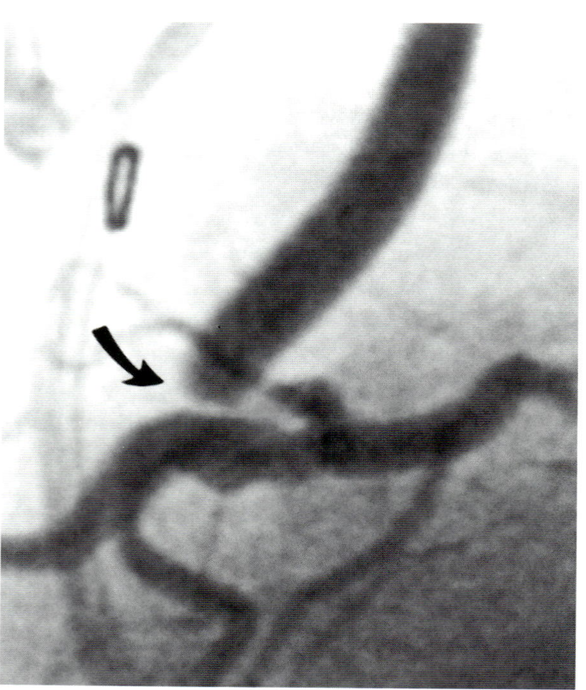

Does this lesion morphology impact your device selection?

Spencer King III, MD, USA: This patient has a severe lesion at the distal anastomosis. Ordinarily, anastomotic lesions respond well to PTCA; they are commonly seen a few months to a year or two after surgery, and probably represent a response to injury during harvesting or during the anastomotic procedure itself. This lesion is over ten years old and I am not sure how it developed or whether the result will be the same as younger lesions (since these lesions at ten years are not common). If this lesion responds like most distal anastomotic lesions, the restenosis rate is quite favorable (the best in vein graft work). I would perform PTCA since that procedure has the best track record, and few other interventions have been tried in this location.

Donald Baim, MD, USA: This patient has a membrane-like stenosis at the distal anastomosis of a ten year old saphenous vein graft. Such older vein grafts respond poorly to conventional PTCA with restenosis rates in excess of 50%. I suspect an even worse long-term outcome given the tendency of membrane-like lesions such as this to be associated with significant recoil. While directional atherectomy is an option for such lesions, and is unlikely to disrupt the suture line this long after surgery, I favor implantation of a Palmaz-Schatz coronary stent.

Masakiyo Nobuyoshi, MD, Japan: This angiogram shows a slit-like anastomotic stenosis of a vein graft to the LAD. Because of the high degree of elastic recoil, vein graft distal anastomotic lesions are often resistant to balloon inflation. I would perform PTCA using a 0.014-inch flexible guidewire and a 4.0 x 20 mm balloon. If recoil occurs, I would use a 4.0 mm Gianturco-Roubin stent. Directional atherectomy is not advisable if there is marked tortuosity, but stenting anastomotic lesions is relatively easy.

Describe your technique.

Spencer King III, MD, USA: I would use a 0.014-inch x 300 cm Hi-torque floppy guidewire and any 3.0 mm balloon at sufficient pressure to eliminate the waist on the balloon. The balloon should match the diameter of the LAD distal to the lesion. Most LAD grafts are entered with a left venous bypass, JR4, or Amplatz guide. The exchange wire is helpful to allow upsizing the balloon, if necessary. It is also helpful to have an over-the-wire system in case the wire needs to be removed and the tip reshaped to cross this lesion. If PTCA is successful, I would stop heparin and continue aspirin.

Donald Baim, MD, USA: Using a 9F JR 4 guiding catheter for optimal visualization, I would place an ACS 0.014-inch Extra-Support guidewire in the distal LAD, and predilate this lesion with a 3.0 mm high-pressure balloon (SciMed NC Bandit or ACS Endura). I would advance a 3.0 mm Palmaz-Schatz coronary stent so the distal portion of the stent is in the native LAD, and the articulation is just proximal to the stenosis. I would dilate the entire stent at high pressure, using the same 3.0 mm balloon. If results are anything but perfect, I would use low-dose

Coumadin (INR ~ 2), aspirin, and ticlopidine.

Masakiyo Nobuyoshi, MD, Japan: The native LAD is 3.0 mm and the vein graft is 4.1 mm in diameter. Accordingly, the initial balloon should be 3.0-3.5 x 20 mm at 8-10 ATM. If the anastomotic site cannot be adequately dilated, I would implant a 4.0 x 20 mm Gianturco-Roubin stent and postdilate at 15 ATM. A 9F JR4 or Cook 8F large-lumen guide (ID = 0.086-inch) is adequate, and I recommend a flexible 0.014-inch x 300 cm guidewire. After implantation of the stent, I would evaluate its full expansion by ultrasound; no additional PTCA is necessary if it is fully expanded. If stenosis persists, additional expansion with a high-pressure noncompliant balloon is necessary. Heparin (10,000-15,000 units/day) is recommend for 3-5 days, and Coumadin and aspirin (81 mg TID) should be continued for 1-3 months.

Describe how you deal with the problem of size-mismatch between the graft and native vessel.

Masakiyo Nobuyoshi, MD, Japan: The diameters of the vein graft and the native coronary artery are different, and therefore the proper size balloon and stent must be selected; a balloon too large for the native LAD may cause dissection. For this case, the proper size balloon is 3.0-3.5 mm.

Donald Baim, MD, USA: It is important to taper the stent to match the 4 mm saphenous vein graft. I would dilate the proximal half of this stent with a 4 mm high pressure balloon, taking care not to allow it to extend into the native LAD. Correctly deployed and postdilated, this stent will have a funnel-like configuration.

What other technical problems might be anticipated?

Spencer King III, MD, USA: Difficulties arise if the vein graft arises with a very superior takeoff; Amplatz guides are useful to achieve good backup and coaxial alignment. Wire manipulation may be aided by placing the balloon into the vein graft just proximal to the lesion, so that the wire can be reshaped to successfully cross the lesion. Caution should be taken not to overinflate this lesion if high pressures are required; rarely this type of lesion can be created by a distal suture problem (I have never seen one ten years out). If pressures exceed 12-14 ATM, I would not inflate at higher pressure, for fear of disrupting the suture line.

<u>Editors' Perspective</u>: The ideal treatment of lesions involving the distal anastomosis is controversial. Important issues to consider include the tortuosity of the vessel proximal and distal to the target lesion, the diameter of the "normal" vessel proximal and distal to the target lesion, the degree of size mismatch between the distal vein graft and native vessel, and the angle of insertion of the vein graft into the native vessel. Anatomic factors favoring PTCA include greater degrees of tortuosity, angulation, and size mismatch. Although it is possible to "mold" balloon-expandable stents, this can be technically challenging, and should be reserved for experienced stent operators. This patient was treated by conventional PTCA with a satisfactory result (30% residual stenosis; see below), and no further intervention has been required for almost 3 years.

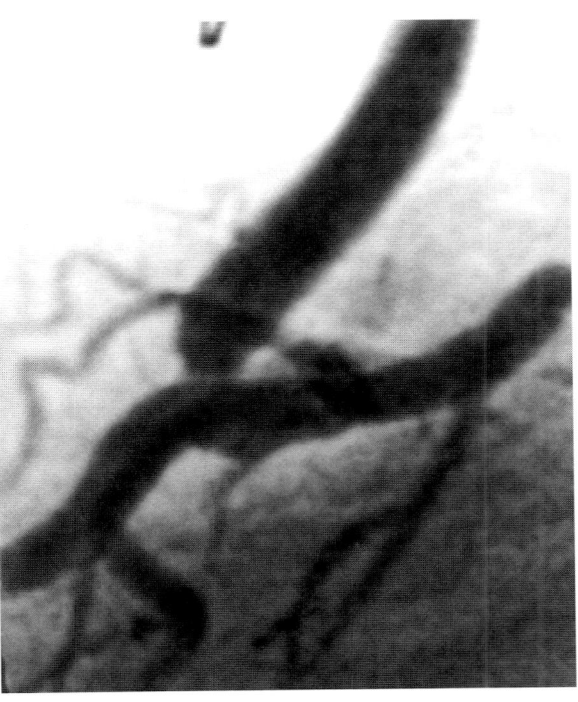

*****

VEIN GRAFT: LARGE THROMBUS

A 70-year-old man with a history of coronary bypass surgery 8 years ago develops stuttering angina and anterior T-wave changes. Coronary angiography reveals a severe stenosis (closed arrowhead) in the vein graft to the LAD (reference vessel diameter = 4.6 mm) with a large intraluminal filling defect (open arrowhead). Other grafts are patent, and left ventricular ejection fraction = 40%.

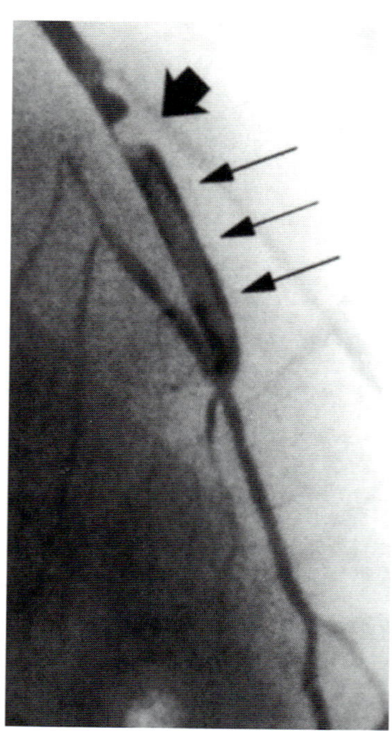

What are your therapeutic options for this patient?

Frank Litvack, MD, USA: This patient represents a difficult therapeutic dilemma. He presents with an unstable ischemic syndrome and an 8-year-old bypass graft with a large burden of angiographic thrombus in the mid- and distal graft. This presents a situation where intervention is associated with a high likelihood of distal embolization and graft thrombosis. Several therapeutic options are possible and include repeat coronary bypass surgery, immediate PTCA, stent placement, and/or thrombolysis. If the patient has significant disease in other vein grafts, I recommend repeat bypass surgery using 2 internal mammary grafts, since this will provide life-long relief. If, on the other hand, this is the only significant problem, I would proceed with cautious intervention.

Antonio Colombo, MD, Italy: There is a large thrombus in this vein graft to the LAD. Due to the age of this graft, the location, and the high risk of distal embolization and myocardial infarction, I would obtain a surgical opinion prior to any intervention. If possible, I recommend redo surgery with arterial revascularization, instead of percutaneous intervention.

Ian Penn, MD, Canada: This patient presents with a vein graft stenosis with a large intraluminal thrombus. The presence of intraluminal thrombus in the vein graft is predictive of poor early and late events, a higher incidence of acute closure and no-reflow, and significant risk of myocardial infarction, cardiogenic shock and death. I recommend repeat CABG.

Assuming that percutaneous intervention is reasonable, what would you recommend?

Frank Litvack, MD, USA: I am not a fan of intragraft urokinase in this setting. If the patient is stable at the time of the procedure, I favor returning him to the Coronary Care Unit and maintaining him on intravenous heparin and aspirin. I would then bring him back to the Cardiac Catheterization Laboratory after several days, with the intent of performing stent placement. Prior to stenting, I would administer intravenous ReoPro to disable the platelets as much as possible. I would pretreat the patient with aspirin (650 mg QD), 2-3 days of ticlopidine (250 mg BID), and Prilosec. Several days of anticoagulation often yields a far better angiographic substrate upon which to perform intervention. Though many operators infuse urokinase in this situation, I would only use it if the thrombus is obstructive, since urokinase itself is prothrombotic.

Antonio Colombo, MD, Italy: Local infusion of urokinase (100,000 units/hr) is possible. Subsequently, Palmaz-Schatz stent or Wallstent implantation should be performed. The decision concerning which type of stent and how many stents will depend on the morphology of the stenosis after urokinase infusion. The use of TEC (without urokinase) followed by stenting is another option.

Ian Penn, MD, Canada: I am very cautious in pre-procedural management of patients with vein grafts and filling defects. I recommend thrombolytic therapy for 12-24 hours before intervention.

Describe your technical approach.

Frank Litvack, MD, USA: I would predilate the lesion with a 3.5 mm balloon over a 0.014-inch Extra-Support wire beginning in the distal portion of the graft, and work proximally. Following PTCA, I would place multiple 4.0 mm Palmaz-Schatz stents. (It is possible that following several days of Heparin therapy, the thrombus will be significantly "cleaned up" and distal stenting may not be necessary.) I would then dilate the stents with a 4.5 mm Total Cross or Schwarten balloon at 8-10 ATM.

Ian Penn, MD, Canada: During the diagnostic angiogram, I would place a Tracker catheter into the LAD graft and instill tPA (50 mg over 45 minutes), forming a well of tPA within the graft. Heparin would be administered with a bolus and infusion to maintain the PTT 70-90 seconds, and the patient would return to the cath lab the following day. Using an AL1 or AL2 guiding catheter and a 0.014-inch wire in the LAD, PTCA would be performed with a single inflation of a 5.0 mm balloon at 4 ATM. A PS204 Palmaz-Schatz biliary stent would be placed on this balloon, deployed in the graft, and postdilated at high pressure. Having obtained an optimal result, I would discharge the patient on aspirin and ticlopidine for one month. If the patient has persistent thrombus despite urokinase infusion, I recommend redo bypass surgery.

Antonio Colombo, MD, Italy: If significant filling defect persists after urokinase infusion, it is likely due to degenerated atherosclerotic material. I would predilate the lesion with a 3.5 mm balloon (or larger, if necessary), and deploy a Wallstent. I would select a stent which is 1 mm larger than the normal vein graft, and postdilate with a 4.5 or 5.0 mm balloon.

What problems do you anticipate?

Frank Litvack, MD, USA: There is a significant chance that distal embolization will occur and I would be prepared to enter the native LAD to break up any embolic clots.

Antonio Colombo, MD, Italy: The risk of distal embolization is high, and it may occur during any phase of revascularization, including during urokinase infusion, predilation, stent deployment, or postdilation. If distal embolization occurs, I would have a low threshold for inserting an intraaortic balloon pump.

Editors' Perspective: The presence of a large thrombus in an otherwise "normal" vein graft represents a difficult therapeutic dilemma. Decision-making about such cases is simplified when other vein grafts are severely diseased, particularly when internal mammary artery grafting remains a viable option. However, redo CABG was not an option for this patient because there were no remaining venous conduits, and the internal mammary arteries were unsuitable as conduits during the original operation. This patient was treated in 1991 before widespread availability of intramural drug delivery devices and stents, and was entered into the original investigational study of TEC atherectomy prior to marketing approval. Several days of intravenous heparin failed to improve the angiographic appearance of the vein graft prior to intervention. TEC was performed with a 7.5F cutter, resulting in considerable thrombus extraction (below) but focal cutoff of the apical portion of the LAD due to distal embolization. Unfortunately, subsequent PTCA resulted in no-reflow (TIMI flow = 1), which improved but did not resolve after administration of intracoronary urokinase and verapamil. After an overnight infusion of heparin, repeat angiography revealed a widely patent graft and distal vessel (next page). Several months later the vein graft was totally occluded.

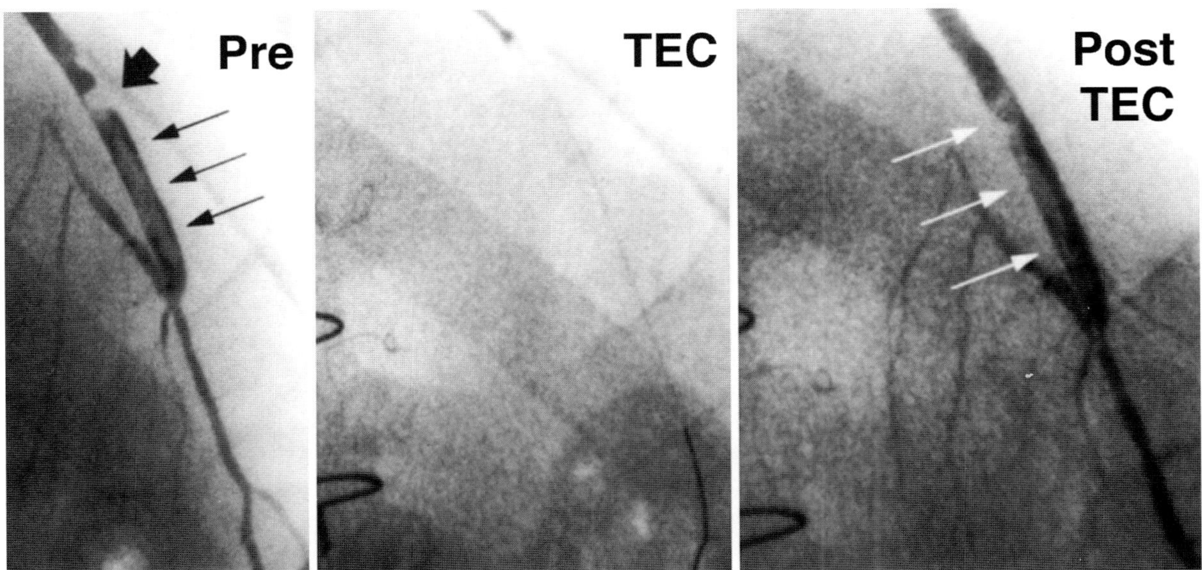

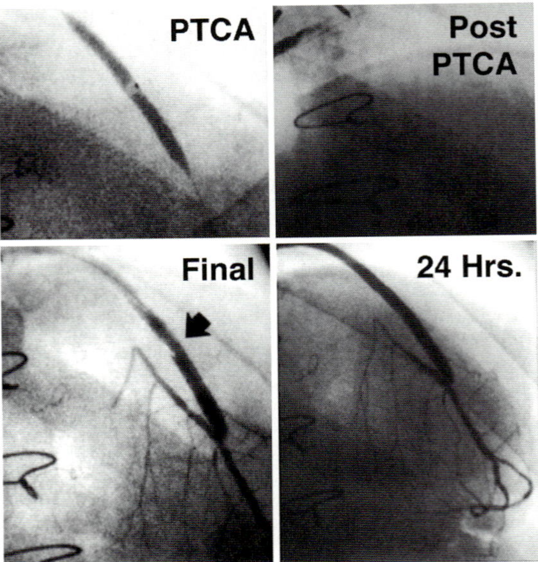

In contemporary interventional practice, there are still no ideal percutaneous approaches for this type of lesion. If CABG is not a good option, our approach to thrombotic vein graft lesions is TEC atherectomy and 2-4 weeks of oral Coumadin (INR ~ 2) or subcutaneous heparin (5000-10,000 units SQ BID) or Lovenox (20-30 mg BID), followed by stent implantation (without predilation) using Palmaz-Schatz coronary stents, Palmaz biliary stents, or Wallstents, depending on the vessel caliber and original lesion length. We avoid immediate stenting (to minimize the risk of distal embolization and no-reflow) unless a high-grade residual stenosis or severe dissection persist after TEC. Wallstents are particularly nice for long lesions, because they minimize multiple entries into the body of the vein graft (thereby minimizing the risk of distal embolization). A potentially useful adjunct for thrombotic vein grafts is the Possis AngioJet, which is currently under investigation in a randomized trial versus an intracoronary infusion of urokinase. Our initial experience with the AngioJet is extremely favorable; if supported by additional data, the AngioJet may become the treatment of choice for thrombotic lesions.

*****

VEIN GRAFT: ULCERATED LESION

A 55-year-old engineer develops progressive angina 5 years after bypass surgery. Coronary angiography demonstrates normal left ventricular function and a high-grade, ulcerated lesion in the mid-body of the vein graft to the PDA (reference vessel = 4.4 mm), and mild proximal tapering (straight arrows). All other grafts are patent.

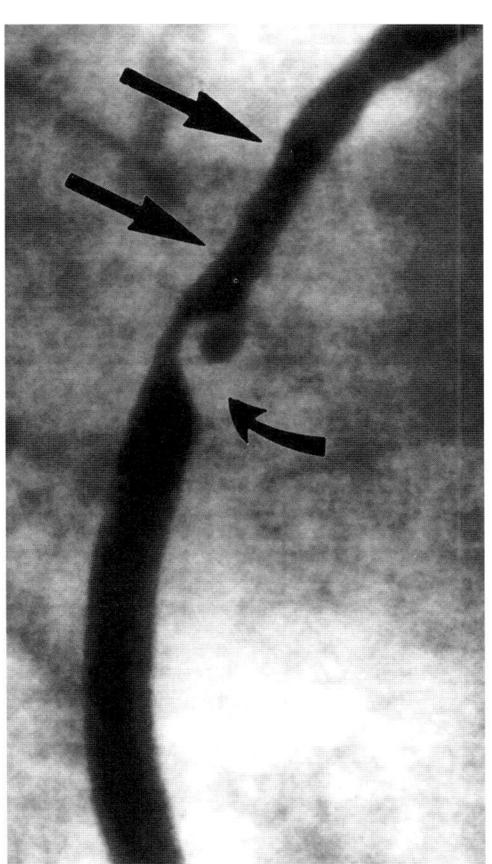

What is your assessment of this lesion?

Bernhard Meier, MD, Switzerland: The patient suffers from angina due to a discrete stenosis in a 5 year old bypass graft to the PDA. The lesion may be caused by plaque originating from a venous valve or by plaque that has partially separated from the graft wall.

John Douglas Jr., MD, USA: The patient has a focal, bulky stenosis with ulceration and a long 20-25% tubular stenosis in the saphenous vein graft to the PDA. There are no excellent options.

What percutaneous approach would you recommend?

Bernhard Meier, MD, Switzerland: I recommend an 8 mm Palmaz-Schatz stent or a 5.5 mm Wallstent without predilation. The stent should cover the entire lesion and should be postdilated with a 4.5 mm balloon.

John Douglas Jr., MD, USA: Since I do not have a long Wallstent, the interventional options narrow to multiple Palmaz-Schatz stents, directional atherectomy, or PTCA.

Gary Roubin, MD, PhD, USA: I would start this case with a 7.5F TEC cutter to debride the surface of this lesion as aggressively as possible prior to additional therapy. Multiple slow passes with a TEC catheter may not make a large difference in the appearance of the lesion, but in my experience allows further therapy with less distal embolization. I would then proceed with the biliary stent placement.

Describe your technique.

Bernhard Meier, MD, Switzerland: I would use an 8F multipurpose guiding catheter, implant a 5.5 mm Wallstent, and postdilate with a 4.5 mm balloon. The mildly diseased segment proximal to the lesion would not be treated. If a good angiographic result is achieved, no heparin is needed after intervention, and the patient would be discharged the next day on aspirin with or without ticlopidine.

John Douglas Jr., MD, USA: Prior to intervention, intracoronary verapamil or diltiazem would be given over 3 minutes to prevent microvascular spasm and no-reflow. I would then implant a 4.0 mm Palmaz-Schatz coronary stent (without predilation), and postdilate with a 5.0 mm Total

Cross at 15 ATM.

Gary Roubin, MD, PhD, USA: After treating the lesion with a 7.5F TEC cutter, I would remove the 10F TEC guiding catheter and replace it with a Cook 8F Lumax multipurpose guiding catheter. I find that stents of all types track better through Cook guides than through the TEC guide. There is usually no problem in re-crossing such a lesion with a guide wire. I would place an extra-support wire, either a Platinum-Plus or a Cook 0.014-0.018-inch Roadrunner, and implant a P154 Palmaz biliary stent on a 5.0 mm Total Cross (Schneider) or Power-Flex balloon (Cordis). Before placing the biliary stent on the balloon, I would inflate the balloon to allow better crimping of the stent. In placing the stent with the Total Cross or Power-Flex, I would deploy the stent cautiously to make sure that the stent is fully apposed to the wall of the graft without necessarily using high inflation pressures. Step-wise increases in inflation pressures are prudent. Following a satisfactory result, I would treat the patient with aspirin (325 mg BID) and ticlopidine (250 mg BID) for four weeks.

What complications do you anticipate?

Bernhard Meier, MD, Switzerland: The risk of significant distal embolization is small in light of the large base of the plaque.

John Douglas Jr., MD, USA: Any intervention will probably result in some distal embolization, a high cardiac event rate within 6-months, and high restenosis rates.

Gary Roubin, MD, PhD, USA: If there is distal embolization, I would treat liberally with nitroglycerin, diltiazem or verapamil. If initial TEC causes distal embolization, I would treat the patient with heparin and defer stenting for twenty-four hours.

Editors' Perspective: Complex, focal lesions in vein grafts are best treated with techniques other than PTCA, to improve immediate lumen enlargement and decrease complications and restenosis. Directional atherectomy and stenting can achieve similar degrees of lumen enlargement, but we generally favor stenting such lesions because of the lower risk of distal embolization and more predictable lumen enlargement (at least in our hands). Issues about debulking are unresolved: Many operators recommend TEC to decrease the risk of embolization, while others do not. We usually stent these lesions without TEC, but further studies are in progress to assess the relative value of TEC and PTCA as adjuncts to stenting in vein grafts (TEC-BEST). The best stent for these lesions is unknown; a randomized trial of the Wallstent versus the Palmaz-Schatz coronary stent is now in progress (WINS). This patient was treated with a Palmaz-Schatz stent by Dr. Marty Leon, with an excellent angiographic result (below).

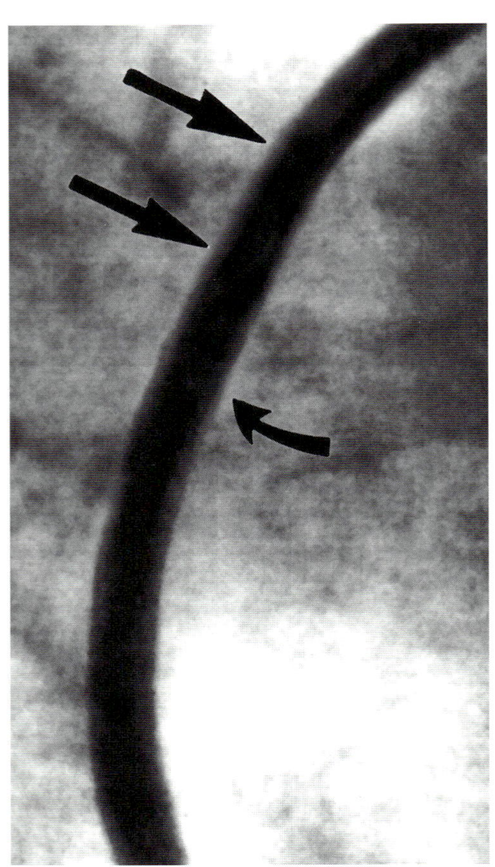

*****

— Section 2 —

Device-Specific Techniques

Directional Atherectomy Techniques

DCA: ECCENTRIC LESION (LAD)

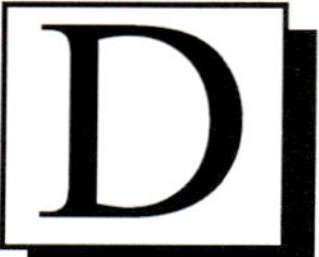
Directional atherectomy of an eccentric lesion in the proximal LAD (reference diameter = 3.4 mm)

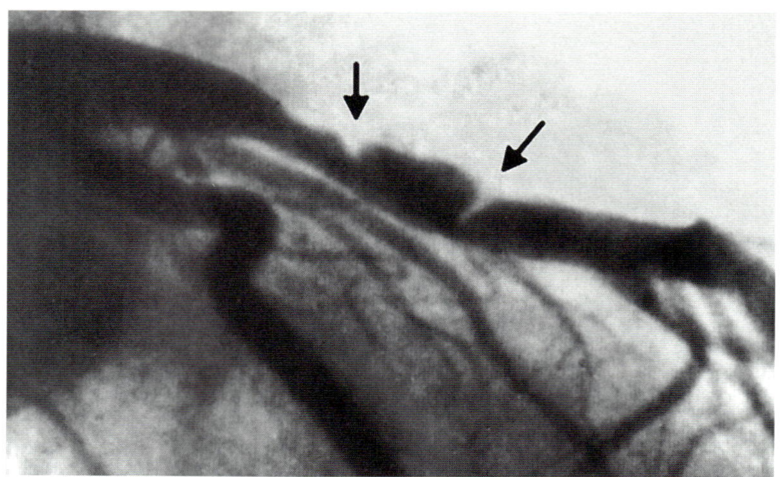

Is directional atherectomy reasonable for this lesion?

David Holmes, MD, USA: Directional atherectomy can be used to treat this lesion, but it is relatively long.

Spencer King III, MD, USA: The LAD lesion is a long lesion with two discrete, very eccentric stenoses. Directional coronary atherectomy is a reasonable way to approach this lesion.

David Foley, MD, The Netherlands: In spite of the focal severity at two points, the entire LAD appears diseased. Although atherectomy can be performed, it is unlikely to be definitive; adjunctive PTCA will be necessary.

Marty Leon, MD, USA: This complex lesion is reasonably approached by directional atherectomy. Although lesion length is a predictor of restenosis and complications with directional atherectomy, the straight appearance and large caliber of the LAD favor a directional atherectomy approach.

Comment on device sizing and important technical tips.

David Holmes, MD, USA: I would use a 7F EX device and perform longitudinal cuts with the AtheroCath oriented superiorly. The vessel appears straight, so guide catheter support will not be an issue. Following atherectomy, I would perform adjunctive PTCA.

Spencer King III, MD, USA: Prior to atherectomy, I would examine this artery with IVUS. If calcification is superficial and involves an arc >180°, I would not perform directional atherectomy. If calcification is deep or the arc is < 180°, I would proceed with directional atherectomy using a DVI guide and a Platinum-Plus or other extra-support wire. I would perform most cuts from the superior surface, but cuts in the proximal vessel would also be taken inferiorly. This is a long lesion and multiple passes will be necessary for adequate tissue removal. I would attempt to achieve a residual stenosis < 10% with or without adjunctive PTCA.

David Foley, MD, The Netherlands: I would perform intravascular ultrasound with motorized pullback to interrogate this vessel for calcium, extent of disease, and true vessel diameter. I would proceed with directional atherectomy using a 7F device and orient my cuts circumferentially. I would perform 8-10 cuts distally and 10-15 cuts proximally, and then repeat quantitative angiography and intravascular ultrasound to optimize the results. I would attempt to achieve an area stenosis < 50% and a diameter stenosis < 20% after atherectomy, followed by adjunctive PTCA with a 3.5 mm compliant balloon at 12 ATM (hoping to achieve a maximal balloon diameter of 3.75-3.8 mm).

Marty Leon, MD, USA: I would perform intravascular ultrasound prior to atherectomy to assess lesion eccentricity, true vessel size, plaque burden in the reference vessel, and lesion length. I would use a 0.014-inch x 300 cm extra-support wire and a DVI 10F guiding catheter; predilation is not necessary. I would begin with a 7F GTO device at low pressure and perform radial cuts, avoiding the inferior margin of the LAD. I would increase pressure to 30 PSI to remove as much tissue as possible. If there is significant residual stenosis after atherectomy, I would not hesitate to use a 7F graft cutter and adjunctive PTCA with a 4.0 mm balloon at low pressure. My goal is to achieve 0% residual stenosis at all sites.

Editors' Perspective: Directional atherectomy of eccentric lesions in large caliber vessels frequently leads to excellent angiographic results. Although earlier randomized trials of directional atherectomy vs. PTCA (CAVEAT and CCAT) did not demonstrate a restenosis advantage for directional atherectomy, patients with highly eccentric lesions were often excluded (since they were not felt to be suitable for PTCA), and contemporary principles of "optimal atherectomy" were not employed. More recent studies (BOAT and OARS) suggest that "stent-like" results can be achieved with optimal atherectomy techniques as follows: First, select an atherectomy device according to the guidelines in Table 36.

Although these sizing recommendations do not conform to those listed in the package insert, they will allow for better lumen enlargement. Second, select an angiographic projection that best displays the eccentricity of the target lesion; spending a little extra time to obtain the ideal view will simplify orientation of the AtheroCath and assessment of results. Third, direct the initial atherectomy cuts toward angiographically-apparent plaque to minimize cutting into normal vessel wall. Since the cutting window allows radial cuts of 120°, it is usually best to rotate the cutting window by 60-90° on either side of the initial cut to ensure plaque excision along the eccentric surface. Fourth, assess the angiographic result in multiple projections to ensure adequate removal of eccentric plaque. Finally, do not hesitate to use adjunctive PTCA (balloon/artery ratio ~ 1.0-1.1) at low pressure (1-4 ATM) to smoothe and enlarge the lumen.

Table 36. Recommendations for DCA Sizing and Normal Vessel Diameter

Size (F)	Vessel diameter (mm)*	Vessel diameter (mm) Practical **
5F	2.5-2.9	≤ 2.5
6F	3.0-3.4	2.5-3.0
7F	3.5-3.9	3.0-3.5
7FG	≥ 4.0	3.5-4.0

Abbreviations: F = French size; G = graft cutter

* These guidelines are based on the product label; recommended by the FDA

** These guidelines are not approved by the FDA, but may allow for more "optimal atherectomy"

This patient was treated by Dr. Gregory Robertson using a 7F AtheroCath without adjunctive PTCA. Final angiography (below) shows no significant residual stenosis and a smooth lumen.

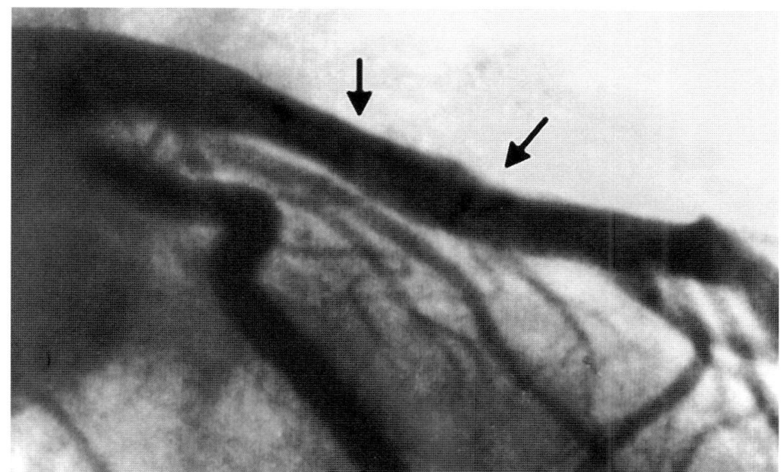

*****

DCA: ECCENTRIC LESION (RCA)

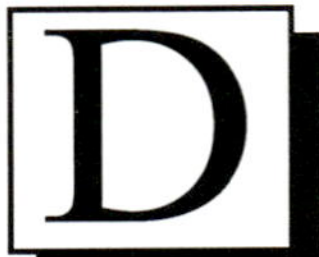

Directional atherectomy of an eccentric lesion in the mid-RCA (reference diameter = 3.2 mm)

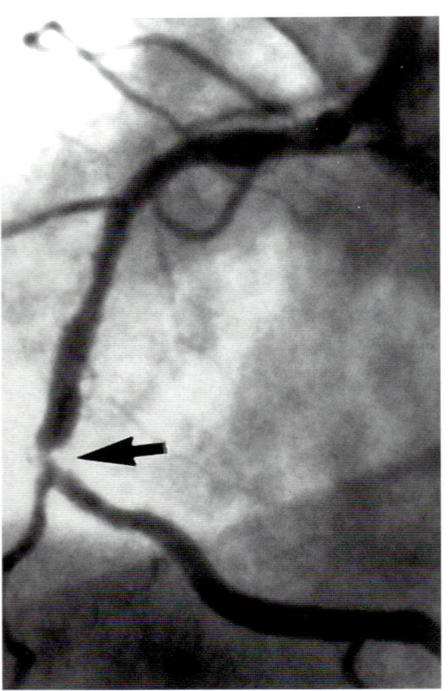

Is directional atherectomy reasonable for this lesion?

David Holmes, MD, USA: This is an angulated, rather diffusely diseased RCA with an eccentric stenosis in its mid-portion. The problems here are diffuse disease and significant angulation. Directional atherectomy is not my first choice for this lesion.

Spencer King III, MD, USA: This RCA lesion is located just before an acute marginal branch and is associated with diffuse disease. I would not choose directional atherectomy for this lesion, since there is significant disease proximal and distal to the severe stenosis.

David Foley, MD, The Netherlands: Directional atherectomy seems reasonable if one concentrates on the focal lesion at the bend. However, the angiogram reveals diffuse disease in the mid and distal RCA.

Marty Leon, MD, USA: This is an interesting eccentric stenosis on a moderate bend. Angulated lesions present special problems for all devices because of a higher risk of dissection, abrupt closure, and major clinical complications. In this case, directional atherectomy is possible, but is not my first choice because of the risk of acute angiographic complications.

Comment on device sizing and important technical tips.

David Foley, MD, The Netherlands: Intravascular ultrasound will be extremely helpful in revealing the true extent of disease. To keep my options open, I would cross the lesion with a 0.014-inch x 300 cm wire to retain the options of directional atherectomy (for focal disease) or Wallstent (for extensive disease). I recommend a 5.0 x 27 mm or a 5.0 x 39 mm Wallstent, and postdilation with a 4.0 mm balloon.

Marty Leon, MD, USA: If directional atherectomy is used, I would begin with a DVI 9.5F short-tip JR4 or a Medtronic 10F JR4 guide and an Extra-Support guidewire to straighten the vessel. I would initially undersize the device, using a 6F GTO or a 7F short-window AtheroCath. I would perform careful cuts at low pressure, with subsequent assessment of angiographic and ultrasound results. I would consider using a 7F GTO device to achieve more optimal tissue removal if there are no complications, followed by adjunctive PTCA with a 3.0-3.5 x 30-40 mm balloon at low pressure. Under these circumstances, I would be willing be accept a "less than perfect" result given the bend in the vessel.

Editors' Perspective: The challenge in treating such a lesion with directional atherectomy is knowing where to begin and where to stop taking cuts, given the proximal and distal disease. Despite the eccentricity, this lesion should probably be treated with other techniques, given the presence of diffuse disease and angulation.

*****

DCA: ULCERATED LESION

Directional atherectomy of an ulcerated lesion in the mid-LAD (reference diameter = 3.2 mm).

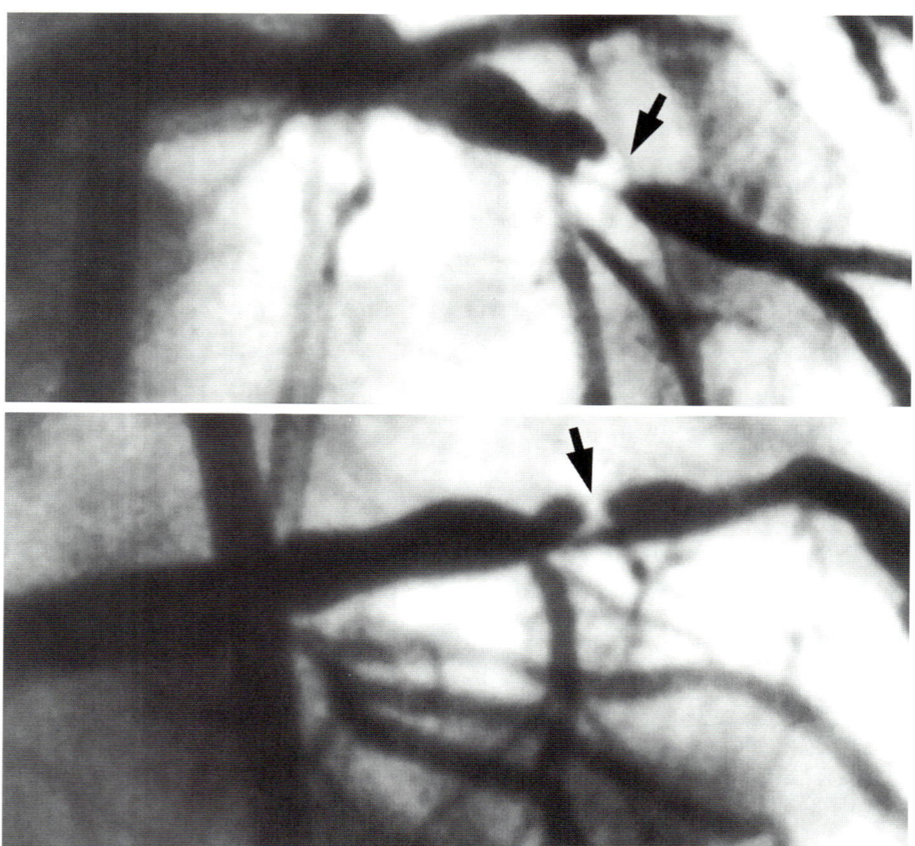

Is directional atherectomy reasonable for this lesion?

David Williams, MD, USA: This patient has a severe, eccentric, and ulcerated lesion in the mid-LAD on a straight segment. The diameter of the LAD is well suited for directional atherectomy. The angulation of the distal LAD is somewhat concerning in terms of potential nosecone injury, although it does not preclude directional atherectomy. The major advantage of directional atherectomy in this setting is selective debulking of plaque that would not respond well to PTCA.

Michael Cowley, MD, USA: There is high-grade eccentric, complex ulceration in the mid-LAD which is ideal for directional atherectomy.

Patrick Serruys, MD, PhD, The Netherlands: This ulcerated lesion in the mid-LAD could certainly be treated by directional atherectomy. However, there is further disease distal to the ulcerated area which may represent a limitation, or may also require treatment. The risk of atherectomy is distal embolization of plaque, which likely consists of a mixture of thrombus and lipid material.

Marty Leon, MD, USA: The lesion is markedly eccentric and ulcerated, with unusual morphologic characteristics and significant tapering. Directional atherectomy is a reasonable choice for this lesion.

Comment on device sizing and important technical tips.

David Williams, MD, USA: I would predilate this lesion, since the minimal lumen diameter is extremely small. I would advance a 7F AtheroCath across the lesion, directing the window superiorly toward the ulcer, making multiple cuts to achieve maximal debulking. Adjunctive imaging modalities are not required for directional atherectomy, but IVUS is helpful if a stent is required. ReoPro is reasonable to reduce the risk of CK elevation.

Michael Cowley, MD, USA: I would perform directional atherectomy using a 7F GTO device, a 0.014-inch Extra-S'port wire, and a DVI 10F JL4 guide catheter. Because of the marked eccentricity of the lesion, I would concentrate cuts away from the inferior surface of the vessel (4-6 cuts at 10 PSI, then increase inflation pressure to 20 PSI, depending on the angiographic response). I would attempt to achieve a residual stenosis of 0-10% and smooth margins. Adjunctive PTCA would be done with a 3.5 mm semicompliant balloon at 1-2 ATM, if needed. Such lesions have uniformly good results with directional atherectomy, and the likelihood of restenosis is low if the final lumen diameter is > 3 mm.

Patrick Serruys, MD, PhD, The Netherlands: I would pretreat with aspirin, ticlopidine for 72 hours, and ReoPro for 12 hours immediately preceding atherectomy. I would proceed with a 7F device and perform 6-10 cuts directed superiorly, followed by IVUS to examine remaining plaque burden and the length of the disease, and assist in decisions regarding further atherectomy or adjunctive PTCA.

Marty Leon, MD, USA: If there is no fluoroscopic calcium, I would begin with a 7F GTO device, directing cuts superiorly at low pressure. If tissue specimens contain thrombus, I would initiate more aggressive treatment with ReoPro. I would use a 0.014-inch Extra-S'port guidewire and a conventional DVI JL4 guiding catheter. I would perform adjunctive PTCA with a slightly oversized perfusion balloon at extremely low pressures (≤ 2 ATM).

Editors' Perspective: The ulcerated lesion in this case could be readily treated with directional atherectomy, but the large plaque burden and moderate disease adjacent to the severe stenosis suggest that extensive atherectomy will be required. Several technical points deserve emphasis: First, a 7F cutter will certainly offer better debulking than a smaller cutter. Second, in the absence of fluoroscopic calcification, predilation will probably be unnecessary. Third, continuous device rotation and gentle forward pressure will facilitate delivery of the AtheroCath to the target lesion. Fourth, an exchange-length guidewire (300 cm) will facilitate exchanges, since multiple passes and adjunctive PTCA (or stenting) will likely be required. Finally, ReoPro may decrease the risk of complications and restenosis when administered according to the recommendations established in the EPILOG trial. Other off-label uses of ReoPro are exciting, but are not yet of proven benefit.

This patient was treated by Dr. Donald Baim using a 7F EX AtheroCath, a 0.014-inch x 300 cm Hi-torque floppy guidewire, and a DVI 11F JCL4 guiding catheter. The final angiogram (below) showed an excellent result, without adjunctive PTCA.

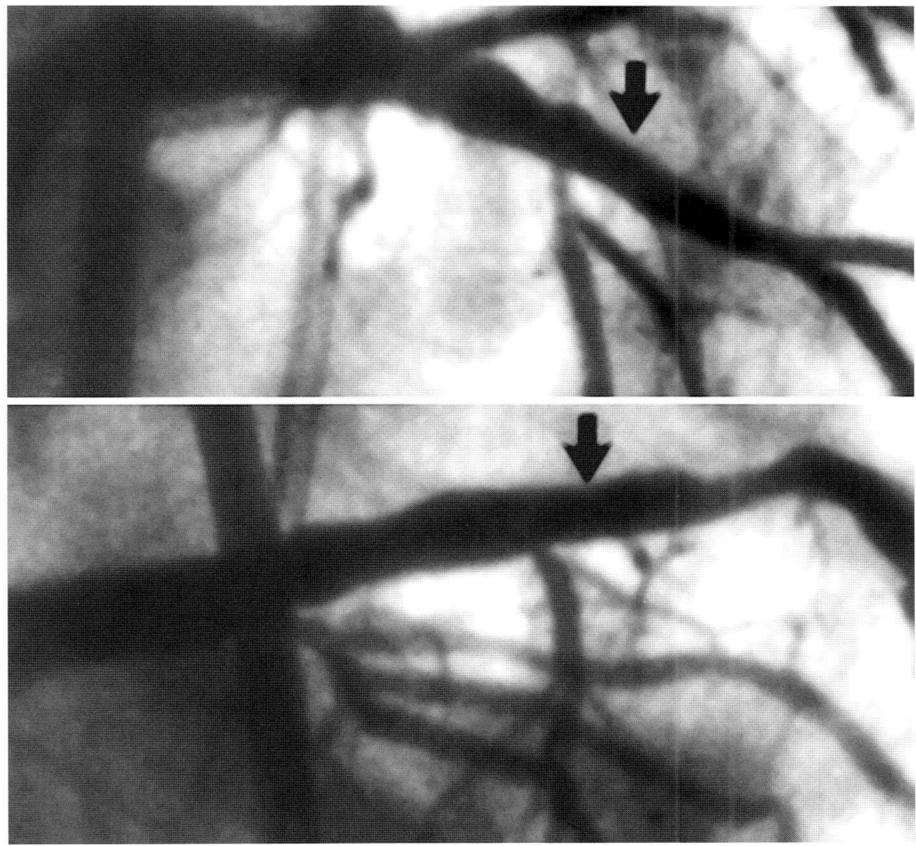

*****

DCA: TUBULAR LESION

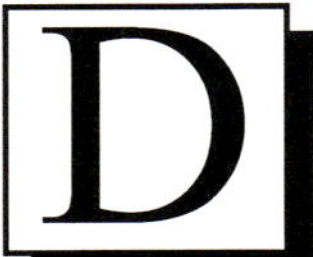irectional atherectomy of a tubular lesion in the mid-RCA (length = 15 mm; reference diameter = 2.5 mm).

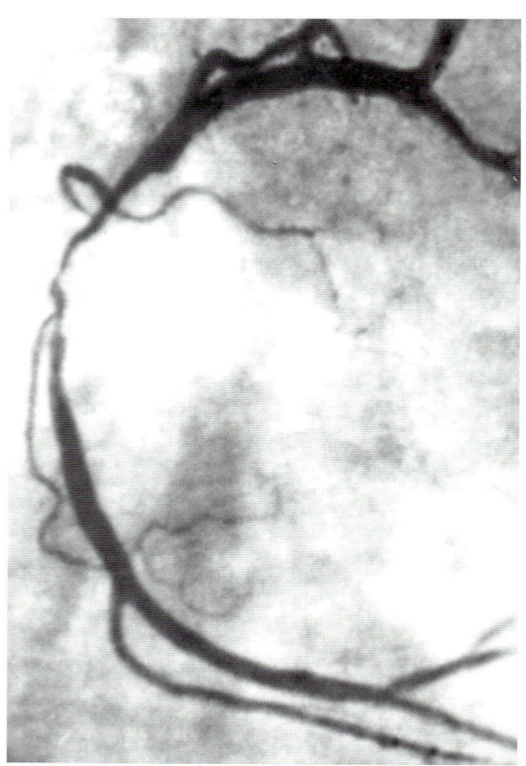

Is directional atherectomy reasonable for this lesion?

Spencer King III, MD, USA: This is a long lesion in the mid-RCA; I would not choose directional atherectomy.

Donald Baim, MD, USA: The stenosis is >20 mm in length, which I do not believe is well suited for directional atherectomy.

David Williams, MD, USA: Directional atherectomy is not a reasonable choice for the mid-RCA; it is simply not a good device for long lesions. An extensive amount of "dottering" would be necessary to advance the device through this lesion, resulting in excessive arterial trauma.

> **Editors' Perspective: The general consensus is that long lesions (> 20 mm) in small vessels (< 3 mm) are unsuitable for directional atherectomy. We agree that directional atherectomy offers no advantages over other techniques and may substantially increase the risk of complications.**

*****

DCA: LONG LESION

Directional atherectomy of a long lesion in the mid-LAD (length = 25 mm; reference diameter = 3.3 mm)

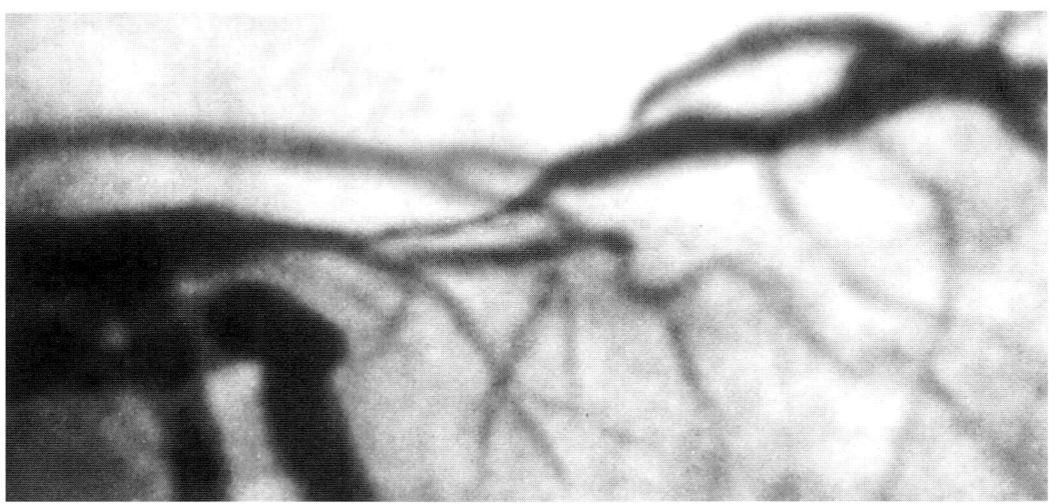

Is directional atherectomy reasonable for this lesion?

Spencer King III, MD, USA: This mid-LAD lesion is too long; I would not use directional atherectomy.

Donald Baim, MD, USA: The stenosis is too long for directional atherectomy.

David Williams, MD, USA: This lesion is not suitable for directional atherectomy because it is too long.

Editors' Perspective: Despite the large caliber of this vessel, the length of the lesion favors an approach using devices other than directional atherectomy. Although atherectomy could be performed, considerable time and effort would be required to adequately treat this lesion.

*****

DCA: FUNCTIONAL TOTAL OCCLUSION

Directional atherectomy of a functional total occlusion in the proximal LAD (reference diameter = 2.7 mm). Assume the occlusion can be crossed with a guidewire.

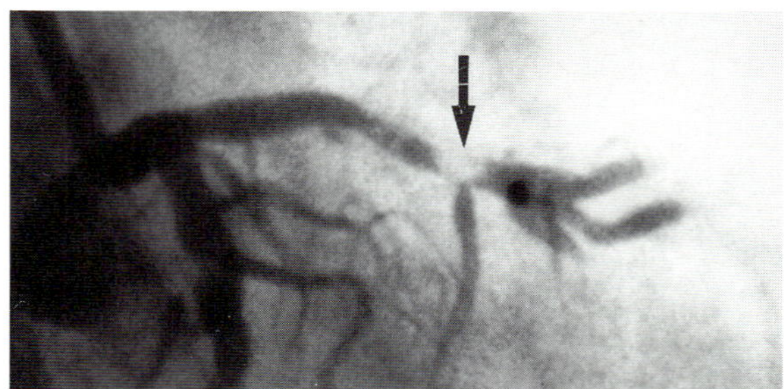

Is directional atherectomy reasonable for this lesion?

Michael Mooney, MD, USA: This lesion represents a functional total occlusion. Given the marked eccentricity, I recommend directional atherectomy.

David Holmes, MD, USA: I would not use directional atherectomy because I cannot determine the size of the distal vessel.

Spencer King III, MD, USA: Directional atherectomy is reasonable for this eccentric, focal lesion, even though additional atheroma must be removed 1 cm proximal to the target lesion. There is a question of intraluminal thrombus, but directional atherectomy is not precluded by this finding. However, if thrombus is present, I recommend ReoPro.

Comment on device sizing and important technical tips.

Michael Mooney, MD, USA: Although the measured reference vessel is 2.7 mm, it is likely that the reference segment itself is diseased. I would use a 7F GTO device, a 0.014-inch x 300 cm Extra-S'port wire, and a 10F JL4 guiding catheter. If the AtheroCath fails to cross the lesion, I would predilate with a 3.0 mm balloon at low pressure. The initial cuts would be taken in the RAO projection, directing the cutter towards the dominant portion of the stenosis. The lesion and the proximal segment must be treated for maximal results. Positioning the device may be challenging; freeze frames are useful to avoid errors in device position. I would perform adjunctive PTCA with a 3.5 x 30 mm balloon at 1-2 ATM for 1-2 minutes. If thrombus is present in the collection chamber, I recommend heparin, 1-2 months of Coumadin, and ReoPro.

Spencer King III, MD, USA: The reference size of 2.7 mm seems small in view of the caliber of the LCX and left main. I would use IVUS to assess calcium and vessel size. I would predilate with a 2.5 mm balloon if there is calcium. If the reference size is 3 mm (as I suspect), I would use a 7F cutter, a DVI guide, and an Extra-Support wire. I would perform multiple cuts from the superior and lateral surface, but not along the septal branch. Based on angiography and IVUS, adjunctive PTCA might be necessary.

Editors' Perspective: Directional atherectomy may be reasonable for this lesion. However, all three experts point out important limitations of directional atherectomy in this setting, including small vessel caliber, the potential for intraluminal thrombus, and the inability to identify the vessel size and morphology beyond the occlusion. These issues may be evaluated in several ways: First, other angiographic projections, on-line QCA, and IVUS can be used to help assess the "true" vessel diameter and lesion length. Second, if the occlusion can be crossed with a guidewire, successful "dottering" with a low-profile balloon or transfer catheter would allow contrast opacification of the distal vessel to assess its caliber, morphology, and extent of disease. Finally, the extent of thrombus can be assessed once there is better flow into the distal vessel. Although small amounts of thrombus do not preclude directional atherectomy, large bulky thrombus is a contraindication. Once the lesion and distal vessel are better defined, directional atherectomy (using "optimal" techniques) can be employed, if appropriate. This patient was treated by Dr. Gregory Pavlides, who chose PTCA over directional atherectomy because of uncertainties about the caliber of the distal vessel. Conventional PTCA was performed and was complicated by severe dissection; directional atherectomy (6F EX AtheroCath) was then used to resect the dissection flap and residual plaque, without further complications.

*****

DCA: TOTAL OCCLUSION

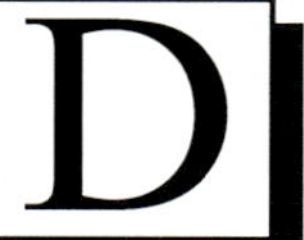

Directional atherectomy of a total occlusion in the proximal RCA (reference diameter = 4.5 mm). Assume the occlusion can be crossed with a guidewire.

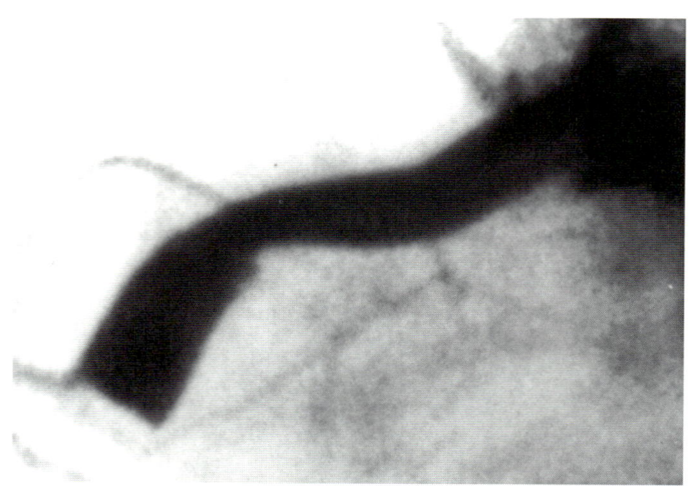

Is directional atherectomy reasonable for this lesion?

Michael Mooney, MD, USA: This proximal RCA has a total occlusion with a blunt cut off, most commonly associated with recent total occlusion. Since it is hard to assess the length of the occlusion and the relative amount of thrombus, directional atherectomy can have an adjunctive and/or rescue role, but I would not use it as primary therapy.

David Holmes, MD, USA: I do not think that directional atherectomy is useful since I cannot be sure of the morphology of the distal vessel and whether there is diffuse disease.

Spencer King III, MD, USA: This RCA has abrupt cutoff in its mid-portion, suggesting thrombotic occlusion. I would not choose directional atherectomy for this lesion.

Editors' Perspective: Directional atherectomy is probably not the primary means of revascularizing this lesion: First, the vessel caliber is extremely large, and it is unlikely that directional atherectomy alone could achieve an adequate angiographic result. Second, the morphology of the occlusion suggests recent thrombotic occlusion, and in a vessel this caliber, the amount of thrombus may be substantial. Third, the length of the occlusion and the caliber of the vessel distal to the target lesion are difficult to assess. On the other hand, directional atherectomy could be used to manage suboptimal results (elastic recoil, focal dissection flaps), if necessary.

*****

DCA: ANGULATED LESION (LAD)

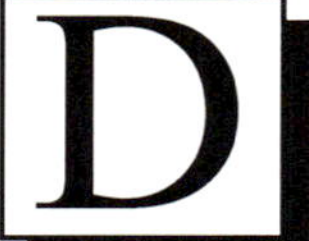irectional atherectomy of an angulated lesion in the proximal LAD (lesion on inner curve; reference diameter = 3.4 mm)

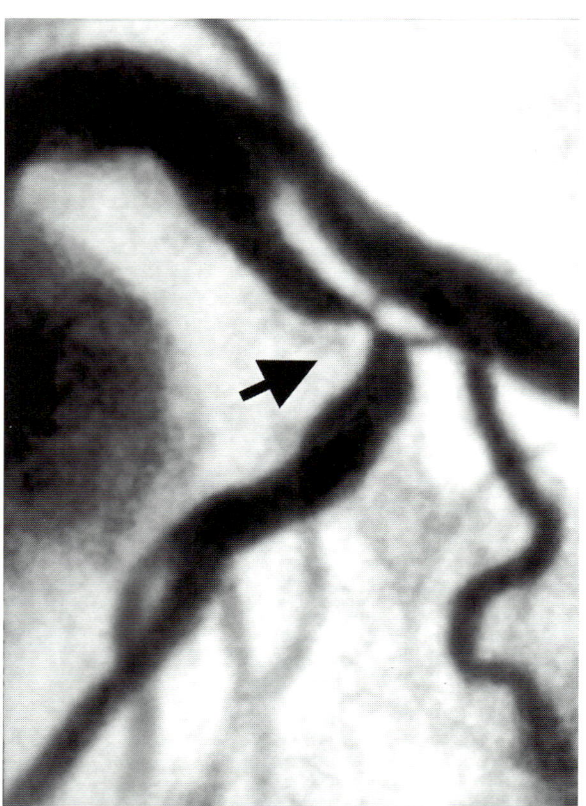

Is directional atherectomy reasonable for this lesion?

David Williams, MD, USA: The LAD lesion is certainly amenable to directional atherectomy. There is some angulation of the LAD, but it is likely foreshortened in this projection.

Michael Cowley, MD, USA: Directional atherectomy is a reasonable choice.

Michael Mooney, MD, USA: In the absence of heavy calcification, I would be quite comfortable with directional atherectomy.

Comment on device sizing and important tips.

David Williams, MD, USA: A 0.014-inch Extra-Support guidewire will help straighten the angulated segment and facilitate passage of a 7F AtheroCath. I would direct cuts toward the eccentric lesion. Adjunctive PTCA will probably be required.

Michael Cowley, MD, USA: With eccentric lesions in a bend, it is often difficult to determine how much of the apparent eccentricity is due to the bend. IVUS would be useful to determine the degree of eccentricity and help direct atherectomy cuts. Lesions of this type are frequently concentric, and circumferential cuts will usually be necessary to achieve optimal results. In the absence of IVUS, directional atherectomy for eccentric lesions in a bend may be associated with deep tissue resection and a more cautious strategy should be used. I recommend frequent angiography after each series of cuts, and slow increments in inflation pressure. I would use a 7F GTO device, a 0.014-inch Extra-Support wire, and a 10F JL4 guide. I would perform initial cuts at 10 PSI with gradual increases in pressure until an optimal result was achieved (with a 3.75 mm balloon, if necessary).

Michael Mooney, MD, USA: I would start with a 7F GTO device at low pressure, perform 20-30 cuts, and postdilate with a 3.5 x 30 mm balloon.

> **Editors' Perspective: In large caliber vessels, directional atherectomy can achieve excellent angiographic results. Optimal technique includes selection of the proper device size (which for this vessel is a 7F AtheroCath) and liberal use of adjunctive PTCA to smoothe the final result, if necessary. In large vessels without calcification, even moderate bends can be sufficiently straightened to facilitate directional atherectomy. A number of excellent guidewires are available to provide extra straightening force, including the ACS Extra-Support guidewire, the ACS S'port wire, the Cordis Stabilizer wire, the Cook Roadrunner wire, and the Meditech Platinum-Plus wire. The Platinum-Plus wire provides the most support, but is the least steerable, and its stiffness may induce coronary artery dissection. Continuous device rotation while advancing the AtheroCath across the lesion is crucial to safe and proper access of a moderately angulated lesion; advancing (without rotating) or jackhammering the AtheroCath through the lesion increases the risk of vessel injury and must be avoided.**

*****

DCA: ANGULATED LESION (RCA)

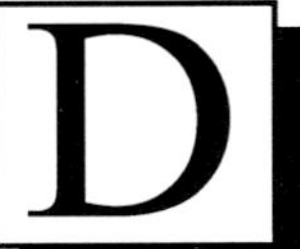

Directional atherectomy of an angulated lesion in the proximal RCA (lesion on outer curve; reference diameter = 3.1 mm).

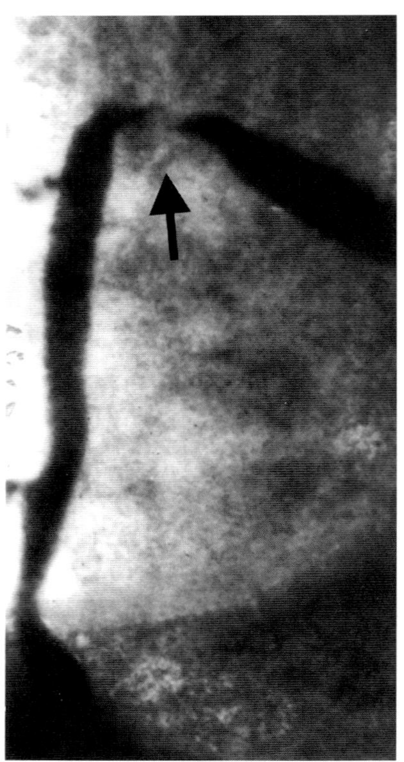

Is directional atherectomy reasonable for this lesion?

David Williams, MD, USA: The RCA lesion is just proximal to an acute angle and is not suitable for directional atherectomy, particulately if calcification is present.

Michael Cowley, MD, USA: Directional atherectomy is reasonable for this lesion, which is highly eccentric, complex, and has a filling defect consistent with thrombus. The lesion is just proximal to a 90° bend and disease extends up to the bend. The complex appearance favors directional atherectomy over other alternatives.

Michael Mooney, MD, USA: This lesion is in an angulated segment at the top of the shepherd's crook, and there is a small ulcer. The artery is moderately diffusely diseased. The shepherd's crook makes directional atherectomy more challenging, but not impossible.

Comment on device sizing and important technical tips.

Michael Cowley, MD, USA: The bend will straighten with the angioplasty guidewire, and directional atherectomy is feasible without predilation. If the proximal vessel is noncompliant (with persistence of the bend after advancing of the wire), predilation with a 2.0 mm balloon and use of a smaller AtheroCath (6F rather than 7F) might be preferable. For this lesion, I would select a 6F GTO device, a 0.014-inch x 300 cm Hi-torque floppy wire, and a DVI 9.5F JCR 4.0 short tip guide catheter. If the AtheroCath does not traverse the lesion, I would predilate with a 2.0 mm balloon. I would perform sequential cuts in the upper and adjacent quadrants at 10 PSI, and avoid cuts along the inferior wall. I would increase pressure to 20-30 PSI as needed, and postdilate with a 3.25 mm balloon at low pressure.

Michael Mooney, MD, USA: I would use a JR4 short tip guiding catheter, an Extra-Support wire, and a 7F short cut device. I would take 20-30 radial cuts throughout this area and postdilate with a 3.5 mm x 30 mm compliant balloon. If the short-cut device does not cross the stenosis, I would predilate with a 3.5 x 30 mm balloon at low pressure.

Editors' Perspective: Directional atherectomy is considered for this lesion because of its marked eccentricity. However, this degree of angulation increases the risk of failure (due to inability to access the target lesion with the AtheroCath) and complications (due to vascular injury from the nosecone or cutter). Useful considerations for increasing the chance of successful delivery of the AtheroCath include the use of extra-support or heavy-duty guidewires to straighten the vessel, the use of short-window devices, and predilation with a 2.0 mm balloon prior to atherectomy. To reduce complications, it may be best to initiate atherectomy with an undersized short-window device, orient initial cuts toward angiographically-apparent plaque, and use adjunctive PTCA (rather than larger AtheroCaths) to achieve greater lumen enlargement. Bolus plus infusion ReoPro is worthwhile to reduce complications and restenosis.

*****

DCA: LARGE THROMBUS

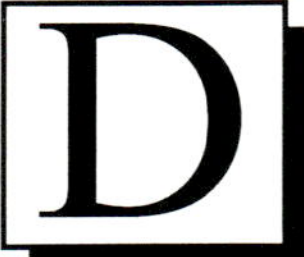

Directional atherectomy of a large thrombus in a degenerated vein graft (reference diameter = 5.2 mm).

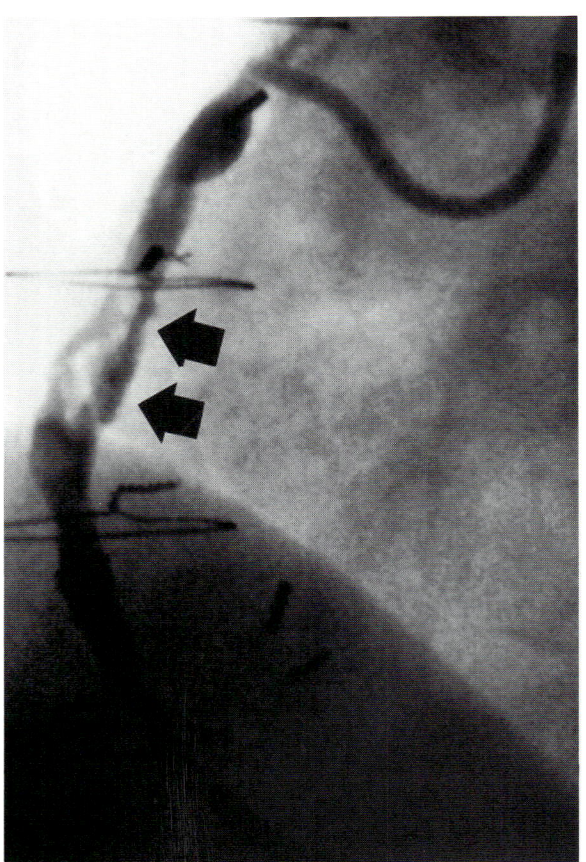

Is directional atherectomy reasonable for this lesion?

Donald Baim, MD, USA: I do not favor primary use of directional atherectomy in thrombus-containing lesions. The risk of distal embolization or no-reflow is unacceptably high.

Spencer King III, MD, USA: This is a large vein graft with bulky thrombus. I would not use directional atherectomy for this lesion because it would dramatically increase the risk of distal embolization.

David Holmes, MD, USA: I would not use directional atherectomy for this degenerated vein graft. The large caliber of the graft limits the degree of lumen enlargement even with the largest AtheroCath, and the large thrombus increases the risk of distal embolization and no-reflow.

> Editors' Perspective: **Although directional atherectomy is an effective tool for tissue removal, it may be associated with a higher risk of distal embolization and CK elevation compared to other devices. Particularly in settings where distal embolization is likely, such as this case, directional atherectomy is best avoided.**

*****

DCA: SMALL THROMBUS

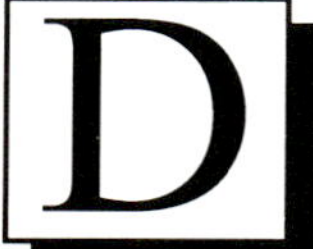irectional atherectomy of a small thrombus in the proximal RCA (reference diameter = 3.4 mm).

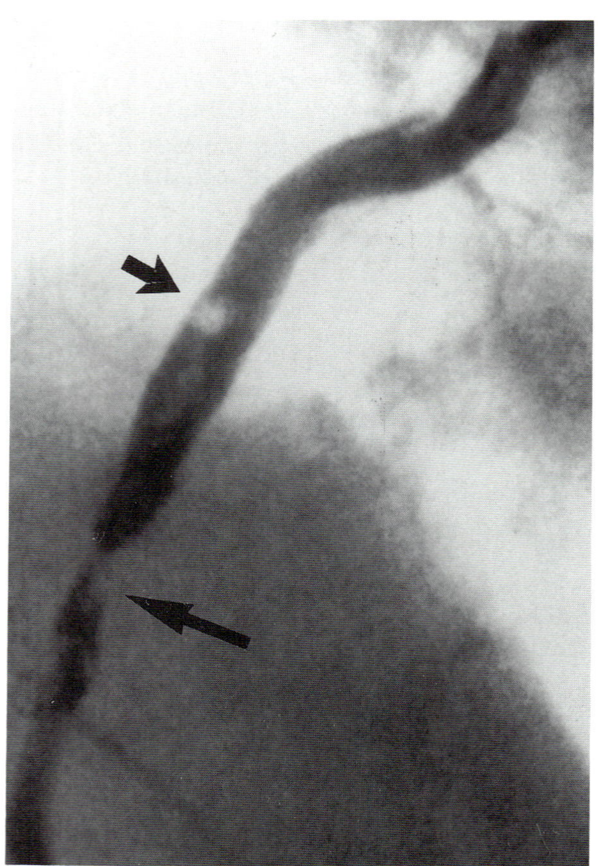

Is directional atherectomy reasonable for this lesion?

Donald Baim, MD, USA: I do not favor primary use of directional atherectomy in thrombus-containing lesions. The risk of distal embolization or "no-reflow" is unacceptably high. Thrombectomy with the Possis AngioJet is a good option for pretreatment, but is still investigational.

Spencer King III, MD, USA: The mid-RCA has a tight lesion with a small proximal thrombus. I would not perform directional atherectomy because of the risk of distal embolization.

David Holmes, MD, USA: Directional atherectomy is not indicated because of the presence of angiographic thrombus.

> Editors' Perspective: **While early studies suggested that directional atherectomy could be used to treat lesions with thrombus, contemporary data indicate that even small amounts of definite thrombus increase the risk of complications. If directional atherectomy is considered for this lesion, intravenous ReoPro is reasonable, to reduce acute ischemic complications and clinical restenosis.**

*****

DCA: TRIFURCATION LESION

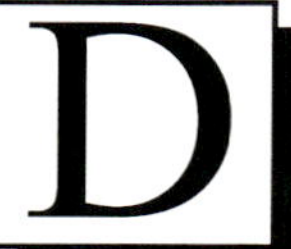
irectional atherectomy of a trifurcation lesion in the proximal LCX (reference diameter of the proximal LCX = 3.4 mm).

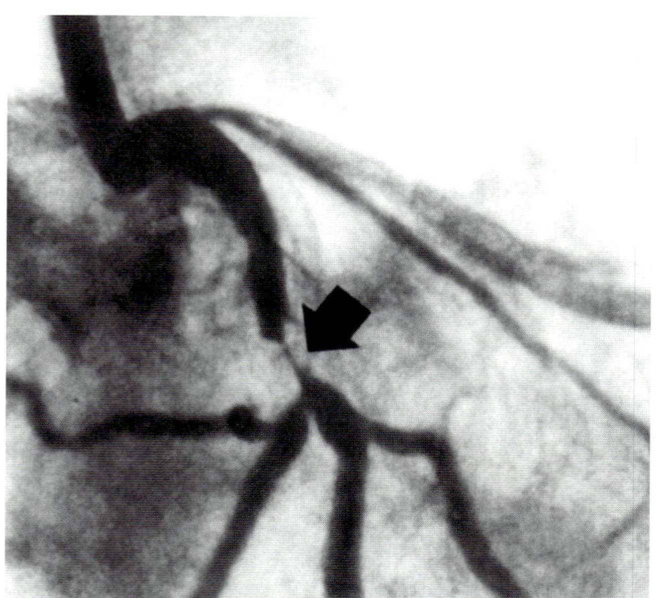

Is directional atherectomy reasonable for this lesion?

David Holmes, MD, USA: Directional atherectomy is very reasonable.

Michael Mooney, MD, USA: This proximal LCX trifurcation stenosis is most reasonably approached with directional atherectomy. The length of the lesion leading up to the trifurcation and the presence of ostial branch stenosis support this approach.

Donald Baim, MD, USA: The short left main makes device delivery relatively easy; directional atherectomy is reasonable.

Comment on device sizing and important technical tips.

David Holmes, MD, USA: I would position a wire in the middle of the trifurcation, through a conventional DVI left guide. I would take circumferential cuts first with a 6F and then with a 7F device. I would place the cutter in the middle branch since nosecone injury might occur if the cutter is placed in the first obtuse marginal. Following a 7F device, adjunctive PTCA is required.

Michael Mooney, MD, USA: I would attempt to pass an Extra-Support wire into the most superior branch and perform directional atherectomy with a 7F AtheroCath. I recommend predilation with a 3.5 x 30 mm balloon due to angulation and lesion length.

Donald Baim, MD, USA: I would place an Extra-Support guidewire in the middle of the three distal branches and use a 7F GTO device to resect the target lesion. I would follow with a 3.5 mm balloon at low pressure.

> **Editors' Perspective: This is a straightforward lesion for a variety of percutaneous interventions, including directional atherectomy. The short left main is especially favorable for directional atherectomy using an EX or GTO device. This patient was treated by Dr. Gregory Robertson using a 6F AtheroCath. An excellent angiographic result was achieved without adjunctive PTCA or IVUS.**

*****

DCA: BIFURCATION LESION

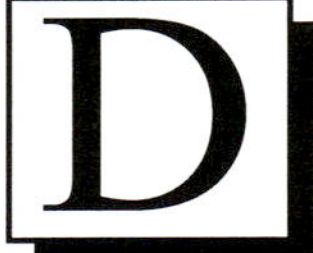

Directional atherectomy of a bifurcation lesion in the distal RCA (reference diameters: RCA = 3.6 mm; PDA= 2.7 mm; PLV = 2.2 mm).

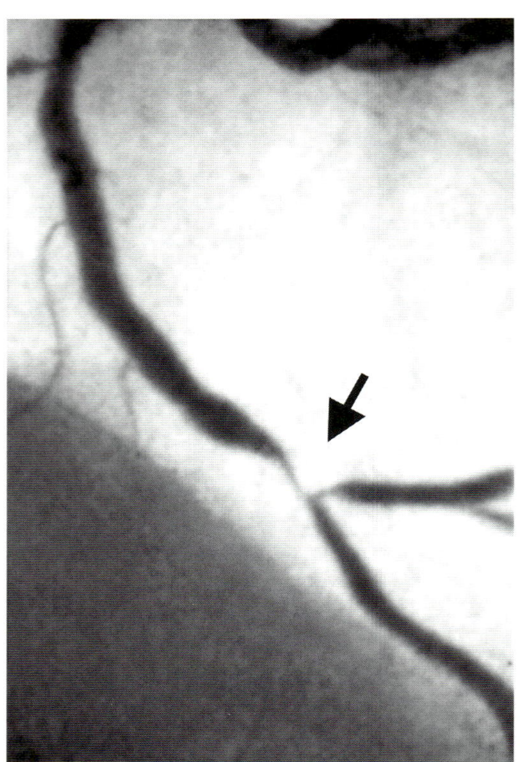

Is directional atherectomy reasonable for this lesion?

David Holmes, MD, USA: Directional atherectomy is an extremely good option for this vessel.

Michael Mooney, MD, USA: This case is ideal for directional coronary atherectomy, where the risk of posterolateral branch occlusion is significant after other devices.

Donald Baim, MD, USA: Directional atherectomy is the treatment of choice.

Comment on device sizing and important technical tips.

David Holmes, MD, USA: I would position a guidewire in the posterolateral segment, rather than in the PDA, and direct cuts superiorly and inferiorly. There appears to be some atheroma on the inferior surface of the vessel. A short cutter might be useful, but is not essential.

Michael Mooney, MD, USA: I would gently predilate the posterolateral branch with a 3.0 mm balloon, and then carry out sequential radial cuts with a 6F GTO device. I would then position the AtheroCath in the PDA and carry out cuts at 5-10 PSI. The posterolateral branch is likely to be significantly larger than 2.2 mm, so I would postdilate with a 3.0 mm compliant balloon.

Donald Baim, MD, USA: To avoid oversizing the distal vessels, I would use a 6F GTO or 7F EX cutter through a DVI 10F JR4 guide. I would perform initial cuts in the posterolateral branch to resect the bulk of the plaque. Even if there is compromise of the ostium of the large PDA, my experience suggests that it is usually fairly simple to gain wire access to such a branch following directional atherectomy. With the guidewire repositioned in the PDA, I would readvance the same AtheroCath and perform cuts spanning the bifurcation. Through the DVI guiding catheter, I would then place a second guidewire in the posterolateral branch, and perform low-pressure, kissing inflations with 3.0 mm (PDA) and 2.5 mm (posterolateral branch) balloons.

Editors' Perspective: Bifurcation lesions are generally unfavorable for many devices, but respond well to directional atherectomy. The distal location of the target lesions and the relatively small caliber of both branch vessels mandate careful selection and placement of the AtheroCath. There are several potential approaches, including atherectomy of the larger posterolateral branch and PTCA of the PDA, or sequential directional atherectomy of both branches. When performing directional atherectomy, a single or double guidewire technique can be employed. The single guidewire technique is easier, but can result in sidebranch occlusion, mandating the need to cross the occluded branch with a guidewire. The double guidewire technique utilizes a Nitinol guidewire in one branch while the other sidebranch is treated with atherectomy. This technique is more cumbersome, particularly in bifurcation lesions located in the distal vessel. As mentioned by Dr. Baim, most operators prefer the single wire technique, since it is virtually always possible to retrieve an occluded branch by PTCA or directional atherectomy.

*****

DCA: CALCIFIED LESION

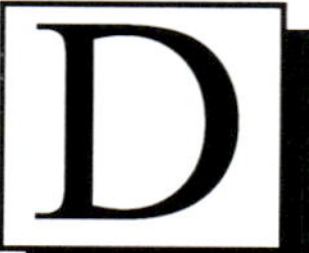

Directional atherectomy of an calcified lesion in the mid-LAD (reference diameter = 2.9 mm).

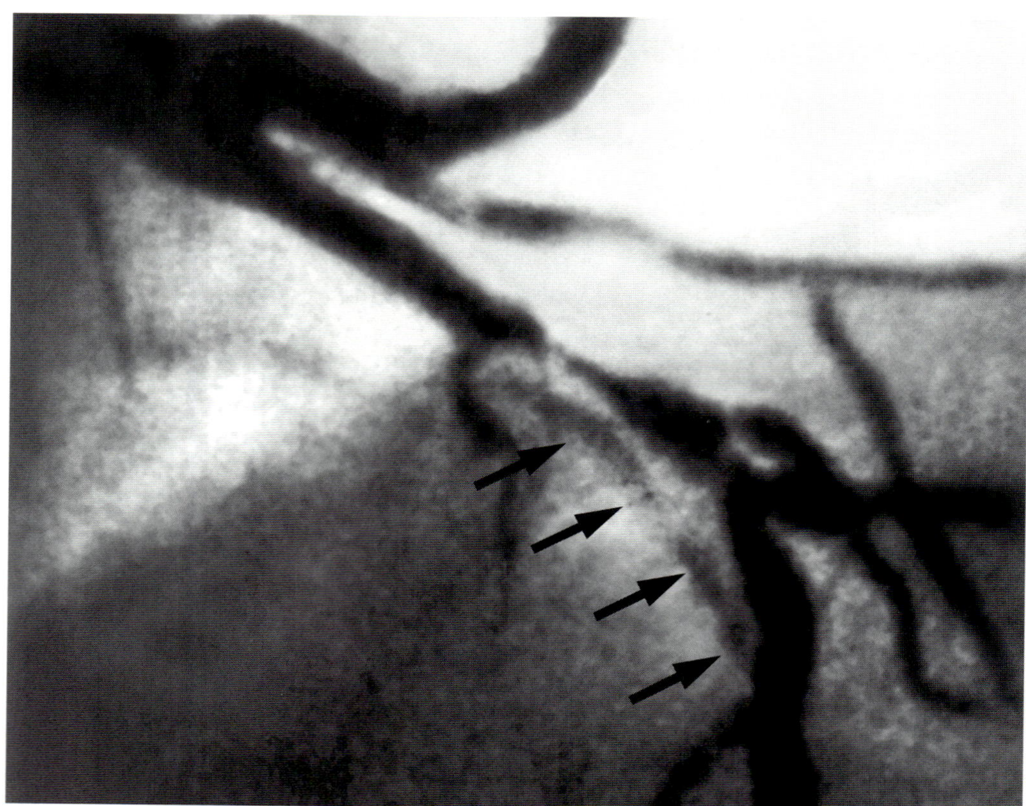

Is directional atherectomy reasonable for this lesion?

Michael Cowley, MD, USA: This concentric mid-LAD lesion is heavily calcified, and the calcification appears to be deep in the vessel wall. IVUS is useful in this setting to determine the extent and localization of lesion calcification and assist with device selection. Deep wall calcification limited to one quadrant does not preclude atherectomy if the lesion is otherwise accessible. However, fluoroscopic calcification is often associated with superficial calcification, which makes atherectomy less feasible.

David Williams, MD, USA: Directional atherectomy is not a good choice for calcified lesions.

Patrick Serruys, MD, PhD, The Netherlands: In order to judge whether directional atherectomy is reasonable for this lesion, intravascular ultrasound is advised to determine the depth and extent of calcification. Clearly, heavy superficial calcification precludes directional atherectomy.

Comment on device sizing and important technical tips.

Patrick Serruys, MD, PhD, The Netherlands: I would begin with a DVI 10F left Judkins guiding catheter, with the assumption that the lesion will be suitable for atherectomy. I would cross the lesion with a 0.014-inch ACS Extra-Support guidewire and perform IVUS with motorized pullback to evaluate plaque burden, degree of calcification, and lesion length. If the angiographic impression of deep calcification in the absence of superficial calcification is correct, I would proceed with directional atherectomy with a 7F AtheroCath. After performing multiple circumferential cuts, I would repeat IVUS to firmly establish my therapeutic goal in terms of luminal dimensions, and postdilate with a 3.5 mm balloon, if necessary.

Editors' Perspective: Vessel calcification is an important correlate of procedural failure and introduces two difficulties for directional atherectomy: First, calcification reduces vessel compliance, and may impair the ability of the AtheroCath to access the target lesion. Second, superficial calcification in the target lesion cannot be resected by current AtheroCath designs (although future calcium-cutters may be able to resect calcified plaque). While IVUS can help differentiate superficial and deep calcium, gross fluoroscopic calcium is frequently associated with superficial and deep calcification in multiple quadrants, and usually identifies vessels that are poorly suited for directional atherectomy.

*****

DCA: CALCIFIED OSTIAL RCA

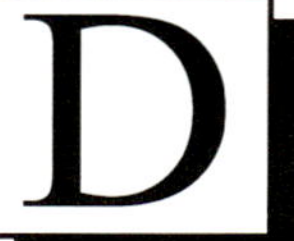

Directional atherectomy of a calcified ostial lesion in the RCA (reference diameter = 2.8 mm).

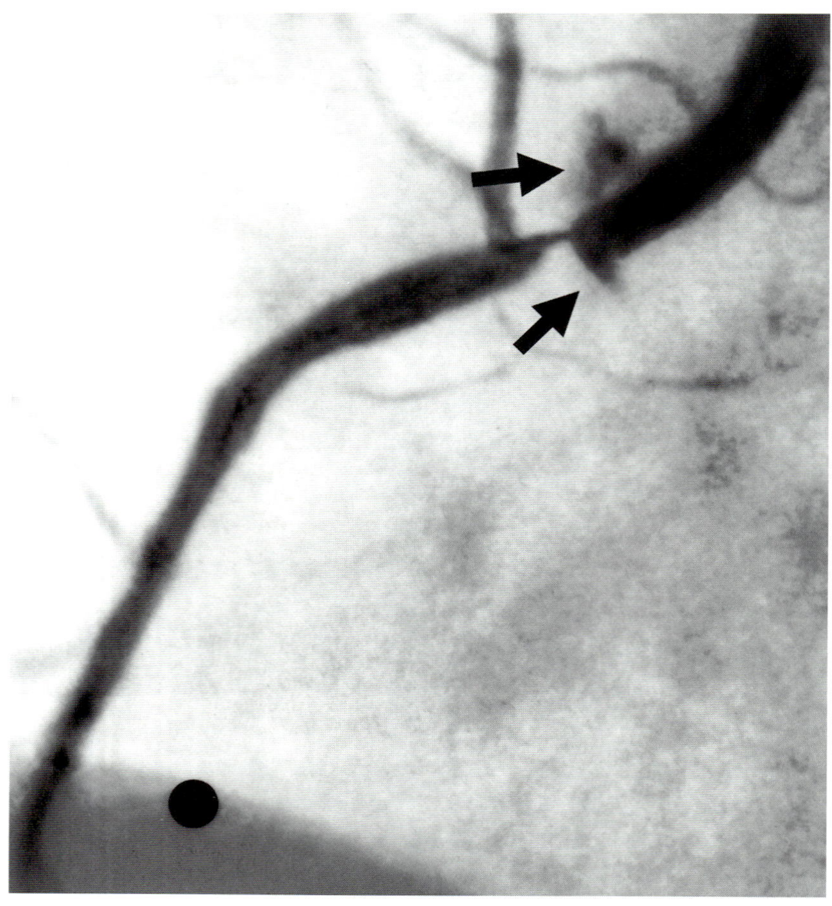

Is directional atherectomy reasonable for this lesion?

Michael Cowley, MD, USA: While directional atherectomy of this lesion may be "reasonable", it is not the approach of choice. This lesion has extensive calcification in the aorta and in the ostium of the RCA.

David Williams, MD, USA: Directional atherectomy is not a good choice for calcified lesions.

David Foley, MD, The Netherlands: This case is not suitable for directional atherectomy.

Comment on device sizing and important technical tips.

Michael Cowley, MD, USA: Directional atherectomy in this setting is technically very difficult. The lesion requires predilation with a 2.5 mm balloon at high pressure to allow passage of the AtheroCath. The vessel size is relatively small for atherectomy, and the eccentric plaque on the lower border of the lesion is more difficult to resect because the usual AtheroCath alignment in the RCA ostium favors plaque removal from the superior wall.

> **Editors' Perspective: Directional atherectomy is problematic for this lesion since extensive ostial calcification will impair guiding catheter engagement and alignment, delivery of the AtheroCath to the target lesion, and ability to resect plaque. Although directional atherectomy is a reasonable approach for some ostial lesions, ostial calcification precludes effective directional atherectomy unless the lesion is pretreated with Rotablator.**

*****

DCA: OSTIAL DIAGONAL

Directional atherectomy of ostial lesion in the diagonal (reference diameter = 3.2 mm).

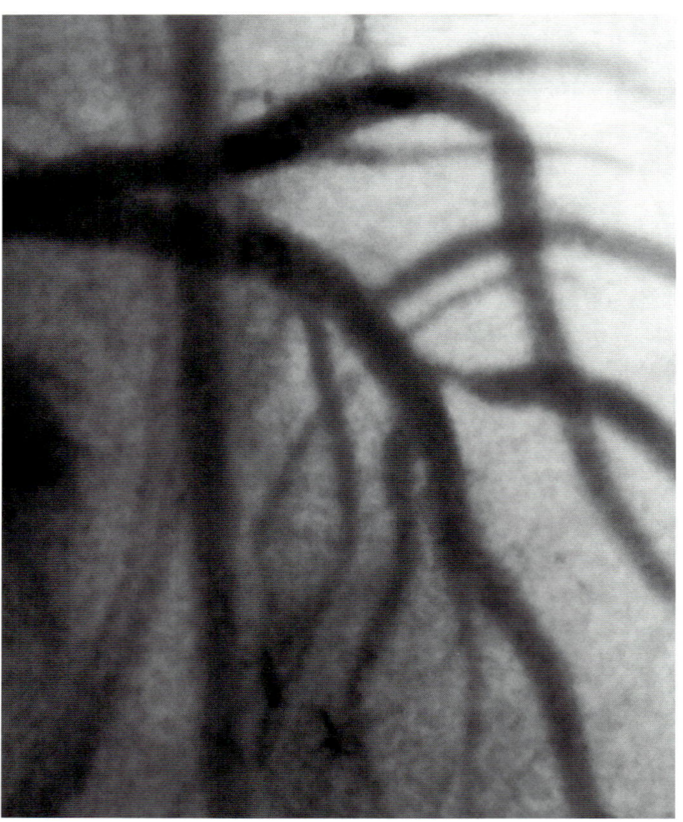

Is directional atherectomy reasonable for this lesion?

Patrick Serruys, MD, PhD, The Netherlands: Directional atherectomy can certainly be successful in this type of ostial lesion.

Donald Baim, MD, USA: I believe that directional atherectomy is an excellent choice.

Spencer King III, MD, USA: This is a large diagonal branch with a high-grade stenosis at its origin. I would select directional atherectomy as my first choice.

Comment on device sizing and important technical tips.

Patrick Serruys, MD, PhD, The Netherlands: I recommend a 7F AtheroCath and adjunctive PTCA with a Chubby balloon, if necessary. IVUS might not provide any additional information in this case, and I would rely on angiographic imaging. The takeoff of the diagonal is not particularly acute and I would not anticipate any major problems delivering the device to the lesion. However, I would still use an Extra-Support guidewire to ease device delivery.

Donald Baim, MD, USA: I would use a 7F GTO through a DVI 10F guiding catheter. I would position the very proximal portion of the window just proximal to the target lesion, to ensure excision of the focal target lesion.

Spencer King III, MD, USA: I would use a DVI guide catheter, an Extra-Support wire, and a 7F cutter with circumferential cuts around the ostium. Ordinarily one pass with 8 to 10 cuts at 15 PSI would be adequate.

Editors' Perspective: Ostial sidebranch lesions are readily treated with directional atherectomy. This patient underwent successful atherectomy, using a DVI 10F JL4 guide, a 0.014-inch x 300 cm Hi-torque floppy guidewire, and a 7F EX AtheroCath. Two passes and 14 cuts were made; adjunctive PTCA was not necessary (below).

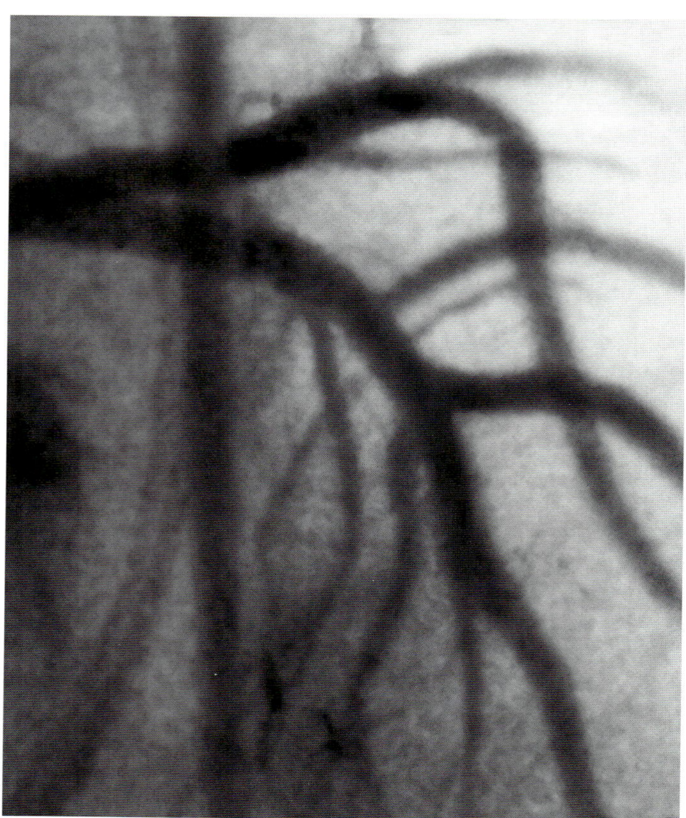

*****

DCA: OSTIAL LAD

Directional atherectomy of an ostial lesion in the LAD (reference diameter = 3.8 mm).

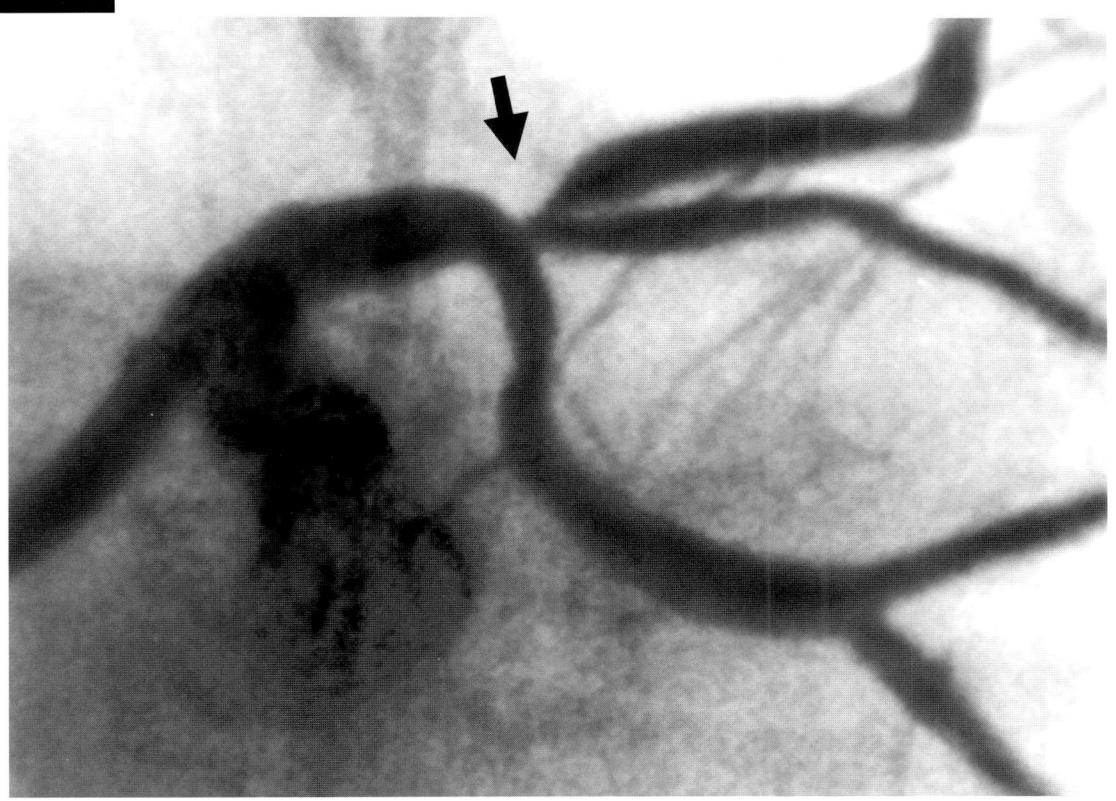

Is directional atherectomy reasonable for this lesion?

David Foley, MD, The Netherlands: I can think of no more suitable therapeutic strategy for this lesion than directional atherectomy.

Donald Baim, MD, USA: I believe that directional atherectomy is an excellent choice.

Spencer King III, MD, USA: This LAD has a significant lesion at its origin. I would select directional atherectomy as my first choice in this eccentric lesion because it is located in the ostium of the LAD. This procedure requires tissue removal from the distal left main coronary artery; therefore, surgery should also be considered.

Comment on device sizing and important technical tips.

David Foley, MD, The Netherlands: I would use a DVI 10F Judkins left guiding catheter and a 7F AtheroCath, performing multiple cuts directed towards the lesion in the most optimal view. I would use intravascular ultrasound to optimize lumen enlargement. The problem with this type of lesion is left main occlusion; cuts must be done very quickly. It is a good idea to place a temporary pacemaker. After performing 5-10 cuts, I would repeat angiography and IVUS to confirm effective plaque removal. I would not hesitate to postdilate with a 4.0 mm compliant balloon at 10 ATM.

Donald Baim, MD, USA: I would use a 7F GTO device advanced through a DVI 10F JL4 guiding catheter, with the very proximal portion of the window just proximal to the target lesion.

Spencer King III, MD, USA: I would use a 7F AtheroCath, a DVI left guide, and a Platinum-Plus guidewire without predilation. If there is any concern about calcium, I would examine this lesion with intravascular ultrasound.

> **Editors' Perspective: This is an ideal lesion for directional atherectomy for several reasons: First, directional atherectomy is the only stand-alone device that can achieve definitive revascularization with excellent angiographic results. Second, the AtheroCath can be positioned to selectively remove plaque from this crucial location, minimizing injury to the adjacent left main coronary artery. Finally, the large vessel caliber, straight approach into the LAD, and lack of calcification favor directional atherectomy over other techniques.**

This patient was treated with directional atherectomy, using a DVI 10F JL4 guide, a 0.014-inch x 300 cm Hi-torque floppy guidewire, and a 7F EX AtheroCath. Residual stenosis was treated with a 7F Graft AtheroCath without adjunctive PTCA, resulting in a smooth lumen, no residual stenosis or dissection, and without injury to the LCX or intermediate branch. The patient has remained asymptomatic for nearly 3 years.

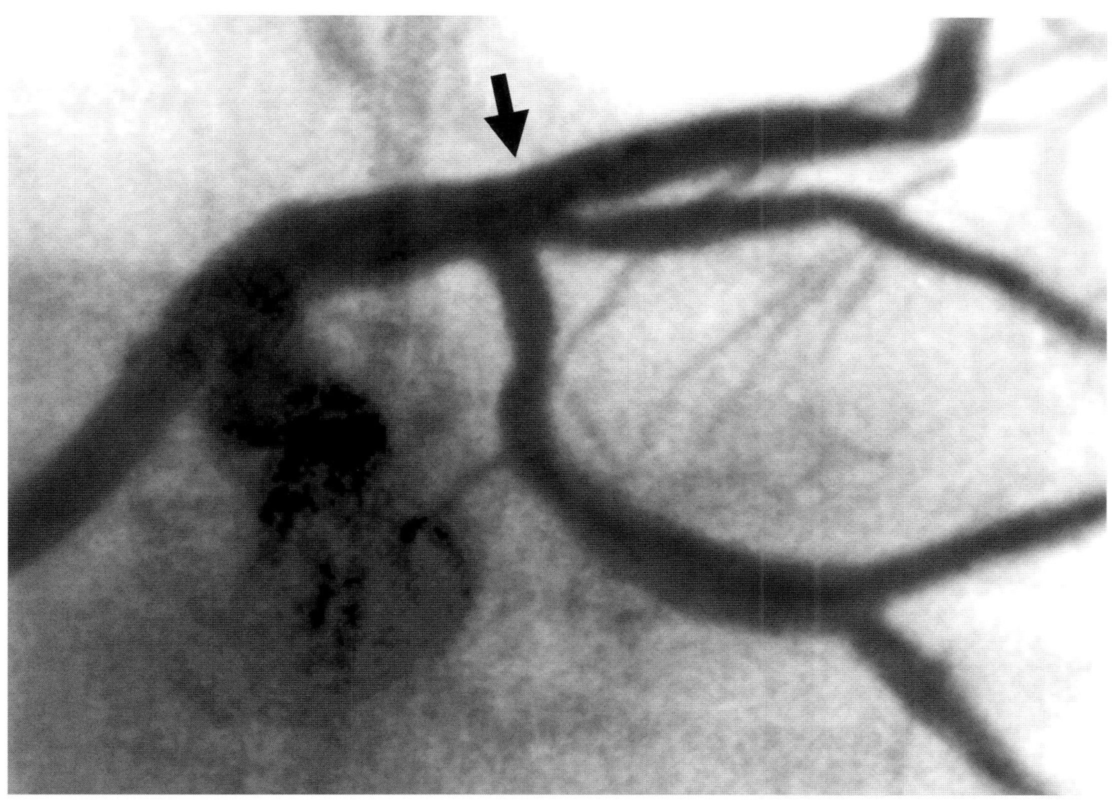

*****

DCA: OSTIAL LCX

Directional atherectomy of an ostial lesion in the LCX (reference diameters: left main = 4.2 mm; LCX = 3.8 mm).

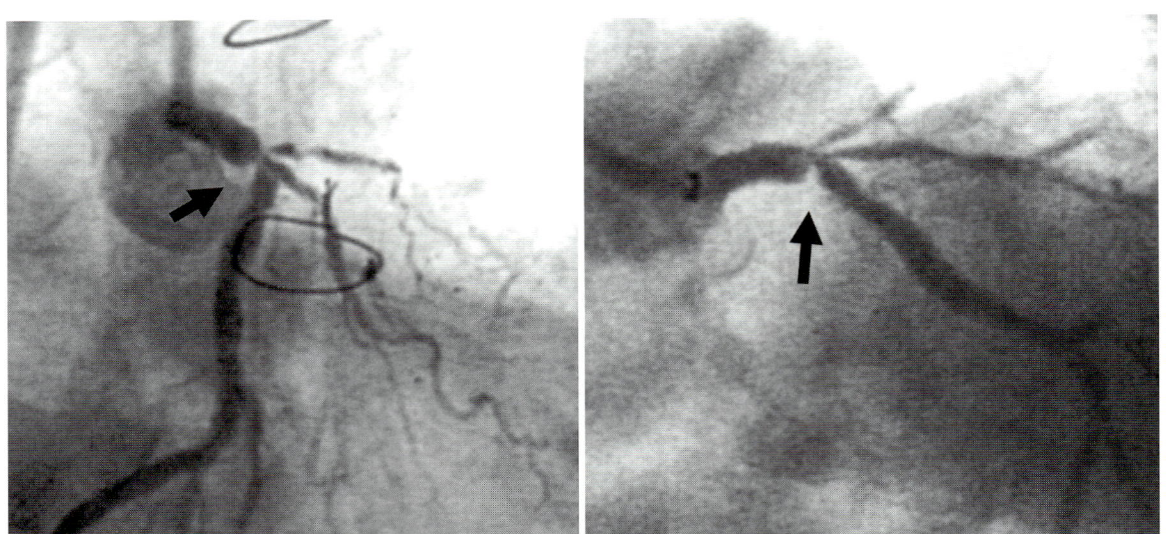

Is directional atherectomy reasonable for this lesion?

Patrick Serruys, MD, PhD, The Netherlands: Directional atherectomy is reasonable for this type of lesion.

Donald Baim, MD, USA: I believe that directional atherectomy is an excellent choice.

Spencer King III, MD, USA: Directional atherectomy is a reasonable approach to this highly eccentric lesion (assuming the LAD bypass is patent).

Comment on device sizing and important technical tips.

Patrick Serruys, MD, PhD, The Netherlands: IVUS is of interest to delineate the extent and distribution of plaque. The takeoff of the LCX is pleasantly gentle so that a DVI 10F Judkins left catheter, a 0.014-inch Extra-Support guidewire, and a 7F AtheroCath will be suitable. Looking for QCA diameter stenosis < 20% and IVUS luminal area 80% of the reference area, I would perform as many cuts as necessary, and also postdilate with a 4.25-4.5 mm compliant or semicompliant balloon.

Donald Baim, MD, USA: I would use a 7F GTO device advanced through a DVI 10F JL4 guiding catheter, with the very proximal portion of the window just proximal to the target lesion.

Spencer King III, MD, USA: I would use a DVI left guide, a Platinum-Plus wire, and a 7F AtheroCath. I would direct multiple cuts towards the plaque (inferior and medial). If there is any concern about complete opening of the vessel, I would follow with a 4.0 mm balloon.

> **Editors' Perspective: Because of the large vessel caliber and lesion eccentricity, directional atherectomy is a reasonable choice. Although a variety of 10F guiding catheters can provide adequate guiding catheter support, the DVI guiding catheters provide the best support. In addition, an extra-support guidewire may be necessary to adequately treat this lesion on a bend. This patient was treated with a 7F EX AtheroCath without adjunctive PTCA.**

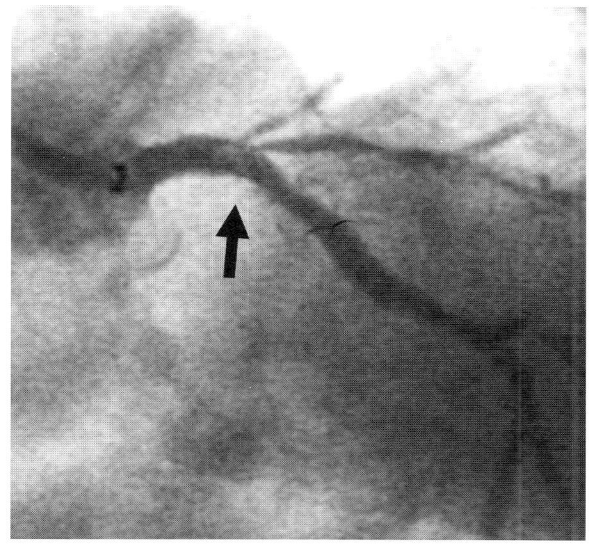

*****

DCA: VEIN GRAFT

Directional atherectomy of a vein graft to the RCA (reference diameter = 3.9 mm).

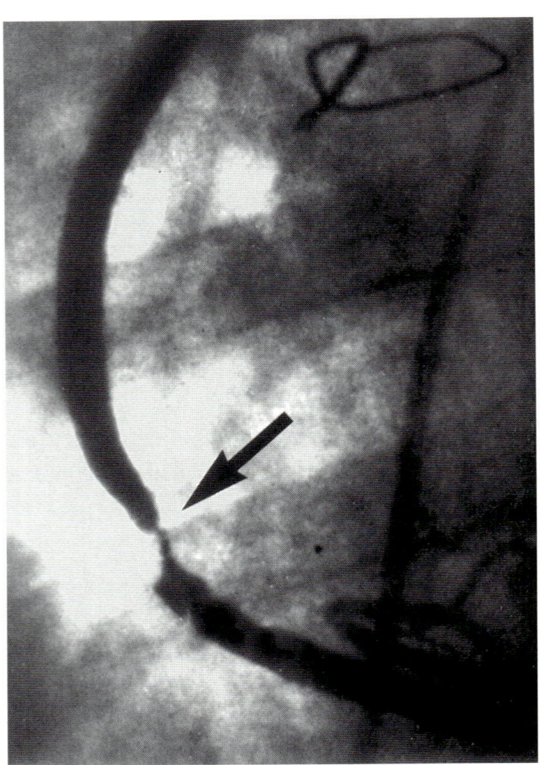

Is directional atherectomy reasonable for this lesion?

Michael Mooney, MD, USA: I do not recommend directional atherectomy due to the irregular appearance of the saphenous vein graft immediately distal to the stenosis.

David Holmes, MD, USA: Directional atherectomy is a superb device for this lesion and will give excellent results.

David Williams, MD, USA: Directional atherectomy is suitable for this lesion.

Comment on device sizing and important technical tips.

David Holmes, MD, USA: I would use a 7F graft device and IVUS.

David Williams, MD, USA: I would perform directional atherectomy with a 7F graft device, followed by PTCA and possibly stenting.

> **Editors' Perspective: Directional atherectomy could be performed with satisfactory results. A multipurpose guiding catheter will provide the best coaxial alignment. Because of the large caliber of the graft, it is unlikely that directional atherectomy alone will provide adequate lumen enlargement, and adjunctive PTCA or stenting will be required.**

*****

DCA: DEGENERATED VEIN GRAFT

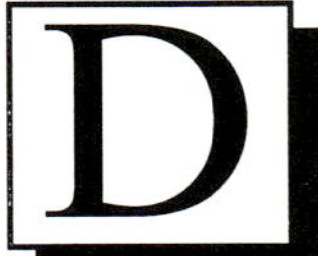

Directional atherectomy of a degenerated vein graft to the OM (reference diameter = 3.9 mm).

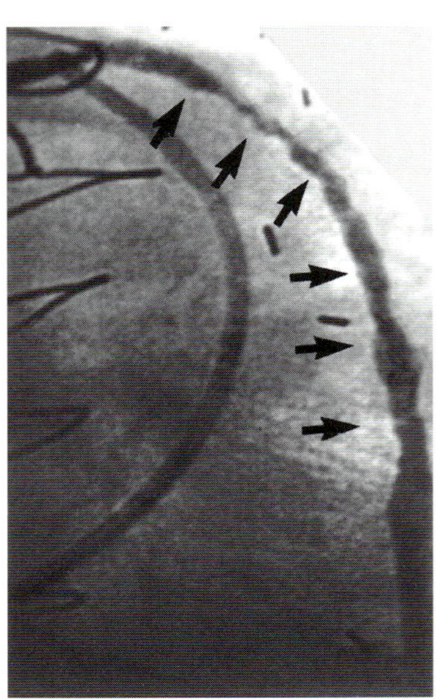

Is directional atherectomy reasonable for this lesion?

Michael Mooney, MD, USA: Good luck with this case! A the present time, I know of no strategy that meaningfully accomplishes long-term revascularization for this type of saphenous vein graft. Any percutaneous attempts on this saphenous vein graft should only be carried out under the most compelling of clinical circumstances, such as refusal of several heart surgeons to perform surgery and/or compelling medical conditions that would not allow for medical management or repeat surgery.

David Holmes, MD, USA: I do not think directional atherectomy is a reasonable option in this degenerated graft.

David Williams, MD, USA: The lesion is extremely long and has a large plaque burden. It is not suitable for directional atherectomy because of the potential for extensive embolization and the inability of directional atherectomy to treat such a long segment.

> **Editors' Perspective: Unfortunately, there are no good choices for percutaneous revascularization of degenerated vein grafts. Directional atherectomy should not be used because of the prohibitively high risk of severe complications (no-reflow, distal embolization), inadequate lumen enlargement, and restenosis.**

*****

DCA: OSTIAL VEIN GRAFT

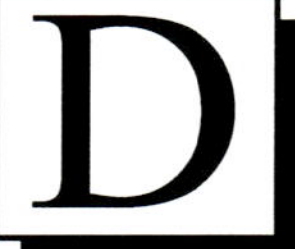

Directional atherectomy of an ostial lesion in a vein graft to the LAD (reference diameter = 3.9 mm).

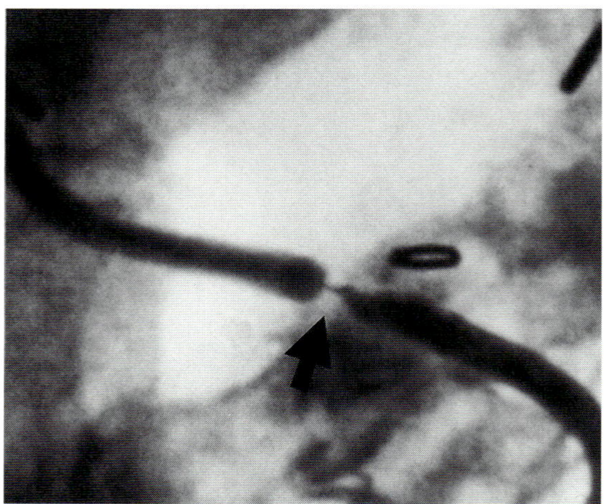

Is directional atherectomy reasonable for this lesion?

Michael Mooney, MD, USA: This ostial stenosis can be most effectively managed by directional atherectomy as an adjunct to biliary stenting.

David Holmes, MD, USA: Directional atherectomy is an excellent approach for this lesion.

David Williams, MD, USA: Directional atherectomy is suitable for this lesion.

Comment on device sizing and important technical tips.

Michael Mooney, MD, USA: I would use an DVI 11F JLG guiding catheter, a 0.014-inch Extra-Support wire, and multiple sequential radial cuts with a 7F AtheroCath to allow maximal debulking. I would mount a PS154 biliary stent on a 4.0 x 20 mm noncompliant balloon. It's too easy to leave the ostium of the vein graft unsupported by the stent; one must make a deliberate attempt to bring the stent back into the aorta almost to the point of being uncomfortable with its position. I choose biliary stenting in this setting simply because of its radial strength and radioopacity.

David Holmes, MD, USA: I would use an Extra-Support wire because of the potential for guide catheter problems, and a 7F AtheroCath to remove as much tissue as possible.

David Williams, MD, USA: I would use a 7F graft device, followed by PTCA and possibly stenting.

Editors' Perspective: **This is an ideal lesion for directional atherectomy because of the horizontal to slightly downward takeoff of the body of the vein graft, the large vessel caliber, and the lack of calcification. Coaxial guiding catheter alignment is crucial, and aggressive intubation must be avoided. Although many vein grafts to the left coronary artery have a vertical upward orientation and are best engaged with a JRG or JLG guiding catheter, this particular graft has a more gentle horizontal takeoff, and might be best engaged with a short-tip JR4 guide. The JR4 configuration will allow coaxial alignment without aggressive intubation, and will allow the operator to retract the guide into the ascending aorta, maximizing tissue resection with the AtheroCath. Even after multiple passes with a 7F graft cutter, residual stenosis may persist, requiring either adjunctive PTCA or stenting. In the near future, modifications of AtheroCath will permit plaque resection in larger caliber vessels. This patient was treated by Drs. Lowell Satler and Jeffrey Popma, using directional atherectomy, adjunctive PTCA, and IVUS guidance (below).**

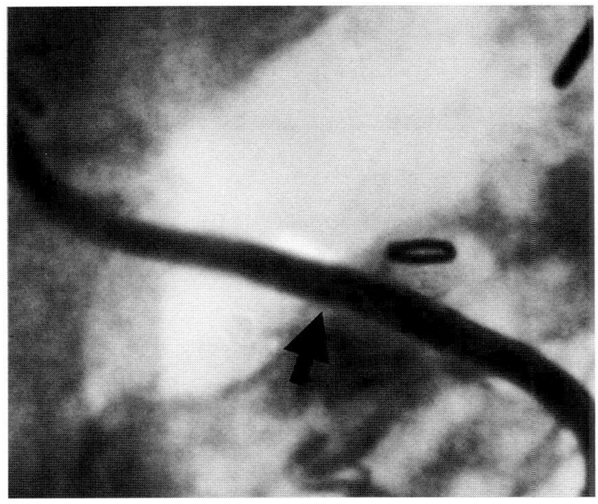

*****

DCA: TORTUOUS LCX

Directional atherectomy of a focal lesion in a tortuous LCX (right angle takeoff; reference diameter = 2.6 mm).

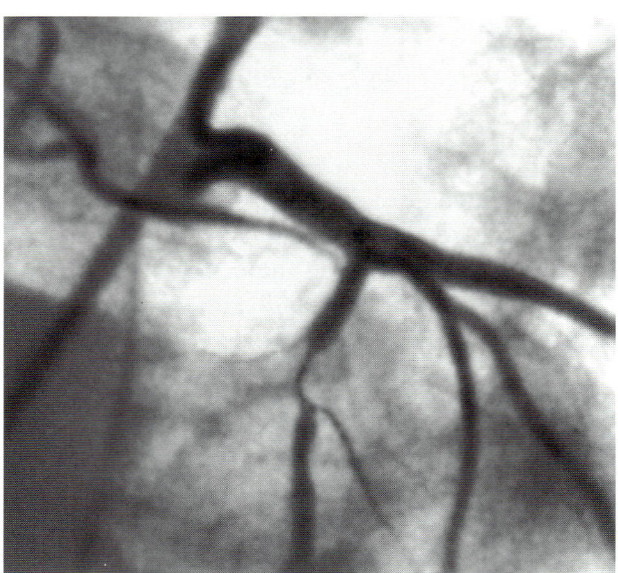

Is directional atherectomy reasonable for this lesion?

Patrick Whitlow, MD, USA: In this case, the difficult angulation of the LCX and the diffuse disease after the severe lesion (and possible nosecone trauma from the AtheroCath) would preclude directional atherectomy.

David Williams, MD, USA: Directional atherectomy is a poor choice. The LCX arises at a 90° angle from the left main and advancing the AtheroCath could result in trauma to the LCX.

Patrick Serruys, MD, PhD, The Netherlands: Atherectomy is not a reasonable choice for this LCX lesion because of the small vessel size and right angle takeoff.

> **Editors' Perspective: Directional atherectomy offers no special value in this lesion, particularly since abnormal lesion contour (marked ulceration or eccentricity) is absent. In addition, the complex anatomy of the target vessel proximal to the stenosis might increase the risk of atherectomy-induced complications. As Dr. Barry George sometimes says, "Why make an easy case difficult?"**

*****

DCA: TORTUOUS RCA

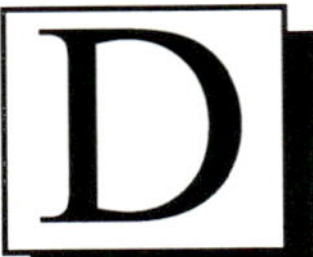

irectional atherectomy of a focal lesion in a tortuous RCA (reference diameter = 3.2 mm).

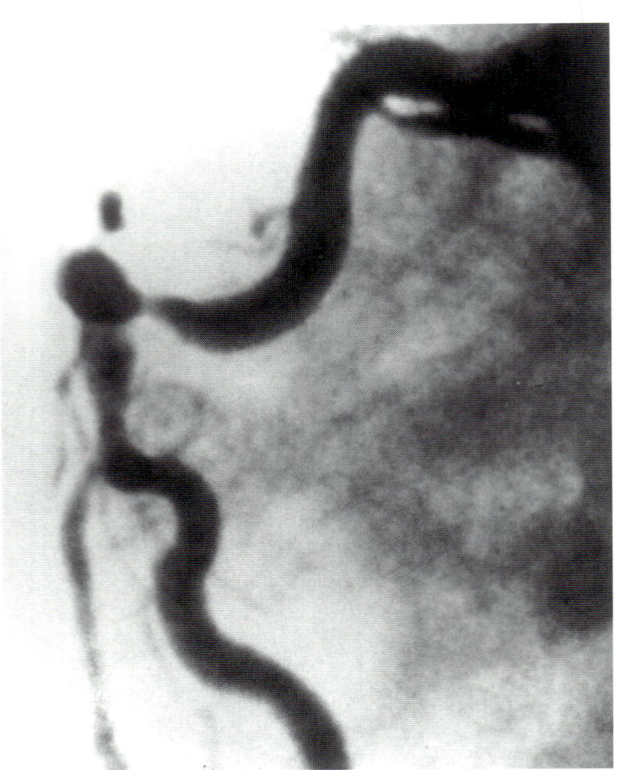

Is directional atherectomy reasonable for this lesion?

Patrick Whitlow, MD, USA: Extreme tortuosity is a relative contraindication to directional atherectomy. Since there is no calcification, I would place an Extra-Support wire to see how the angle straightens out. If the lesion straightens remarkably, directional atherectomy might be reasonable. However, if the tortuosity remains, directional atherectomy would be extremely difficult and possibly complicated.

David Williams, MD, USA: Directional atherectomy is a poor choice because the RCA is extremely tortuous.

David Foley, MD, The Netherlands: The proximal RCA is extremely tortuous, with a focal lesion in a horizontal portion and further disease more distally. With a 90° bend in this case, atherectomy would not be helpful since the more distal disease could not be treated. Furthermore, atherectomy might cause dissection in the tortuous segment. This is actually an extremely challenging problem to tackle.

Comment on device sizing and important technical tips.

Patrick Whitlow, MD, USA: I would utilize a Medtronic 10F short tip JR4 guide and a 0.014-inch Extra-S'port wire or Traverse wire. If the wire straightens the curves, I would utilize a 6F GTO device and cut along the inferior surface of the artery. If the wire straightens the artery, it is extremely important to use contrast injections to establish the exact lesion location, since the anatomy changes when the tortuous vessel is straightened.

Editors' Perspective: This type of lesion is extremely challenging for virtually all devices — there are no perfect solutions. Directional atherectomy could be performed, but several technical points must be considered: First, coaxial guiding catheter alignment is best achieved with a JR4 or hockey stick configuration. Second, extra-support guidewires are useful to straighten the tortuous vessel, including the Platinum-Plus, Stabilizer, Roadrunner, or S'port wire; when these heavy-duty guidewires are used, the operator should anticipate the creation of multiple pseudolesions. Third, since standard devices may have significant difficulty "cornering" around the bends, short-window AtheroCaths may be useful to access the lesion. Finally, if adjunctive PTCA is necessary, a short (9-10 mm) balloon (to avoid the bends in the vessel) or a long (30-40 mm) balloon (to conform to the bends) could be used to smoothe the result and improve lumen diameter.

This patient was initially treated with conventional PTCA, which failed to result in significant lumen enlargement. The patient remained symptomatic despite medical therapy, and was referred to us for further evaluation and treatment. Directional atherectomy was performed using a 9.5F JR4 guide, a 0.014-inch x 300 cm Extra-Support guidewire, and a 7F EX short-window AtheroCath. After 2 series of passes and multiple circumferential cuts, there was no residual stenosis or dissection. Adjunctive PTCA was not necessary.

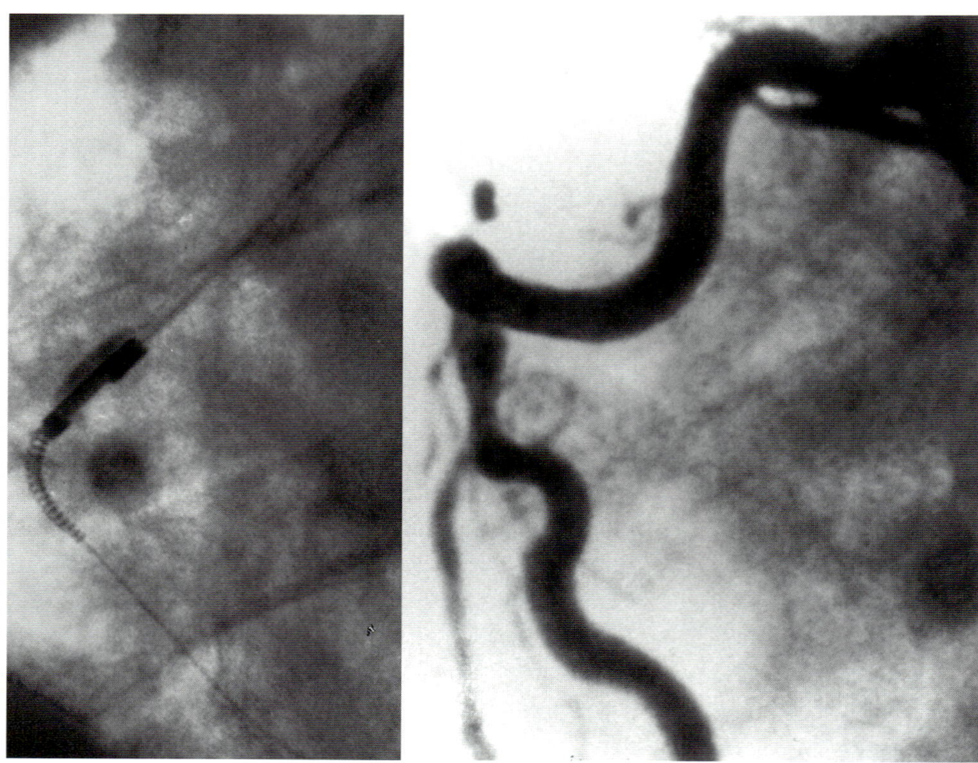

*****

TEC Atherectomy Techniques

TEC: ECCENTRIC LESION (LAD)

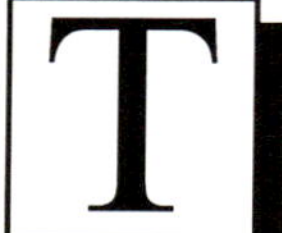

TEC atherectomy of an eccentric lesion in the proximal LAD (reference diameter = 3.4 mm).

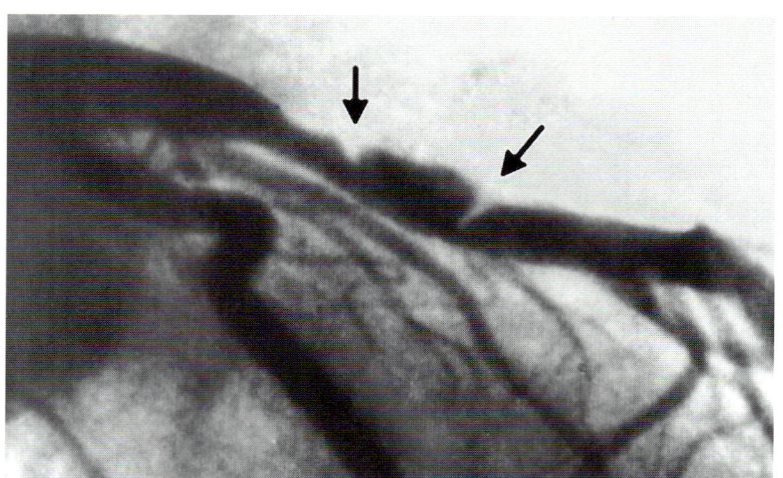

Is TEC reasonable for this lesion?

William O'Neill, MD, USA: The vessel size is adequate and the lesion is in a straight portion of the artery. This lesion can be safely and easily treated with TEC.

Barry George, MD, USA: This complex, eccentric, ulcerated lesion can be treated with TEC, but a more acceptable result is likely with directional atherectomy.

Cindy Grines, MD, USA: This large vessel has tandem eccentric, ulcerated lesions and is suitable for TEC atherectomy.

Comment on device sizing and important technical tips.

William O'Neill, MD, USA: I would use an IVT 10F JL4 guiding catheter, start with a 6.5F cutter, and then increase to a 7.5F cutter. I would complete the procedure with a 3.5 x 40 mm balloon at low pressure.

Cindy Grines, MD, USA: I would start with a 9F giant lumen JL4 guiding catheter and cross the lesion with a steerable 300 cm wire. The TEC atherectomy wire is difficult to steer, and due to the complexity of the lesion, I am worried about subintimal passage. After passing a steerable wire, I would exchange for a TEC wire, and perform atherectomy with a 5.5-6F cutter (which results in damped pressure and difficulty injecting contrast when using a 9F guide). I would position the TEC cutter just proximal to the first stenosis, and fill several vacuum bottles while slowly advancing through both lesions, assuring continuous flow. I would perform adjunctive PTCA with a 3.5 mm balloon, and possibly place a stent.

Editors' Perspective: In most practices, TEC would not be employed for such lesions. Nevertheless, TEC atherectomy may be useful for lesions with irregular margins, because of its ability to remove thrombus. If used in native coronary arteries, it is best to use relatively undersized cutters (cutter/artery ratio < 0.7) to minimize dissection; adjunctive PTCA or stenting is virtually always required. Dr. Grines mentions an important point about the TEC guidewire being stiff and difficult to steer, particularly in native coronary arteries. When exchanging a conventional PTCA guidewire for the TEC wire, it is important to remember that the tip of the TEC wire has a 0.021-inch ball; therefore, transfer catheters with internal diameters > 0.021 inches must be used. Another important point about the TEC guidewire is that it frequently causes "pseudolesions."

*****

TEC: ECCENTRIC LESION (RCA)

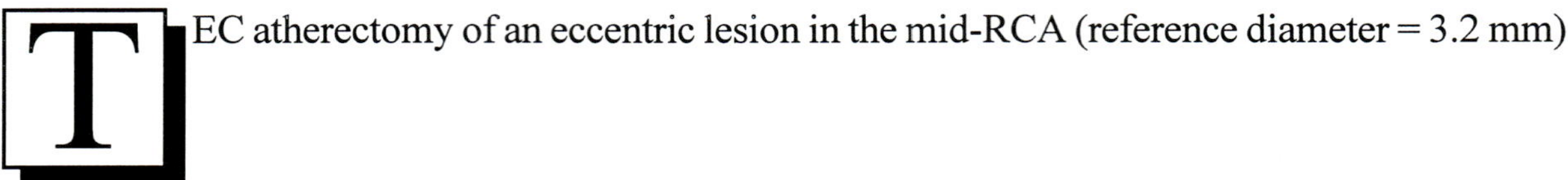

TEC atherectomy of an eccentric lesion in the mid-RCA (reference diameter = 3.2 mm).

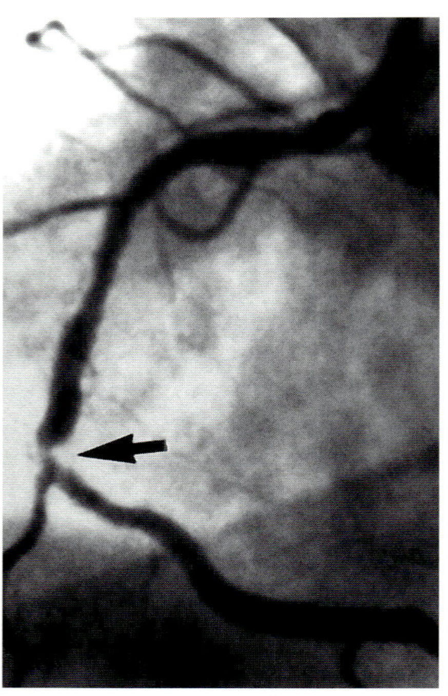

Is TEC reasonable for this lesion?

William O'Neill, MD, USA: This lesion is very poorly suited for TEC due to the extremely high risk for perforation.

Barry George, MD, USA: TEC is technically feasible, but not recommended for this lesion.

Cindy Grines, MD, USA: This lesion is not ideal for TEC atherectomy since the curvature of the bend will direct the cutter into the normal vessel, increasing the risk of perforation. Furthermore, TEC-induced perforations of native vessels occur more commonly at bend points.

> **Editors' Perspective: TEC offers no advantage over other techniques for this type of lesion. Although the TEC catheter is quite flexible and can negotiate significant tortuosity, lesion angulation is a relative contraindication because of the risk of dissection and perforation.**

*****

TEC: ULCERATED LESION

TEC atherectomy of an ulcerated lesion in the mid-LAD (reference diameter = 3.2 mm).

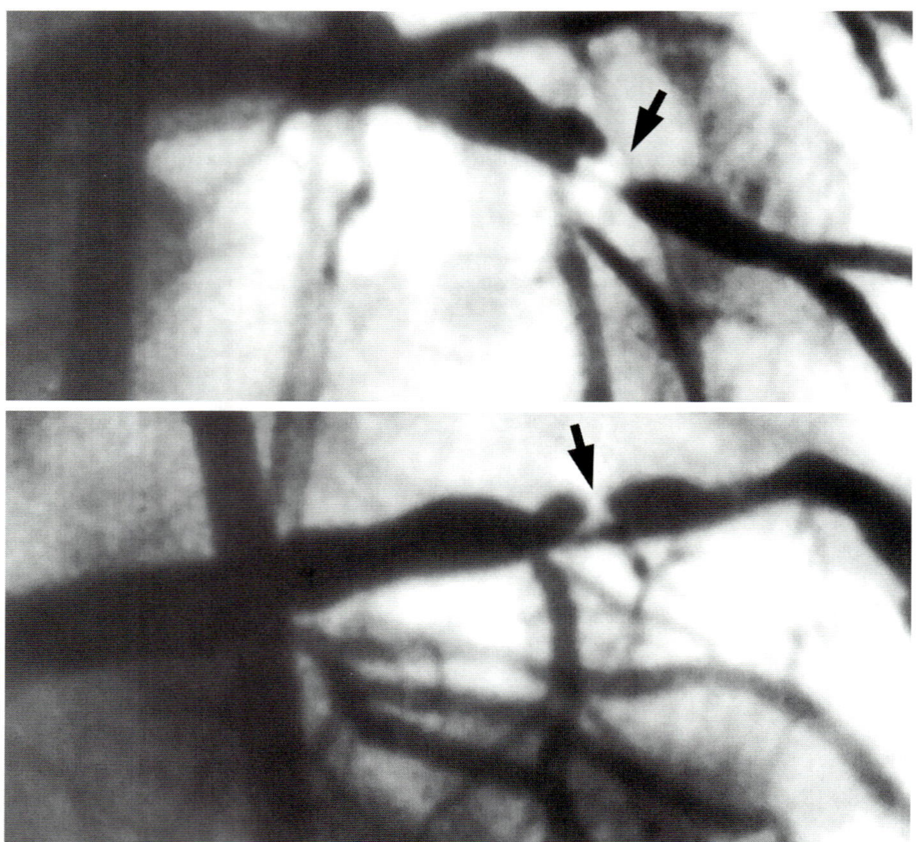

Is TEC reasonable for this lesion?

William O'Neill, MD, USA: TEC is suitable for this ulcerated plaque. The lesion is in a straight segment of the vessel; although it is very eccentric, it probably contains thrombus.

Barry George, MD, USA: This lesion is complex and ulcerated; probably riddled with thrombus; and is associated with a high likelihood of distal embolization, non-Q-wave myocardial infarction, recurrent thrombosis, and restenosis. TEC is the appropriate first choice for debulking and thrombectomy.

Cindy Grines, MD, USA: TEC atherectomy is reasonable for this lesion, due to the large vessel caliber, the absence of angulation, and the presence of an ulcerated stenosis that is probably soft.

Comment on device sizing and important technical tips.

William O'Neill, MD, USA: I would start with an IVT 10F FL4 guide and a TEC guidewire. If I have difficulty crossing the lesion, I would exchange for a 0.018-inch soft Reflex wire. I would start with a 5.5F cutter, upsize to a 6.5F cutter, and complete the procedure with a 3.0 x 40 mm balloon.

Barry George, MD, USA: I would choose a 6.5F TEC cutter, a 0.014-inch TEC guidewire, and a 10F JL4 guiding catheter. Extremely slow passes are recommended, and uninterrupted suction will minimize distal embolization. Following debulking, I would use a 3.5 x 20 mm Lifestream perfusion balloon for 5 minutes. I would continue heparin for 48 hours.

Cindy Grines, MD, USA: I would start with a 9F giant lumen catheter and cross the lesion with a TEC wire. I would undersize the device in a native vessel, and start with a 5.5-6F cutter. Then, I would perform PTCA with a 3.0 x 20 mm compliant balloon. If the result is suboptimal, I would increase the balloon inflation pressure or upsize to a 3.5 mm tapered balloon at 3-4 ATM.

> **Editors' Perspective: Complex lesions such as this may be associated with occult thrombus, a scenario for which TEC may be useful. In fact, several angioscopy studies have demonstrated that TEC is very efficient at removing fresh thrombus, and preliminary data from a large multicenter trial (TOPIT) suggest that TEC may be associated with less asymptomatic CK release than PTCA. However, in our experience, TEC in native coronary arteries is virtually always associated with dissection, and its ability to cut and remove atheroma is limited. If TEC is performed, we recommend cutters ≤ 6.5F to aspirate thrombus and minimize dissection; larger cutters should be avoided due to the risk of vessel injury. As in virtually all TEC cases, PTCA, directional atherectomy, or stenting will be needed for definitive lumen enlargement.**

*****

TEC: TUBULAR LESION

TEC atherectomy of a tubular lesion in the mid-RCA (length = 15 mm; reference diameter = 2.5 mm).

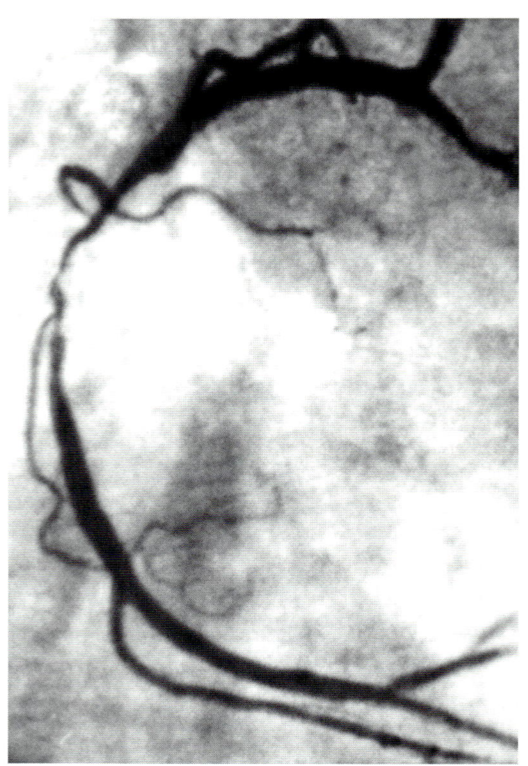

Is TEC reasonable for this lesion?

William O'Neill, MD, USA: This lesion is not suitable for TEC; the lesion is too long.

Barry George, MD, USA: This lesion is likely fibrotic and dense; Rotablator is better.

Cindy Grines, MD, USA: This is a small vessel with a long lesion; TEC is not the best approach.

Editors' Perspective: TEC offers no advantage over other techniques for treating long lesions without thrombus. Tissue removal is minimal and the risk of dissection is high.

*****

TEC: LONG LESION

TEC atherectomy of a long lesion in the mid-LAD (length = 25 mm; reference diameter = 3.3 mm).

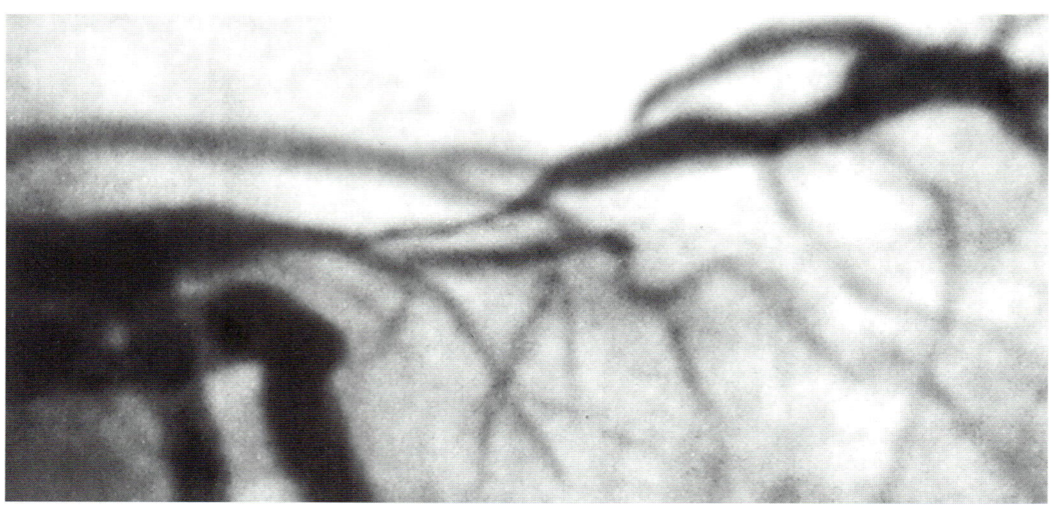

Is TEC reasonable for this lesion?

William O'Neill, MD, USA: This lesion is not suitable for TEC; it is too long.

Barry George, MD, USA: This lesion is likely fibrotic and dense; Rotablator is better.

Cindy Grines, MD, USA: The length, eccentricity, tortuosity and lack of thrombus preclude TEC.

Editors' Perspective: **In the absence of thrombus, TEC has no role for this lesion.**

*****

TEC: TORTUOUS RCA

TEC atherectomy of a focal lesion in a tortuous RCA (reference diameter = 3.2 mm).

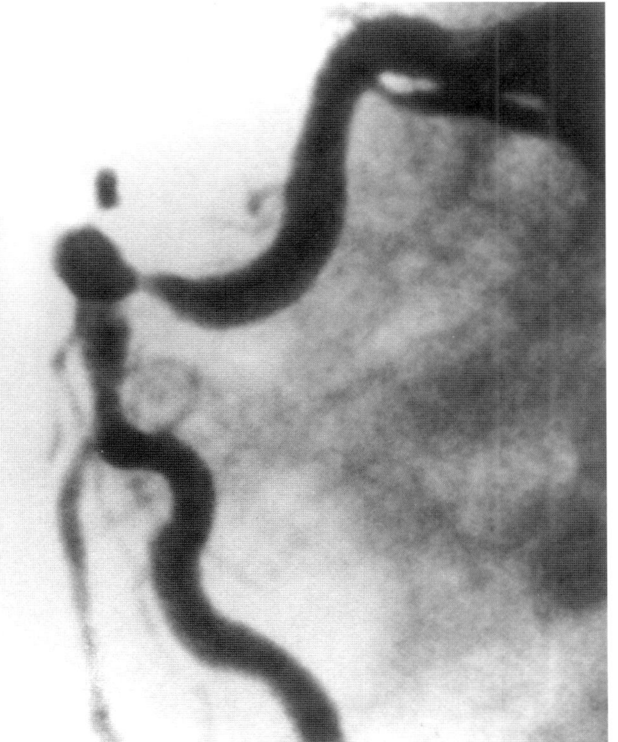

Is TEC reasonable for this lesion?

Barry George, MD, USA: There is "obscene" tortuosity, which is unsuitable for TEC. Only highly experienced operators (100 cases/year) should take on this case.

William O'Neill, MD, USA: TEC atherectomy can be done, but I see no advantage over PTCA.

Cindy Grines, MD, USA: I would not perform TEC due to the risk of perforation.

> **Editors' Perspective: In the absence of thrombus, TEC has no role for this type of lesion due to the risk of dissection and perforation.**

*****

TEC: TORTUOUS LCX

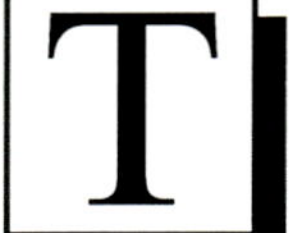

TEC atherectomy of a focal lesion in a tortuous LCX (right angle takeoff; reference diameter = 2.6 mm).

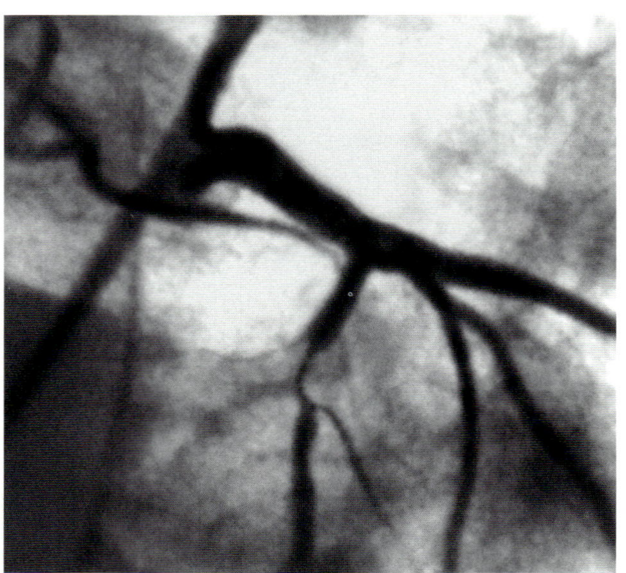

Is TEC reasonable for this lesion?

William O'Neill, MD, USA: This vessel is not suitable for TEC. The left main has a severe bend, increasing the risk of dissection.

Barry George, MD, USA: The LCX lesion, because of its sharp takeoff from the left main, presents a technical challenge. The guidewire may prolapse into the LAD before achieving good purchase in the LCX. I do not recommend TEC.

Cindy Grines, MD, USA: Although the TEC cutter is flexible, I would not use it here because of the right angle takeoff of the LCX and the risk of dissection.

> **Editors' Perspective: TEC has no advantage in this lesion, and the risk of dissection is increased because of proximal vessel tortuosity.**

*****

TEC:FUNCTIONAL TOTAL OCCLUSION

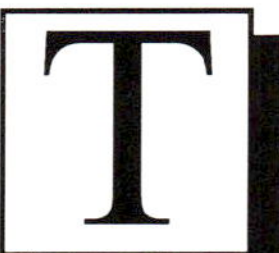EC atherectomy of a functional total occlusion in the proximal LAD (reference diameter = 2.7 mm). Assume the occlusion can be crossed with a guidewire.

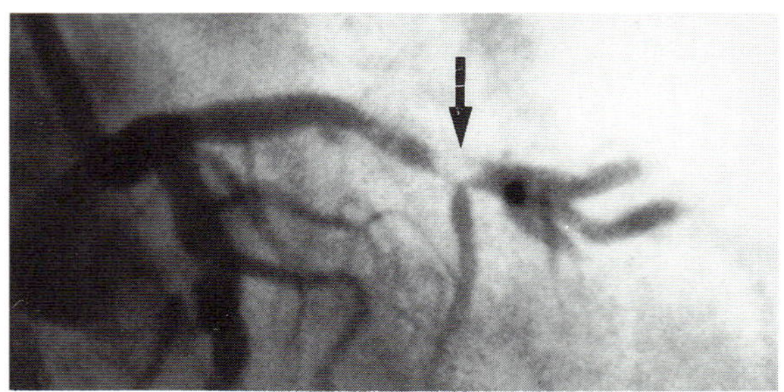

Is TEC reasonable for this lesion?

William O'Neill, MD, USA: This lesion is very well suited for TEC because of intraluminal thrombus. Although the lesion is eccentric, it is on a straight segment and should respond nicely.

Barry George, MD, USA: The arteriogram shows a thrombus-laden vessel, with the appearance of recent occlusion. It is suitable for TEC.

Patrick Whitlow, MD, USA: This thrombus-containing lesion is in a relatively straight portion of the LAD. I can clearly see the downstream anatomy to avoid passing the front-cutting TEC device around a bend. If there is no calcification, TEC atherectomy is reasonable for this lesion.

Comment on device sizing and important technical tips.

William O'Neill, MD, USA: I would use a 9F giant lumen guiding catheter with sideholes and a 5.5F cutter, which will provide excellent aspiration. After the thrombus is removed, the procedure could be completed with a 2.5 mm balloon. Angioscopy could be performed to confirm clot removal if a stent is contemplated after TEC.

Barry George, MD, USA: I would proceed with an IVT 10F FL4 guiding catheter and a 5.5F cutter to debulk the lesion. I would not use a larger cutter because of the slight bend in the LAD. I would then perform PTCA with a 3.0 x 30 mm Lifestream perfusion catheter for 5-minutes at 4-6 ATM. I would administer a bolus and 12 hour infusion of ReoPro and weight adjusted heparin, achieving an ACT of 300 seconds.

Patrick Whitlow, MD, USA: This type of patient has fewer complications when pretreated with ReoPro. Although TEC was not included in the EPIC trial, I would extrapolate those data to this setting. A bolus (0.25 mg/kg) plus infusion (10 mcg/min for 12 hours) of ReoPro with weight adjusted heparin (70 units/kg) would be given prior to instrumentation of the artery. I would start with a 5.5F cutter (no more) and a 10F guide. The larger the cutter, the more efficient the suction, but the greater the risk of dissection. I would use TEC to partially debulk the lesion, but mainly to remove the loose thrombotic elements, in hopes of decreasing distal embolization and recurrent thrombosis.

> **Editors' Perspective: Despite TEC's ability to remove fresh thrombus, its widespread use has been limited by the inability to remove atheroma (it is a poor atherectomy device), frequent development of vessel dissection, and absolute need for adjunctive lumen enlargement with PTCA, directional atherectomy, or stents. To minimize the risk of dissection, it is best to start with small cutters in native vessels (device/artery ratio ~ 0.5-0.6), reserving larger cutters for definite residual thrombus.**

*****

TEC: TOTAL OCCLUSION

TEC atherectomy of a total occlusion in the proximal RCA (reference diameter = 4.5 mm). Assume the occlusion can be crossed with a guidewire.

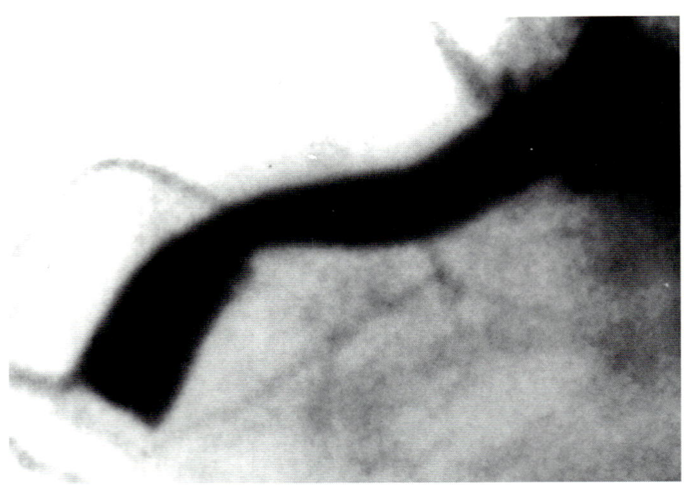

Is TEC reasonable for this lesion?

William O'Neill, MD, USA: This is a very large vessel. The clinical setting is very important. If this patient presents with an acute MI, thrombolytic failure, or post-infarction angina, I assume extensive clot burden is present. In this setting, TEC is my strongly preferred treatment option.

Barry George, MD, USA: The arteriogram shows a thrombus-laden vessel, with the appearance of recent occlusion. It is suitable for TEC.

Patrick Whitlow, MD, USA: Based on the convex filling defect in the proximal RCA, I expect that this lesion is an acute occlusion. Without visualizing the vessel distal to the occlusion, I would not utilize TEC atherectomy, which may disrupt the vessel in a curve. I do not utilize TEC if I cannot clearly visualize the anatomy distal to the lesion.

Comment on device sizing and important technical tips.

William O'Neill, MD, USA: I would start with an IVT 10F FR4 guide and a 7F cutter to aspirate thrombus, followed by adjunctive PTCA with a 4.0 mm compliant balloon. If I cannot cross with a guidewire, I would infuse urokinase for 8 hours.

Barry George, MD, USA: I would use an IVT FR4 guiding catheter and a 0.014-inch Choice-PT guidewire, which is far and away the most user-friendly guidewire to cross total occlusions. Following passage of the guidewire, I would assess the tortuosity and the caliber of the distal vessel, and the extent of thrombus. I would exchange for the 0.014-inch TEC guidewire and a 7.5F TEC catheter, perform slow passes through the occlusion to ensure thrombus extraction, and administer a bolus and 12 hour infusion of ReoPro. Following TEC, I would use a 4.5 x 20 mm Sub-4 balloon at 4-8 ATM.

Editors' Perspective: TEC is the only device approved by the FDA with significant thrombectomy capability. However, as stated by Dr. Whitlow, cutting devices (such as TEC or directional atherectomy) must be used cautiously (if at all) in anatomic situations where the distal vessel size and morphology cannot be visualized. In this situation, it is worthwhile to "dotter" the occlusion first using a transfer catheter over a conventional angioplasty guidewire; the transfer catheter can then be used to exchange the PTCA wire for the TEC wire (remember: the TEC wire has a 0.021" ball-tip, so a suitable transfer catheter must be employed). Further contrast injections will define the length of the occlusion, thrombus burden, and vessel caliber distal to the occlusion, facilitating selection of the proper size TEC cutter. In native coronary arteries, cutter/artery ratios < 0.6 are recommended to minimize dissection even though larger cutters (> 6.5F) may have better ability to aspirate thrombus. If in doubt about cutter selection, it is best to select a smaller cutter first, followed by larger cutters for residual thrombus. This patient was treated with conventional PTCA techniques, but the occlusion could not be crossed with a guidewire. This patient was referred to Dr. William O'Neill, who administered an overnight infusion of intracoronary urokinase, which successfully recanalized the total occlusion. TEC atherectomy was then performed with a 7F cutter followed by adjunctive PTCA without incident.

*****

TEC: ANGULATED LESION (LAD)

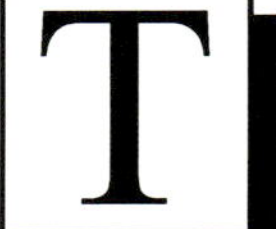

TEC atherectomy of an angulated lesion in the proximal LAD (lesion on inner curve; reference diameter = 3.4 mm).

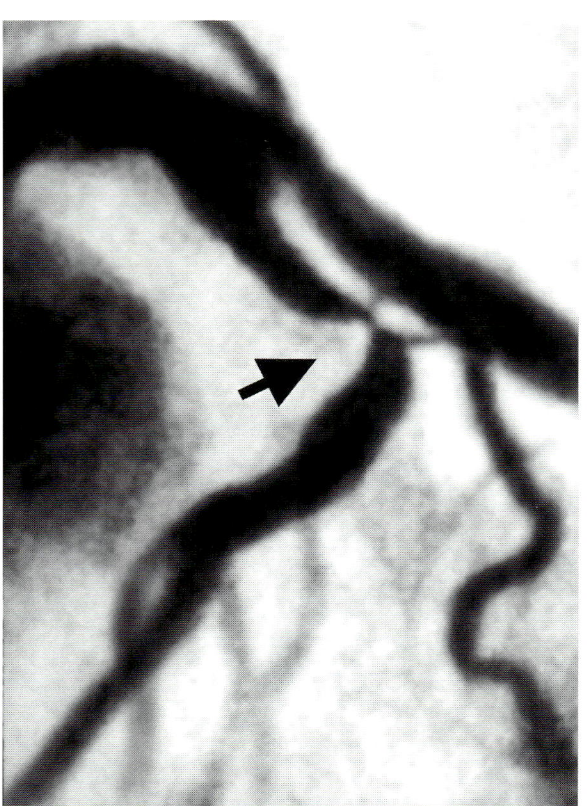

Is TEC reasonable for this lesion?

William O'Neill, MD, USA: This vessel is not suitable for TEC. It is too high-risk for perforation since the lesion is on the inner curve of the bend.

Barry George, MD, USA: Because of the bend and eccentricity, there is a higher incidence of dissection and procedural complications. My enthusiasm for atherectomy (Rotablator, TEC or directional atherectomy) is low because of the risk of perforation. I would not try to make an easy case difficult.

Patrick Whitlow, MD, USA: I do not recommend TEC atherectomy for a lesion in a native coronary artery near a bend because of the risk of vessel disruption.

> **Editors' Perspective: The risk of dissection and perforation preclude the use of TEC atherectomy for moderately angulated lesions.**

*****

TEC: ANGULATED LESION (RCA)

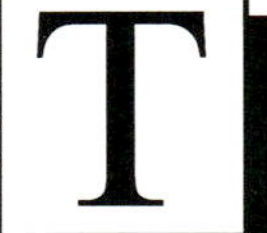

TEC atherectomy of an angulated lesion in the proximal RCA (lesion on outer curve; reference diameter = 3.1 mm).

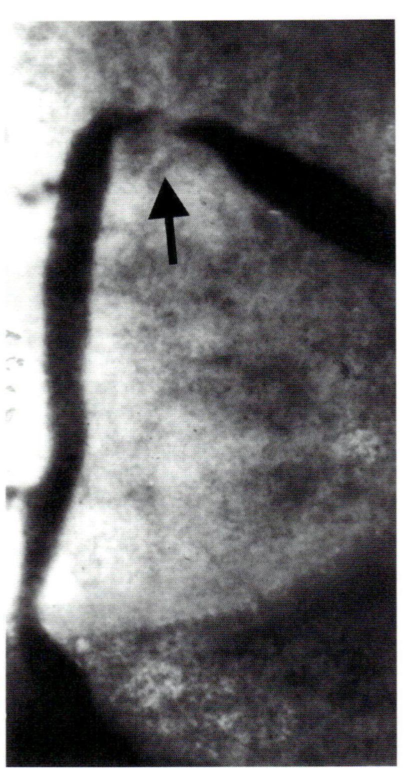

Is TEC reasonable for this lesion?

William O'Neill, MD, USA: This lesion is excellent for TEC. The lesion is eccentric but the plaque is on the outer aspect of the bend.

Barry George, MD, USA: Because of the bend and eccentricity, there is a higher risk of dissection, complications, and perforation, despite appropriate execution and sizing of devices. I would not try to make an easy case difficult.

Patrick Whitlow, MD, USA: To completely debulk this thrombotic lesion, the front-cutting TEC catheter would have to be advanced into the acute bend in the RCA. Since the TEC cutter could lead to intimal disruption, I do not recommend TEC atherectomy in this case.

> Editors' Perspective: **Acutely angulated lesions should be approached cautiously with TEC and other devices that ablate or remove tissue. The merits of TEC (thrombus extraction) must be weighed against the risk of complications (dissection, perforation); potentially safer intervention with other devices (PTCA, stents) should be strongly considered.**

*****

TEC: TRIFURCATION LESION

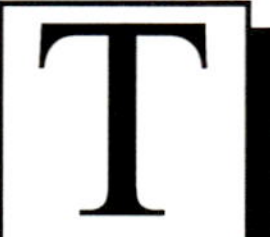

TEC atherectomy of a trifurcation lesion in the proximal LCX (reference diameter of proximal LCX = 3.4 mm).

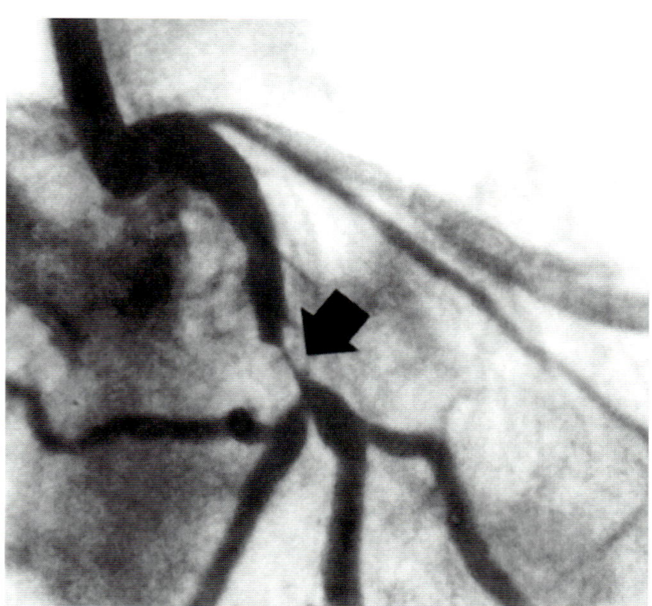

Is this device reasonable for this lesion?

William O'Neill, MD, USA: I see no advantage to TEC in this setting.

Barry George, MD, USA: TEC is not indicated for this lesion.

Patrick Whitlow, MD, USA: I would not utilize TEC because other devices are safer.

> **Editors' Perspective: TEC has no particular role for this lesion in the absence of thrombus.**

*****

TEC: BIFURCATION LESION

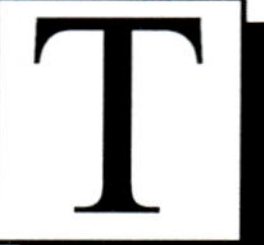EC atherectomy of a bifurcation lesion in the distal RCA (reference diameters: RCA = 3.6 mm; PDA = 2.7 mm; PLV = 2.2 mm).

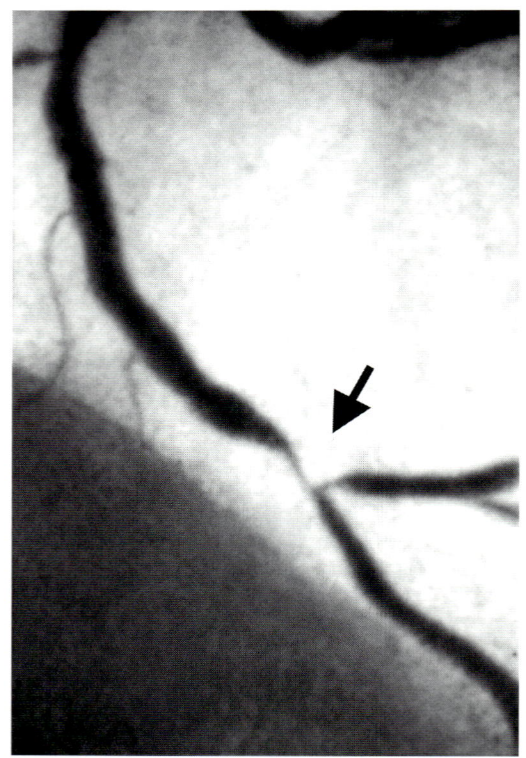

Is this device reasonable for this lesion?

William O'Neill, MD, USA: This vessel is well-suited for TEC. There appears to be a filling defect in the vessel which is probably thrombus.

Barry George, MD, USA: The RCA shows a lesion at the bifurcation. TEC is not indicated.

Patrick Whitlow, MD, USA: I would not consider TEC atherectomy for this lesion.

Comment on device sizing and important technical tips.

William O'Neill, MD, USA: I would use a 9F guiding catheter with sideholes, a 5.5F cutter, and place the TEC wire in the posterolateral branch. There is no risk of sidebranch occlusion because the TEC cutter will not "snow-plow" the lesion if the cutter is advanced slowly. Once thrombus is removed, I would leave the TEC wire in the PDA and place another guidewire in the posterolateral branch. I would then dilate with a 2.5 mm balloon.

> **Editors' Perspective: In the absence of thrombus, TEC has no particular role for this type of lesion. If thrombus is present at or near the bifurcation, TEC may be reasonable to extract thrombus, rather than debulk plaque. Because of the risk of dissection, small (cutter/artery ratio < 0.6) cutters should be employed, followed by "kissing" balloon angioplasty.**

*****

TEC: CALCIFIED LESION

TEC atherectomy of a calcified lesion in the mid-LAD (reference diameter = 2.9 mm).

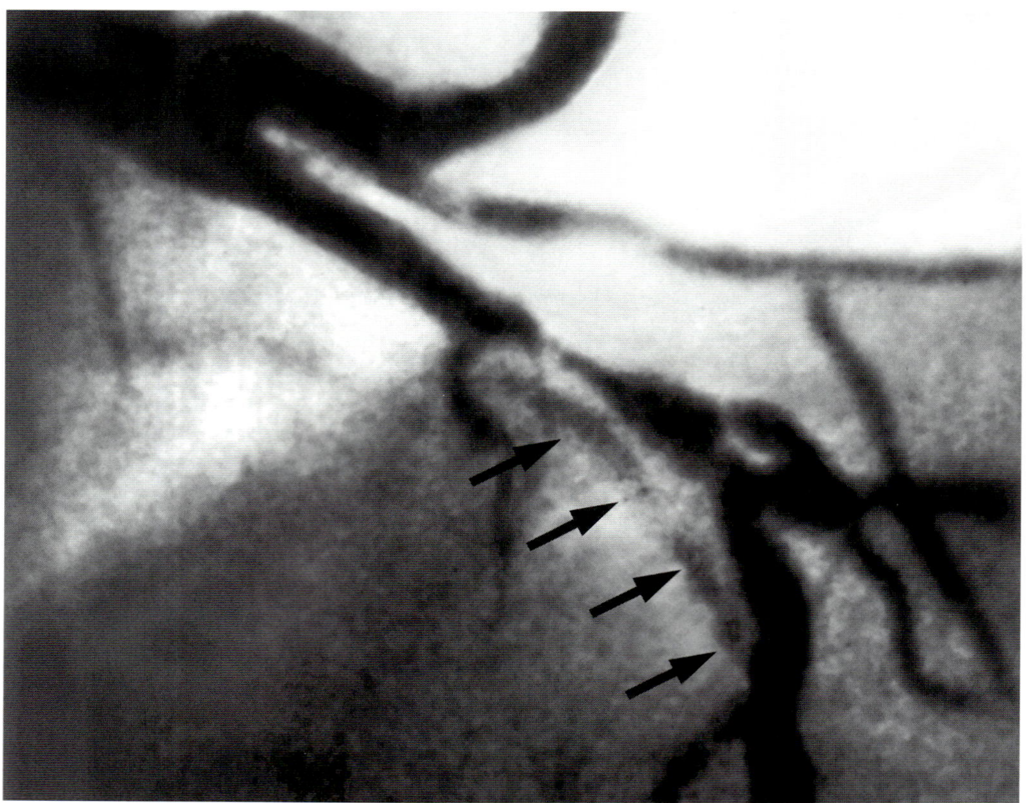

Is TEC reasonable for this lesion?

William O'Neill, MD, USA: This lesion could be treated with TEC, but no advantage exists.

Barry George, MD, USA: The angiogram shows a calcified LAD lesion, which is not suitable for TEC.

Patrick Whitlow, MD, USA: TEC atherectomy is not a serious consideration for calcified lesions.

> **Editors' Perspective: TEC has limited ability to cut calcium and has no role in the treatment of calcified lesions.**

*****

TEC: CALCIFIED OSTIAL RCA

TEC atherectomy of a calcified ostial lesion in the RCA (reference diameter = 2.8 mm).

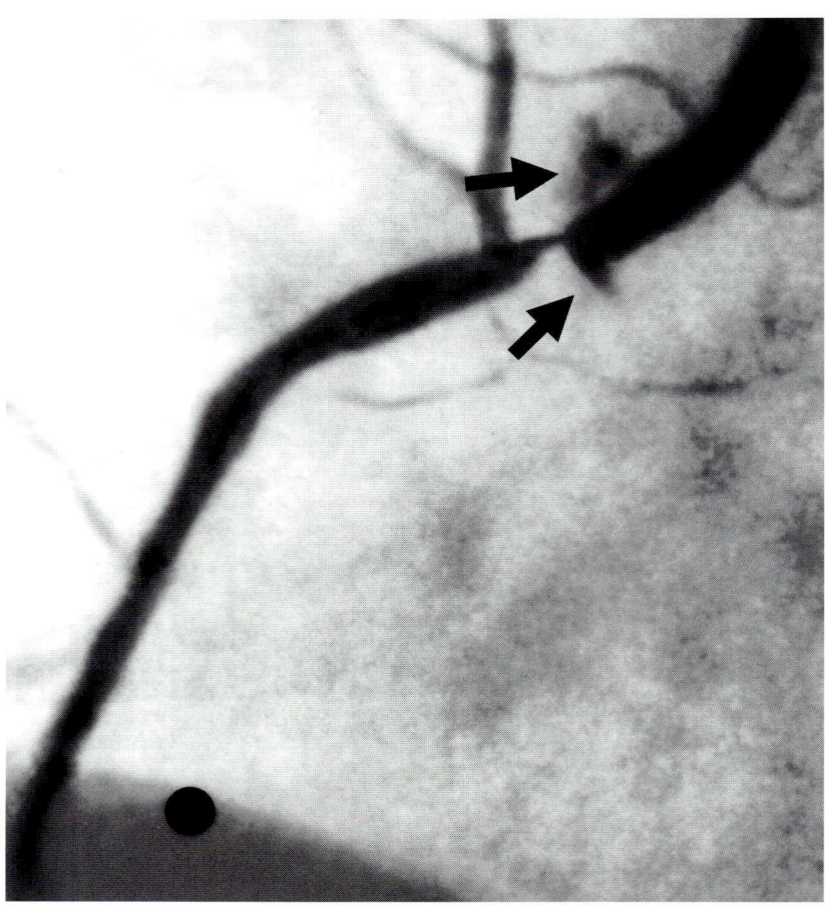

Is TEC reasonable for this lesion?

William O'Neill, MD, USA: Great caution must be used in treating this eccentric plaque with TEC, since the cutter will be directed inferiorly. Fortunately, this is where the bulk of the plaque exists.

Barry George, MD, USA: This ostial, calcified lesion is not suitable for TEC.

Patrick Whitlow, MD, USA: TEC atherectomy is contraindicated in this type of lesion.

Comment on device sizing and important technical tips.

William O'Neill, MD, USA: I would use a 10F guiding catheter, followed by a 5.5F, a 6.5F and, if possible, a 7.5F cutter to aggressively remove as much plaque as possible (but stop if a dissection occurs).

> **Editors' Perspective: TEC is relatively ineffective as an atherectomy device, despite its ability to aspirate thrombus, and should not be used by inexperienced operators when lesion calcium is present.**

*****

TEC: OSTIAL DIAGONAL

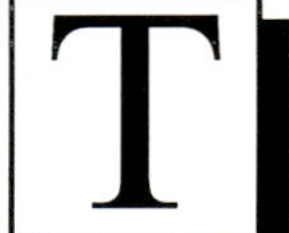

EC atherectomy of an ostial lesion in the diagonal branch (reference diameter = 3.2 mm).

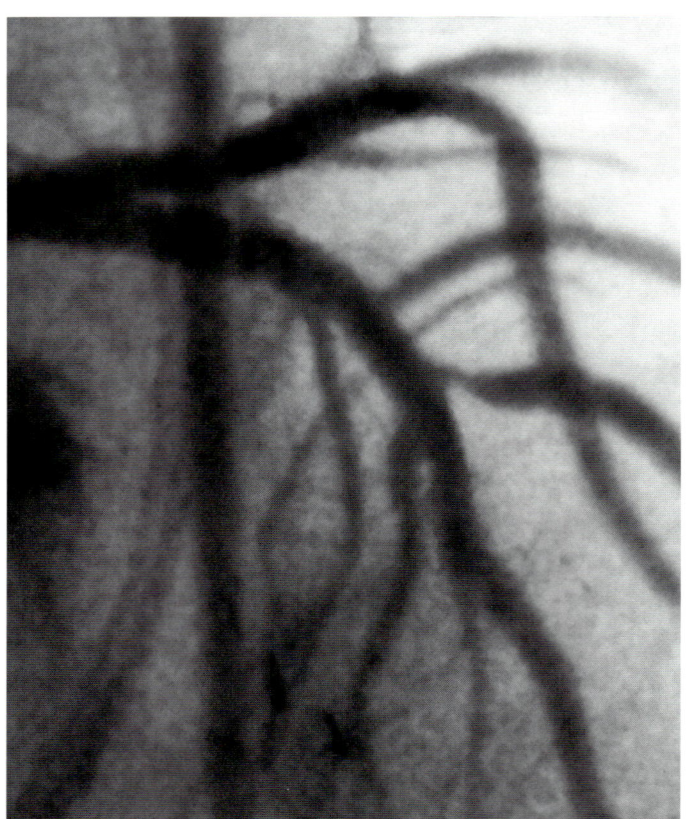

Is TEC reasonable for this lesion?

Barry George, MD, USA: Although TEC atherectomy is reasonable, I prefer stenting.

Cindy Grines, MD, USA: This ostial diagonal lesion is amenable to TEC atherectomy, but I do not recommend TEC in the absence of thrombus.

> **Editors' Perspective: In the absence of thrombus, TEC has no advantage over other techniques for this lesion.**

*****

TEC: OSTIAL LAD

TEC atherectomy of an ostial lesion in the LAD (reference diameter = 3.8 mm).

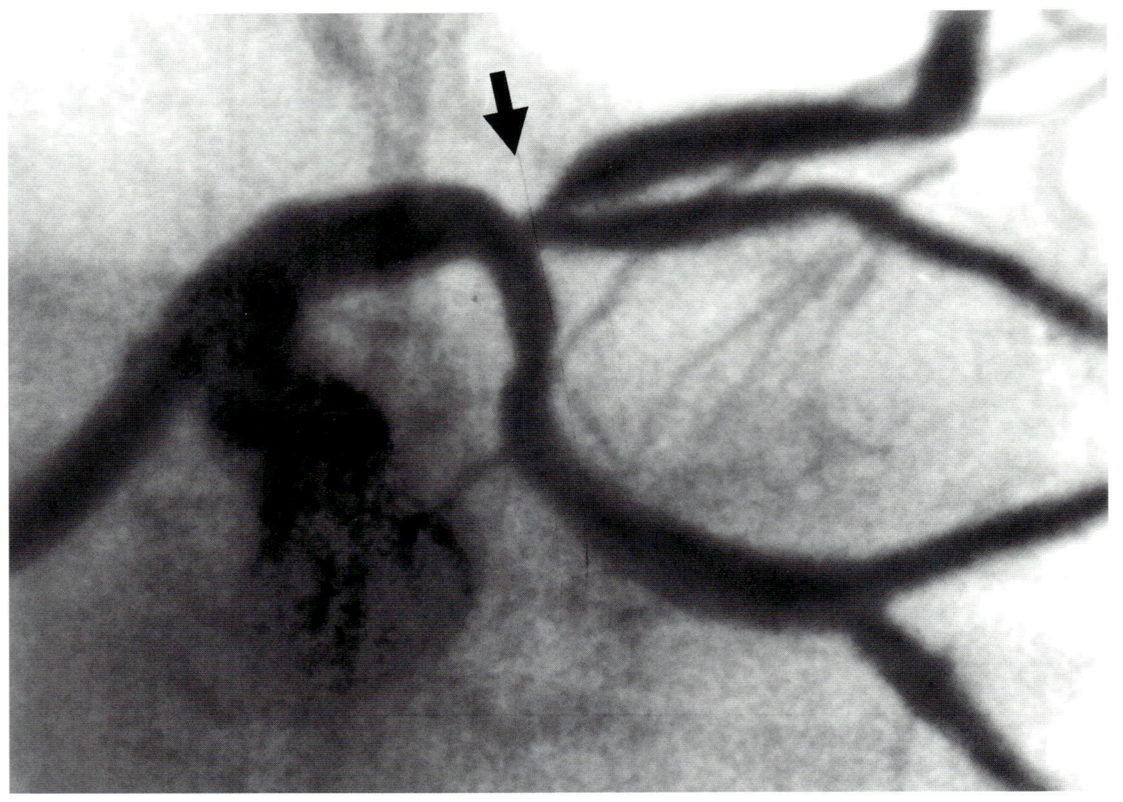

Is TEC reasonable for this lesion?

Barry George, MD, USA: TEC atherectomy is reasonable but less user-friendly than directional atherectomy.

Cindy Grines, MD, USA: Although TEC atherectomy can be performed in this lesion, the largest TEC device will be too small, and will not achieve significant lumen enlargement. I would use directional atherectomy or stenting.

> **Editors' Perspective: TEC in native coronary arteries is often associated with dissection, which in this particular location, could be problematic. In the absence of thrombus, these lesions should not be treated with TEC.**

*****

TEC: OSTIAL LCX

TEC atherectomy of an ostial lesion in the LCX (reference diameters: left main = 4.2 mm; LCX = 3.8 mm).

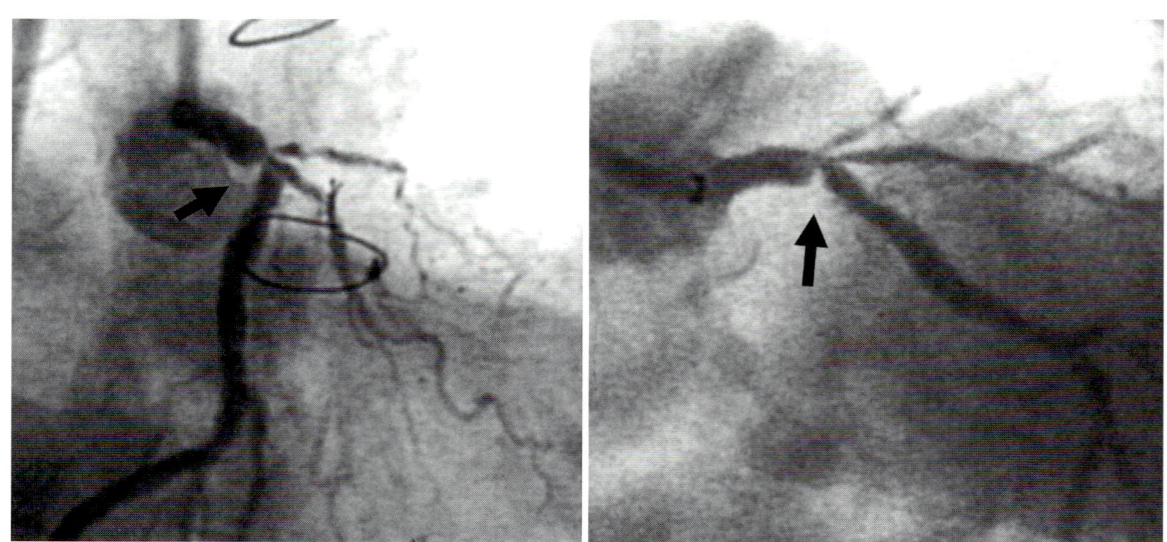

Is TEC reasonable for this lesion?

Barry George, MD, USA: I would choose the least complicated approach to achieve the best result. Although TEC could be done, I prefer directional atherectomy

Cindy Grines, MD, USA: I would not choose TEC as my first approach. The fact that the patient has had previous bypass surgery indicates that this is most likely a very rigid lesion.

Editors' Perspective: It is unlikely that TEC will offer any benefit for this lesion.

*****

TEC: DEGENERATED VEIN GRAFT

TEC atherectomy of a degenerated vein graft to the OM (reference diameter = 3.9 mm).

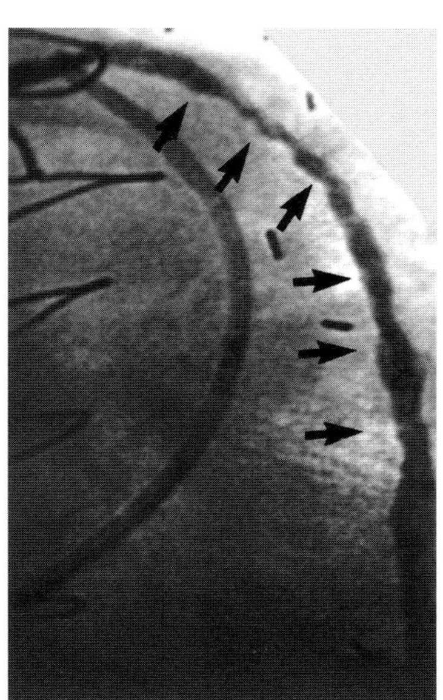

Is TEC reasonable for this lesion?

William O'Neill, MD, USA: This is excellent case for TEC.

Barry George, MD, USA: The angiogram shows a saphenous vein graft to the OM, which is markedly degenerated over 6-8 cm. There is substantial risk of distal embolization, myocardial infarction, and restenosis. This is where TEC shines.

Patrick Whitlow, MD, USA: These diffusely degenerated saphenous vein grafts have a significant chance of distal embolization no matter what modality is chosen for intervention. However, I believe that TEC atherectomy offers the lowest chance of distal embolization.

Comment on device sizing and important technical tips.

William O'Neill, MD, USA: I would use a 10F guide and a 7.5F cutter. The graft needs extensive debulking for 3-5 minutes, and at least five biliary stents to achieve definitive lumen enlargement.

Barry George, MD, USA: The saphenous vein graft to the OM has a very high "cheese index". I would use a 10F JR4 guiding catheter, a 0.014-inch TEC guidewire, and a 7.5F cutter. Careful attention to continuous suction is extremely important to minimize distal embolization. If residual stenosis is < 50%, I would not further instrument the graft. Truly, in this type of anatomy, perfection is the enemy of success. There is an extremely high likelihood of distal embolization if this lesion is treated further, and I advise against PTCA. I strongly recommend indefinite Coumadin therapy (INR 2.0-2.5) in addition to aspirin.

Patrick Whitlow, MD, USA: The TEC Amplatz guide generally fits very well into LCX vein grafts. The TEC wire can be easily negotiated into diffusely degenerated grafts. I would initially use a 6F TEC cutter, allowing a great deal of time to remove any loose material in the graft. I would follow with a 7.5F cutter. As long as flow is normal, and there are no signs of distal embolization, I would place sequential P204 biliary stents in this degenerated graft from the end of the diffuse disease all the way back to the ostium. I would utilize a 4.0 mm Schwarten balloon to deploy each stent with the same guiding catheter and TEC guidewire. I would use a 4.0 x 40 mm PET balloon to postdilate the stents at 16-18 ATM. I choose the Palmaz biliary stent because it is much easier to see, is 5 mm longer than the coronary stent, and costs half as much as the Palmaz-Schatz coronary stent.

> **Editors' Perspective: TEC is the least likely of all the percutaneous techniques to cause distal embolization and no-reflow in this situation. Unfortunately, TEC alone cannot achieve adequate lumen enlargement, and adjunctive PTCA after TEC is associated with a high risk of no-reflow and restenosis. Because of the extensive degenerative changes throughout the body of this graft, we favor TEC atherectomy with a 7-7.5F cutter, followed by 2 weeks of subcutaneous heparin to "clean-up" the graft, followed by readmission, repeat angiography, and definitive stenting. The choice of stents is largely at the discretion of the operator, but the Wallstent has the advantage of covering long segments of disease with a single stent. Alternatively, multiple biliary stents could be implanted. Redo bypass surgery should be strongly considered and may offer the best long-term result.**

This patient was treated before the availability of stents. Initial TEC atherectomy was performed with a 7.5F cutter, and was followed by adjunctive PTCA using multiple overlapping inflations with a 4.0 x 40 mm compliant balloon. There were no complications (below).

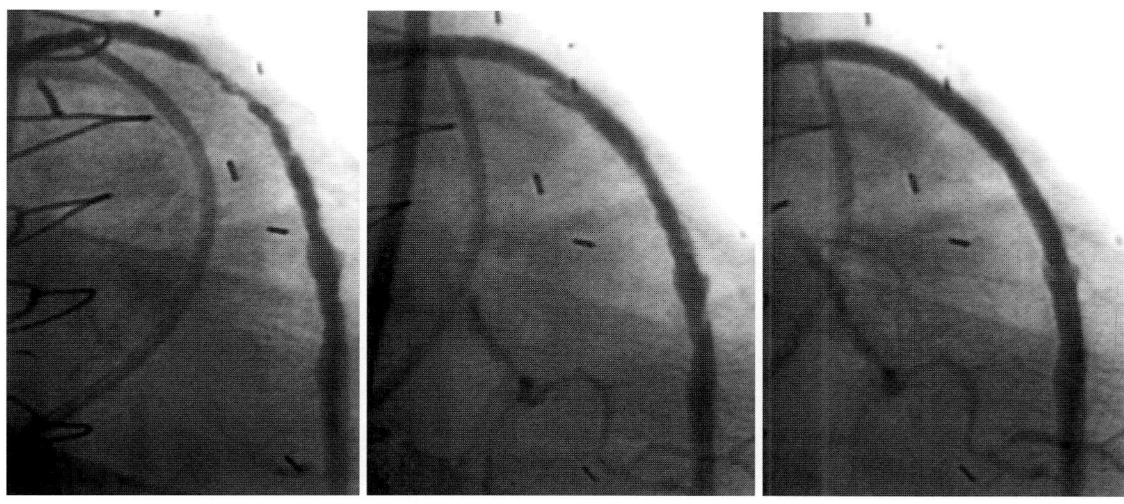

*****

TEC: OSTIAL VEIN GRAFT

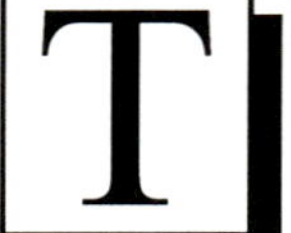

EC atherectomy of an ostial lesion in a vein graft to the LAD (reference diameter = 3.9 mm).

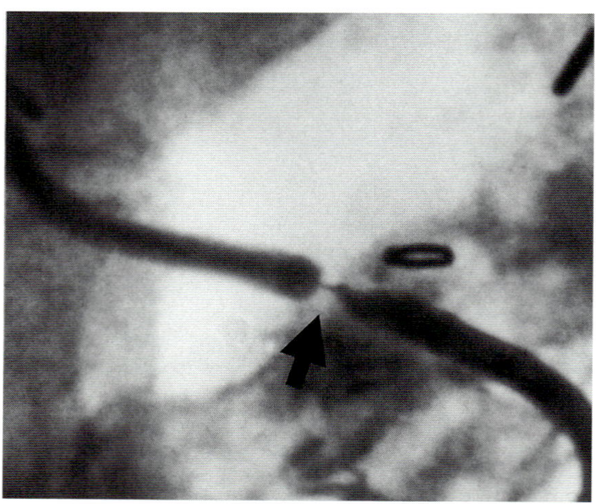

Is TEC reasonable for this lesion?

William O'Neill, MD, USA: This is an excellent lesion for TEC.

Barry George, MD, USA: TEC is reasonable for this aortoostial lesion.

Patrick Whitlow, MD, USA: Aortoostial lesions are frequently very fibrotic and hard. I have not found TEC atherectomy to be very helpful in this situation, because the cutter is not very efficient in fibrotic, hard lesions.

Comment on device sizing and important technical tips.

William O'Neill, MD, USA: I would use a 9F guide, a 6.5F cutter, and an articulated biliary stent.

Barry George, MD, USA: I would use an IVT 10F JR4 guiding catheter, a 7.5F TEC cutter, and make slow deliberate passes with careful attention to continuous suction. Following this, I would remove the TEC guidewire and leave the guiding catheter in place. I would then take a 4.5 x 20 mm Cordis Opti-5 peripheral balloon preloaded with a 0.035-inch Magic torque exchange guidewire. I would premount a 15 mm biliary stent on the Opti-5 balloon and deploy it with special care to leave 1-2 mm of the stent in the aorta. I would inflate the Opti-5 balloon at 12-14 ATM. I would be very aggressive in using the biliary stent in this aortoostial lesion because of its radial strength. I would not use Coumadin following stent deployment.

> Editors' Perspective: **TEC is most useful for aspirating thrombus. Although it could be used prior to definitive lumen enlargement using other techniques, its ability to debulk ostial lesions such as this is unpredictable. If stenting is considered for this lesion, it is important to adequately expand the ostium before stent implantation, which can be better achieved with techniques such as PTCA, Rotablator, or directional atherectomy.**

*****

TEC: VEIN GRAFT

TEC atherectomy of a vein graft to the RCA (reference diameter = 3.9 mm).

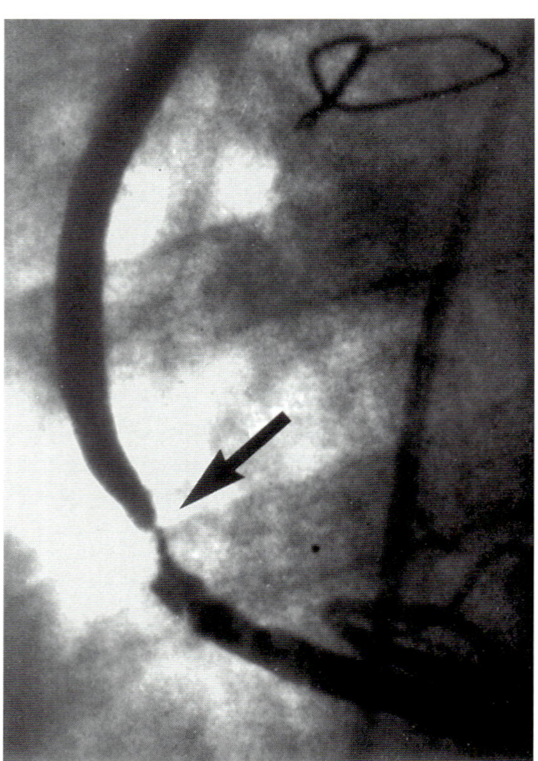

Is TEC reasonable for this lesion?

William O'Neill, MD, USA: This is an excellent case for TEC.

Barry George, MD, USA: The angiogram shows a lesion in the saphenous vein graft to the RCA, with irregular borders consistent with grumous and thrombus. This is a setup for distal embolization and procedural complications such as myocardial infarction and restenosis. I am very aggressive in stating that this is where TEC shines.

Patrick Whitlow, MD, USA: TEC atherectomy is quite effective in saphenous vein grafts because of the soft material frequently encountered in these lesions.

Comment on device sizing and important technical tips.

William O'Neill, MD, USA: I would use a 9F guide, a 6.5F cutter, and then implant an articulated PS204 biliary stent.

Barry George, MD, USA: I would use an IVT 10F JR4 guiding catheter, a 0.014-inch TEC guidewire, and a 7.5F cutter. After multiple slow passes, I would place a 4.0 x 15 mm Palmaz-Schatz coronary stent in the body of the vein graft, and postdilate with a 4.0 x 15 mm Titan at 16-18 ATM. The likelihood of distal embolization in this particular vein graft lesion is low because of the small volume of grumous and thrombotic material.

Patrick Whitlow, MD, USA: For RCA grafts, the IVT JR4 or multipurpose guide usually provides a stable platform for any intervention. The TEC guidewire could easily be placed across this lesion and provides a good rail for almost any coronary intervention. I would choose a 6F TEC cutter to allow easy passage of a 4.0 mm Palmaz-Schatz stent. After placement, I would postdilate with a 4.0 mm high-pressure balloon. TEC atherectomy followed by stenting has become my procedure of choice for saphenous vein graft lesions such as this.

> **Editors' Perspective: Saphenous vein graft lesions are frequently associated with thrombus, and as such, are ideal candidates for initial treatment with TEC. Because of the large caliber of this graft, TEC cutters ≥ 6.5F should be used to achieve maximal thrombus extraction. Since this lesion will ultimately be stented, the concern over dissection from larger TEC cutters is minimal.**

*****

TEC: SMALL THROMBUS

TEC atherectomy of a small thrombus in the proximal RCA (reference diameter = 3.4 mm).

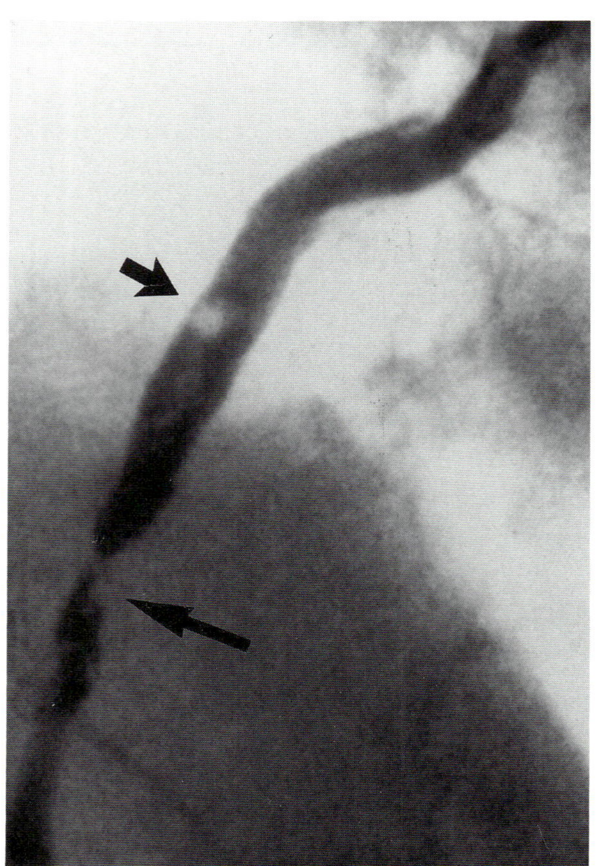

Is TEC reasonable for this lesion?

William O'Neill, MD, USA: This lesion is extremely well-suited for TEC atherectomy.

Barry George, MD, USA: There is a filling defect with intraluminal thrombus just proximal to the severe stenosis, which increases the risk of procedural complications and restenosis. TEC is feasible for this lesion.

Cindy Grines, MD, USA: This ulcerated stenosis with globular thrombus is ideal for TEC.

Comment on device sizing and important technical tips.

William O'Neill, MD, USA: I would first place a 10F JR4 or hockey stick guiding catheter and a TEC guidewire, and perform angioscopy to differentiate clot and plaque. If clot is present, I would start with a 7.5 TEC cutter and slowly advance the cutter for 2-5 minutes. I would repeat angioscopy to confirm clot removal and place two or three articulated biliary stents.

Barry George, MD, USA: I would use an IVT 10F FR4 guiding catheter over a 0.063-inch J-guidewire to reduce the likelihood of cholesterol embolization from the abdominal aorta. I would use a 0.014-inch TEC guidewire and a 7F TEC cutter. It is important to advance the device slowly. If significant resistance is encountered, I would not force the cutter, but I would perform PTCA. If the cutter passes without resistance, I would follow with a prolonged inflation with a 3.5 x 20 mm Lifestream perfusion balloon.

Cindy Grines, MD, USA: Since this is a native vessel, I would undersize the cutter. I would select a 9F JR4 and cross the lesion using the TEC wire. I would use a 6F cutter, followed by prolonged inflations with a 3.5 x 40 mm balloon.

> **<u>Editors' Perspective</u>: TEC atherectomy is an effective device for aspirating fresh thrombus from lesion such as this. The large caliber and gentle takeoff of the vessel suggest that TEC will be straightforward. Although larger cutters may achieve better aspiration of thrombus, they are also associated with more dissection in native coronary arteries. It is probably reasonable to initiate TEC with a 6F cutter (cutter/artery ratio ~ 0.6-0.7), with larger devices reserved for incomplete thrombus extraction. In our experience, TEC is extremely efficient at thrombus removal, but adjunctive stenting is frequently required to tack-up dissection and achieve definitive lumen enlargement.**

*****

TEC: LARGE THROMBUS

TEC atherectomy of a large thrombus in a degenerated vein graft (reference diameter = 5.2 mm).

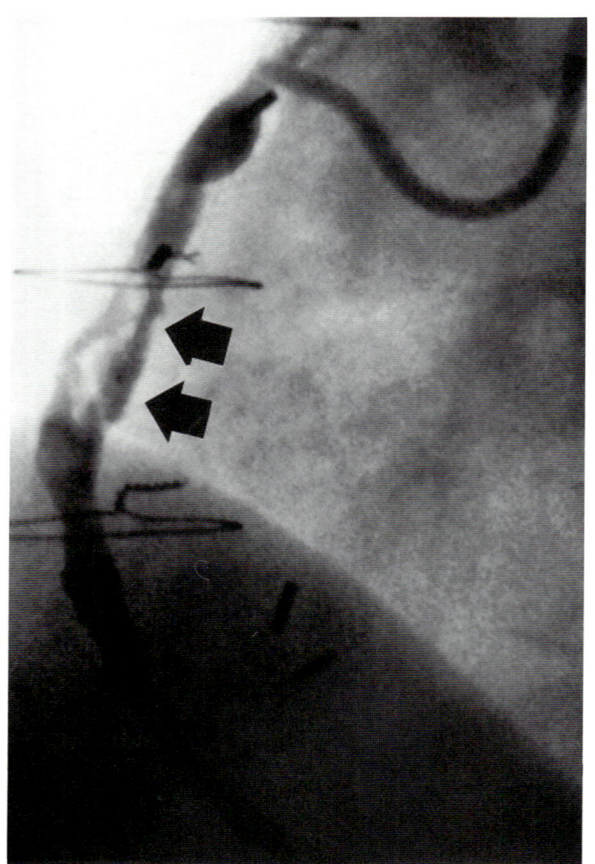

Is TEC reasonable for this lesion?

William O'Neill, MD, USA: This degenerated vein graft with a filling defect is suited for TEC atherectomy. However, it is impossible to know if thrombus is present based solely on angiographic criteria. If the patient has a recent acute ischemic syndrome, then thrombus is inevitably present.

Barry George, MD, USA: There is extensive filling defect in the mid-body of the vein graft, and the angiographic appearance is one of classic degeneration with subsequent thrombus formation. Because of the amount of thrombus and grumous material, the likelihood of distal embolization is extremely high. In addition, restenosis rates are significantly higher in the degenerated saphenous vein graft. Because of the inadequacies of our hardware, complete extraction of material cannot be achieved. In my opinion, this type of lesion remains a difficult challenge. Nevertheless, I would proceed with TEC.

Cindy Grines, MD, USA: This angiogram demonstrates a degenerated saphenous vein graft to the RCA, with an extremely large thrombus. This case is ideal for TEC atherectomy.

Comment on device sizing and important technical tips.

William O'Neill, MD, USA: I would place a 10F JR4 or hockey stick guiding catheter and definitely perform angioscopy to differentiate clot from grumous. If clot is present I recommend a 7.5F TEC cutter, slowly advancing through the proximal half of the graft. The cutter will be activated for 2-5 minutes, and I would repeat angioscopy to confirm clot extraction. Then I would place two or three articulated biliary stents in the proximal vessel, all the way to the ostium. If extensive thrombus persists after TEC, I would place the patient on Coumadin, and defer further intervention and stent implantation for 4-6 weeks.

Barry George, MD, USA: I would place a TEC guidewire into the distal vessel, and make slow deliberate passes with a 7F and then a 7.5F cutter. If there is substantial debulking, I would then smoothe the body of the graft with a 5.0 x 40 mm Sub-4 peripheral balloon at low pressure, to reduce the likelihood of distal embolization. If there is concern about residual thrombotic material after using the 7.5F cutter, I would not proceed with PTCA, but would administer intracoronary urokinase (120,000 units/hour for 6-12 hours). The patient would be discharged on Coumadin and aspirin. If there is recurrent stenosis, I recommend biliary stenting. A very common pitfall in attacking these degenerated saphenous vein grafts is to keep "pounding" the body of the graft with balloons. Many times, this causes more distal embolization, no reflow, and myocardial infarction. A fundamental rule that I always use when dealing with degenerated vein graft disease is always assess the feasibility of native vessel restoration, to reduce procedural complications and restenosis.

Cindy Grines, MD, USA: I would use an IVT 10F JR4 guiding catheter, a TEC wire, and a 7-7.5F cutter. I would omit the flush solution to reduce the chance of distal embolization. It is important to perform slow passes and take the necessary time to fill at least 10 vacuum bottles. If thrombus is adequately excised, I would consider stent placement.

> **Editors' Perspective: There is no perfect solution to this problem; all devices are associated with significant risk of distal embolization and no-reflow. Nevertheless, if percutaneous revascularization is indicated, TEC is a reasonable device for thrombus extraction, which can be maximized by making slow passes with a large (≥ 7F) cutter. Dr. Grines makes an interesting point about omitting the flush solution to prevent distal embolization; although this technique has not been evaluated in detail, the flush solution may not be necessary for aspiration of fresh thrombus. The timing of adjunctive PTCA, directional atherectomy, and especially stenting following TEC atherectomy of degenerated vein grafts is a matter of debate. Observational data suggest that it may be reasonable to defer further intervention if the residual stenosis after TEC is < 50%. Our bias is to discharge the patient on subcutaneous heparin for 2 weeks, then readmit the patient for implantation of a Wallstent. TEC atherectomy was performed in this case using a 10F multipurpose guide and a 7.5F TEC cutter, but was complicated by refractory no-reflow, which failed to respond to intracoronary nitrates, verapamil, and urokinase delivered directly into the distal vessel. Hypotension and bradycardia ensued, necessitating insertion of an intraaortic balloon pump and temporary pacemaker. The patient was ultimately discharged from the hospital, but only after a stormy hospital course complicated by Q-wave myocardial infarction, bleeding, and blood transfusions.**

*****

Rotablator Techniques

ROTABLATOR: ECCENTRIC LESION (LAD)

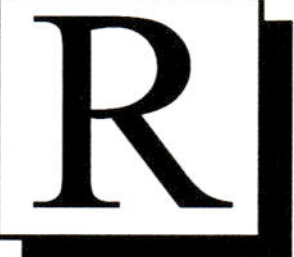otablator atherectomy of an eccentric lesion in the proximal LAD (reference diameter = 3.4 mm).

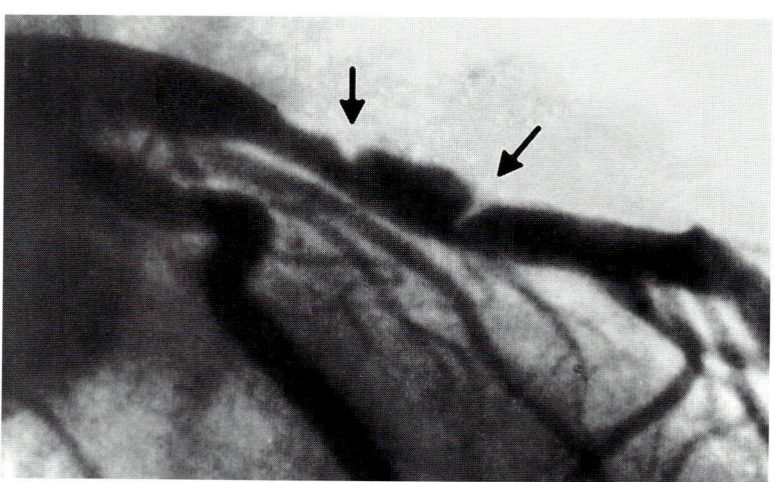

Is Rotablator reasonable for this lesion?

Michael Cowley, MD, USA: The proximal LAD has a moderate eccentric narrowing of 50% and there is a severe, highly eccentric "shelf-like" narrowing in the adjacent segment. The lesion morphology is not well suited for Rotablator because the proximal narrowing would require a very large burr to achieve any lumen enlargement, and the shelf-like narrowing is better treated with other devices (in the absence of calcification).

Nicolaus Reifart, MD, Germany: The Rotablator is reasonable since it produces a more predictable acute result in this type of morphology.

Raimund Erbel, MD, Germany: The lesion should not be treated with Rotablator, because it is a Type C lesion (eccentric and unstable). If IVUS demonstrates severe calcification, the Rotablator is my first choice.

Comment on device sizing and important technical tips.

Nicolaus Reifart, MD, Germany: I recommend a 1.75 mm burr (175,000-190,000 RPM for 10-15 seconds) and upsize to a 2.0 mm burr, followed by a 3.5 x 40 mm Europass at 2-3 ATM. If this balloon is not fully inflated at 4 ATM, I would exchange the balloon for a 2.25 mm burr to debulk more plaque, and then dilate again at low pressure. A long perfusion balloon (ACS Lifestream) may be very helpful after rotablation because it allows prolonged inflations at low pressure. I prefer a cautious burr strategy (burr/artery ratio ~ 0.5-0.6), short spinning intervals (10-15 seconds), 10-20 seconds between runs, and a rotaflush cocktail of saline (500 cc), verapamil (5 mg), and nitroglycerin (2 mg) to prevent spasm and no-reflow.

Editors' Perspective: The value of Rotablator for eccentric lesions is a matter of controversy. In our practice, we would not consider Rotablator for this type of lesion unless fluoroscopy (or IVUS) demonstrates significant calcification that might prevent adequate lumen enlargement by PTCA, directional atherectomy, or stenting. For operators who would perform Rotablator, the ideal burr/artery ratio is unknown. It is possible that burrs > 2.38 mm could be used as a "stand-alone" strategy, but it is more likely that adjunctive devices will be needed for definitive lumen enlargement.

*****

ROTABLATOR: ECCENTRIC LESION (RCA)

Rotablator atherectomy of an eccentric lesion in the mid-RCA (reference diameter = 3.2 mm).

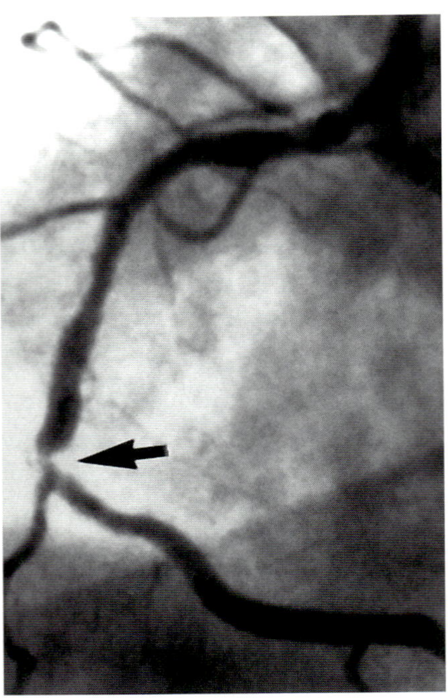

Is Rotablator reasonable for this lesion?

Michael Cowley, MD, USA: Rotablator is a reasonable device for this lesion. Although the lesion is eccentric and located in a bend, the degree of angulation is mild and should not be associated with technical difficulties.

Nicolaus Reifart, MD, Germany: This patient has diffuse disease with an eccentric lesion in a bend in the mid-RCA. The Rotablator is reasonable for this lesion.

Raimund Erbel, MD, Germany: The Rotablator is ideal.

Comment on device sizing and important technical tips.

Michael Cowley, MD, USA: Rotational ablation would involve debulking with sequential burrs to a final burr/artery ratio of 0.75-0.80. Since the lesion is not extremely tight, I would start with a 1.75 mm or 2.0 mm burr, followed by a 2.25 mm burr. Depending on the angiographic result, a 2.38 mm or 2.50 mm burr might be used for further debulking. Larger burrs may not be needed with eccentric lesions due to preferential ablation of eccentric plaque. When the burr/artery ratio is ~ 0.8, PTCA is often not necessary. However, if the final burr/artery ratio is < 0.7, adjunctive PTCA is usually necessary to achieve a satisfactory final result.

Nicolaus Reifart, MD, Germany: Since the significant lesion is focal, I would start with a 2.0 mm burr and follow with a 3.5 x 35 mm Speedy. In RCA lesions, I use prophylactic atropine and short (5-10 seconds) ablation sequences to avoid AV block.

> **Editors' Perspective: Use of the Rotablator for this lesion is straightforward. However, optimal burr size, burr/artery ratio, and adjunctive PTCA technique are currently under evaluation. Because of the relatively long segment of moderate disease proximal to the target lesion, it may be necessary to adjust the platform speed in the proximal RCA (about 3-5 mm from the tip of the guiding catheter) to avoid engaging the moderate lesion with the Rotablator burr.**

*****

ROTABLATOR: ULCERATED LESION

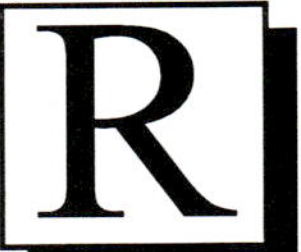

Rotablator atherectomy of an ulcerated lesion in the mid-LAD (reference diameter = 3.2 mm).

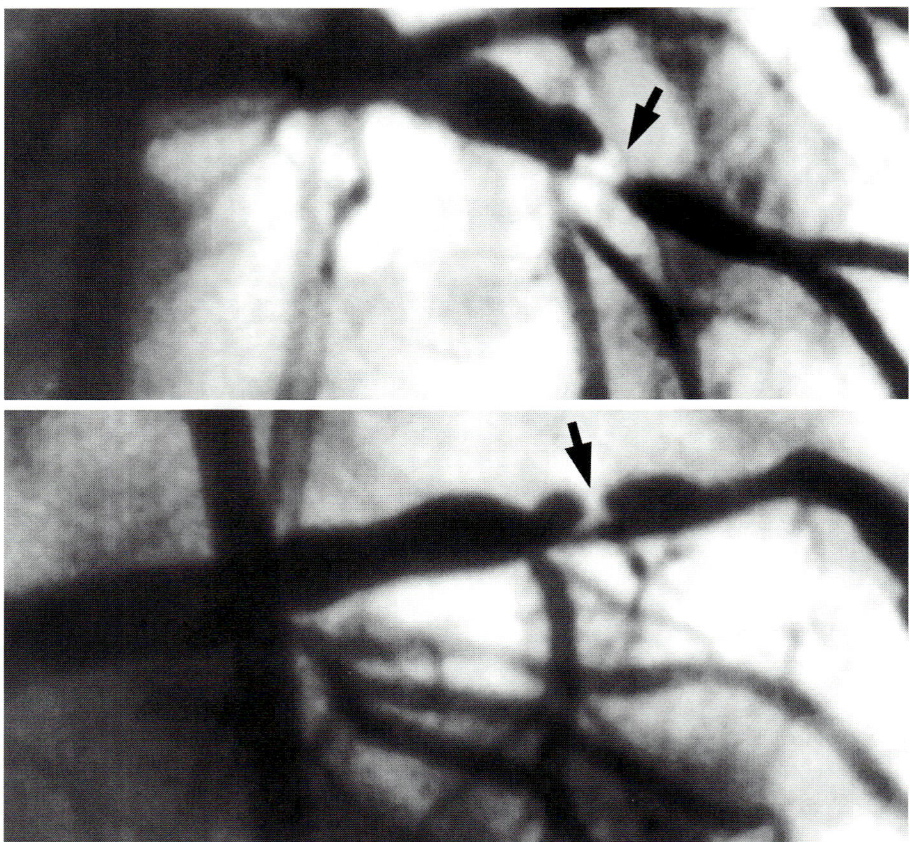

Is Rotablator reasonable for this lesion?

Raimund Erbel, MD, Germany: The Rotablator is the ideal device for this lesion.

Paul Teirstein, MD, USA: The lesion is an ulcerated, eccentric stenosis in the LAD. If moderate calcification is noted on fluoroscopy, I would proceed with Rotablator.

Michael Mooney, MD, USA: This proximal LAD has a complex ulcerated stenosis at a bifurcation, adding to already significant complexity. This is not a case for rotational atherectomy due to the inability to protect the sidebranch and the complexity of the lesion.

Comment on device sizing and important technical tips.

Paul Teirstein, MD, USA: I would use an 8F JL4 guide catheter with sideholes, and start with 1.5 mm and 2.0 mm burrs to debulk this lesion. I would then place a 3.0 mm balloon across the stenosis to predilate it, and exchange for a 0.014-inch Extra-S'port guidewire. I would then deploy a 3.0 mm Palmaz-Schatz coronary stent, and postdilate with a 3.5 x 9-10 mm balloon at 16 ATM. I would use IVUS.

Editors' Perspective: Our experts disagree about the value of Rotablator atherectomy for this lesion. In the absence of significant calcification, we see little advantage to the Rotablator in this setting, especially since the markedly abnormal contour increases the likelihood that directional atherectomy or stenting will be necessary. On the other hand, if studies in progress demonstrate that debulking with Rotablator facilitates stenting, then "Rotastent" may be valuable. In our practice, we currently limit the use of Rotastenting to ostial and/or calcified lesions in vessels that are otherwise suitable for stenting.

*****

ROTABLATOR: TUBULAR LESION

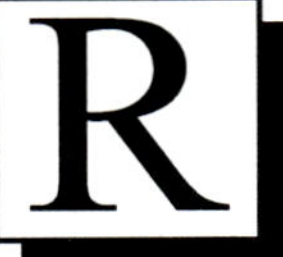
Rotablator atherectomy of a tubular lesion in the mid-RCA (length = 15 mm; reference diameter = 2.5 mm).

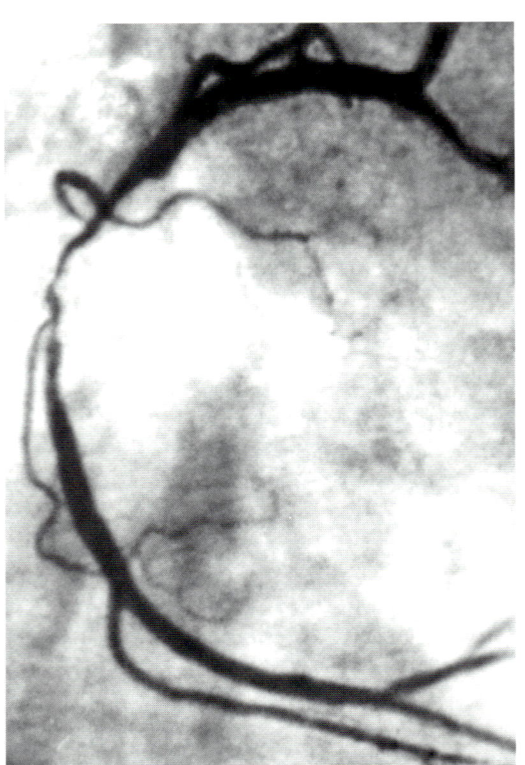

Is Rotablator reasonable for this lesion?

Michael Mooney, MD, USA: This is an ideal lesion for the Rotablator, because it is a long stenosis in a relatively small artery. Rotational atherectomy is clearly the best strategy here.

Patrick Whitlow, MD, USA: The Rotablator is an excellent device for debulking long lesions, and is definitely my device of choice for this lesion.

Richard Myler, MD, USA: Rotablator atherectomy is suitable for this lesion

Comment on device sizing and important technical tips.

Michael Mooney, MD, USA: I would pretreat this patient with intracoronary diltiazem (2 mg over 12 minutes up to a total of 10 mg) to prevent microvascular spasm, and definitely place a temporary pacemaker. I use a step-burr approach with a Rotablator-C wire, and 1.75 mm and 2.0 mm burrs. I would then postdilate at low pressure with a 3.0 x 40 mm balloon.

Patrick Whitlow, MD, USA: In the early Rotablator experience, these lesions were associated with increased complications. My experience in the last few years has taught me to use small and then progressively larger burrs, to limit runs to 15-30 seconds, to advance the burr slowly, not let the speed decrease by more than 5,000 RPM, and use verapamil and nitroglycerin in the flush solution. With this newer and gentler technique, the Rotablator is associated with very high success and low complication rates, even with long lesions. I would use a 9F FR4 guiding catheter, a Rotablator-C wire, a temporary pacing catheter, and make sure that the patient is well hydrated. I would start with a 1.5 mm burr, and then step-up by quarter sizes to a final burr size of 2.0 mm. I would then use a 3.0 mm noncompliant balloon at 1-2 ATM. It is important to assess coronary flow by contrast injection during and after each Rotablator run. If flow decreases, the Rotablator should be parked in the guiding catheter until the ST segments return to normal, the patient's chest pain resolves, and the TIMI flow is normal. Nitroglycerin should be used liberally, and intracoronary verapamil is helpful for slow-flow.

Richard Myler, MD, USA: I would use slow passes with a 1.5 mm burr over a 0.009-inch Rotablator-C wire via an 8F large lumen JR4 guiding catheter, upsizing to a 2.0 mm burr. IVUS may indicate whether a 2.15 mm burr or adjunctive PTCA is necessary with a 2.5 x 30 mm PET balloon at low-pressure.

> **Editors' Perspective: Early reports of Rotablator for long lesions were disappointing, due to the high incidence of no-reflow and non-Q-wave myocardial infarction. However, as described by Dr. Whitlow, appreciation for the nuances of Rotablator technique have decreased the risk of complications and improved immediate results. When performing rotational atherectomy in long lesions, it is important to be patient — excessive haste can lead to suboptimal results. Several technical points are worth emphasizing: First, short (< 30 seconds) ablation runs are preferred to minimize particulate debris and**

embolization; it is not necessary to traverse the entire length of the lesion during the initial pass. Second, it is best to allow ample time between passes for resolution of chest pain, ECG changes, and impaired flow; liberal use of intracoronary nitrates and calcium channel blockers will help promote flow. Third, the addition of nitrates, a calcium channel blocker, and heparin to the Rotablator flush bag may attenuate flow disturbances during the procedure. Fourth, the burr should be slowly and gently advanced into the lesion using RPM surveillance; burr deceleration > 5000 RPM indicates that burr advancement is too aggressive. Fifth, frequent injections of contrast during rotablation can help the operator assess burr advancement and position, and can promote distal runoff by inducing reactive hyperemia. Antegrade flow of contrast should always be evident during ablation; if not, the burr should be retracted slightly. Finally, it is best to start with small burrs and work up to larger burrs in 0.25-0.5 mm increments. The operator should be willing to accept the increased procedural cost in lieu of better immediate results. Although these recommendations may improve acute procedural success rates, their impact on late outcome is unknown; clear superiority to PTCA with a long balloon has not yet been demonstrated.

*****

ROTABLATOR: LONG LESION

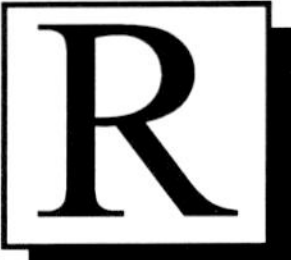

Rotablator atherectomy of a long lesion in the mid-LAD (length = 25 mm; reference diameter = 3.3 mm).

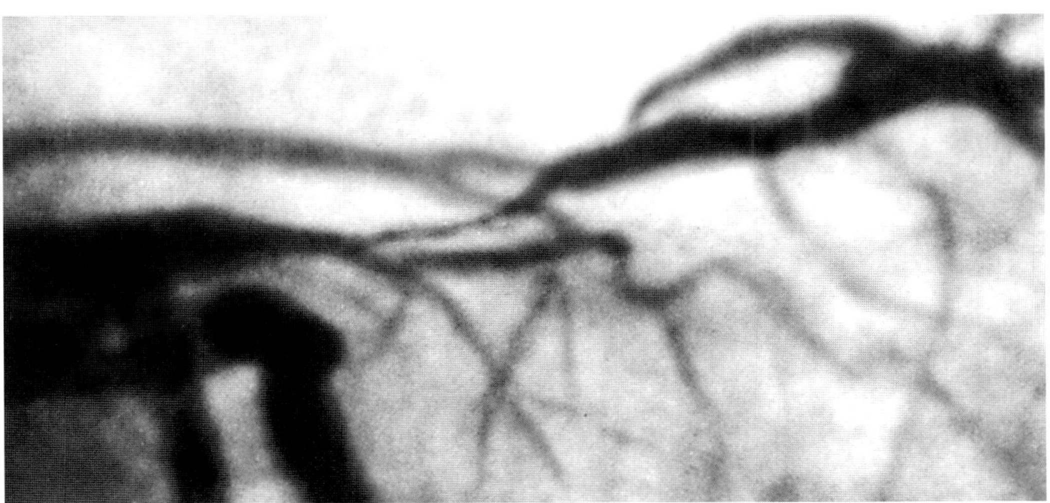

Is Rotablator reasonable for this lesion?

Michael Mooney, MD, USA: This long lesion is optimally managed with Rotablator atherectomy only if the artery is heavily calcified on fluoroscopy.

Patrick Whitlow, MD, USA: The Rotablator is reasonable; it is my first choice for this long lesion.

Richard Myler, MD, USA: This lesion is suitable for Rotablator atherectomy.

Comment on device sizing and important technical tips.

Michael Mooney, MD, USA: A routine pitfall is to assess the degree of calcification on cine; fluoroscopy is much more accurate. In this setting, intravascular ultrasound is clearly helpful to identify superficial calcification, which most strongly impacts both the acute and long term outcome. If significant calcification is present, rotablation followed by stenting is the most appropriate strategy.

Patrick Whitlow, MD, USA: The LAD has an excellent runoff bed, and rotablation of long lesions is better tolerated in the LAD than in the LCX or RCA. With the technique modifications noted previously, complications are unusual. I would use a 9F short tip JL4 guiding catheter with sideholes, to point the barrel of the guiding catheter toward the LAD without deeply intubating the left main. Sideholes allow adequate flow into the LCX. A Rotablator-C wire would easily negotiate this long and straight lesion (I rarely use the type A wire because of its stiff distal tip). I would begin with a 1.5 mm burr and step-up in 0.25 mm increments to avoid rapid release of debris in the distal bed. Burr advancement should be extremely slow, with sufficient time between each run for normalization of ST segments, resolution of chest pain, and restoration of TIMI-3 flow. The final burr size is likely to be 2.25 mm, followed by PTCA with a 3.5 x 40 mm noncompliant balloon at 1-2 ATM.

Richard Myler, MD, USA: I would start with a 1.5 mm burr using very slow passes with incremental increases in burr size to 2.25 mm, via a 9F large lumen JL4 guiding catheter. IVUS before (to evaluate the lesion) and afterwards (to assess the need for further therapy) is recommended. I would use adjunctive PTCA with a 3.5 x 30 mm PET balloon at low pressure.

Editors' Perspective: Even in large caliber vessels, Rotablator is frequently applied to debulk the lesion prior to more definitive therapy to enlarge the lumen. Several studies suggest that pretreatment with Rotablator can facilitate subsequent enlargement with PTCA, although a restenosis benefit has not yet been confirmed with this approach. "Rotastenting" is gaining popularity among interventionalists, but has not yet been shown to be superior to PTCA alone, Rotablator plus PTCA, or stenting. In the presence of significant calcification by fluoroscopy or IVUS, "Rotastenting" seems a reasonable approach.

In treating long lesions with the Rotablator, several points should be emphasized: First, the risk of distal embolization, no-reflow, and myocardial infarction can be reduced by using small burrs, brief ablation runs, and 30-60 second intervals between runs. Second, burr deceleration should never be allowed to exceed 5,000 RPM; if this occurs, the burr should be retracted to minimize dissection, large particulate embolization, and burr stalling. Third, it is not necessary to traverse the entire length of the lesion in the first pass; a slow, gentle pecking motion is preferred. Fourth, liberal use of intracoronary nitrates and calcium antagonists will promote vasodilation and attenuate spasm. Fifth, increases in burr size should be limited to 0.25-0.50 mm increments; smaller increments are recommended when burrs > 2.0 mm are employed. Finally, adjunctive PTCA with low-pressure inflations using noncompliant balloons are useful to minimize barotrauma and dissection.

*****

ROTABLATOR: FUNCTIONAL TOTAL OCCLUSION

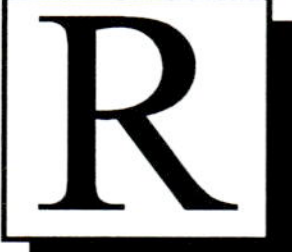

Rotablator atherectomy of a functional total occlusion in the proximal LAD (reference diameter = 2.7 mm). Assume the occlusion can be crossed with a guidewire.

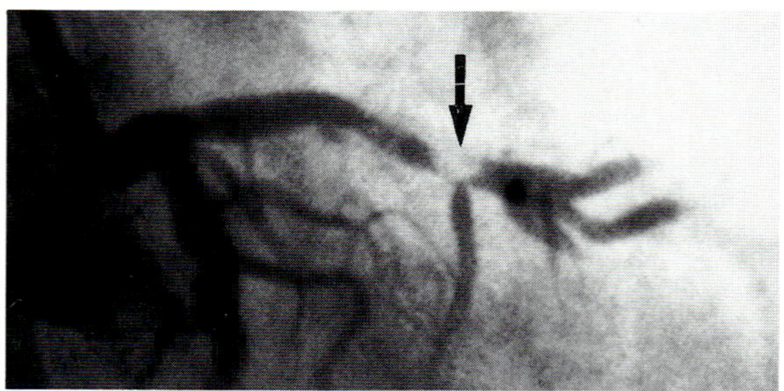

Is Rotablator reasonable for this lesion?

Richard Myler, MD, USA: Rotablator is not reasonable for this lesion because thrombus (probably associated with an unstable fissured plaque) adversely affects outcome, due to embolic debris, no-reflow, spasm and dissection.

Michael Cowley, MD, USA: Rotablator should not be used because it is ineffective in debulking soft thrombotic material, and it will likely cause distal embolization and no-reflow.

Nicolaus Reifart, MD, Germany: This LAD lesion probably contains thrombotic material; Rotablator is not indicated in this case.

Editors' Perspective: Conventional wisdom suggests that Rotablator should be avoided in lesions with thrombus due to the risk of no-reflow.

*****

ROTABLATOR: TOTAL OCCLUSION

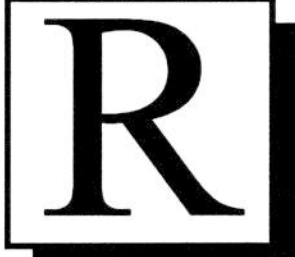
otablator atherectomy of a total occlusion in the proximal RCA (reference diameter = 4.5 mm). Assume the occlusion can be crossed with a guidewire.

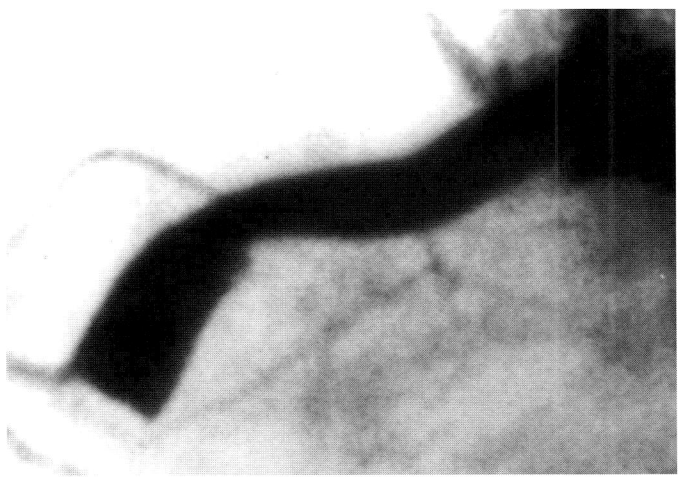

Is Rotablator reasonable for this lesion?

Richard Myler, MD, USA: Rotational atherectomy is not reasonable; the sharp cut-off strongly suggests acute or subacute thrombus (and an acute ischemic syndrome).

Michael Cowley, MD, USA: Rotablation is not appropriate for this vessel which has the angiographic appearance of a large, fresh thrombotic total occlusion.

Nicolaus Reifart, MD, Germany: Rotablator is not recommended because the lesion looks very much like a recent thrombotic occlusion.

Editors' Perspective: Rotablator should not be used for thrombotic lesions because of the risk of no-reflow and distal embolization.

*****

ROTABLATOR: ANGULATED LESION (LAD)

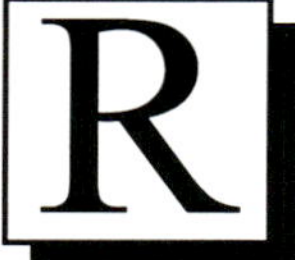

Rotablator atherectomy of an angulated lesion in the proximal LAD (lesion on inner curve; reference diameter = 3.4 mm).

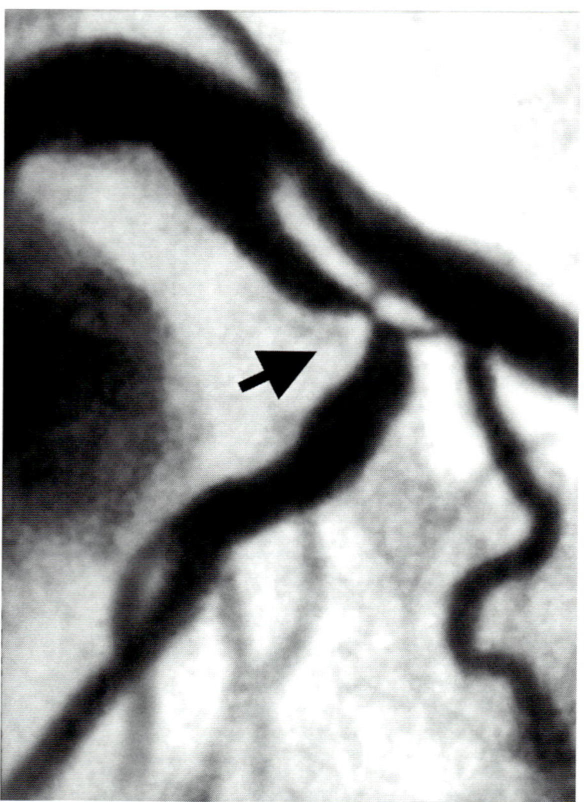

Is Rotablator reasonable for this lesion?

Nicolaus Reifart, MD, Germany: This proximal LAD lesion on the inner curve may be treated by Rotablator and adjunctive PTCA.

Paul Teirstein, MD, USA: The proximal LAD contains a concentric lesion located on a significant bend. If the lesion is calcified, I would proceed with rotational atherectomy.

Comment on device sizing and important technical tips.

Nicolaus Reifart, MD, Germany: After insertion of an 8F JL4 guiding catheter and a Rotablator-C wire, I would use 1.75 mm and 2.0 mm burrs. I would not select a larger burr because of the risk of perforation. I would perform adjunctive PTCA with a 3.5 x 20 mm balloon expanded to 1-2 ATM.

Paul Teirstein, MD, USA: I would select a 9F JL4 catheter with sideholes and use sequential 1.75 mm and 2.0 mm burrs to debulk this lesion. I would then use a 3.0 mm balloon, exchange for a 0.014-inch Extra-S'port guidewire, deploy a 3.5 mm coronary stent, and use a 4.0 mm short high-pressure balloon to optimally expand the stent. I would use intravascular ultrasound.

Editors' Perspective: Moderate angulation has little or no influence on the ability of the Rotablator to access the lesion, as might occur with rigid stents or directional atherectomy. The Rotablator drive shaft is extremely flexible and the high-speed burr rotation reduces friction, thus facilitating access to moderately angulated lesions. In severely angulated lesions, however, the drive shaft may become compressed, precluding successful access to the lesion. For angulated lesions located on the *inner* curve, Rotablator should be used cautiously (if at all), since the Rotablator burr may deflect off the plaque and into the outer normal wall, increasing the risk of dissection or perforation. If necessary, small burrs (burr/artery ratio < 0.6) should be employed, and definitive lumen enlargement should be achieved with balloons or stents, rather than with larger burrs. In contrast, plaque located on the *outer* curve of an angulated lesion can be treated with the Rotablator, since the burr will deflect off plaque and into the center of the vessel lumen. Again, relatively small burrs should be used.

*****

ROTABLATOR: ANGULATED LESION (RCA)

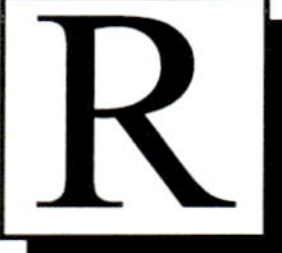

Rotablator atherectomy of an angulated lesion in the proximal RCA (lesion on outer curve; reference diameter = 3.1 mm).

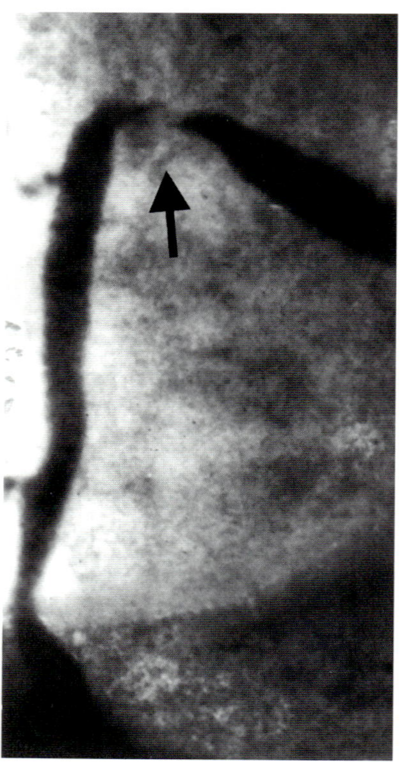

Is Rotablator reasonable for this lesion?

Nicolaus Reifart, MD, Germany: This proximal, very eccentric, and subtotal RCA lesion with plaque on the outer curve will respond nicely to Rotablator.

Paul Teirstein, MD, USA: The lesion is on a bend; if calcified, Rotablator is reasonable.

Comment on device sizing and important technical tips.

Paul Teirstein, MD, USA: If the lesion is calcified, I would use an 8F JR4 or hockey stick guide with sideholes, a 1.5 mm followed by a 2.0 mm burr, and a 3.0 mm balloon. While the balloon is across the stenosis, I would exchange for a 0.014-inch Extra-S'port or Platinum-Plus guidewire, and then deploy a 3.0 mm Palmaz-Schatz stent. I would use a 3.5 mm x 10 mm balloon at 16 ATM to expand the stent. I would use intravascular ultrasound.

Patrick Whitlow, MD, USA: Care is necessary to pass the burr extremely slowly so that it does not "jump" through the lesion and into the normal wall. However, with care, the Rotablator should effectively debulk this lesion without complication. I would utilize a 9F guiding catheter with sideholes, at Rotablator-C wire, and a 1.75 mm burr. I would follow with a 2.25 mm burr and finish the procedure with a 3.25 mm noncompliant balloon inflated to 1-2 ATM.

> **Editors' Perspective: In angulated lesions with plaque located on the outer curve, Rotablator atherectomy may be considered, particularly if the target lesion is calcified. Atherectomy should be initiated with a small (e.g., 1.5 mm) burr. Larger burrs may be used cautiously, but a final burr/artery ratio < 0.7 will enhance the safety of the procedure in such complex lesions. In addition, slow passes should be performed to allow optimal contact of the burr with the plaque.**

*****

ROTABLATOR: TORTUOUS LCX

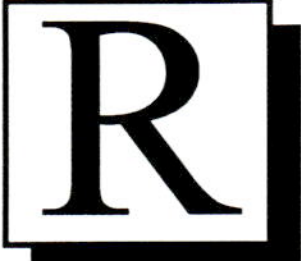
otablator atherectomy of a focal lesion in a tortuous LCX (right angle takeoff; reference diameter = 2.6 mm).

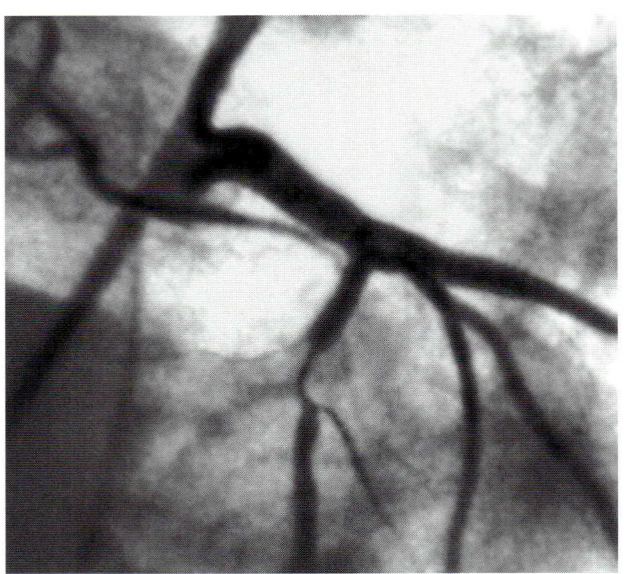

Is Rotablator reasonable for this lesion?

Paul Teirstein, MD, USA: The lesion is relatively discrete and concentric. If there is calcium, I favor Rotablator. If not, I favor PTCA.

Michael Mooney, MD, USA: There is no specific indication or contraindication for rotational atherectomy in this type A lesion.

Michael Cowley, MD, USA: Rotational ablation is a reasonable approach for this tubular LCX lesion, which is about 7-8 mm in length. The angulation will not present technical difficulties, and rotational ablation is usually highly effective for these lesions whether or not calcium is present.

Comment on device sizing and important technical tips.

Paul Teirstein, MD, USA: If this lesion is calcified, I would use 1.5 mm and 2.0 mm burrs, followed by a 2.5 mm balloon at 3 ATM.

Michael Cowley, MD, USA: I would use an 8F large lumen (0.086-inch ID) JL4 guide, a Rotablator-C wire, a 1.5 mm and a 2.0 mm burr, and a slow pass technique with ablation runs of 30-60 seconds, being very careful to avoid a decrease in rotational speed > 5,000 RPM. This technique minimizes thermal injury and spasm. A final burr of 2.0 mm will achieve a burr/artery ratio 0.75, which represents excellent debulking. If the angiogram shows smooth luminal margins, postdilation might not be necessary. However, I would perform adjunctive PTCA for residual narrowing or spasm, using a 3.0 mm balloon at 1 ATM.

> **<u>Editors' Perspective</u>: This target lesion is readily treated by Rotablator atherectomy if so desired by the operator. The right angle takeoff of the LCX from the left main is not a contraindication to the Rotablator, since the target lesion is distal to this angulated segment. In the absence of proximal vessel calcification, the proximal vessel will "yield" to the advancing burr without difficulty.**

*****

ROTABLATOR: TORTUOUS RCA

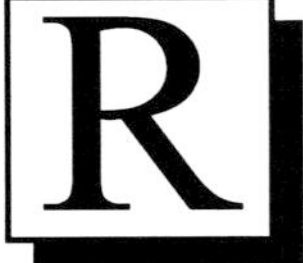

otablator atherectomy of a focal lesion in a tortuous RCA (reference diameter = 3.2 mm).

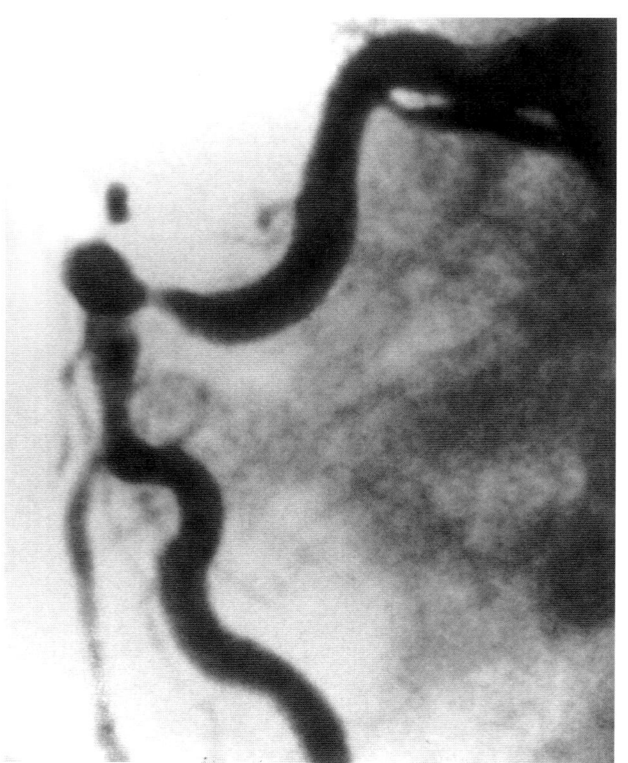

Is Rotablator reasonable for this lesion?

Paul Teirstein, MD, USA: Although the RCA is extremely tortuous, I favor Rotablator atherectomy.

Michael Mooney, MD, USA: This highly tortuous artery is best handled by an experienced operator. I would not use rotational atherectomy in this setting due to the difficulty in passing a Rotablator-C wire through multiple zones of tortuosity. When going through these angulated segments, the burr is likely to cause dissection.

Michael Cowley, MD, USA: Rotational ablation of this lesion is reasonable but is not my preferred approach due to prominent tortuosity, large vessel size, and lack of calcification or other morphologic features for which Rotablator is particularly useful. There is no clear reason to select Rotablator, in preference to PTCA or another device.

Comment on device sizing and important technical tips.

Paul Teirstein, MD, USA: I would use an 8F JR4 guide with sideholes, a Rotablator-C guidewire, and a 1.5 mm followed by a 2.0 mm burr. I would then use a 2.75 mm balloon at 3 ATM, being careful to avoid overdilating this very tortuous vessel. I am concerned about dissection because stent deployment in this tortuous vessel would be very difficult.

Editors' Perspective: In this case, Rotablator atherectomy is technically feasible but challenging. There are several points worth emphasizing: First, coaxial guiding catheter alignment is absolutely crucial. Second, it may be impossible to steer the Rotablator wire through the tortuous segments and into the distal vessel, even with the new flexible Rotablator wire. The best approach to wiring this lesion is to use a conventional flexible angioplasty wire and exchange it for the Rotablator wire using a suitable transfer catheter. If the transfer catheter can be adequately positioned in the straight segment of the distal RCA, the stiffer Type A Rotablator wire may be superior to the Type C wire from the standpoint of straightening the vessel, although pseudolesions should be expected. Third, cautious Rotablation should be employed, starting with a 1.5 mm burr. Because of considerable vessel tortuosity proximal to the target lesion, compression of the drive shaft may lead to significant loss of rotational speed, mandating that an ideal platform speed be achieved before advancing the burr into the lesion.

*****

ROTABLATOR: LARGE THROMBUS

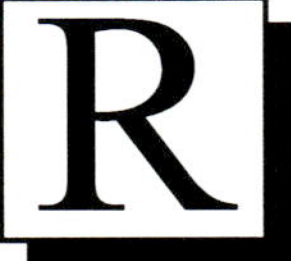

Rotablator atherectomy of a large thrombus in a degenerated vein graft (reference diameter = 5.2 mm).

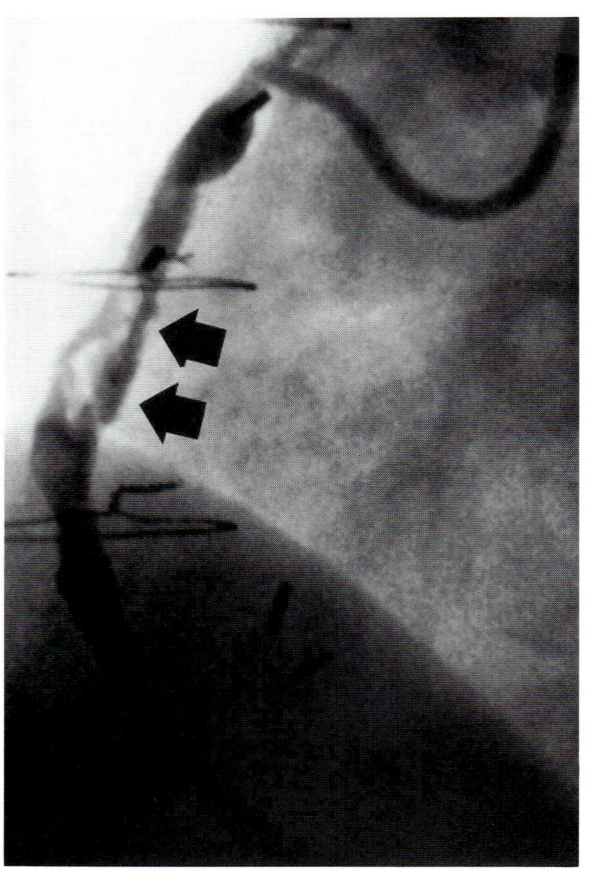

Is Rotablator reasonable for this lesion?

Patrick Whitlow, MD, USA: The Rotablator is not reasonable for this type of thrombus-laden lesion in a degenerated vein graft. The Rotablator will cause distal embolization, slow flow, and disaster.

Richard Myler, MD, USA: Rotablator is not reasonable for this lesion. Thrombus and friable debris adversely affect Rotablator procedural outcome, with a high likelihood of distal embolization and no-reflow.

Michael Cowley, MD, USA: Rotablator is not appropriate for this degenerated vein graft.

> **Editors' Perspective: Rotablator atherectomy is absolutely contraindicated in this setting because of the risk of distal embolization and no-reflow.**

*****

ROTABLATOR: SMALL THROMBUS

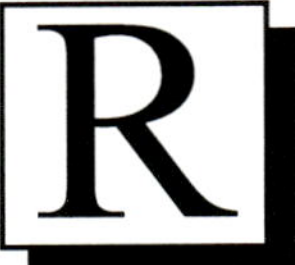

Rotablator atherectomy of a small thrombus in the proximal RCA (reference diameter = 3.4 mm).

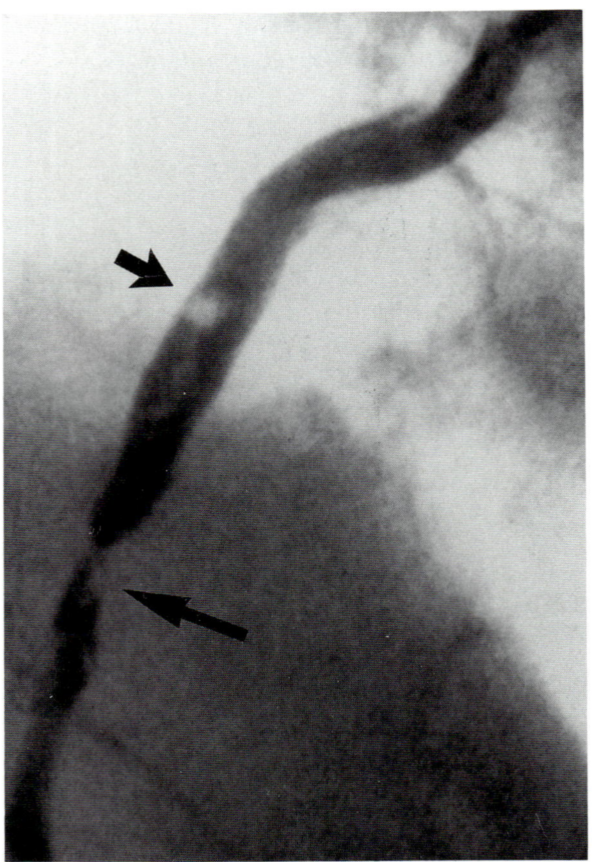

Is Rotablator reasonable for this lesion?

Patrick Whitlow, MD, USA: I would not use Rotablator in an ulcerated lesion with thrombus. Rotational ablation will be associated with slow-flow even if optimal technique is utilized.

Richard Myler, MD, USA: Rotablator is not reasonable for this lesion.

Michael Cowley, MD, USA: Rotational atherectomy is not appropriate for this vessel unless there is heavy calcification in the lesion, or the lesion is rigid and fails to dilate with a balloon. Thrombus is a relative contraindication to the Rotablator because of the increased incidence of no-reflow, which is likely due to release of clot bound thrombin and other vasoactive substances.

Editors' Perspective: Rotablator should be avoided in thrombus-containing lesions because of the risk of major complications.

*****

ROTABLATOR: TRIFURCATION LESION

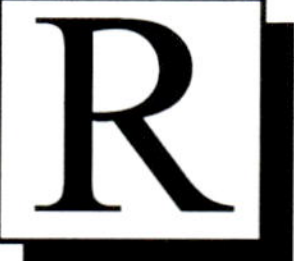

Rotablator atherectomy of a trifurcation lesion in the proximal LCX (reference diameter of proximal LCX = 3.4 mm).

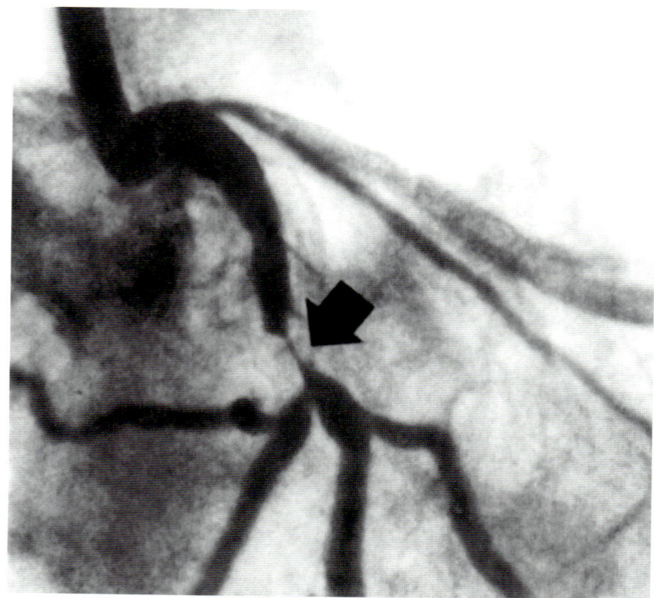

Is Rotablator reasonable for this lesion?

Michael Cowley, MD, USA: The LCX has an irregular proximal narrowing and a complex appearance, suggesting possible thrombus. In view of the large vessel size and the possibility of thrombus, Rotablator atherectomy is not the preferred treatment (unless there is heavy calcification).

Nicolaus Reifart, MD, Germany: The Rotablator is reasonable for this lesion at a trifurcation, since it helps avoid high inflation pressures and dissection beyond the trifurcation.

Comment on device sizing and important technical tips.

Nicolaus Reifart, MD, Germany: To assure good guiding catheter support, I would use an 8F DC or Voda guiding catheter, a Rotablator-C wire, and a 1.75 mm burr. I would operate the burr at 180,000 RPM for 10-15 seconds per run. After rotablation, I would follow with a 3.5 x 40 mm monorail balloon at 2 ATM.

Editors' Perspective: In the absence of thrombus, Rotablator atherectomy is certainly feasible, particularly if significant calcification is present.

*****

ROTABLATOR: BIFURCATION LESION

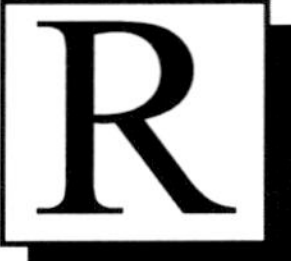

otablator atherectomy of a bifurcation lesion in the distal RCA (reference diameters: RCA = 3.6 mm; PDA= 2.7 mm; PLV = 2.2 mm).

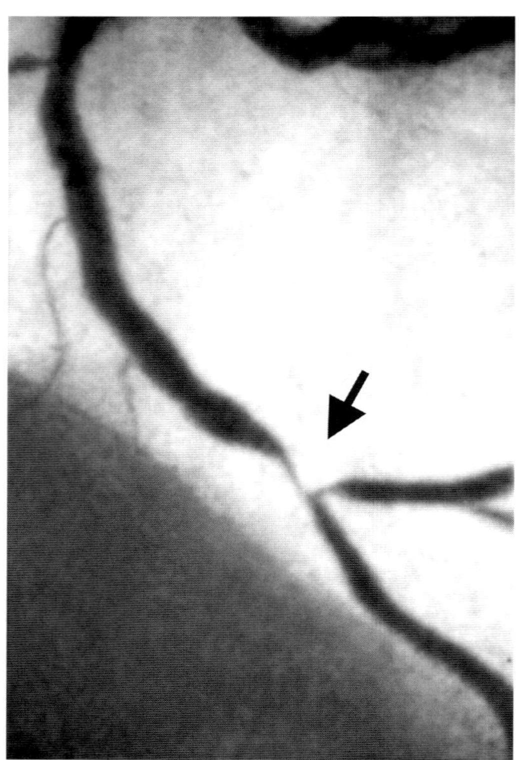

Is Rotablator reasonable for this lesion?

Michael Cowley, MD, USA: This complex lesion is eccentric and irregular. Rotational ablation is reasonable for this lesion, although I prefer directional atherectomy. Accumulating clinical experience suggests that bifurcation lesions are best treated with debulking, and directional atherectomy and Rotablator are highly effective in treating bifurcation lesions.

Nicolaus Reifart, MD, Germany: This is a true bifurcation lesion of the distal RCA. The Rotablator might be used, but has no advantages compared to PTCA. The likelihood of sidebranch occlusion is similar.

> **Editors' Perspective: Experience with Rotablator in bifurcation lesions is quite variable and unpredictable. It is not possible to protect the sidebranch, and Rotablator can result is sidebranch occlusion, dissection, spasm, and no-reflow. In other cases, Rotablator of both branches can lead to beautiful results. If Rotablator is considered for this lesion, it is best to treat both branches with a small burr (burr/artery ratio < 0.6) before using a larger burr in either branch, to minimize the chance of sidebranch occlusion. Alternatively, the sidebranch can be predilated with a small balloon to decrease the chance of occlusion after Rotablator of the parent vessel. Adjunctive PTCA with "kissing" balloons at low pressure will usually lead to excellent results.**

*****

ROTABLATOR: CALCIFIED LESION

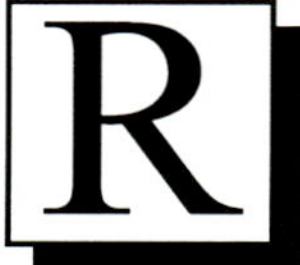

Rotablator atherectomy of a calcified lesion in the mid-LAD (reference diameter = 2.9 mm).

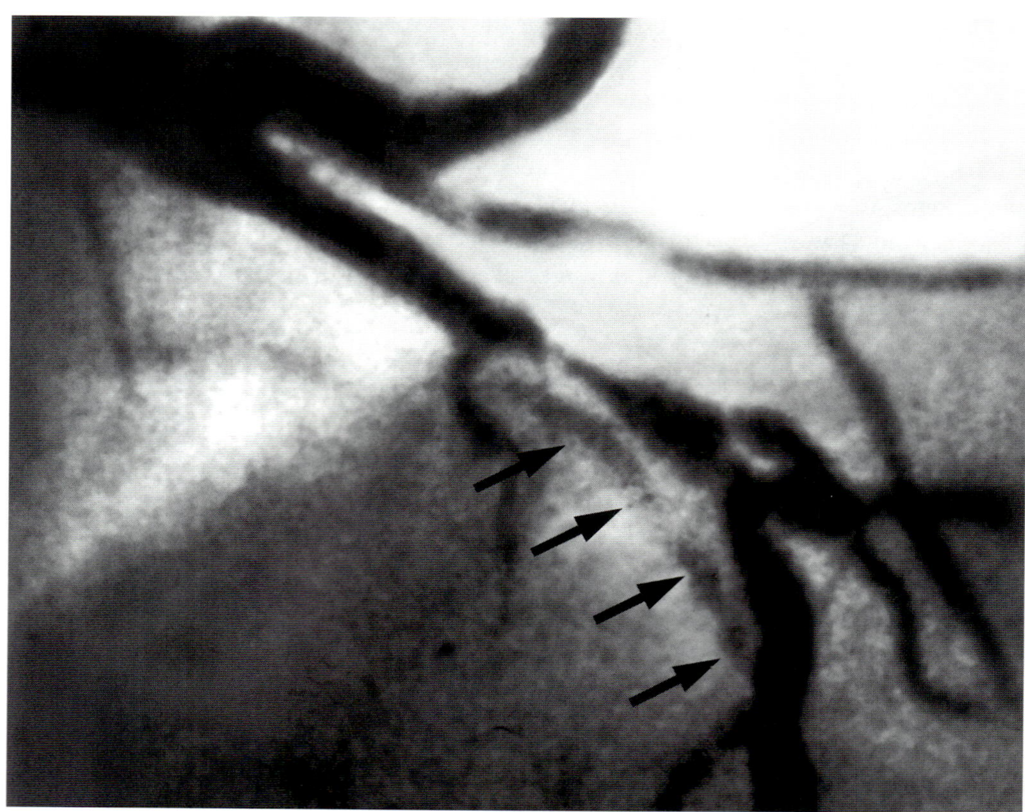

Is Rotablator reasonable for this lesion?

Raimund Erbel, MD, Germany: Rotablator is an ideal device, since heavy calcification is present.

Paul Teirstein, MD, USA: The mid-LAD contains a long, calcified stenosis. I would not attempt to use any modality other than Rotablator.

Michael Mooney, MD, USA: This mid-LAD lesion is reasonably approached with the Rotablator.

Comment on device sizing and important technical tips.

Raimund Erbel, MD, Germany: I would use a 1.5 mm burr and a 2.0 mm burr, followed by a 3.0 mm balloon. If chest pain occurs during Rotablator, burr activation should be discontinued, and PTCA should be performed.

Paul Teirstein, MD, USA: I would approach this patient with an 8F JL4 catheter with sideholes. I would use 1.5 mm, 2.0 mm, and possibly 2.15 mm burrs, followed by a 3.0 x 30 mm balloon at 3 ATM for 3 minutes.

Michael Mooney, MD, USA: I would use a DVI 10F JL4 guiding catheter, a Rotablator-C wire, and a 2.0 mm burr. I would be extremely patient with burr advancement, being certain not to allow rotational speed to fall by more than 5,000 RPM. I would give Diltiazem (2 mg IC), upsize to a 2.5 mm burr, and postdilate with a 3.0 mm noncompliant balloon.

Editors' Perspective: This is an ideal lesion for Rotablator atherectomy. The only issue is whether to follow with PTCA, directional atherectomy, or stenting. Although optimal Rotablator technique has not been defined, it is probably reasonable to use a stepped-burr approach; because of the severity of the stenosis and extent of calcification, it may be best to begin with a 1.5 mm burr, using progressively larger burrs in 0.25-0.5 mm increments (up to a burr/artery ratio of 0.6-0.8) to achieve maximal debulking and calcium ablation. Slow passes and short runs (< 30 seconds) are desirable to minimize complications and ensure the burr engages the plaque. It is crucial to slowly peck at the lesion, not allowing the burr to decelerate more than 5,000 RPM. Many operators routinely use nitroglycerin, verapamil, and heparin in the Rotaflush solution to maximize vasodilation and minimize flow disturbances. It is also important to use frequent contrast injections to assess runoff during ablation runs (the contrast can also induce reactive hyperemia).

This patient underwent successful Rotablator atherectomy and adjunctive PTCA, guided by IVUS. Interventional hardware included a 9F JL4 guide with sideholes, a Rotablator-C wire, and sequential 1.5 mm and 2.0 mm burrs. A 3.0 x 40 mm noncompliant balloon was used to smoothe the final result (below).

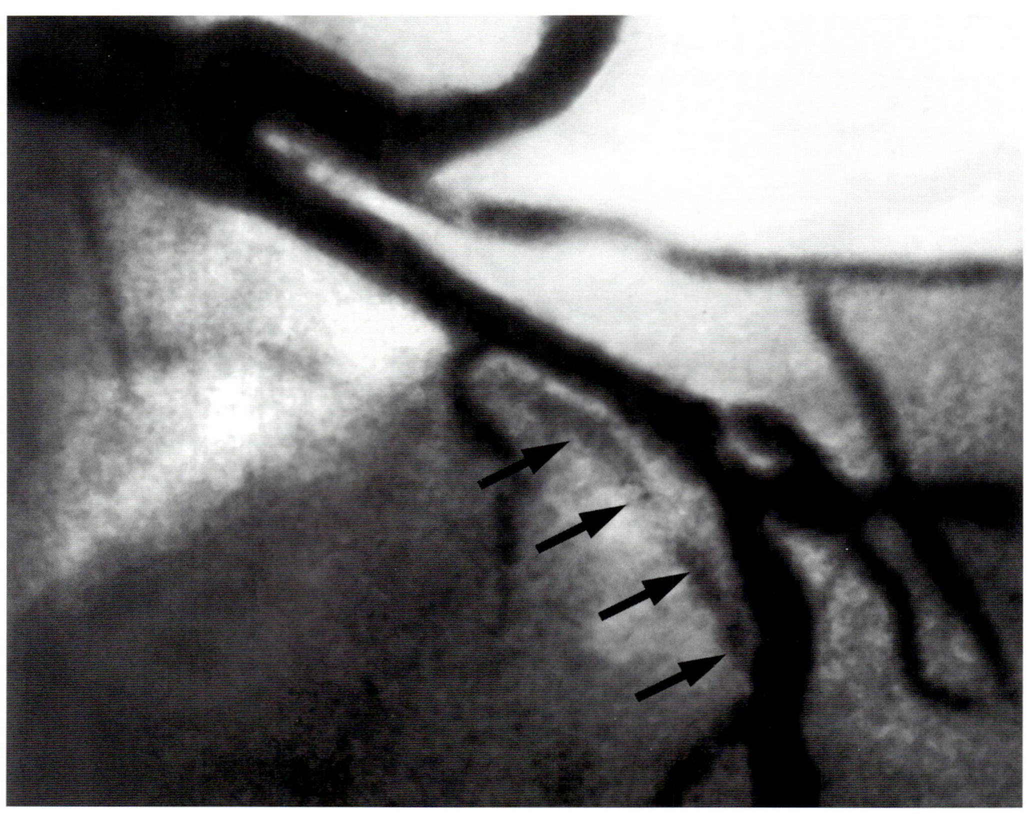

*****

ROTABLATOR: CALCIFIED OSTIAL RCA

Rotablator atherectomy of a calcified ostial lesion in the RCA (reference diameter = 2.8 mm).

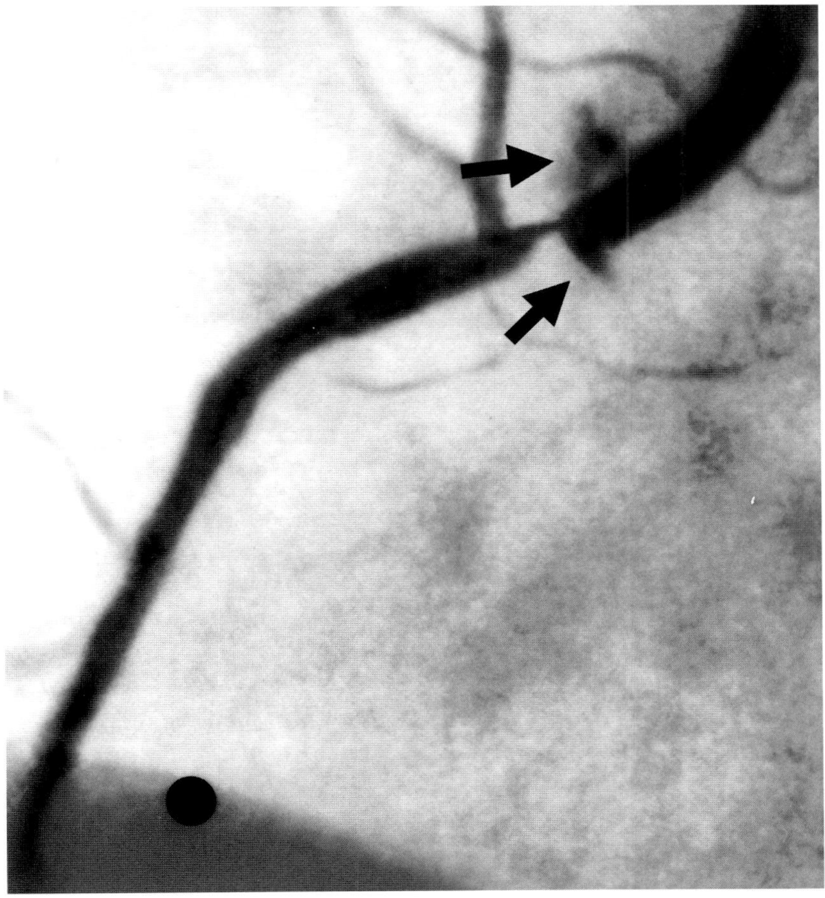

Is Rotablator reasonable for this lesion?

Raimund Erbel, MD, Germany: The ostial RCA lesion is ideal for Rotablator.

Paul Teirstein, MD, USA: The ostial RCA is perfect for Rotablator.

Michael Mooney, MD, USA: Rotablation is an acceptable initial strategy.

Comment on device sizing and important technical tips.

Raimund Erbel, MD, Germany: Because of the severity and calcification of the stenosis, I would use sequential 1.25 mm, 1.75 mm, and 2.0 mm burrs, followed by PTCA, if necessary. I would administer prophylactic atropine, and limit the duration of burr rotation to 10-20 seconds.

Paul Teirstein, MD, USA: I recommend an 8F JL4 catheter with sideholes. I would use 1.5 mm, 2.0 mm, and perhaps 2.15 mm burrs, and then a 3.0 mm balloon to better "predilate" the lesion. While the balloon is across the lesion, I would exchange for an ACS Extra-S'port guidewire, and then deploy a 3.0 mm Palmaz-Schatz coronary stent in the ostium. I believe coronary stenting will provide the best chance of avoiding restenosis. My final inflation would be with a 3.5 mm balloon at 22 ATM. The patient would be discharged the following day on aspirin and ticlopidine (250 mg BID). I would use intravascular ultrasound.

Michael Mooney, MD, USA: I would use a 9F JR4 guiding catheter, a Rotablator-C wire, and sequential 1.75 mm and 2.25 mm burrs. I would then place a 3.0 mm Palmaz-Schatz stent, and postdilate with a 3.0 mm balloon. I would perform IVUS to verify correct positioning of the stent, stent geometry, and apposition.

> **Editors' Perspective: The Rotablator has certainly simplified the percutaneous approach to calcified ostial lesions, and is undoubtedly the treatment of choice. However, several important points must be emphasized: First, coaxial guiding catheter support is crucial, to minimize "guidewire bias" and ensure coaxial presentation of the burr to the target lesion; an oblique presentation of the burr can lead to coronary or aortic dissection. Aggressive guiding catheter intubation increases the risk of ostial injury and is not recommended. Second, slack in the guidewire must be reduced completely before advancing the burr into the target lesion, to avoid kinking the wire. Third, the platform speed must be set in the guiding catheter, since there is no "platform segment" with aortoostial lesions. Fourth, it is extremely important to be patient when engaging the lesion with the burr. Aggressive burr advancement should be avoided because of the risk of creating large microparticle debris, no-reflow, and**

vessel dissection; if burr rotational speed falls by more than 5000 RPM, the burr should be withdrawn from the lesion. Finally, Rotablator of the RCA may be associated with severe bradycardia and/or high-degree AV block. Pretreatment with atropine and a prophylactic temporary pacemaker are useful, and limiting each pass to 20-30 seconds may also attenuate bradyarrhythmia. After successful Rotablator, further lumen enlargement can be achieved with PTCA, directional atherectomy, or stenting. This patient underwent conventional PTCA with a 3.0 mm balloon. Despite inflation pressures up to 14 ATM, there was a persistent waist in the balloon and no luminal improvement after repeat inflations. The patient was referred to us, and successful Rotablator atherectomy was performed using a 9F JR4 guide with sideholes; 1.5 mm, 1.75 mm, and 2.0 mm burrs; and a Rotablator-C guidewire. After the 2.0 mm burr, there was transient slow-flow and ST segment elevation, which resolved after intracoronary verapamil (500 mcg). Final lumen enlargement was achieved with a 3.0 x 40 mm noncompliant balloon at 8 ATM (below). Today, we would also stent this lesion after adjunctive PTCA.

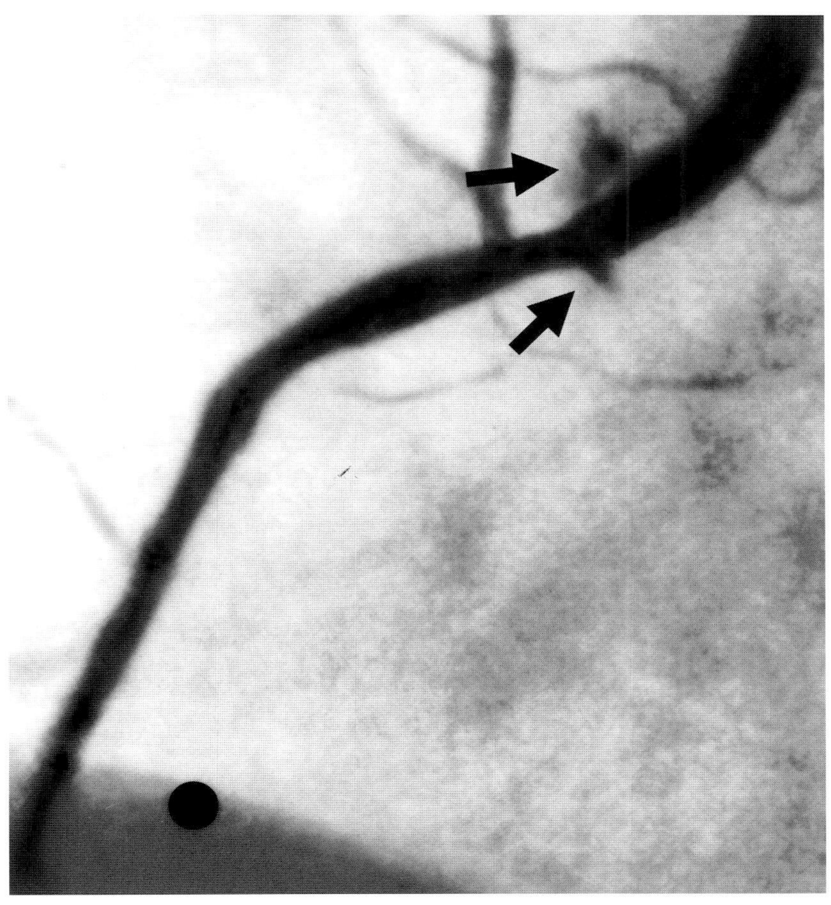

*****

ROTABLATOR: OSTIAL DIAGONAL

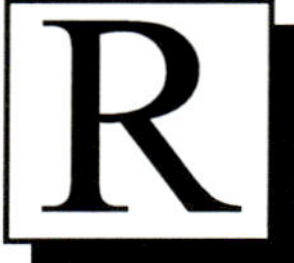otablator atherectomy of an ostial lesion in the diagonal (reference diameter = 3.2 mm).

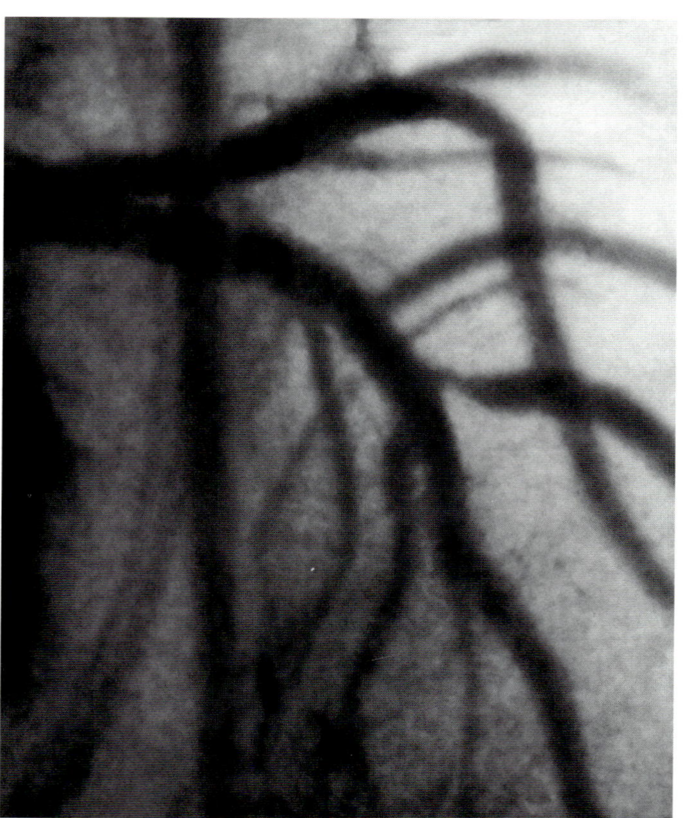

Is Rotablator reasonable for this lesion?

Michael Mooney, MD, USA: Rotablator or other debulking techniques are reasonable.

Patrick Whitlow, MD, USA: The Rotablator is my first choice and is a very reasonable device for debulking this ostial lesion, especially since the predominant plaque burden is located on the inferior aspect of the vessel. The Rotablator will track into the lesion rather than into the normal wall.

Richard Myler, MD, USA: Rotablator is quite reasonable.

Comment on device sizing and important technical tips.

Richard Myler, MD, USA: I recommend a slow pass technique, with increase in burr size from 2.0 mm to 2.25 mm burr, over a Rotablator-C wire, through a 9F JL4 guide. Low-pressure adjunctive PTCA (3.25 x 20 mm PET balloon) or stenting (3.5 mm Palmaz-Schatz stent) will be needed.

> **Editors' Perspective: This is a straightforward lesion for Rotablator atherectomy using standard techniques and equipment.**

*****

ROTABLATOR: OSTIAL LAD

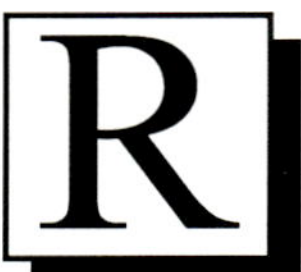
Rotablator atherectomy of an ostial lesion in the LAD (reference diameter = 3.8 mm).

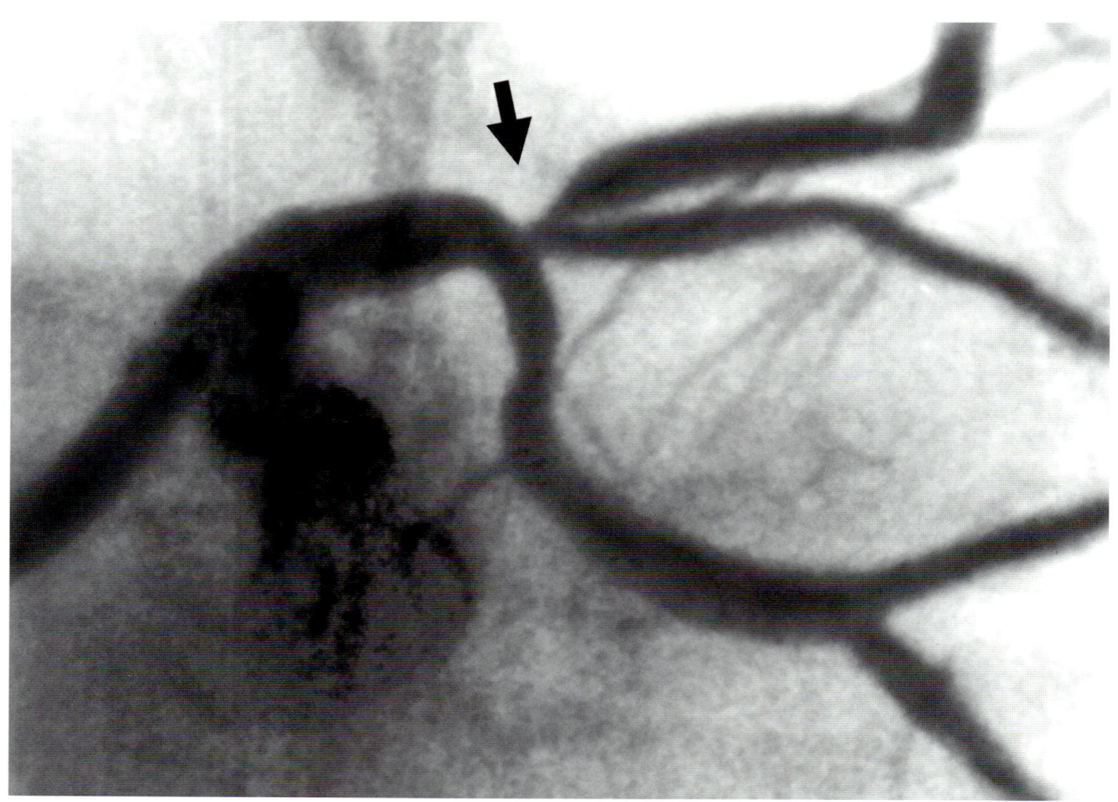

Is Rotablator reasonable for this lesion?

Michael Mooney, MD, USA: It is difficult to envision the merits of rotational atherectomy in the absence of calcification, particularly in a large vessel. I recommend directional atherectomy.

Patrick Whitlow, MD, USA: The Rotablator is reasonable to debulk this lesion prior to PTCA, if there is calcification.

Richard Myler, MD, USA: Rotablator is reasonable for this lesion (especially if calcified).

Comment on device sizing and important technical tips.

Richard Myler, MD, USA: I recommend a slow pass technique with sequential use of 2.0 mm and 2.25 mm burrs over a Rotablator-C wire, via a 9F JL4 guide. I also recommend adjunctive PTCA (4.0 x 20 mm PET balloon) or stenting (4.0 mm Palmaz-Schatz stent).

> **Editors' Perspective: Rotablator atherectomy is technically feasible, but must be followed by adjunctive therapy to achieve definitive lumen enlargement. In the absence of calcification, there is no particular value of Rotablator compared to other techniques.**

*****

ROTABLATOR: OSTIAL LCX

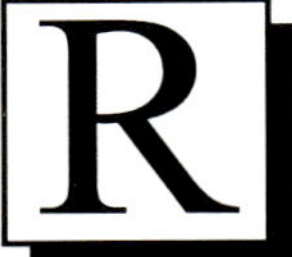
Rotablator atherectomy of an ostial lesion in the LCX (reference diameters: left main = 4.2 mm; LCX = 3.8 mm).

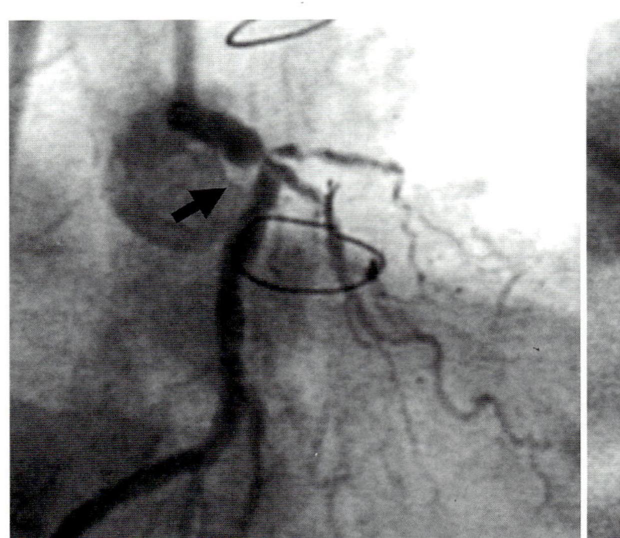

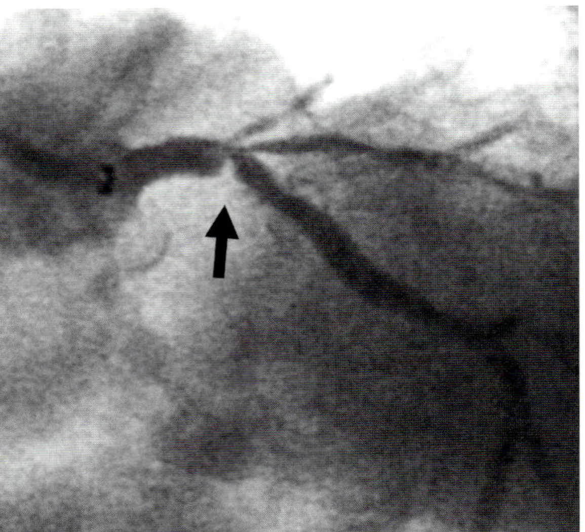

Is Rotablator reasonable for this lesion?

Michael Mooney, MD, USA: The left main and LCX are involved. If calcium is present, Rotablator is reasonable.

Patrick Whitlow, MD, USA: Rotational atherectomy could be done, but is not my first choice. The eccentric orientation of the lesion would bias passage of the burr into the normal wall.

Richard Myler, MD, USA: Rotablator is reasonable for this eccentric, angulated lesion.

Comment on device sizing and important technical tips.

Michael Mooney, MD, USA: I would image first with intravascular ultrasound. If calcium is identified, I would use a 1.75 mm burr and then deliver a 10 mm biliary stent (biliary stents have more radial strength than coronary stents). I would postdilate with a 4.0 mm noncompliant balloon at 18 ATM and use intravascular ultrasound to assess the adequacy of stent deployment.

Patrick Whitlow, MD, USA: The LCX is a very large artery, and rotablation with a 2.5 mm burr might not yield optimal debulking. I would use a 10F Amplatz guide so it can be withdrawn from the ostium and pointed down the barrel of the LCX, allowing Rotablator to make more effective contact with the plaque. The lesion is discrete, and I would start with a 2.0 mm burr, increasing up to 2.25 mm and 2.5 mm burrs. Adjunctive PTCA is necessary with a 4.0 mm balloon at 2-4 ATM. If the final residual stenosis is > 20%, I would implant a 4.0 mm Palmaz-Schatz stent.

Richard Myler, MD, USA: I recommend incremental increases in burr size from 1.75 mm to 2.25 mm, a Rotablator-C wire, and a 9F JL4 guide. Low-pressure adjunctive PTCA (4.0 x 20 mm PET balloon) or stenting (4.0 mm Palmaz-Schatz stent) is necessary.

> **Editors' Perspective: Rotablator atherectomy could be performed, but definitive lumen enlargement will be required with subsequent PTCA, directional atherectomy, or stenting. If the lesion has significant superficial calcification, Rotablator is likely to provide better lumen enlargement than other techniques, particularly if followed by stenting.**

*****

ROTABLATOR: VEIN GRAFT

Rotablator atherectomy of a vein graft to the RCA (reference diameter = 3.9 mm).

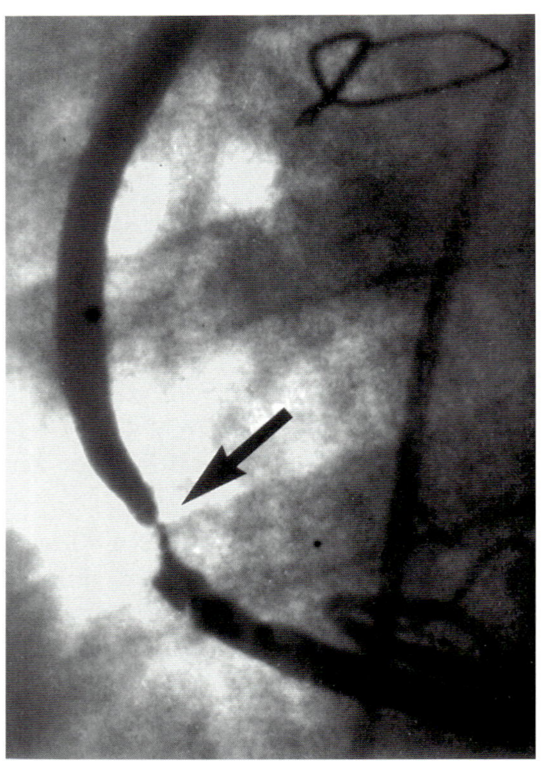

Is Rotablator reasonable for this lesion?

Richard Myler, MD, USA: Rotablator is not a reasonable choice for this vein graft lesion.

Michael Cowley, MD, USA: Rotablator atherectomy is not appropriate for lesions in the body of a vein graft, although it can be used for rigid vein graft lesions which fail to dilate despite high pressure.

Nicolaus Reifart, MD, Germany: I do not consider Rotablator a good choice for this type of lesion.

Editors' Perspective: Rotablator is a poor choice in vein grafts, unless there is reason to be concerned about lesion rigidity. The most important limitations of Rotablator in this setting are distal embolization, no-reflow, and myocardial infarction.

*****

ROTABLATOR: DEGENERATED VEIN GRAFT

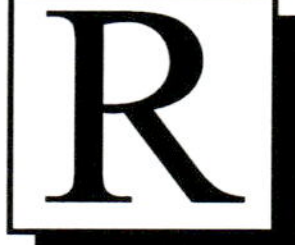otablator atherectomy of a degenerated vein graft to the OM (reference diameter = 3.9 mm).

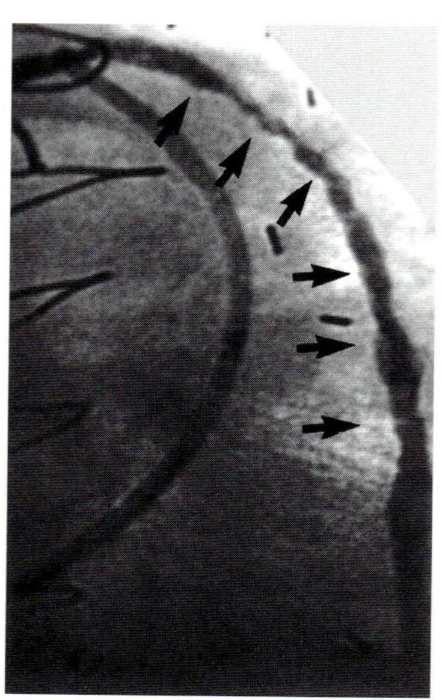

Is Rotablator reasonable for this lesion?

Richard Myler, MD, USA: Rotablation is contraindicated in this diffusely diseased vein graft with friable plaque, because it will be associated with embolic debris and no-reflow.

Michael Cowley, MD, USA: Rotablator is inappropriate for this diffusely degenerated vein graft.

Nicolaus Reifart, MD, Germany: This is certainly a contraindication for Rotablator, since thrombotic material will be dislodged, resulting in catastrophe.

Editors' Perspective: This is a poor case for Rotablator atherectomy because of the risk of distal embolization, no-reflow, and myocardial infarction.

*****

ROTABLATOR: OSTIAL VEIN GRAFT

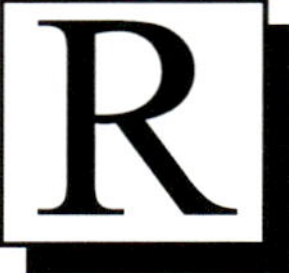otablator atherectomy of an ostial lesion in a vein graft to the LAD (reference diameter = 3.9 mm).

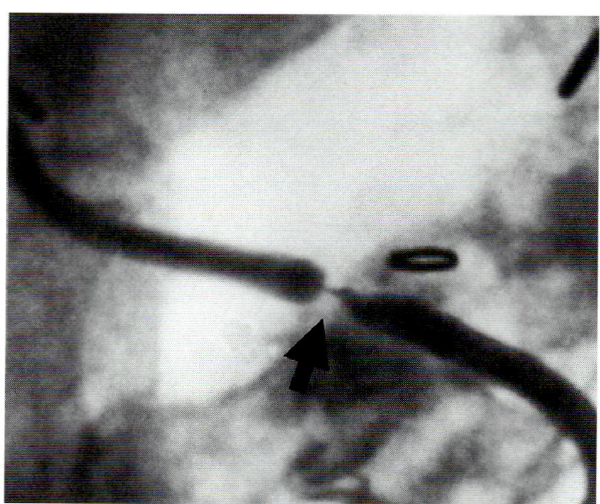

Is Rotablator reasonable for this lesion?

Richard Myler, MD, USA: Rotablation is reasonable, especially if the lesion is calcified.

Michael Cowley, MD, USA: Rotablator is feasible in this setting, but there is little clinical information regarding its use in aortoostial vein graft lesions.

Nicolaus Reifart, MD, Germany: Like for any other aortoostial lesion, the Rotablator is a good choice. The success rate is very high, and the complication rate in ostial vein grafts is very low.

Comment on device sizing and important technical tips.

Richard Myler, MD, USA: I recommend IVUS to evaluate calcium. If calcium is present, I recommend Rotablator and stenting. I use a slow pass Rotablator technique with increases in burr size from 2.0 mm to 2.25 mm over a Rotablator-C wire, through a 9F large-lumen JR4 guide. Adjunctive PTCA (4.0 x 20 mm PET balloon) and stenting may be necessary.

Michael Cowley, MD, USA: The Rotablator is well suited for ostial vein graft lesions, which are frequently elastic and respond poorly to PTCA. I use rotational ablation for treating ostial vein graft lesions in selected cases, and the technique works well for initial debulking. However, even with the 2.5 mm burr, there will be significant residual narrowing, for which further directional atherectomy or stenting will be needed.

Nicolaus Reifart, MD, Germany: I would select an 8F AL2 or AL3 guiding catheter, a Rotablator-C wire, and a 2.0 mm burr. I would follow with a 4.0 mm balloon at 2 ATM. If the residual stenosis is > 20 %, the lesion has to be stented, preferably with a biliary stent.

Editors' Perspective: Rotablator is not routinely recommended in lesions in the body of saphenous vein grafts because of the risk of distal embolization and no-reflow. Exceptions to this general rule include calcified or fibrotic vein graft lesions that fail to expand despite other techniques. In general, aortoostial vein graft stenoses tend to be rigid, elastic, fibrotic, and occasionally calcified; Rotablator is a reasonable technique to increase lesion compliance and "prepare" the lesion for stenting. Safe rotablation can be accomplished with large burrs (burr/artery ratio ≥ 0.7), and other rules about Rotablator technique should be followed, including coaxial guiding catheter alignment and optimal burr speed. Since stenting is commonly employed after Rotablator, it is best to exchange the Rotablator wire for a more suitable extra-support guidewire, particularly if biliary stenting is considered. It is not known whether Rotablator is superior to PTCA before definitive stenting.

*****

Excimer Laser Techniques

ELCA: ECCENTRIC LESION (LAD)

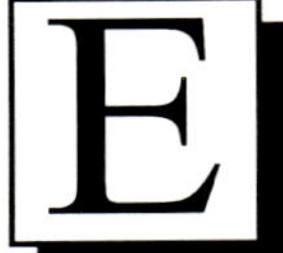

Excimer laser angioplasty of an eccentric lesion in the proximal LAD (reference diameter = 3.4 mm).

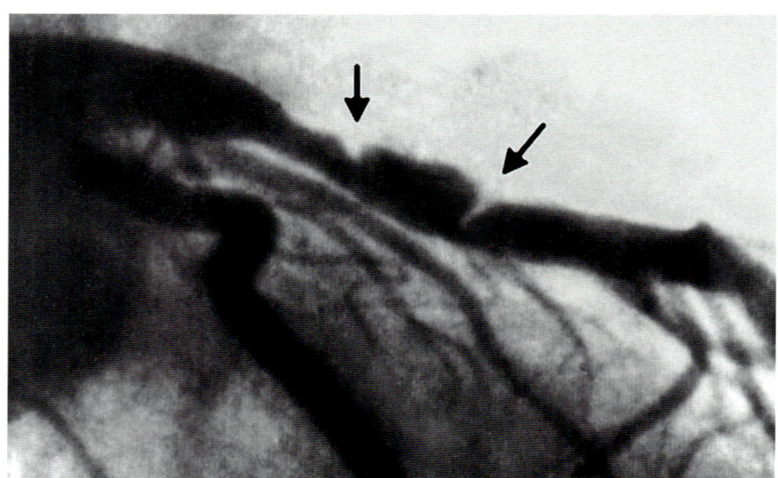

Is ELCA reasonable for this lesion?

John Bittl, MD, USA: ELCA is not suitable for this eccentric lesion because of the increased risk of dissection and major complications. It is not clear if the eccentric laser catheter has overcome this limitation.

Frank Litvack, MD, USA: This lesion is not appropriate for ELCA, since it provides no benefit compared to other interventional approaches. This type of morphology is not favorable for ELCA.

Timothy Sanborn, MD, USA: ELCA is not very effective for this type of lesion.

> **Editors' Perspective: There is general agreement that ELCA has little role in the treatment of eccentric lesions. Although the directional laser could be applied, adjunctive PTCA, directional atherectomy, or stenting is mandatory.**

*****

ELCA: ECCENTRIC LESION (RCA)

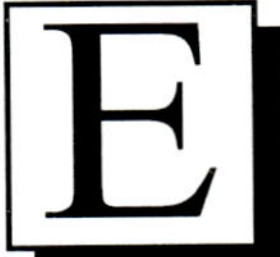
xcimer laser angioplasty of an eccentric lesion in the mid-RCA (reference diameter = 3.2 mm).

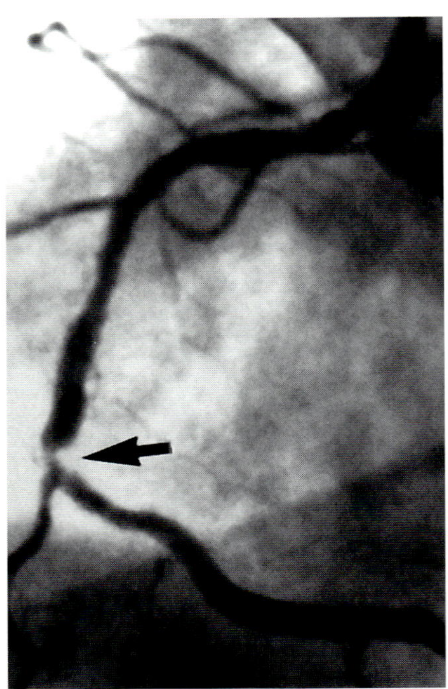

Is ELCA reasonable for this lesion?

John Bittl, MD, USA: ELCA is not suitable for this eccentric lesion because of the risk of dissection, perforation, and major complications.

Frank Litvack, MD, USA: I do not favor ELCA for this lesion. ELCA is associated with a higher complication rate than conventional PTCA for this type of lesion.

Timothy Sanborn, MD, USA: ELCA is not indicated, since the risk of perforation is much higher in such lesions.

> **Editors' Perspective: Experienced laser operators do not recommend use of the concentric ELCA catheter for this lesion, because of the risk of severe complications. Some data suggest that the directional laser might be safer, but adjunctive PTCA, directional atherectomy, or stenting is mandatory.**

*****

ELCA: ULCERATED LESION

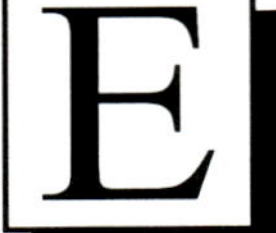xcimer laser angioplasty of an ulcerated lesion in the mid-LAD (reference diameter = 3.2 mm).

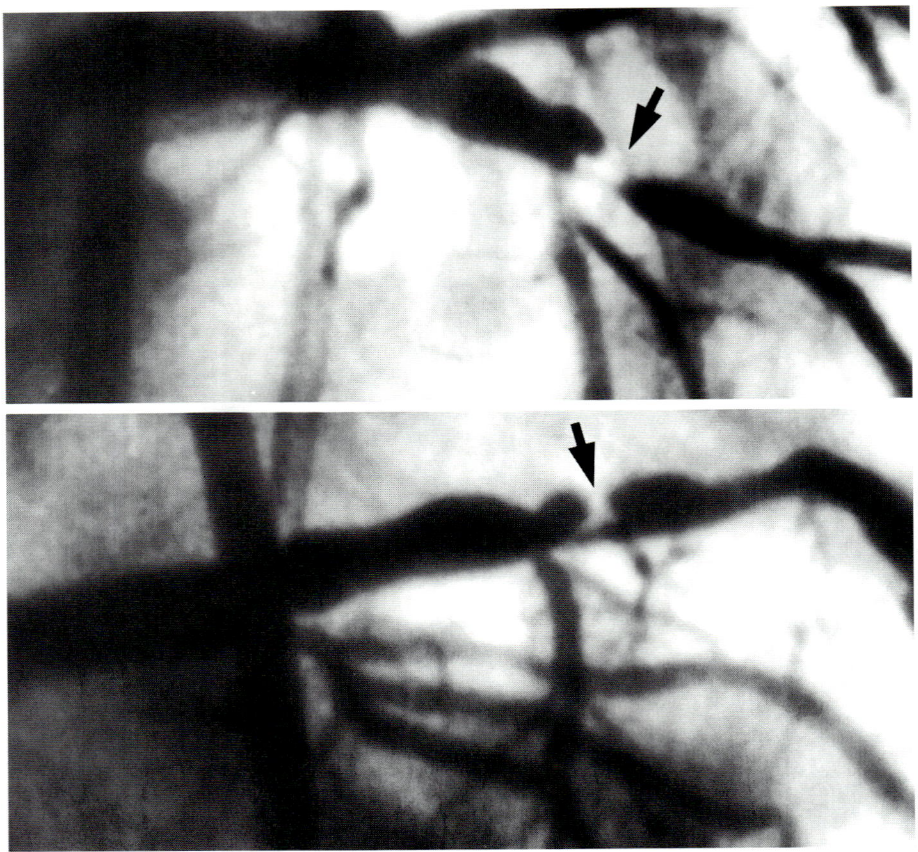

Is ELCA reasonable for this lesion?

John Bittl, MD, USA: ELCA is contraindicated in ulcerated lesions because of the increased risk of dissection and major complications.

Frank Litvack, MD, USA: I do not believe that ELCA is the treatment of choice for this lesion. Though it could be traversed with ELCA, I do not expect any benefit compared to other therapies.

Timothy Sanborn, MD, USA: I do not recommend ELCA for ulcerated lesions.

Editors' Perspective: ELCA has little or no value for this lesion.

*****

ELCA: TUBULAR LESION

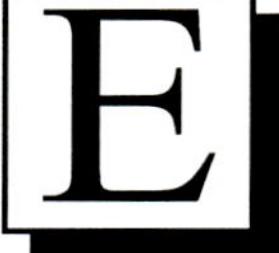

Excimer laser angioplasty of a tubular lesion in the mid-RCA (length = 15 mm; reference diameter = 2.5 mm).

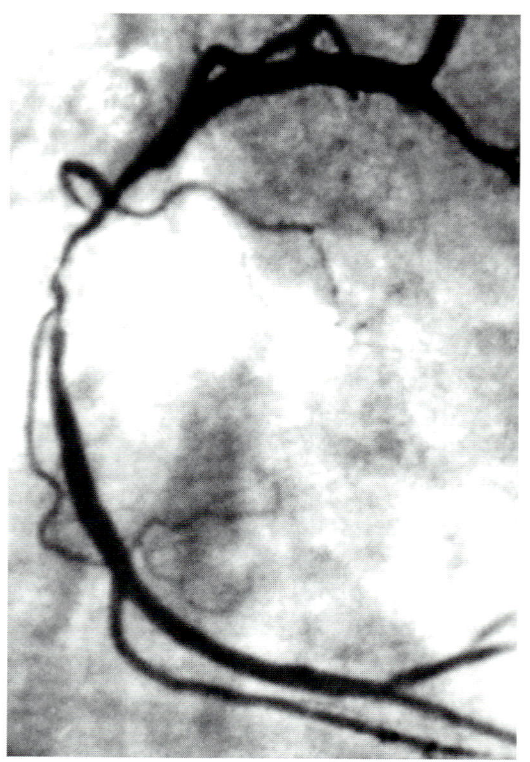

Is ELCA reasonable for this lesion?

John Bittl, MD, USA: ELCA is not indicated for this long lesion. ELCA failed to achieve any benefit over conventional PTCA in the AMRO trial (randomized comparison of ELCA and PTCA for long lesions). Several registries have demonstrated worse results after ELCA for long lesions compared to discrete lesions.

Frank Litvack, MD, USA: This is an excellent lesion for ELCA, since the lesion is long and the reference diameter is only 2.5 mm.

Timothy Sanborn, MD, USA: This long lesion could certainly be treated by ELCA.

Comment on device sizing and important technical tips.

Frank Litvack, MD, USA: I would use an 8F JR4 or hockey stick guide, and cross the lesion with an Extra-Support wire. I would use a 1.4 mm laser catheter followed by 1.7 mm catheter. I would be extremely attentive to saline infusion via the guide catheter, so that laser energy is emitted in a blood- and contrast-free environment. I would perform adjunctive PTCA with a 3.0-3.5 mm x 30 mm balloon. Without saline infusion, there is significant risk of dissection.

> **Editors' Perspective: During the initial development of laser technology, there was tremendous hope that long lesions would become prime targets for excimer laser revascularization. Unfortunately, the "great light hope" has been dimmed. Although ELCA could be performed easily with few complications in this lesion, available studies suggest no benefit compared to conventional PTCA. However, it is important to remember that the saline infusion technique, which has been shown to decrease laser-induced acoustic effect and dissection, was not employed in earlier laser studies; contemporary studies using the saline infusion technique are needed.**

*****

ELCA: LONG LESION

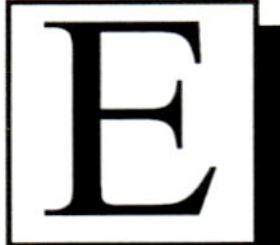

Excimer laser angioplasty of a long lesion in the mid-LAD (length = 25 mm; reference diameter = 3.3 mm).

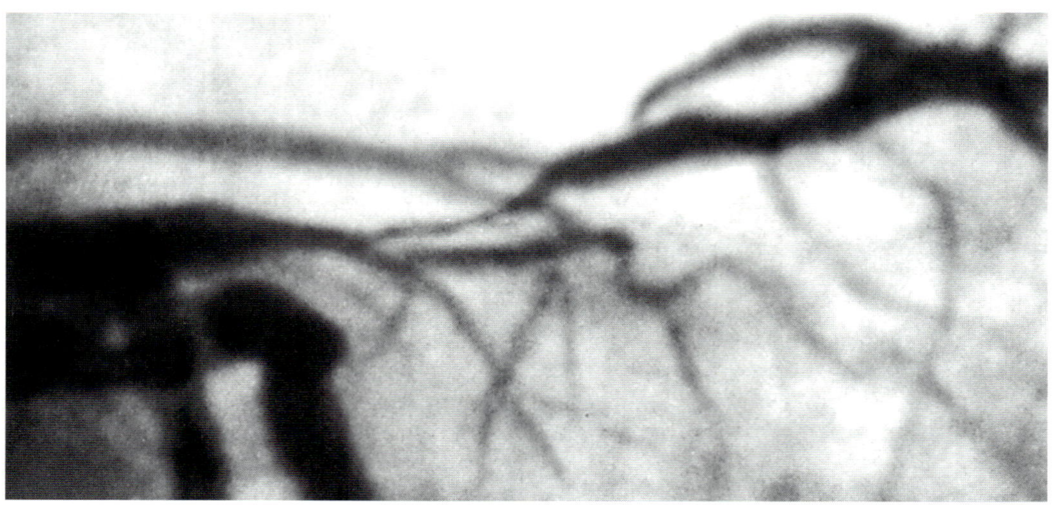

Is ELCA reasonable for this lesion?

John Bittl, MD, USA: ELCA is not indicated for this long lesion. ELCA failed to achieve any benefit over conventional PTCA in the AMRO trial, which compared ELCA to PTCA for long lesions. Several registries have demonstrated worse results after ELCA in long lesions than in discrete lesions.

Frank Litvack, MD, USA: This lesion is appropriate for ELCA.

Timothy Sanborn, MD, USA: This long lesion is amenable to ELCA.

Comment on device sizing and important technical tips.

Frank Litvack, MD, USA: I would use a 1.4 mm laser catheter and then go directly to adjunctive PTCA or to a 1.7 mm catheter followed by adjunctive PTCA. I would use an 8F JL4 guide and cross the lesion with an Extra-Support wire. I would use vigorous saline infusion to assure that the artery is clear of contrast and blood during lasing. Laser energy would be applied at 45 mJ/mm^2.

Timothy Sanborn, MD, USA: Laser energies of 50-60 mJ/mm^2 may be required to cross this long, high-grade stenosis.

> **Editors' Perspective: Most interventionalists no longer use ELCA for long lesions in large vessels, since available studies suggest no benefit over conventional PTCA alone. Nevertheless, the saline infusion technique may improve laser results, and should be employed if ELCA is considered.**

*****

ELCA: FUNCTIONAL TOTAL OCCLUSION

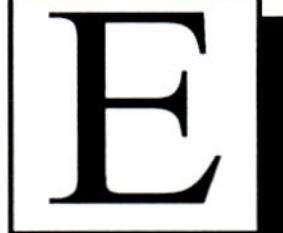

Excimer laser angioplasty of a functional total occlusion in the proximal LAD (reference diameter = 2.7 mm). Assume the occlusion can be crossed with a guidewire.

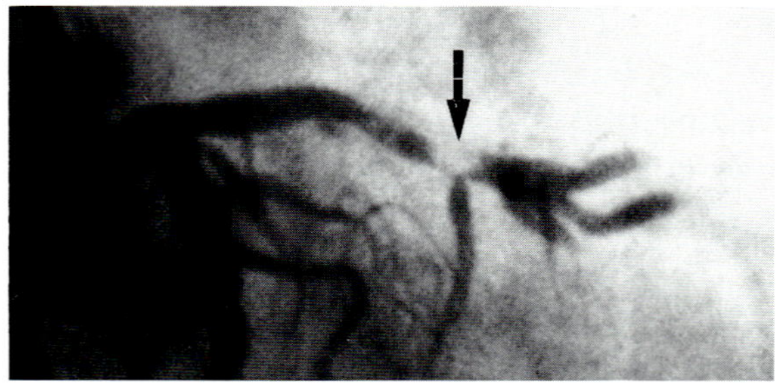

Is ELCA reasonable for this lesion?

John Bittl, MD, USA: The lesion is associated with a globular filling defect surrounded by contrast on three sides; this is the angiographic hallmark of intracoronary thrombus. ELCA is associated with an increased risk of embolic phenomena, and should not be considered.

Frank Litvack, MD, USA: The angiogram has evidence for proximal thrombus and total occlusion. If the occlusion is chronic, I would consider debulking with ELCA. On the other hand, if there is fresh thrombus and the occlusion is recent, I see no benefit with ELCA.

Timothy Sanborn, MD, USA: This subtotal occlusion in a small vessel will benefit from debulking with ELCA.

Comment on device sizing and important technical tips.

Frank Litvack, MD, USA: I would use a 1.4 mm laser catheter prior to adjunctive PTCA.

Timothy Sanborn, MD, USA: I would "bare wire" the lesion with a 0.014-inch Hi-torque floppy guidewire and then use a 1.7 mm monorail ELCA catheter to debulk the lesion. I would exchange for a 3.0 mm Monorail balloon, and quickly perform adjunctive PTCA. ReoPro may be useful if this is an "acute" lesion.

> **Editors' Perspective: Fresh thrombus is a relative contraindication to ELCA, because of the risk of embolization. ELCA probably has no advantages over other techniques for total occlusion.**

*****

ELCA: TOTAL OCCLUSION

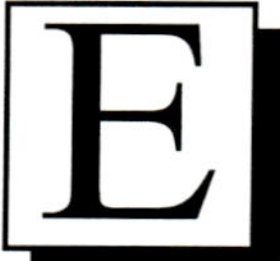xcimer laser angioplasty of a total occlusion in the proximal RCA (reference diameter = 4.5 mm). Assume the occlusion can be crossed with a guidewire

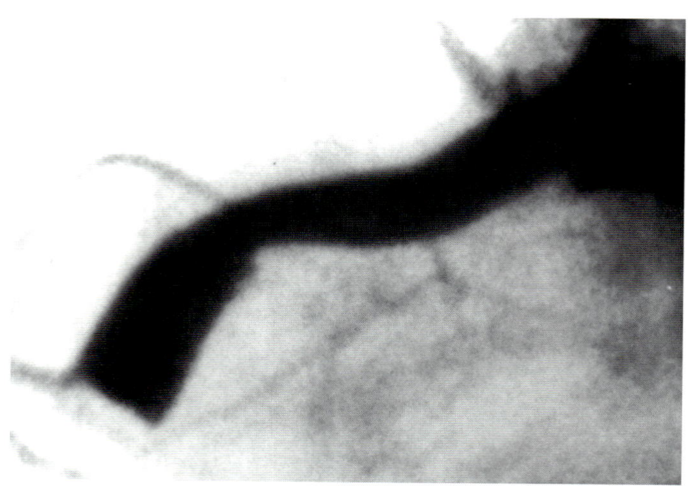

Is ELCA reasonable for this lesion?

John Bittl, MD, USA: This total occlusion has an abrupt cutoff. Although it is difficult for angiography to provide definitive evidence for thrombus (especially in the setting of total occlusions), this angiographic appearance strongly suggests that thrombus is present. ELCA is associated with an increased risk of embolic phenomena and should not be considered.

Frank Litvack, MD, USA: This is an abrupt thrombotic occlusion. ELCA has no value in fresh thrombus or short total occlusions.

Timothy Sanborn, MD, USA: This total occlusion in a large vessel has significant plaque/clot burden; it will benefit from debulking with ELCA.

Comment on device sizing and important technical tips.

Timothy Sanborn, MD, USA: After crossing the occlusion with a guidewire, I would debulk with a 1.7 mm eccentric laser catheter using the saline infusion technique. ReoPro may be useful if there is a persistent filling defect after crossing the lesion with a guidewire.

> **Editors' Perspective: Although ELCA could be used for this lesion, it is difficult to imagine why an operator would select ELCA over other devices.**

*****

ELCA: ANGULATED LESION (LAD)

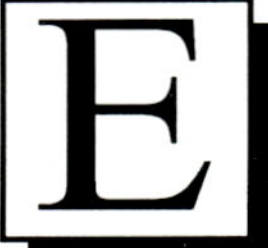

Excimer laser angioplasty of an angulated lesion in the proximal LAD (lesion on inner curve; reference diameter = 3.4 mm).

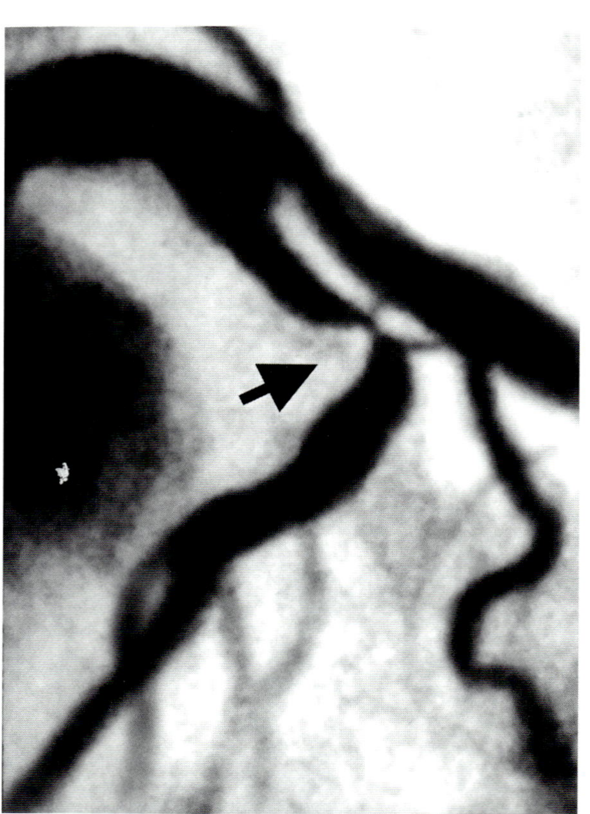

Is ELCA reasonable for this lesion?

John Bittl, MD, USA: This eccentric, angulated lesion in the proximal LAD should not be treated with ELCA because of the increased risk of vessel dissection, perforation, and major complications.

Frank Litvack, MD, USA: The angiogram reveals a discrete lesion in a bend. This is not an appropriate lesion for ELCA, not because the lesion is in a bend, but because ELCA has no benefit in focal lesions.

Timothy Sanborn, MD, USA: I am concerned about vessel perforation and dissection in this angulated lesion, and I do not recommend ELCA.

> **Editors' Perspective: Concentric excimer laser catheters have no role in the treatment of angulated lesions because of poor lumen enlargement and the risk of complications. The directional laser may be safer, but experience in angulated lesions is limited, and definitive lumen enlargement requires adjunctive PTCA, directional atherectomy, or stenting.**

*****

ELCA: ANGULATED LESION (RCA)

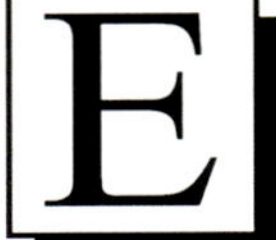xcimer laser angioplasty of an angulated lesion in the proximal RCA (lesion on outer curve; reference diameter = 3.1 mm).

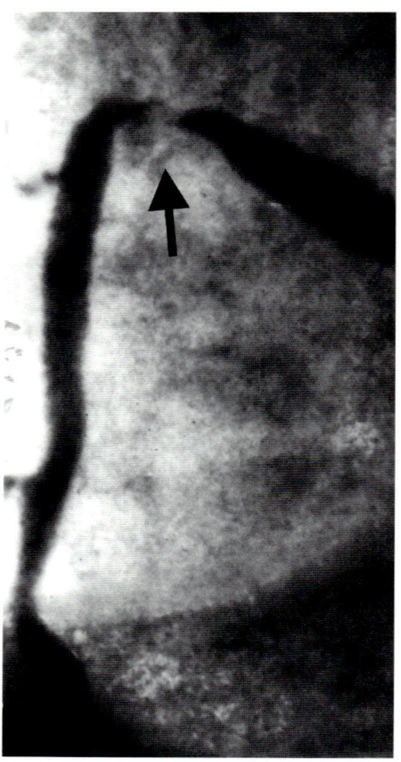

Is ELCA reasonable for this lesion?

John Bittl, MD, USA: This discrete lesion in the proximal RCA should not be treated with ELCA.

Frank Litvack, MD, USA: The lesion in the RCA is extremely discrete. I see no advantage in utilizing ELCA.

Timothy Sanborn, MD, USA: I am concerned about perforation and dissection. I do not recommend ELCA in angulated lesions.

Editors' Perspective: There is no particular value for ELCA in this lesion, and complications are potentially increased.

*****

ELCA: TORTUOUS LCX

Excimer laser angioplasty of a focal lesion in a tortuous LCX (right angle takeoff; reference diameter = 2.6 mm).

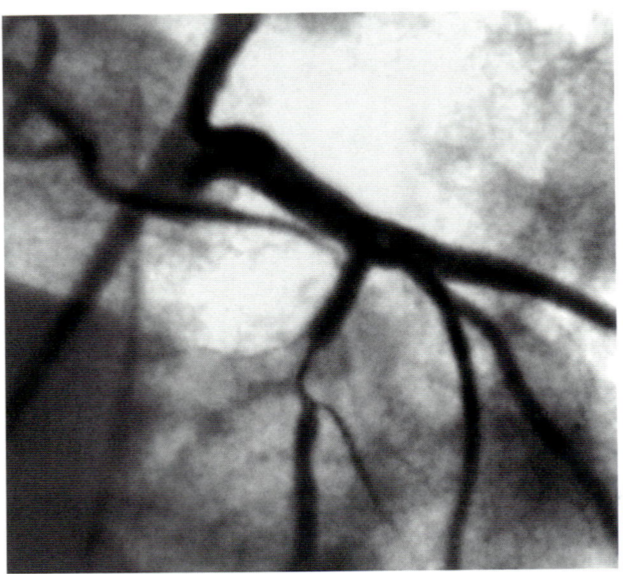

Is ELCA reasonable for this lesion?

John Bittl, MD, USA: Although currently available ELCA catheters are flexible and can negotiate this tortuous vessel, ELCA is not recommended since it failed to show any benefit over conventional PTCA in the randomized trial comparing ELCA with PTCA (AMRO).

Frank Litvack, MD, USA: This lesion is suitable for ELCA.

Comment on device sizing and important technical tips.

Frank Litvack, MD, USA: I would use an 8F JL4 guide and an Extra-Support wire. The 1.4 mm or 1.7 mm ELCA catheters will have no difficulty making the right angle bend and can be used to debulk the artery prior to adjunctive PTCA.

Timothy Sanborn, MD, USA: A 1.4 mm or 1.7 mm ELCA catheter will traverse the 90° turn at the origin of LCX, and should be followed by adjunctive PTCA.

Editors' Perspective: Because of the flexibility of the excimer laser catheters, the angulated takeoff of the LCX does not represent a significant technical challenge for ELCA. However, operation of the laser should be limited to the relatively straight portion of the circumflex distal to its takeoff from the left main. Recent data suggest that the saline infusion technique will decrease acoustic shock and dissection, and should be used if ELCA is performed. Thus far, ELCA has failed to show a favorable impact on restenosis compared to other techniques.

*****

ELCA: TORTUOUS RCA

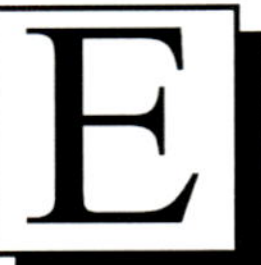

Excimer laser angioplasty of a focal lesion in a tortuous RCA (reference diameter = 3.2 mm).

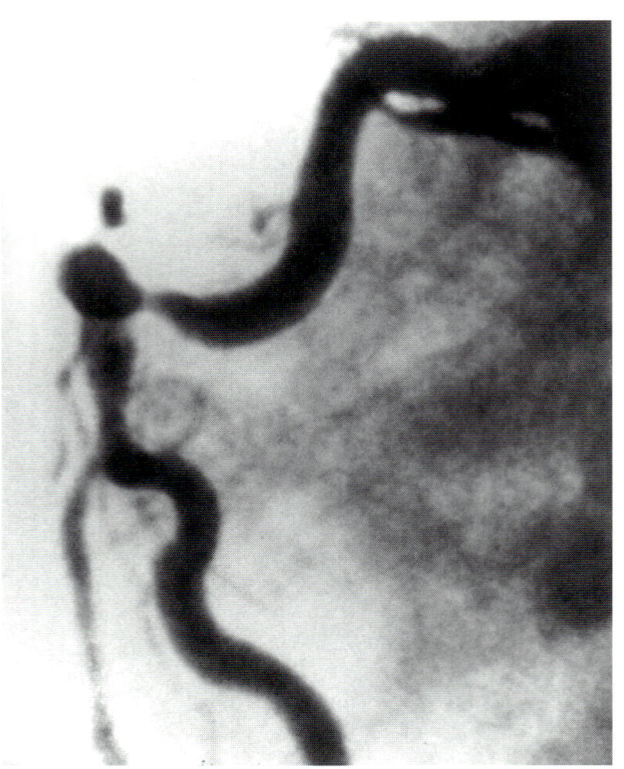

Is ELCA reasonable for this lesion?

John Bittl, MD, USA: ELCA is contraindicated in angulated lesions.

Frank Litvack, MD, USA: I do not favor ELCA for this lesion. Although the ELCA catheter could reach the lesion, I would not use ELCA because there is no proven benefit for ELCA in concentric, discrete lesions.

Timothy Sanborn, MD, USA: The sharp angle distal to the lesion raises my concern about vessel perforation and dissection with ELCA.

> **Editors' Perspective: The risk of dissection and perforation preclude safe use of ELCA in this type of anatomy.**

*****

ELCA: LARGE THROMBUS

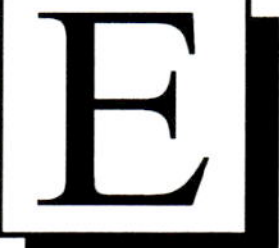

Excimer laser angioplasty of a large thrombus in a degenerated vein graft (reference diameter = 5.2 mm).

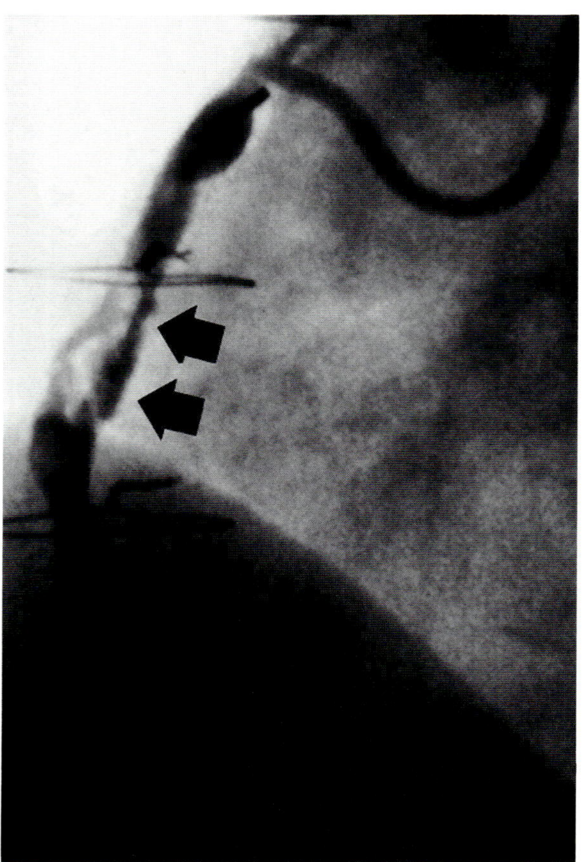

Is ELCA reasonable for this lesion?

John Bittl, MD, USA: I would not perform any percutaneous intervention because of the risk of embolization.

Frank Litvack, MD, USA: There is a large mass of thrombus in the shaft of the graft. ELCA is quite feasible in this situation and can be used with adjunctive PTCA.

Timothy Sanborn, MD, USA: ELCA is unlikely to aid in debulking this lesion.

> **Editors' Perspective: As Dr. Bittl suggests, percutaneous intervention on this vein graft would be associated with significant risk of major complications. Although ELCA is technically feasible and some operators utilize ELCA in degenerated vein grafts, its advantage over other percutaneous techniques has not been demonstrated.**

*****

ELCA: SMALL THROMBUS

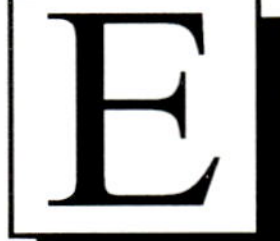

Excimer laser angioplasty of a small thrombus in the proximal RCA (reference diameter = 3.4 mm).

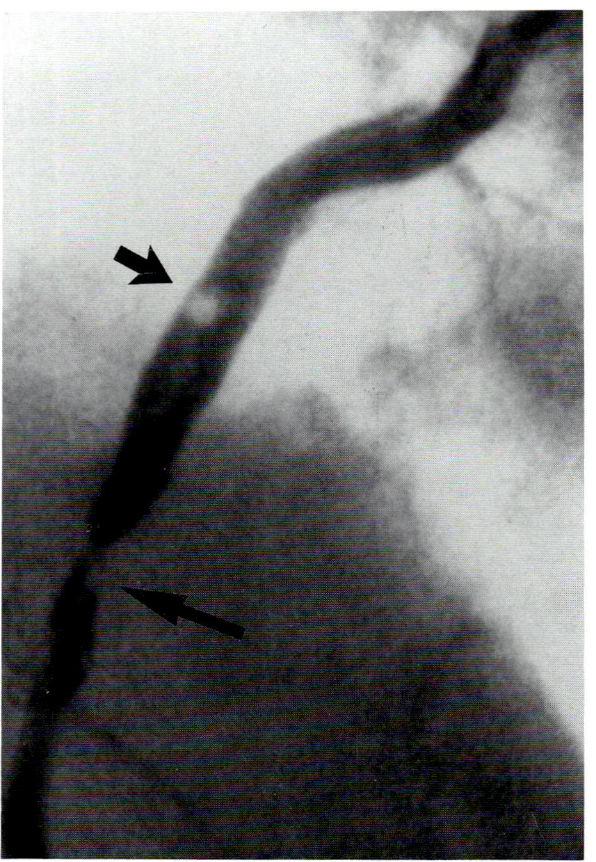

Is ELCA reasonable for this lesion?

Frank Litvack, MD, USA: The angiogram reveals the typical "meatball" appearance of intracoronary thrombus. I do not favor ELCA for this lesion.

Timothy Sanborn, MD, USA: ELCA is unlikely to aid in debulking this lesion.

> **Editors' Perspective: ELCA is associated with an increased risk of complications in thrombus-containing lesions, and should probably be avoided.**

*****

ELCA: TRIFURCATION LESION

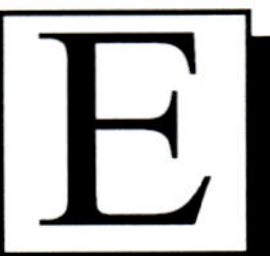
Excimer laser angioplasty of a trifurcation lesion in the proximal LCX (reference diameter of proximal LCX = 3.4 mm).

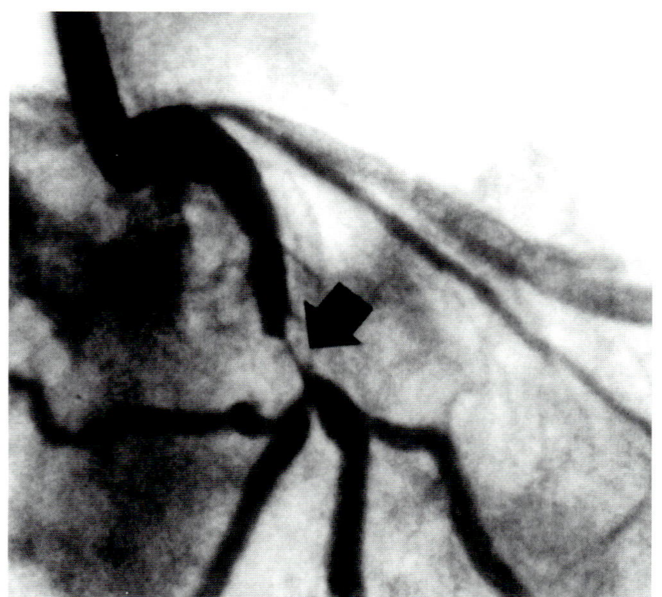

Is ELCA reasonable for this lesion?

John Bittl, MD, USA: ELCA is contraindicated because of increased complications and reduced success in bifurcation lesions.

Frank Litvack, MD, USA: ELCA is reasonable to debulk the lesion before PTCA or stent placement. I am not worried about perforation because the lesion is well before the trifurcation.

Timothy Sanborn, MD, USA: Bifurcation lesions are among the strongest predictors of complications and perforation after ELCA, which should be avoided.

Comment on device sizing and important technical tips.

Frank Litvack, MD, USA: I would place the guidewire in the large middle branch, so the laser catheter "sees" a straight shot into the LCX.

Editors' Perspective: Given the unpredictability of ELCA for this type of lesion, other percutaneous methods are preferred.

*****

ELCA: BIFURCATION LESION

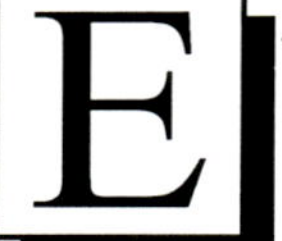

Excimer laser angioplasty of a bifurcation lesion in the distal RCA (reference diameters: RCA = 3.6 mm; PDA = 2.7 mm; PLV = 2.2 mm).

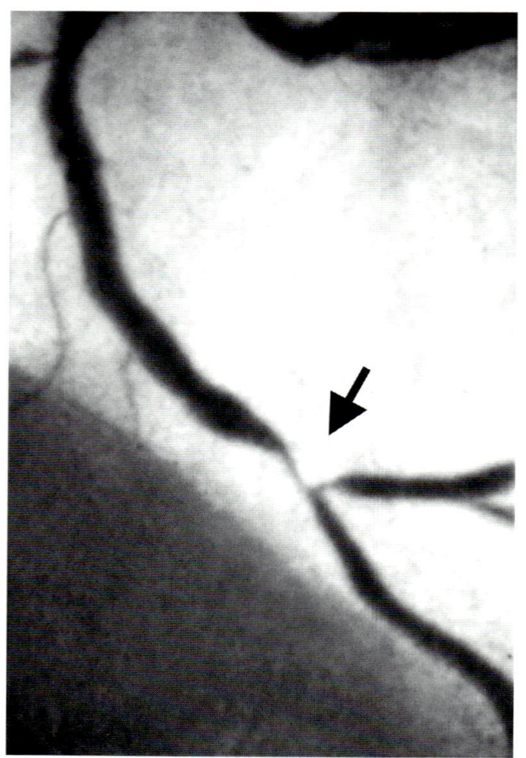

Is ELCA reasonable for this lesion?

John Bittl, MD, USA: ELCA is contraindicated in bifurcation lesions.

Frank Litvack, MD, USA: This is not a good case for concentric ELCA, since laser energy could perforate the carina. This is an excellent lesion for the directional laser catheter.

Timothy Sanborn, MD, USA: Bifurcation lesions are among the strongest predictors for complications and perforation after ELCA.

> **Editors' Perspective: Concentric excimer laser fibers should not be used to treat bifurcation lesions due to the risk of dissection and perforation. It is uncertain whether the directional laser will provide safer revascularization in this setting.**

*****

ELCA: CALCIFIED LESION

Excimer laser angioplasty of a calcified lesion in the mid-LAD (reference diameter = 2.9 mm).

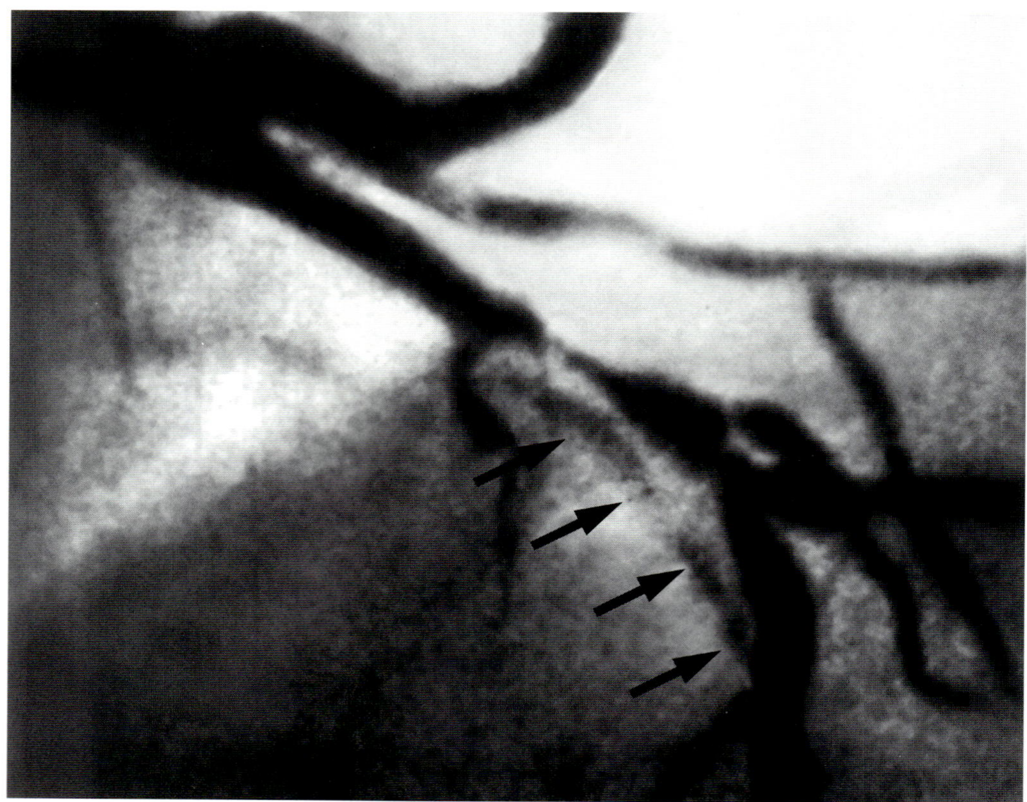

Is ELCA reasonable for this lesion?

John Bittl, MD, USA: ELCA is not recommended for calcified lesions because of reduced likelihood of successful catheter passage and increased risk of dissection.

Frank Litvack, MD, USA: I do not favor ELCA for discrete lesions, since there is no reason to assume that ELCA will provide any advantage compared to other techniques.

Timothy Sanborn, MD, USA: ELCA is quite reasonable for this long, calcified segment.

Comment on device sizing and important technical tips.

Timothy Sanborn, MD, USA: I would start with a 1.4 mm catheter and follow with a 1.7 mm catheter (f there is no dissection), followed by PTCA to optimize the angiographic result.

> **Editors' Perspective: Although calcified lesions were originally targeted by excimer lasers, recent data suggest that lasers have little ability to adequately ablate calcified plaque. However, these data may reflect inadequate power density and failure to use the saline infusion technique, which has been shown to improve laser results. Nevertheless, most operators prefer the Rotablator for calcified lesions, since it is more predictable than the excimer laser.**

*****

ELCA: CALCIFIED OSTIAL RCA

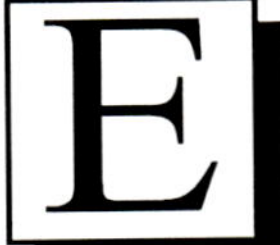

Excimer laser angioplasty of a calcified ostial lesion in the RCA (reference diameter = 2.8 mm).

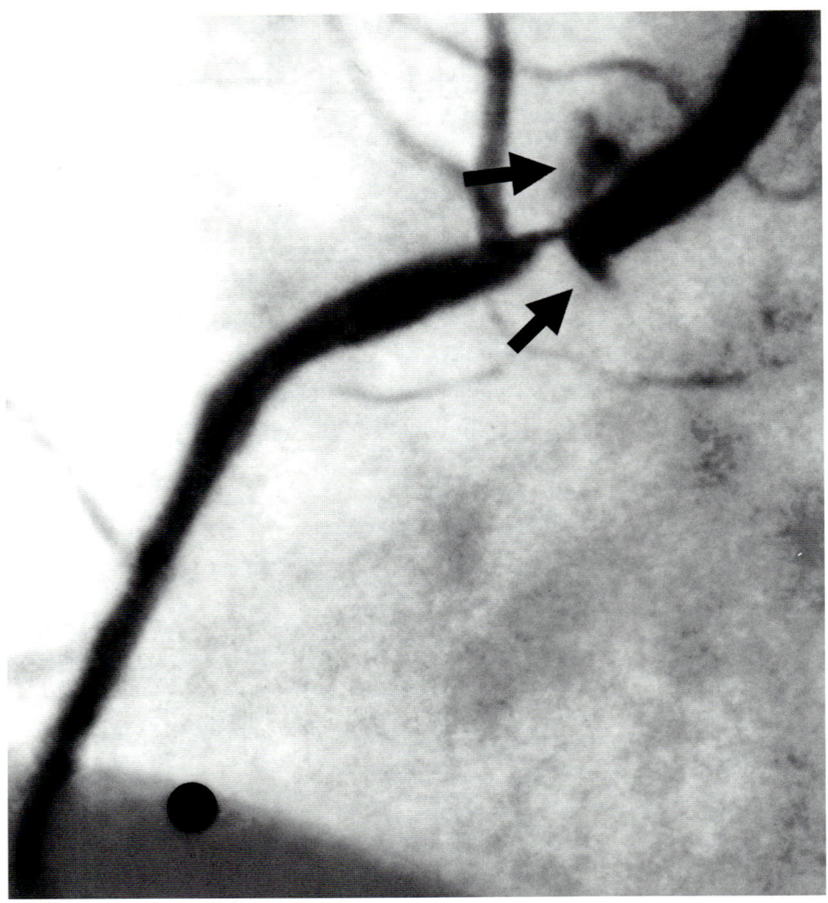

Is ELCA reasonable for this lesion?

John Bittl, MD, USA: ELCA is recommended for this calcified ostial lesion.

Frank Litvack, MD, USA: This represents a perfect case for ELCA.

Timothy Sanborn, MD, USA: This an ideal case for ELCA.

Comment on device sizing and important technical tips.

John Bittl, MD, USA: I recommend ELCA with a 9F JR4 guide, a 0.014-inch Extra-S'port wire, and a 1.4 mm Monorail ELCA catheter at a fluence of 50 mJ/mm^2. Coaxial alignment of the guide catheter must be ensured in both the LAO and RAO projections before advancing the laser catheter. If an initial attempt to pass the laser catheter is unsuccessful, the fluence should be increased to 60 mJ/mm^2. If an inadequate lumen is obtained after passage of the small laser catheter, I would increase to a 2.0 mm laser catheter. For all laser treatments, the saline infusion technique must be employed. After laser, I would perform PTCA with a 3.0 mm Lifestream.

Frank Litvack, MD, USA: I would approach this lesion with a 9F JR4 or Amplatz guide with sideholes, and cross the lesion with an extra-support wire. I would perform ELCA using vigorous saline flush with a 1.4 mm and then with a 1.7 mm or 2.0 mm catheter. I would perform multiple passes, and reorient the guide to redirect the laser beam and achieve a larger lumen. I would then perform adjunctive PTCA.

Timothy Sanborn, MD, USA: I would use a 1.4 mm catheter followed by a 1.7 mm catheter. Adjunctive PTCA will be needed to optimize the result.

Editors' Perspective: ELCA can be used for calcified ostial lesions, but Rotablator may achieve more predictable results. If ELCA is used, the saline infusion technique must be employed to minimize complications and improve plaque ablation.

*****

ELCA: OSTIAL DIAGONAL

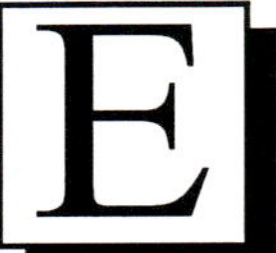xcimer laser angioplasty of an ostial lesion in the diagonal (reference diameter = 3.2 mm).

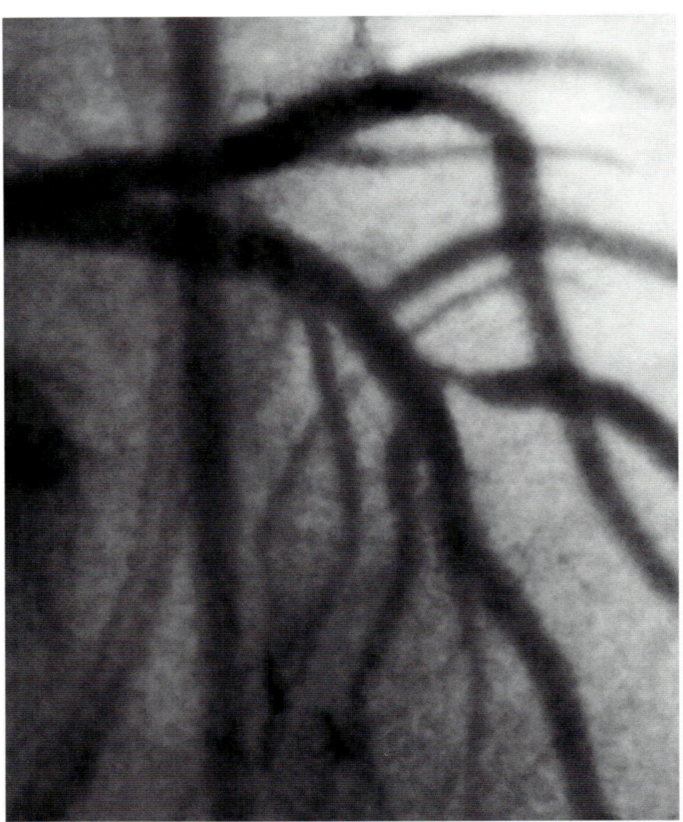

Is ELCA reasonable for this lesion?

John Bittl, MD, USA: ELCA is not recommended because of the abrupt angle of origin of the diagonal branch from the LAD.

Frank Litvack, MD, USA: I do not favor ELCA because of the risk of perforation at the carina.

Comment on device sizing and important technical tips.

Timothy Sanborn, MD, USA: I would pretreat this lesion with a 1.7 mm ELCA catheter prior to PTCA with a 3.0 mm compliant balloon.

Editors' Perspective: The results of ELCA for this lesion type are unpredictable.

*****

ELCA: OSTIAL LAD

Excimer laser angioplasty of an ostial lesion in the LAD (reference diameter = 3.8 mm).

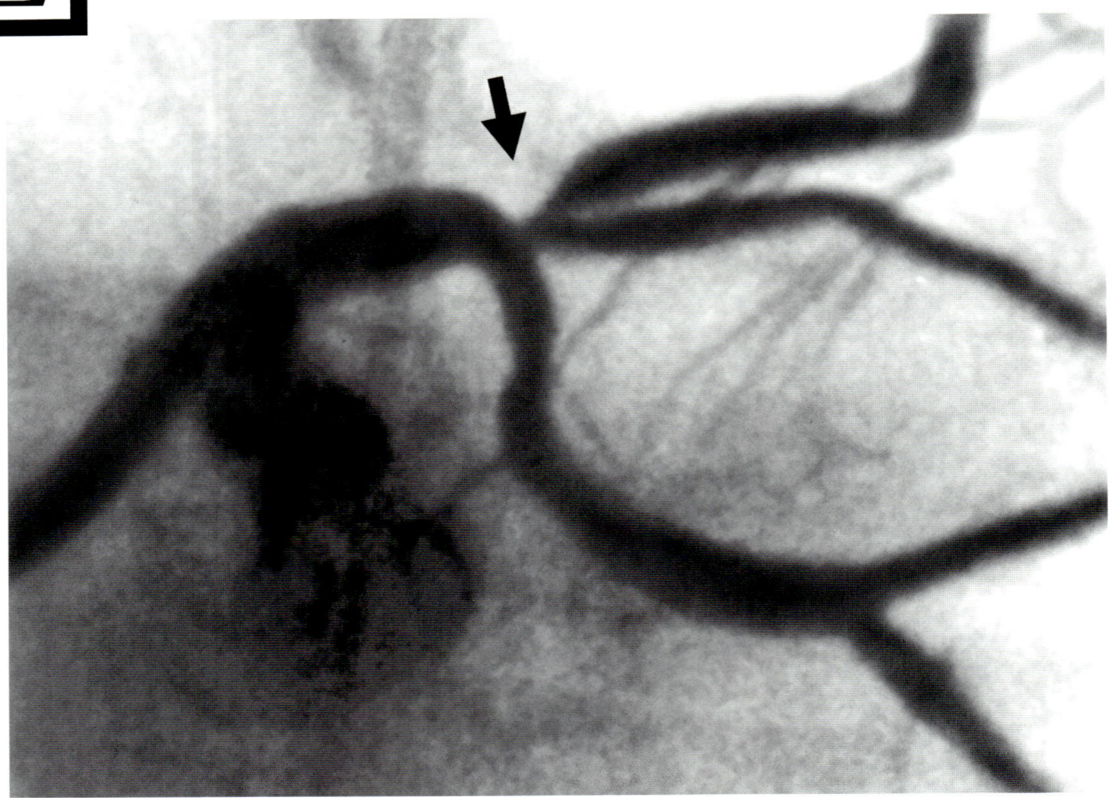

Is ELCA reasonable for this lesion?

Frank Litvack, MD, USA: I do not favor ELCA.

<u>Editors' Perspective</u>: **ELCA has no role for this lesion.**

*****

ELCA: OSTIAL LCX

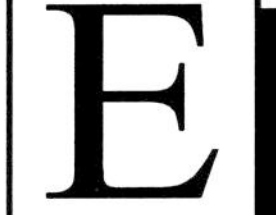

xcimer laser angioplasty of an ostial lesion in the LCX (reference diameters: left main = 4.2 mm; LCX = 3.8 mm).

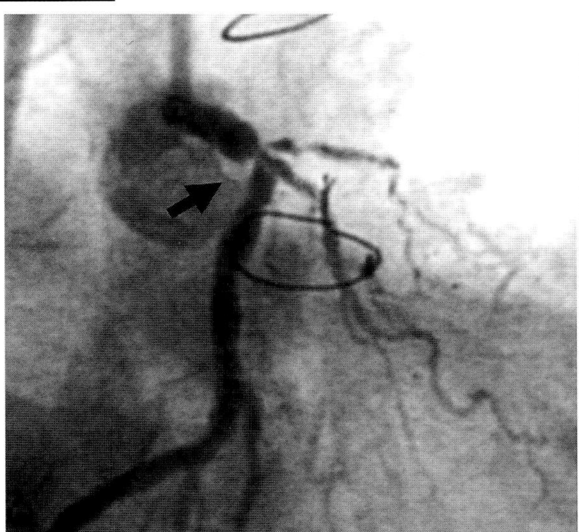

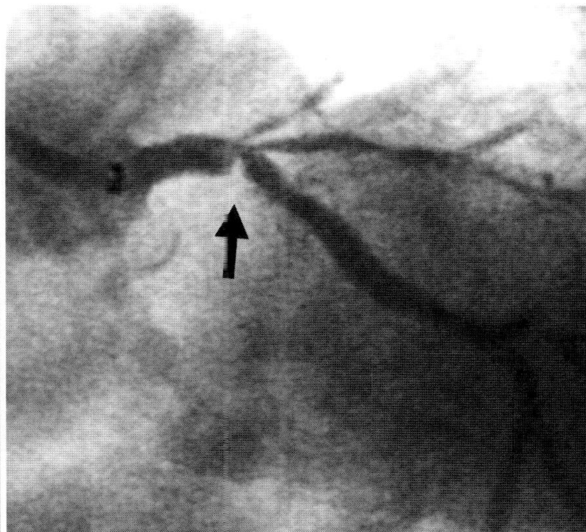

Is ELCA reasonable for this lesion?

Frank Litvack, MD, USA: The lesion is eccentric and involves the origin of two small obtuse marginal branches. I do not favor ELCA since the lesion is very discrete.

> **<u>Editors' Perspective</u>: ELCA with concentric laser catheters has virtually no role for this lesion. Because of marked eccentricity, the role of the directional laser catheter is uncertain. Although the initial plan was to perform directional atherectomy, a DVI 10F guiding catheter could not be positioned in the ostium of the left main. ELCA was performed by using a 9F JL4 guide, a 0.018-inch Extra-Support guidewire, and a 1.8 mm AIS directional laser catheter (before the availability of stents and Rotablator). Adjunctive PTCA was performed with a 3.5 x 40 mm balloon without complication.**

*****

ELCA: VEIN GRAFT

Excimer laser angioplasty of a vein graft to the RCA (reference diameter = 3.9 mm).

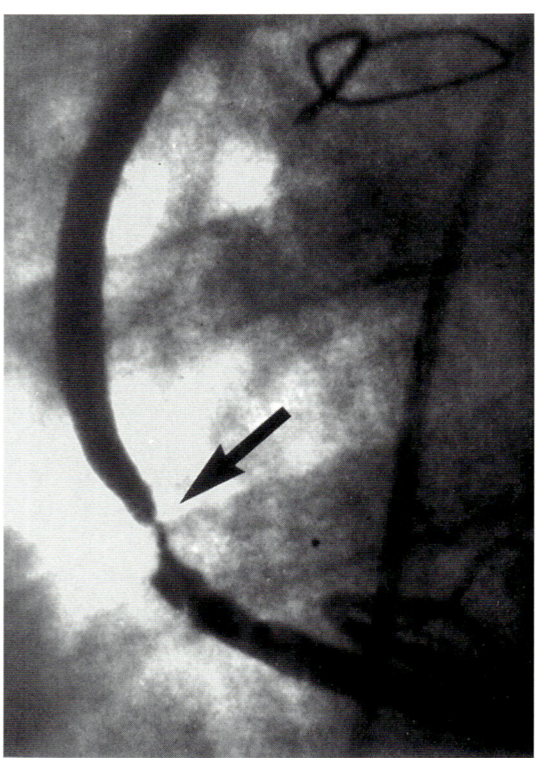

Is ELCA reasonable for this lesion?

John Bittl, MD, USA: This discrete lesion in the mid-portion of the graft to the RCA can be pretreated with ELCA.

Frank Litvack, MD, USA: This is an excellent case for ELCA and adjunctive PTCA.

Comment on device sizing and important technical tips.

John Bittl, MD, USA: I would use a 2.0 mm ELCA catheter through a 9F JR4 or IMA guide. I would then implant several 4.0 mm Palmaz-Schatz stents, and postdilate with a 4.0 x 18 mm Titan. ReoPro may reduce the likelihood of CK elevation from distal embolization.

Frank Litvack, MD, USA: I would debulk with a 1.4 mm and then a 2.0 mm laser catheter, follow by adjunctive PTCA and multiple stent placement. One must be prepared to accept the risk of distal embolization and no-reflow in this situation.

> **Editors' Perspective: ELCA could be employed in this situation, but its value compared to other techniques such as TEC or PTCA is unknown. Several centers have favorable experience with ELCA in degenerated vein grafts, but definitive lumen enlargement with PTCA or stenting is always required.**

*****

ELCA: OSTIAL VEIN GRAFT

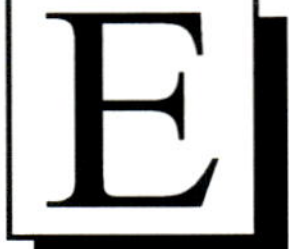xcimer laser angioplasty of an ostial lesion in a vein graft to the LAD (reference diameter = 3.9 mm).

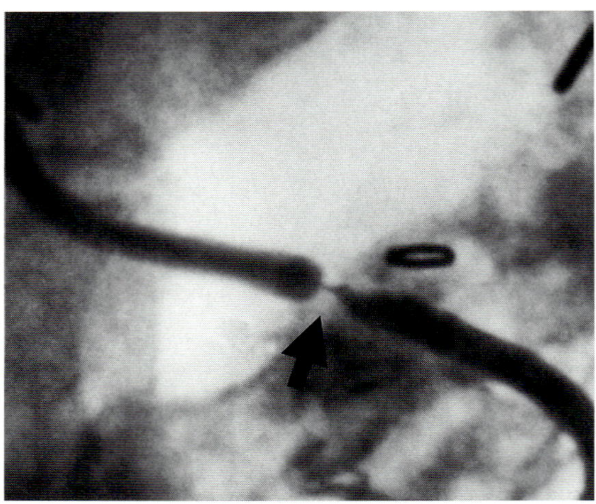

Is ELCA reasonable for this lesion?

John Bittl, MD, USA: ELCA is reasonable to reduce the likelihood of distal embolization and no-reflow.

Frank Litvack, MD, USA: This lesion can be treated with ELCA followed by adjunctive PTCA or stent placement.

Timothy Sanborn, MD, USA: ELCA is very successful in debulking these ostial vein graft lesions.

Comment on device sizing and important technical tips.

John Bittl, MD, USA: I would insert a 2.0 mm laser catheter through a 9F JR4 guide catheter. I would deploy a 4.0 mm Palmaz Schatz coronary stent and postdilate with a 4.0 x 18 mm Titan.

Timothy Sanborn, MD, USA: This is an excellent case for device synergy (ELCA followed by stent), to obtain the optimum angiographic result. I would use the 1.7 mm eccentric laser catheter rather than the stiffer 2.0 mm laser catheter. Multiple passes and catheter rotation will allow the most debulking prior to stent deployment.

Editors' Perspective: As with Rotablator atherectomy, ELCA can be used quite effectively to debulk such lesions before definitive stenting. Larger excimer laser fibers are required to sufficiently debulk the ostium before stenting, and the saline infusion technique is mandatory.

*****

Stent Techniques

STENT: ECCENTRIC LESION (LAD)

Stent of an eccentric lesion in the proximal LAD (reference diameter = 3.4 mm).

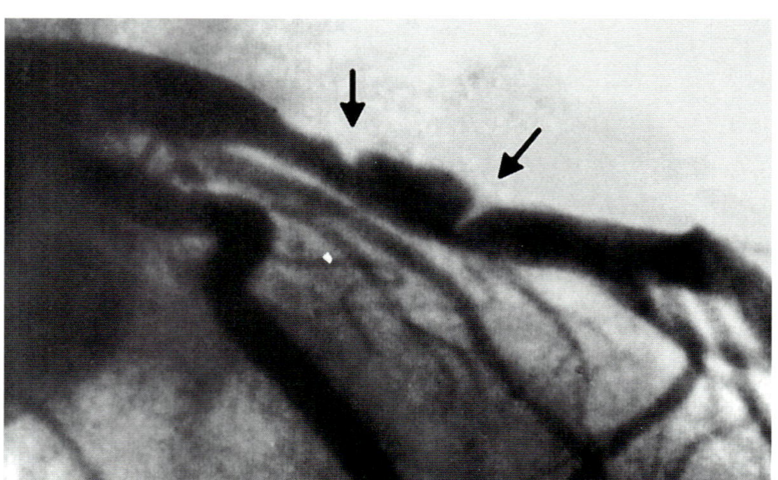

Is stenting reasonable for this lesion?

Donald Baim, MD, USA: The LAD lesion is well treated by stenting.

Antonio Colombo, MD, Italy: Stenting is reasonable and appropriate; multiple stents are required.

Ian Penn, MD, Canada: Stenting is entirely reasonable for this tandem eccentric stenosis in the LAD. The length, eccentricity, and complexity of the stenosis suggest that the optimal therapy is stenting.

Comment on device sizing and important technical tips.

Donald Baim, MD, USA: I would cover both lesions with two Palmaz-Schatz coronary stents or a single PS 204 biliary stent. My usual approach is to place the distal stent first. In this case, the proximal stent could be placed first and postdilated to 3.5 mm.

Antonio Colombo, MD, Italy: I would start with an 8F JL4 guiding catheter, a 0.014-inch Hi-torque floppy guidewire, a 3.5 mm balloon for predilation, and two 3.5 mm Palmaz-Schatz stents. Final dilation may require a 4.0 mm balloon. The lesion is ulcerated and probably soft, suggesting that good stent expansion will be achieved. IVUS is important to confirm an optimal result. Aspirin with optional ticlopidine would be prescribed.

Ian Penn, MD, Canada: The reference diameter is 3.4 mm, but the proximal vessel may be larger. This is important, since stenting a tapering vessel requires certain technical modifications. I would place one or two 3.5 mm Palmaz-Schatz stents or a 30 mm Nir stent in this eccentric stenosis, followed by a 3.5 mm balloon at 16-20 ATM. A short balloon may be needed to taper the stent. A stent without an articulation is ideal here, but if unavailable, the articulation should be placed between the two lesions. This can be accomplished by crimping the stent onto a single-marker balloon such as a Titan or NC Express, which could be used for predilating, stent delivery, and postdilation.

> **Editors' Perspective: For many interventional cardiologists, stenting is the procedure of choice for eccentric lesions in large vessels. There are a variety of stents to choose from, but the only approved stent for this lesion in the United States is the Palmaz-Schatz coronary stent. Several technical points are worthy of special emphasis: First, it is very important to ensure complete coverage of this lengthy segment, even if multiple stents are required. Second, since there is significant vessel tapering, it is important to "mold" the stents with high-pressure balloons to match the proximal and distal reference segments. Third, it is best to avoid placing the articulation in the most severe portion of the stenosis, if possible. A special technique for "eliminating" the articulation involves cutting the Palmaz-Schatz stent at the articulation and remounting the two half-stents on the delivery balloon so they overlap by 1-1.5 mm; the delivery balloon can then be pulled back into the delivery sheath, followed by stent deployment and high-pressure PTCA. Other stents without articulations could be used quite effectively (AVE Microstent, Cook GR-II stent, ACS MultiLink stent, etc). The Schneider Wallstent is extremely conformable, and may be useful in long segments of disease in tapered vessels.**

*****

STENT: ECCENTRIC LESION (RCA)

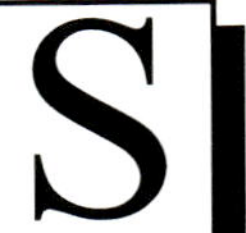tent of an eccentric lesion in the mid-RCA (reference diameter = 3.2 mm).

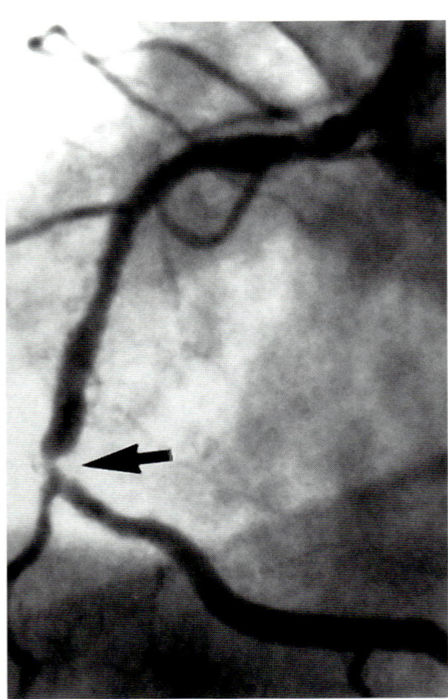

Is stenting reasonable for this lesion?

Donald Baim, MD, USA: This RCA lesion is not well suited for Palmaz-Schatz stenting, given anticipated delivery problems around the acute angle in the mid- and distal RCA. Although a Gianturco-Roubin stent might pass around this angle over a stiff guidewire, the focal lesion might protrude through the coils of the stent. Newer, more flexible slotted-tube designs (MultiLink stent, Nir stent) might be more suitable.

Antonio Colombo, MD, Italy: Stenting is reasonable and appropriate; multiple stents are required.

Ian Penn, MD, Canada: This patient has diffuse disease, ectasia, and a severe stenosis in a bend. Although diffuse disease argues against stenting, I consider the RCA a conduit to the nutrient branches, and as such can tolerate moderate disease as long as there is no significant focal stenosis. The focal stenosis should be stented.

Comment on device sizing and important technical tips.

Ian Penn, MD, Canada: The approach to stenting is straightforward. I would use a JR4 guide, a 0.014-inch Extra-S'port wire, and a flexible 3.5 mm Cordis or GR-II stent. For all flexible coil stents, rigorous predilation is necessary with high pressure inflations with a slightly undersized balloon (0.25-.5 mm less than the reference diameter), ensuring that there are no segments resistant to expansion. Another approach is to use a short (8 mm) or half (7 mm) Palmaz-Schatz stent to cover the focal stenosis, and postdilate with a 3.5 mm x 8-10 mm Titan or High Energy.

> **Editors' Perspective: The vessel caliber certainly favors stenting, although the acute bend in the mid-RCA may impair stent delivery. However, use of extra-support or heavy-duty guidewires, such as the Platinum-Plus, has greatly simplified the stent approach to such lesions. Although the Wallstent is not available in the United States, experience in Europe suggests that it is extremely trackable and may be useful in this setting.**

*****

STENT: ULCERATED LESION

Stent of an ulcerated lesion in the mid-LAD (reference diameter = 3.2 mm).

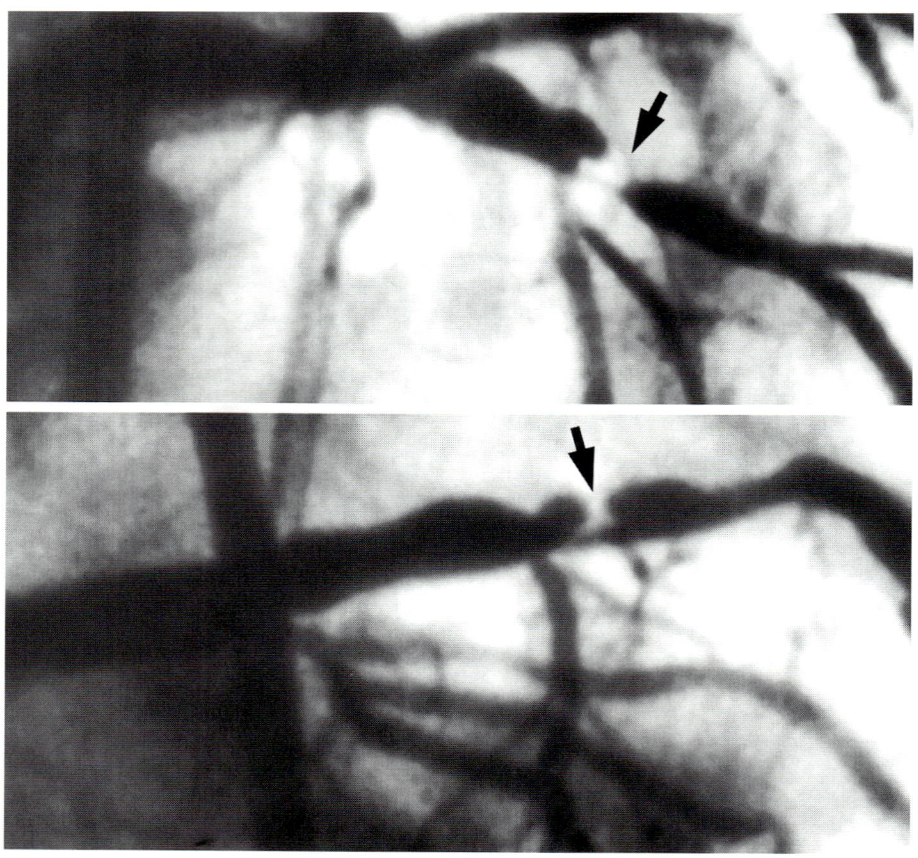

Is stenting reasonable for this lesion?

Antonio Colombo, MD, Italy: Stenting is appropriate.

Gary Roubin, MD, PhD, USA: This tapering LAD is suitable for stent placement.

Comment on device sizing and important technical tips.

Antonio Colombo, MD, Italy: I would initially predilate the large septal branch with a 2.0-2.5 mm ACE, and predilate the LAD with a 3.0 mm balloon. I would implant a 3.0 mm Palmaz-Schatz stent (with a delivery sheath) and then dilate at 17-18 ATM with a 3.5 x 9-10 mm balloon. I would use a short balloon for the final high-pressure dilation because the distal vessel tapers. At the end, it may be necessary to further dilate the large septal through the stent.

Gary Roubin, MD, PhD, USA: My strategy is to start with a 3.5/3.0 x 25 mm tapered balloon and predilate at low pressure, prior to placing a 3.5 x 20 mm Gianturco-Roubin stent. I would carefully rewrap the tapered balloon before the high-pressure inflation, but if it does not advance easily, I would change to an Olympix-II or Mighty. If there is compromise of the distal diagonal or septal prior to stent placement, I would dilate with a 2.0 mm Bandit over a 0.014-inch wire, prior to high-pressure inflation.

<u>Editors' Perspective</u>: Because of the large caliber of this vessel and the abnormal contour of the lesion, stenting is an attractive therapeutic option. However, there are several issues to consider: First, it is likely that two Palmaz-Schatz coronary stents or a single 20 mm Gianturco-Roubin stent will be required to fully cover the lesion. Second, there is significant vessel tapering, which introduces uncertainty about the "true" vessel diameter and the technique of "optimal" stenting; accurate vessel sizing (and assessment of lesion length) are readily achieved with IVUS and/or on-line QCA. If necessary, the proximal and distal aspects of the stent(s) can be "molded" with high-pressure balloons of appropriate diameter, or by tapered balloons (the proximal end is 0.5 mm larger than the distal end, with gentle transition from end to end). This "molding" technique is important to minimize the chance of marginal dissection from overexpanding the distal end of the stent, and inadequate stent apposition from underexpanding the proximal end of the stent. Finally, a large septal perforator and diagonal will be traversed by the stent(s) in the LAD and possibly "jailed." When stenting across sidebranches, it is important to consider the diameter and distribution of the sidebranch, the extent of ostial sidebranch disease, and the likelihood that percutaneous revascularization of the sidebranch is (or could be) clinically important. Although sidebranches can be retrieved after stenting, it is not always possible, and even when successful, retrieval can be technically challenging. In general, it is best not to stent across large sidebranches which themselves could be considered suitable for bypass surgery. Smaller branches rarely lead to significant clinical problems, even if permanently trapped in "stent-jail." As mentioned by Dr. Roubin, if sidebranch occlusion is anticipated after stenting, predilation of the sidebranch before stenting (either before or after predilation of the target lesion in the parent vessel) may help preserve sidebranch patency.

*****

STENT: TUBULAR LESION

Stent of a tubular lesion in the mid-RCA (length = 15 mm; reference diameter = 2.5 mm).

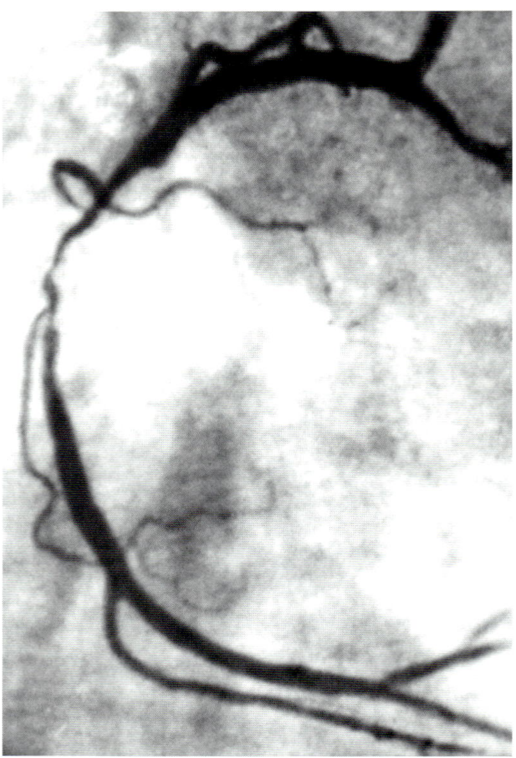

Is stenting reasonable for this lesion?

Marie-Claude Morice, MD, France: Stenting long lesions in small arteries does not offer any benefit in terms of restenosis, and probably increases the risk of stent thrombosis. I would stent this lesion only if the PTCA result is suboptimal.

Masakiyo Nobuyoshi, MD, Japan: The vessel diameter is too small for a stent.

Richard Schatz, MD, USA: The angiogram shows a long, severe lesion in a vessel which is not tortuous. This lesion is ideal for stenting due to the excellent "nondiseased" smooth inflow and outflow. The morphology of the lesion is irrelevant when considering a patient for stenting; one need only consider the inflow, outflow, and vessel diameter (3.0 mm stent is a minimum).

Comment on device sizing and important technical tips.

Marie-Claude Morice, MD, France: If PTCA is suboptimal, I would perform IVUS to accurately size the vessel diameter. If appropriate, this lesion could be treated with a 32 mm Nir stent mounted on a 36 mm Viva balloon.

Richard Schatz, MD, USA: Since the lesion is long, I would place at least two stents, with the distal one first in the most "normal" part of the vessel, to avoid the unfortunate situation where more distal disease needs to be stented. If there is any doubt at all, I always err on the side of placing an extra stent distally, since adding proximal stents is easier than adding distal stents. Each stent should overlap the other by 1-2 mm. I would postdilate with a 3.0 mm NC Bandit at 20 ATM. If the familiar "step-up" and "step-down" is visible in two projections, intravascular ultrasound is not required. If absent, I would use a 3.25 mm or 3.5 mm NC Bandit at 18-20 ATM.

> **Editors' Perspective: The use of multiple stents in vessels < 3 mm is a matter of some controversy. Early stent experience suggested that stenting small vessels was associated with an increased risk of stent thrombosis and restenosis. Furthermore, many stents that are manufactured in the United States are not available in diameters < 3 mm (particularly those that are premounted on a delivery balloon). Nevertheless, preliminary studies in Europe and Japan suggest that stenting small vessels may have real benefit, particularly if optimal stent technique is employed. Several observational and randomized studies are planned or in progress to assess the relative merits of stenting small vessels. For users of the Palmaz-Schatz stent, the delivery balloon (and stent) can be removed from the delivery sheath, the stent remounted on a 2.5 mm balloon, and the stent delivered with or without the delivery sheath. High-pressure PTCA should follow, as usual. The GR-II and Microstents will be available in diameters < 3 mm.**

*****

STENT: LONG LESION

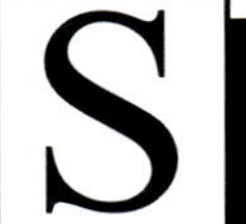

tent of a long lesion in the mid-LAD (length = 25 mm; reference diameter = 3.3 mm).

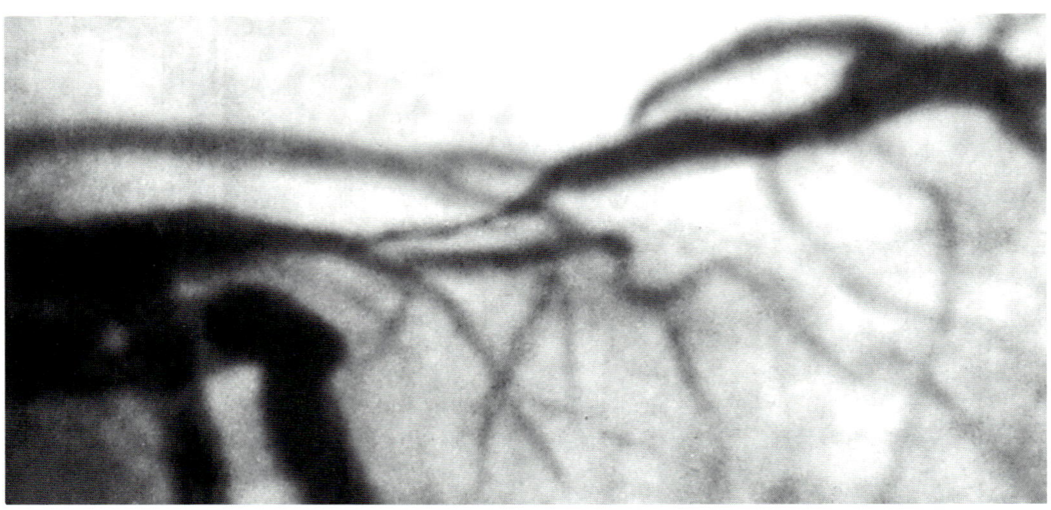

Is stenting reasonable for this lesion?

Marie-Claude Morice, MD, France: Stenting a long lesion in a large vessel is reasonable to decrease the risk of the procedure. However, there are no data on long-term restenosis after stenting long lesions.

Masakiyo Nobuyoshi, MD, Japan: This lesion in a large vessel is suitable for stenting.

Richard Schatz, MD, USA: The length of the lesion is irrelevant, as long as there is excellent inflow and outflow, and at least a 3.0 mm stent can be implanted. The cuff in the proximal LAD is extremely favorable since it will permit safe stenting without encroaching upon the left main or LCX.

Comment on device sizing and important technical tips.

Marie-Claude Morice, MD, France: In this case, my choice is to stent with two 3.5 x 20 mm Gianturco-Roubin stents to completely cover the lesion. Two Palmaz Schatz stents will not be long enough to cover the whole lesion. Alternatively, 3.5 x 32 mm and 3.5 x 16 mm Nir stents can be used to cover the entire lesion. I do not routinely use IVUS.

Masakiyo Nobuyoshi, MD, Japan: I would first predilate with a 3.0 x 40 mm balloon, using an 8F JL4 guide and a 0.014- inch guidewire. I would place a 3.5 x 20 mm Palmaz-Schatz stent in the distal part of the lesion, and then place a second stent in the more proximal part of the lesion. I would dilate both stents with a 3.5 x 20 mm noncompliant balloon at 15 ATM. If two stents don't cover the entire lesion, I would implant a third stent.

Richard Schatz, MD, USA: I would make some assessment of calcification by angiography or ultrasound. If calcium is present, I would perform rotational atherectomy first, followed by two tandem 3.5 mm Palmaz-Schatz stents (the distal one first). I would make sure they overlap 1-2 mm, the distal end of the distal stent is in contact with "normal" wall, and the proximal end of the proximal stent is up to the left main. I would postdilate with a 3.5 mm NC Bandit at 20 ATM, looking carefully in multiple projections for the familiar "step-up" and "step-down", to confirm optimal deployment. Since this vessel tapers, there is a chance that the proximal end of the stents may need to be dilated with a 4.0 x 9 mm Titan or a 4.0/3.5 x 25 mm tapered balloon.

Editors' Perspective: Long lesions in large vessels are readily treated with stents or other devices. Although Palmaz-Schatz stents have been shown to achieve better immediate and late results than PTCA in focal lesions, similar studies in long lesions have not yet been completed. Bill O'Neill frequently refers to the pretty angiograms produced by stenting as the "pursuit of luminal cosmetology;" further studies are clearly needed to confirm the benefits of stenting these lesions. If stenting is performed, plan for multiple stents, ensuring 1-2 mm of stent overlap and that unstented gaps do not occur between stents. Since there is often significant tapering of vessels containing long lesions in such vessels, it is extremely important to ensure optimal stent apposition, particularly at the ends of the proximal and distal stents.

*****

STENT: FUNCTIONAL TOTAL OCCLUSION

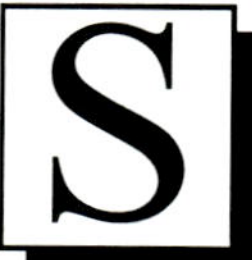

Stent of a functional total occlusion in the proximal LAD (reference diameter = 2.7 mm). Assume the occlusion can be crossed with a guidewire.

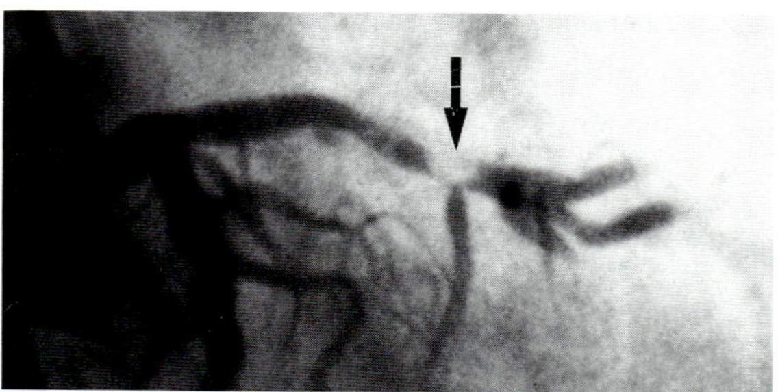

Is stenting reasonable for this lesion?

Masakiyo Nobuyoshi, MD, Japan: Stenting is not recommended because of the risk of occlusion of the diagonal branch.

Marie-Claude Morice, MD, France: Stenting this total occlusion is a good choice; the artery is 2.7 mm, but it can be "stretched" to 3.0 mm with a stent.

Ulrich Sigwart, MD, England: I assume there is thrombus which overlies the first septal branch. I cannot see the distal vessel and there may be debris, as well. A stent is not my first choice in this situation.

Comment on device sizing and important technical tips.

Marie-Claude Morice, MD, France: Because of tortuosity, I would select an 8F JL4 guiding catheter, cross the lesion with a 0.018-inch Extra-Support wire, and dilate with a 3.0 mm Cobra balloon. I would place a 3.0 mm x 12 mm Gianturco-Roubin stent to maintain access to the large septal branch. One question in this case is whether to protect the septal branch with a wire, since the risk of embolizing thrombus to the septal branch is not negligible. For simplicity, I would not protect it; in case of occlusion of the septal branch, crossing it with a wire will be easy. However, I would not cover the origin of the septal branch with a Palmaz-Schatz stent. IVUS is not necessary.

> **Editors' Perspective: Stenting this lesion shares some of the issues concerning directional atherectomy, including uncertainty about the size and morphology of the vessel distal to the occlusion, the "true" size of the normal reference vessel, and the extent of thrombus in the lesion. Additional considerations include stenting across septal and diagonal sidebranches.**

*****

STENT: TOTAL OCCLUSION

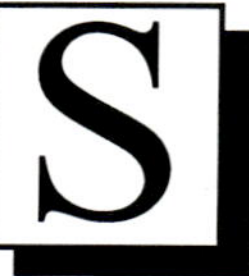

Stent of a total occlusion in the proximal RCA (reference diameter = 4.5 mm). Assume the occlusion can be crossed with a guidewire.

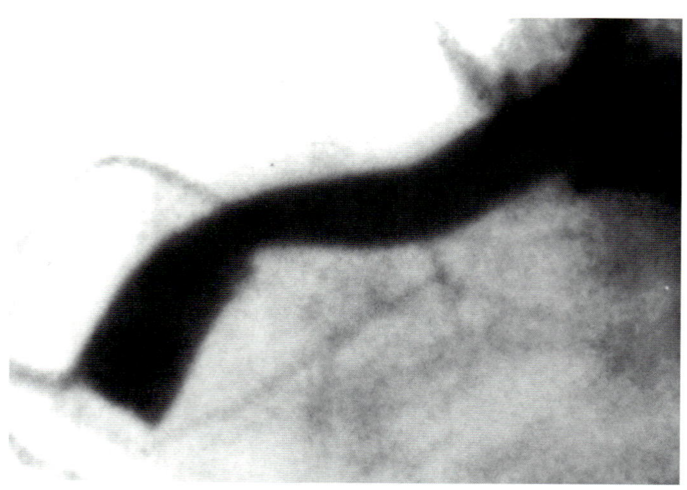

Is stenting reasonable for this lesion?

Masakiyo Nobuyoshi, MD, Japan: This is a large artery; if PTCA is successful, it should be followed by stenting.

Marie-Claude Morice, MD, France: Primary stenting is reasonable in this lesion because the RCA is so large, and stenting will probably prevent restenosis. However, since I do not know the precise length of the occlusion, indications for stenting are uncertain.

Ulrich Sigwart, MD, England: This looks like fresh thrombus. I am not terribly worried about dilating this lesion with a 3.5 mm or larger balloon at low pressure and seeing what the distal artery looks like. A stent is no problem in this situation, if the artery doesn't look perfect after

PTCA. Intracoronary urokinase can be added, if necessary.

Comment on device sizing and important technical tips.

Masakiyo Nobuyoshi, MD, Japan: Since biliary stents are not available in Japan, I would use a 4.0 mm Palmaz-Schatz stent expanded with a 4.5 x 20 mm noncompliant high-pressure balloon, an 8F JR4 guide, and a 0.014-inch wire. It is important to remember that the lesion is long; multiple stents are necessary. If there is a large thrombus, intravenous urokinase (96,000 units over 24 hours) should be given after stenting.

Marie-Claude Morice, MD, France: I would select a 6F right Amplatz guiding catheter because the occlusion is very proximal and good guide support is needed. I would use a 0.014-inch Extra-Support wire and a 3.5 mm balloon; intermediate or standard wires are too stiff and are as likely to cross the occlusion as perforate the artery. I would inflate the balloon for a few seconds, inject intracoronary nitrates, and assess the distal bed, lesion length, and additional stenoses. For a single short lesion, I would place a Palmaz-Schatz stent crimped on the same balloon, and dilate with a 4.5 mm high-pressure, noncompliant balloon. For a lesion longer than 20 mm or for multiple lesions, I would perform PTCA alone or implant multiple stents. Since IVUS has not been shown to decrease stent restenosis, I routinely use high-pressure adjunctive PTCA without IVUS.

> Editors' Perspective: **In large caliber vessels, stents may offer the best opportunity for lumen enlargement and prevention of restenosis. However, stenting a total occlusion raises the issues about thrombus burden, length of the occlusion, and diameter of the target vessel beyond the occlusion. If stenting is considered for this lesion, there are several considerations: First, single or multiple stents must be employed to cover the entire length of the lesion. Second, the operator must select the appropriate type and size stent (e.g., the large caliber of this vessel would mitigate against the Gianturco-Roubin or MultiLink stents, but would favor the Palmaz-Schatz coronary stent, the Palmaz biliary stent, the Microstent, or the Wallstent). Third, if there is significant thrombus burden, adjunctive therapies may be warranted before and/or after stenting including bolus or prolonged intracoronary infusion of urokinase, local drug delivery with the Ultramed or Dispatch catheter, prolonged intravenous infusion of heparin, and/or bolus plus infusion of ReoPro.**

*****

STENT: ANGULATED LESION (LAD)

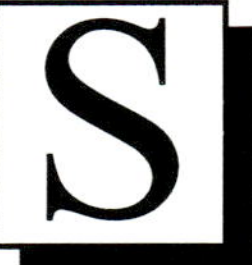tent of an angulated lesion in the proximal LAD (lesion on inner curve; reference diameter = 3.4 mm).

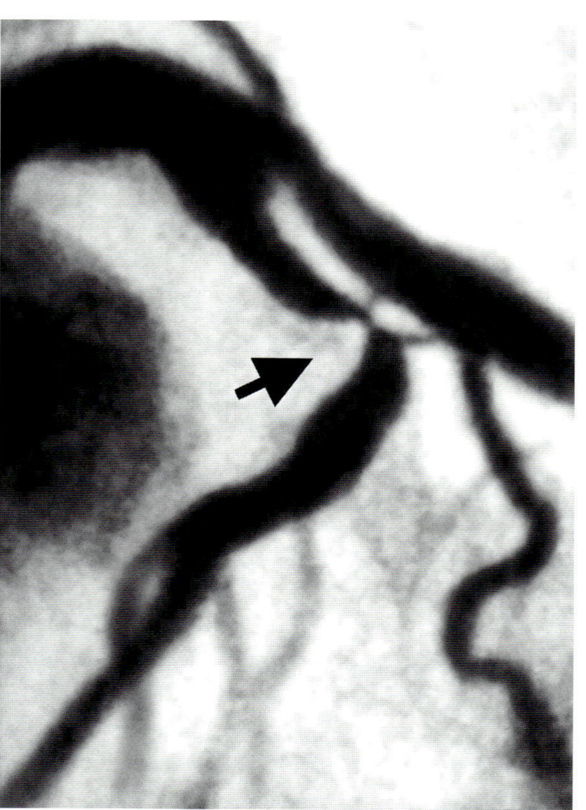

Is stenting reasonable for this lesion?

Ian Penn, MD, Canada: The use of short disarticulated stents for focal stenoses has been associated with excellent short-term results, although the long-term benefit is unknown. This approach is attractive since angulated lesions are often difficult to cross with longer, rigid stents, and coil separation is frequent with flexible stents. The disadvantage of a short stent is that the area of disease is often more extensive than suggested by angiography. Therefore, other potentially useful stents include a flexible tubular stent (e.g. Nir stent) or a flexible coil stent (GR-II, Cordis stent).

Gary Roubin, MD, PhD, USA: I would approach this lesion with elective stenting.

Patrick Serruys, MD, PhD, The Netherlands: The first question in approaching this lesion is whether the diagonal branch, which appears to be emerging from the lesion, is important. If the diameter of the diagonal is ≥ 2.5 mm, I recommend stenting the ostium of the diagonal prior to stenting the LAD.

Comment on device sizing and important technical tips.

Ian Penn, MD, Canada: Good coaxial guiding catheter support is required, and a Voda or left Amplatz guide should be inserted prior to stent placement. The use of an Extra-Support wire or a 0.018-inch wire will facilitate stent passage around this severe bend. I rarely stent in the LAO view, but prefer the AP cranial view to straighten the proximal LAD. I would predilate with a double marker high-pressure balloon, then place the stent using the same view, making sure to have the proximal margin of the stent just beyond the origin of the LAD and the distal margin of the stent in the ectatic distal reference segment (3-4 mm distal to the lesion). IVUS is helpful (given the tapering of the proximal LAD) to determine the true reference size.

Gary Roubin, MD, PhD, USA: I would use a 0.018-inch compatible balloon, a 0.018-inch Roadrunner wire in the distal LAD, and a short tip JL3 or JL4 guiding catheter. A 4.0 x 12 mm Gianturco-Roubin stent is much more trackable than the 20 mm stent and should easily cover the lesion. After deploying the stent at 5-6 ATM, I would withdraw the balloon 2-3 mm inside the stent and inflate to 8-9 ATM to embed the coils in the vessel. A 3.5 x 4.0 mm tapered balloon or short Titan is suitable for postdilation. I would discharge the patient on aspirin and ticlopidine.

Patrick Serruys, MD, PhD, The Netherlands: In order to facilitate the use of 2 wires and kissing balloons, I recommend an 8F giant-lumen JL4 guiding catheter, a 300 cm wire in the LAD, a 175 cm wire in the diagonal, a 2.0 mm compliant balloon in the diagonal, and a 3.0 mm compliant balloon in the LAD. I would perform kissing balloon inflations at low pressure. One approach is to then carefully implant a half Palmaz-Schatz stent or an AVE Microstent precisely in the ostium of the diagonal. The entire procedure can be jeopardized if the stent in the diagonal protrudes into the LAD. Having successfully implanted the diagonal stent, I would cross the LAD with the 3.0 mm balloon to ensure that the diagonal stent is not interfering, and inflate it at this site. Having done this, I would choose a 5.0 x 18 mm Wallstent, and postdilate using a 4.0 mm noncompliant balloon at 16 ATM. More recently, my approach is to predilate both lesions with kissing balloons, and then deploy a flexible coil stent (e.g. Nir stent, Bistent, or Microstent) in the LAD, maintaining guidewire access in the diagonal branch. A third wire is then advanced into the diagonal, and the original wire in the diagonal is removed. A low-profile stent (e.g. Nir stent, Bistent) is deployed in the diagonal. I would treat this patient with aspirin (100 mg QD) and Ticlopidine (250 mg BID for 1 month).

Editors' Perspective: A number of technical points are worth emphasizing when stenting angulated lesions in large vessels: First, excellent guidewire and guiding catheter support should be achieved prior to stent implantation. This is readily accomplished with a variety of left coronary guiding catheters, such as a left Amplatz, XB (extra backup), EBU (extra backup), left Voda, or GL (geometric left), which derive their power support from the left sinus of Valsalva (left Amplatz) or the opposite wall of the aorta (XB, EBU, Voda, GL). Extra-Support, Platinum-Plus, Roadrunner, and Stabilizer guidewires are particularly useful for stenting angulated lesions. Second, there may be important differences in performance between stents. For example, flexible coil stents such as the Gianturco-Roubin stent are very conformable; however, Extra-Support guidewires and power guides are required to access the angulated lesion and prevent telescoping of the stent. The short (12 mm) stent may be particularly useful in focal, angulated stenoses, and the flatwire construction of the new GR-II will eliminate most of the problems with earlier designs. Rigid tubular stents such as the Palmaz-Schatz stent may have difficulty accessing angulated lesions; the "buddy-wire" and "stentless delivery sheath" techniques (p. 74), and use of disarticulated half-stents may enhance success. With excellent guidewire and guiding catheter support, "bare" stents can be employed, but there is a significant risk of premature stent delivery. Both the Gianturco-Roubin and Palmaz-Schatz stents share the potential problem of prolapse of atheroma through the coils (Gianturco-Roubin stent) or articulation in the angle vertex (Palmaz-Schatz stent), necessitating placement of an overlapping stent. Other stents such as the Microstent or the MultiLink stent may be particularly useful because of their flexibility and ease of insertion. The Wallstent is extremely flexible and trackable, and may be useful for such lesions, as well.

*****

STENT: ANGULATED LESION (RCA)

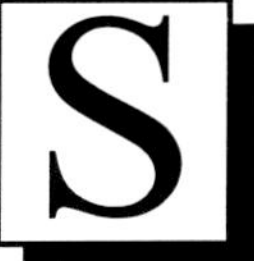

Stent of an angulated lesion in the proximal RCA (lesion on outer curve; reference diameter = 3.1 mm).

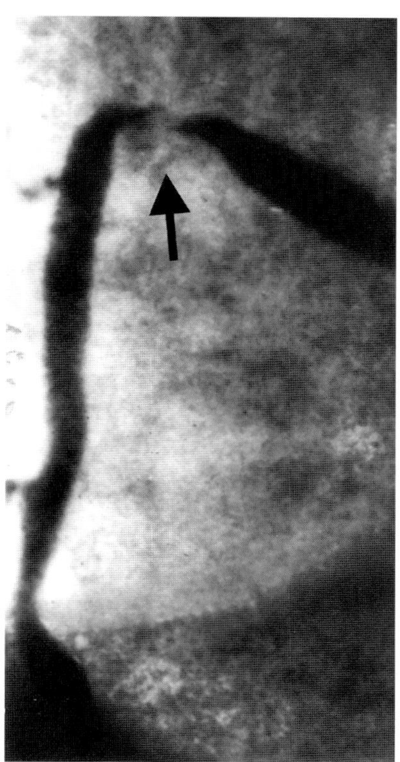

Is stenting reasonable for this lesion?

Ian Penn, MD, Canada: This patient has an eccentric stenosis in the proximal RCA with diffuse irregularity beyond the marginal branch. This lesion is suitable for stenting; the only issue is which one.

Gary Roubin, MD, PhD, USA: This lesion will be challenging with a Palmaz-Schatz stent or the first generation Gianturco-Roubin stent. However, stenting is readily accomplished with a GR-II stent.

Patrick Serruys, MD, PhD, The Netherlands: Many stents may be used in this lesion; the only dilemma is choosing which one.

Comment on device sizing and important technical tips.

Ian Penn, MD, Canada: Excellent guiding catheter support is mandatory, using a left Amplatz guide with sideholes. I also recommend a 0.014-inch or 0.018-inch Extra-Support wire and a 7-10 mm tubular stent to improve the chance of successful delivery and reduce the chance of distal dissection. I would predilate with a 3.0 x 8 mm high-pressure balloon, deliver the stent, and postdilate at 20 ATM. I recommend ultrasound to determine the adequacy of stent deployment. Another approach is to use a flexible coil stent (e.g. Cordis, Gianturco-Roubin stent) because of its flexibility, conformability and good radial support.

Gary Roubin, MD, PhD, USA: I would start with a Lumax left Amplatz guiding catheter for excellent support, an undersize Bandit balloon, and a flexible guidewire. After predilating the lesion, I would advance the balloon into the distal RCA, and exchange the flexible wire for a 0.014-inch Platinum-Plus wire. I would assess the lesion and vessel size for choice of a stent. A 12 mm Gianturco-Roubin stent should take care of this lesion and will certainly be easier to track around the bend than the 20 mm Gianturco-Roubin stent. I would deploy the stent at 4-5 ATM to ensure full stent expansion prior to deflating the delivery balloon. I would then withdraw the balloon 2-3 mm and reinflate at 8 ATM for as long as possible to ensure good stent apposition. I would place a Mighty or Olympix-II balloon through the stent, and inflate at 3-4 ATM to get a good idea of where the distal end of the balloon is relative to the distal end of the stent. I would then bring the balloon back to the stent and inflate at 14-16 ATM. If the GR-II is available, it will easily track over a 0.014-inch guidewire through standard Judkins guiding catheters. The stent can be deployed at 4-5 ATM. Further high-pressure (12-14 ATM) inflations can be performed using the same balloon after withdrawing it into the stent; additional balloons are not necessary. I would discharge the patient on aspirin and ticlopidine.

Patrick Serruys, MD, PhD, The Netherlands: My strategy is to use a 9F Amplatz guide, a Schneider 0.014-inch x 300 cm guidewire to cross the lesion, and predilate with a short undersize balloon to avoid dissection. I would then implant a 4.5 x 20 mm Wallstent in the distal lesion, halfway between the acute marginal branch and the atrial branch. I would postdilate with a 3.5-4.0 mm noncompliant balloon at 16-18 ATM (size depends on online QCA). Alternative stent choices are a 20 mm GR-II stent to preserve the curve or a 16 mm Nir stent. I would postdilate using a balloon determined by online QCA.

Editors' Perspective: Technical considerations about stenting this lesion are similar to those described in the previous case. Trackable, conformable, and non-articulated stents will enhance procedural success and are preferred for this case.

*****

STENT: TORTUOUS LCX

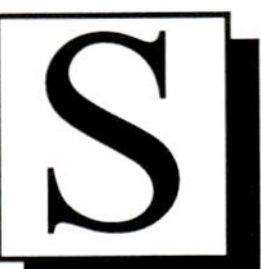
Stent of a focal lesion in a tortuous LCX (right angle takeoff; reference diameter = 2.6 mm).

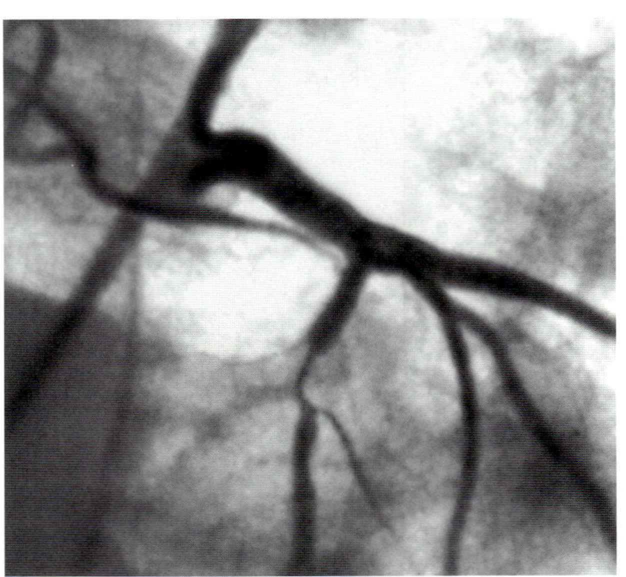

Is stenting reasonable for this lesion?

Ian Penn, MD, Canada: This case illustrates the problem of stenting an angulated lesion in the LCX which has a right angle takeoff after a long left main; stenting will not be easy.

Donald Baim, MD, USA: Stenting a LCX which originates at a right angle from a long left main segment is quite difficult even with current second generation stent technology.

Comment on device sizing and important technical tips.

Gary Roubin, MD, PhD, USA: I would approach this lesion with a trackable balloon, such as a 2.5 mm Bandit or Predator, and a 0.014-inch Traverse or a 0.014-inch Hyperflex wire. After predilating, I would place the balloon into the distal LCX, and exchange the flexible wire for a Platinum-Plus wire. I would then stent the dilated segment with one or two 3.0 x 12 mm Gianturco-Roubin stents to ensure tracking down the LCX. My guiding catheter of choice is a Cook short-tip JL3.5 or JL4. If the stent does not track, I would exchange for a 0.018-inch Roadrunner wire and attempt again to place the stent. I would postdilate with a 3.0 mm Olympix or Bandit at 16-18 ATM.

Ian Penn, MD, Canada: I would select a 0.014-inch or 0.018-inch Extra-Support wire (double bend in the tip of the wire to negotiate the sharp angulation) and a left Amplatz, Voda, or Geometric left guide for support. I may have problems crossing the lesion, so several guidewires may be required; an over-the-wire balloon or a tracking catheter is my first choice. After crossing with a guidewire, I would predilate with a low profile Europass to get an idea as to the difficulty of stent placement. My first choice of stents is a flexible stent, such as a Nir stent, GR-II, or Cordis stent. The Cordis stent can negotiate severe angulation with relative ease due its low profile and flexibility. Also, the stent is so radiopaque that undetected stent embolization is unlikely.

Donald Baim, MD, USA: This requires a highly supportive guiding catheter such as a 9F Voda, and extra-support guidewires. I would cross this lesion and predilate with conventional guidewire and balloon technology, and then exchange for a 0.014-inch Platinum-Plus guidewire for extra support. Delivery of a Palmaz-Schatz stent might then be possible, despite the unfavorable angulation. If difficulties are encountered advancing the delivery sheath around the bend into the LCX, I would resist the temptation to advance a bare stent beyond the sheath, since failure to deliver the bare stent may result in stent embolization. Better alternatives might be to hand mount a Palmaz-Schatz stent on a Bandit balloon, or to use a more flexible second generation stent, such as the MultiLink stent or the GR-II.

<u>Editors' Perspective</u>: Important technical considerations include the use of extra-support or heavy-duty guidewires, and power guides for optimal coaxial alignment and support. Stents with enhanced flexibility are preferred, such as the Microstent, the MultiLink stent, the Cordis stent, and the Wallstent. Early reports of the Nir stent suggest that it is extremely flexible, and may be useful for such lesions. The GR-II maybe particularly useful because of its flatwire construction and extreme flexibility. As mentioned by Dr. Baim, the Palmaz-Schatz stent may be difficult to deliver to the target lesion because of its inflexibility. In addition to power guides and extra-support wires, additional techniques to facilitate delivery of the Palmaz-Schatz stent include the "buddy-wire" and "stentless delivery sheath" technique (p. 74), and the use of half disarticulated stents. Further modifications of the Palmaz-Schatz stent (spiral articulation) may improve the success of stent delivery.

*****

STENT: TORTUOUS RCA

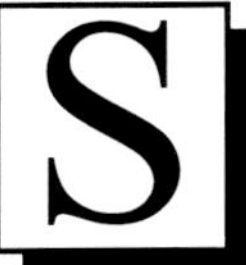
tent of a focal lesion in a tortuous RCA (reference diameter = 3.2 mm).

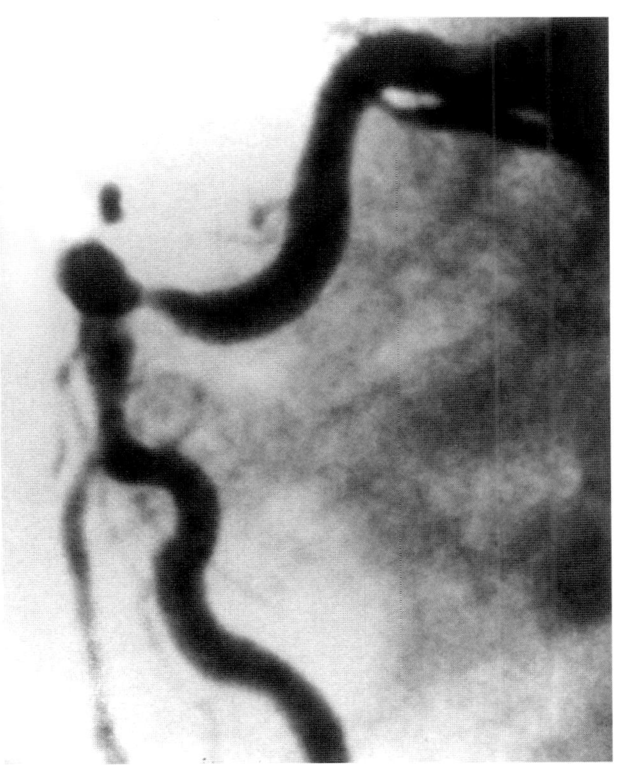

Is stenting reasonable for this lesion?

Ian Penn, MD, Canada: This lesion in an extremely tortuous vessel is suitable for a flexible coil or short tubular stent.

Donald Baim, MD, USA: The RCA is too tortuous for a Palmaz-Schatz stent, but might be suitable for a GR-II or MultiLink stent.

Gary Roubin, MD, PhD, USA: Stenting is feasible, but will be difficult.

Comment on device sizing and important technical tips.

Donald Baim, MD, USA: I would use a 9F AL 0.75 guide, an Extra-Support guidewire, and a flexible MultiLink or GR-II stent.

Gary Roubin, MD, PhD, USA: I would start this case with a Lumax 8F JR4 guiding catheter and a trackable balloon such as a Bandit, Olympix-II, or Predator. After passing a flexible 0.014-inch wire through this lesion, I would predilate and then exchange for a 0.014-inch Platinum-Plus wire. I would start distally with a 3 x 12 mm Gianturco-Roubin stent, being sure to cover the entire segment of disease. If the stent does not track over the Platinum-Plus wire, I would exchange for a 0.018-inch Roadrunner wire, perform additional inflations with a 2.5 mm balloon, and then place multiple 3-3.5 x 12 mm stents in the proximal vessel. Given the extreme tortuosity of this vessel, an irregular appearance is likely after stenting. If this is the case, I would discharge the patient on aspirin, ticlopidine, and subcutaneous Lovenox (30 mg BID for 10 days).

Ian Penn, MD, Canada: I would ensure strong guide support with an Amplatz or hockey stick guide, and cross the lesion with an Extra-Support wire, which might straighten the proximal segment. Pseudolesions are extremely common with stiff wires, and should be ignored for the time being. My first choice for stenting this lesion is a 7-8 mm tubular stent. However, the short stent should be deployed on a 20 mm balloon to reduce the chance of "melon-seeding" at the bend. I would predilate with a 3.0 mm semicompliant balloon with a single central marker, mount the stent across the central marker, and inflate at 18 ATM. If there is a clear step-up and step-down, I would not perform intravascular ultrasound. This is an excellent example where a second half stent may be required for the distal 50% lesion. The proximal vessel tortuosity is difficult for a rigid 15 mm stent (despite the best guide and guidewire support), but a short rigid stent or a flexible coil stent can be used successfully. My advice is to place a stent proximally, assess the results, and put in a second stent distally only if necessary. High-pressure inflation will be required with 9-10 mm balloons to avoid dissection.

Editors' Perspective: Although the target lesion is suitable for stenting, the tortuosity of the target vessel will make stenting very difficult. There are several important technical points to consider: First, coaxial guiding catheter support with a "power" guide is crucial. Potentially useful guiding catheter configurations include a left Amplatz, right Voda, Hockey stick, or El Gamal. Second, extra-support guidewires will be needed to straighten the vessel for stent implantation. Since some of these wires may be difficult to steer into the distal vessel it may be best to position a flexible angioplasty wire in the distal vessel, and exchange it for a heavy-duty guidewire such as the Platinum-Plus wire, the S'port wire, or the Roadrunner wire. Third, the choice of stents is clearly important, since flexible stents (12 mm Gianturco-Roubin stent or GR-II stent, Microstent, MultiLink stent, Nir stent, and Wallstent) have greater ability to access the target lesion. Many of these flexible stents are not yet widely available in the United States. Useful techniques for successful deployment of the Palmaz-Schatz stent include the "buddy-wire" and "stentless delivery sheath" technique (p. 74), and use of covered or bare half (disarticulated) stents.

*****

STENT: TRIFURCATION LESION

Stent of a trifurcation lesion in the proximal LCX (reference diameter of proximal LCX = 3.4 mm).

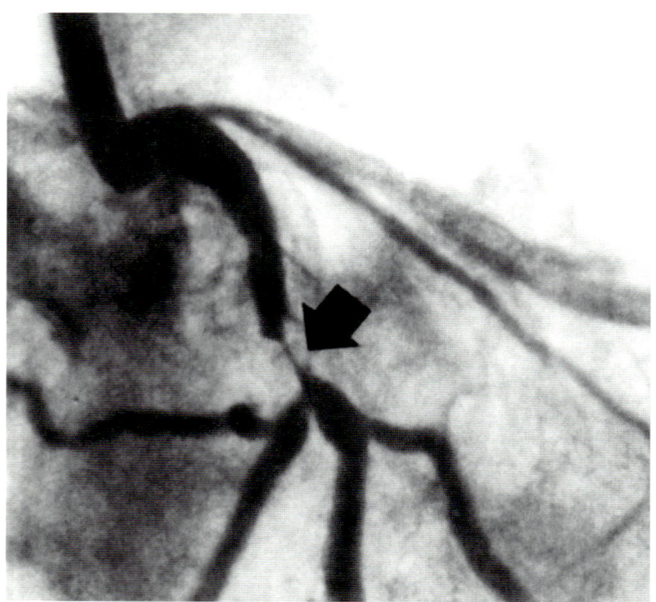

Is stenting reasonable for this lesion?

Ulrich Sigwart, MD, England: This is a large LCX with a lesion just proximal to the takeoff of the AV branch. Virtually any device is acceptable, but the greatest chance of long-term success is with stent implantation.

Richard Schatz, MD, USA: Stenting is reasonable if the LCX is nondominant.

Comment on device sizing and important technical tips.

Richard Schatz, MD, USA: I would predilate with a 3.5 mm NC Bandit, place a 3.5 mm Palmaz-Schatz stent, and postdilate at 20 ATM with the same NC Bandit. If the LCX is lost, I would wire it directly through the stent, and pass a low-profile balloon through the stent struts and try to keep it open. This strategy has a high success rate and a low complication rate. If the LCX is large enough, I would place a half stent at the ostium of the LCX and then place a full stent across the lesion creating a "T" effect. This has the advantage of protecting the ostium of the LCX, as well as treating the proximal LCX.

Editors' Perspective: Stenting can be accomplished using a variety of stents without much difficulty. The target lesion is associated with a "cuff" of nondiseased vessel on either side, so anchoring the stent in relatively normal tissue will be possible.

*****

STENT: BIFURCATION LESION

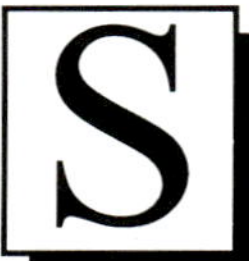

tent of a bifurcation lesion in the distal RCA (reference diameters: RCA = 3.6 mm; PDA = 2.7 mm; PLV = 2.2 mm).

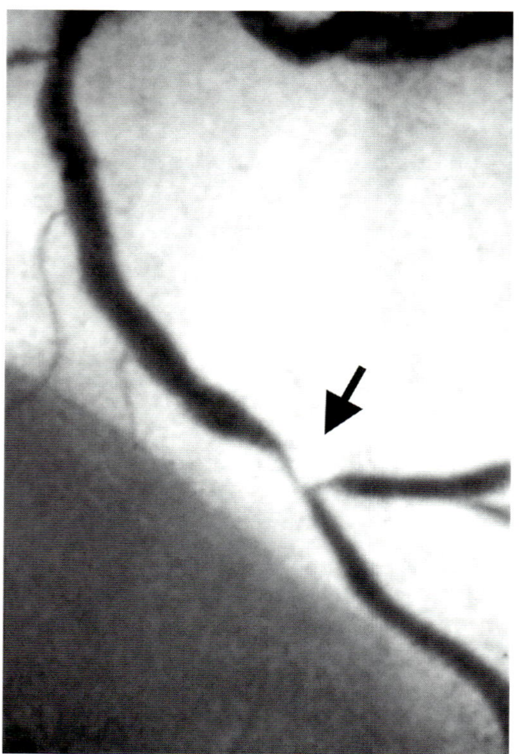

Is stenting reasonable for this lesion?

Ulrich Sigwart, MD, England: A good long-term result in this situation is difficult to achieve. Bifurcational stenting is not a good idea because of the distal location of the lesion and the reduced visibility.

Richard Schatz, MD, USA: Coronary stenting is not my first choice due to the relatively small branches. This is a very complex, eccentric bifurcation lesion.

Editors' Perspective: The branches of the distal RCA may be too small for stenting in this case. However, when the diameter of both branches exceeds 2.8 mm, bifurcation stenting can be considered, although the various approaches are technically demanding and are best reserved for experienced stent operators. One approach is to dilate the branch vessel (to decrease the chance of stent-induced sidebranch narrowing) and then stent the parent vessel; if stenting results in sidebranch narrowing, the sidebranch can be redilated through the stent. A second approach is to stent the parent vessel and then retrieve the sidebranch if necessary; in true bifurcation lesions, it will virtually always be necessary to dilate the sidebranch. A third approach is to place a stent at the ostium of the branch, followed by a stent in the parent vessel. This creates a "T-stent," which can lead to excellent results when the branch originates at a right angle from the parent vessel, and minimizes the chance that all or part of the proximal end of the stent will reside in the parent vessel. When T-stenting is performed, it is absolutely imperative that the operator position both stents perfectly, so that the sidebranch stent completely covers the sidebranch lesion, but does not protrude into the parent vessel. The likelihood of suboptimal stent alignment is increased when the branch does not originate at a right angle (as is the case in most bifurcation lesions). A fourth approach is to place "kissing" stents in the bifurcation, which is a more favorable approach when the sidebranch originates from the parent vessel at an angle $< 90°$. Adequate guiding catheter support, stent alignment, and contrast visualization are of paramount importance. Finally, some stent types allow a second stent to be deployed in the sidebranch through the stent in the parent vessel; "kissing" balloon inflations can then be performed to achieve optimal stent deployment. This technique cannot be accomplished with stents protected by a delivery sheath, and coil stents work better than slotted tubular stents.

*****

STENT: CALCIFIED LESION

Stent of a calcified lesion in the mid-LAD (reference diameter = 2.9 mm).

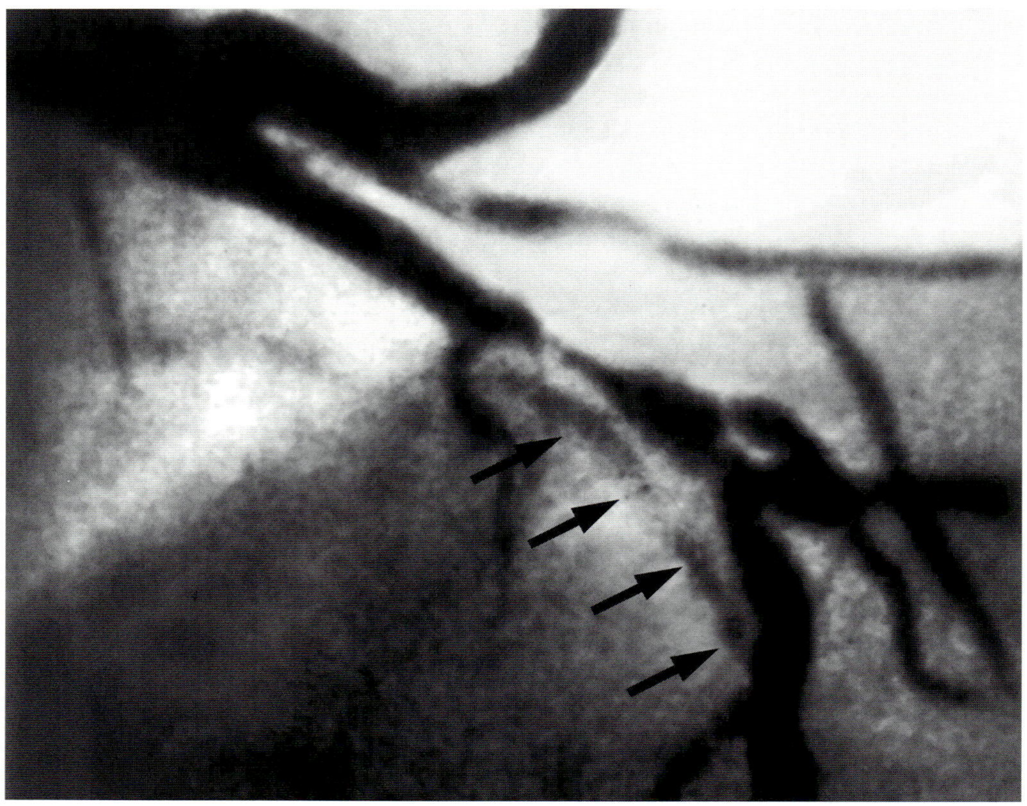

Is stenting reasonable for this lesion?

Donald Baim, MD, USA: This calcified lesion is amenable to stenting, perhaps after pretreatment with Rotablator to improve lesion compliance.

Antonio Colombo, MD, Italy: Coronary stenting in calcified lesions requires prior rotational atherectomy to facilitate lumen enlargement.

Marie-Claude Morice, MD, France: Stenting this lesion is a good strategy. The lesion is short, concentric, and does not involve major branches (the septal branch is very small).

Comment on device sizing and important technical tips.

Donald Baim, MD, USA: Initial treatment with rotational atherectomy is preferable. I have found that a 1.75 mm burr will provide significant enhancement of lesion compliance, making stent delivery and full expansion easier. I would then place a single 3.0 mm Palmaz-Schatz coronary stent, and postdilate with a high-pressure balloon of appropriate size.

Antonio Colombo, MD, Italy: I would pretreat with a 1.75 mm Rotablator burr and then dilate with a 3.0 mm balloon. I would implant a 3.0 mm Palmaz-Schatz stent and postdilate with a 3.5 mm high-pressure balloon. Two stents may be needed. If the vessel is not tortuous, stenting can be performed over the Rotablator wire. If there is any doubt, the Rotablator wire should be exchanged for a 0.014-inch Extra-Support wire. IVUS should be performed in calcified lesions because of the higher risk of focal underexpansion of the stent. Due to the use of adjunctive rotational atherectomy, I would continue heparin for at least 12 hours prior to sheath removal.

Marie-Claude Morice, MD, France: I would perform this case in a very simple way using a 6F JL4 guiding catheter, a 0.014-inch Extra-Support wire, and a 3.0 mm high-pressure balloon. If there is a persistent waist on the balloon during predilation at 12-13 ATM, I would pull everything out and exchange for an 8F giant-lumen JL4 guiding catheter, a Rotablator wire, and "prepare" the lesion with a 2.0 mm burr. The risk of severe dissection when applying high pressure to a calcified lesion is very high. However, the risk is minimized by pretreating with Rotablator. I would implant a Palmaz-Schatz 154 stent at 16-18 ATM with the same 3.0 mm balloon. This is a low-cost approach (the same balloon is used for predilation and stenting), without IVUS.

Editor's Perspective: The approach to stenting calcified lesions is similar to that of stenting noncalcified lesions. However, two ancillary issues may impact procedural success: First, calcification of the vessel segment proximal to the lesion may impair stent delivery because of decreased vessel compliance. This is especially true for rigid stents, such as the covered Palmaz-Schatz stent and Palmaz biliary stents. Techniques that can enhance procedural success include the use of power guiding catheters and extra-support guidewires. Second, lesion calcification may decrease lesion compliance and impair full stent expansion, particularly when there is extensive superficial calcification in multiple quadrants. IVUS may be useful to identify the extent and distribution of calcium; superficial multi-quadrant calcification is readily treated by the Rotablator, which can facilitate optimal stent deployment. If Rotablator is not available (or the operator prefers not to use it), predilation of the target lesion should be performed with a noncompliant full-size balloon, to ensure full balloon expansion without a residual waist.

*****

STENT: CALCIFIED OSTIAL RCA

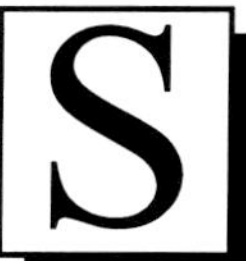tent of a calcified ostial lesion in the RCA (reference diameter = 2.8 mm).

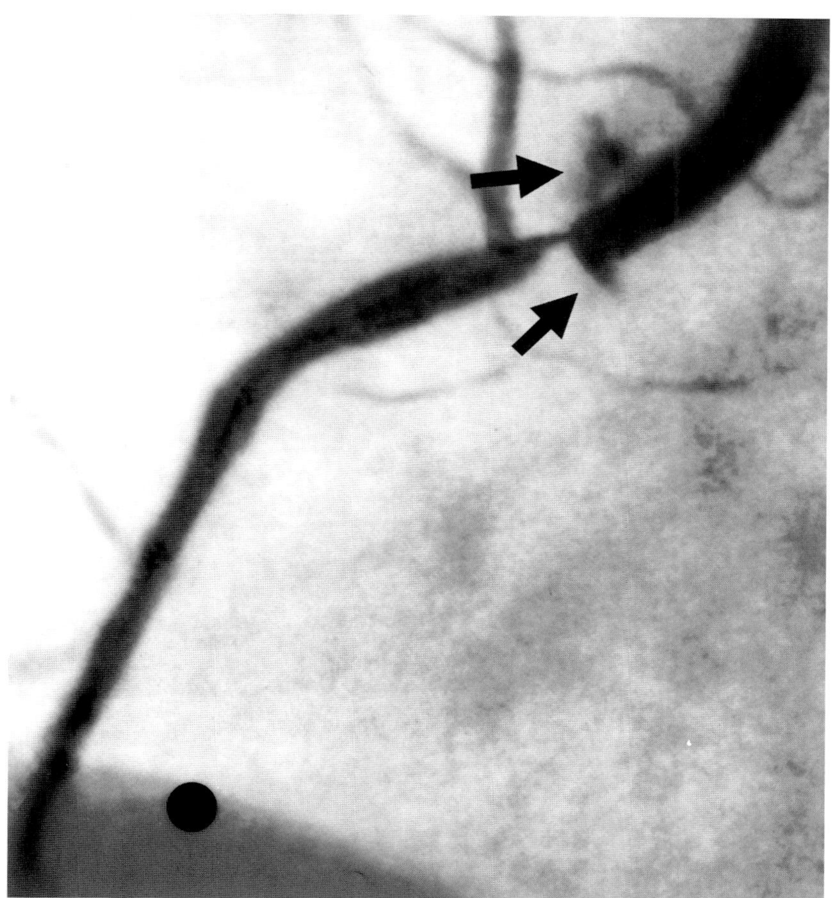

Is stenting reasonable for this lesion?

Donald Baim, MD, USA: This calcified lesion is amenable to stenting.

Antonio Colombo, MD, Italy: Coronary stenting in calcified lesions requires initial rotational atherectomy to facilitate lumen enlargement.

Marie-Claude Morice, MD, France: Yes, stenting is a reasonable approach for this lesion. The restenosis rate is very high in calcified ostial lesions, and stenting can decrease acute complications and restenosis.

Comment on device sizing and important technical tips.

Antonio Colombo, MD, Italy: I would use two sequential Rotablator burrs to maximize the lumen before stenting. I would use a 3.0 mm Palmaz-Schatz stent (better for calcified lesions in the ostial location) and postdilate with a 3.5 mm high-pressure balloon. IVUS is important to verify optimal stent deployment. Subsequent management includes aspirin and optional ticlopidine.

Marie-Claude Morice, MD, France: Because of ostial calcification, I would treat this lesion with rotational atherectomy (8F guiding catheter and a 2.0 mm burr). I don't implant pacemakers anymore during rotational atherectomy (even for the RCA), but use liberal doses of atropine and fluids, and multiple short debulking runs. I would then dilate at low pressure with a 3.0 mm noncompliant balloon, and then implant a Palmaz-Schatz 84 stent with the same balloon at high pressure. The challenge with stenting the ostium is precision in positioning the stent, to be certain the ostium is completely covered. In my opinion, the best stent for such precision is the Palmaz-Schatz stent.

Editors' Perspective: Stenting of ostial lesions is technically challenging, particularly in the presence of severe calcification. Several considerations impact on procedural outcome: First, the ostium must be adequately "prepared" to accommodate the stent;

this usually involves the use of Rotablator, which will ablate calcium, increase lesion compliance, and facilitate subsequent stent expansion. If Rotablator is not employed, predilation should be performed with a full-size noncompliant balloon. Failure to fully expand the balloon is an absolute contraindication to stenting. Second, the ideal stent should have excellent radial strength and radioopacity; unfortunately, such a stent is not yet available. The best stent for ostial stenting in vessels > 4 mm is the Palmaz biliary stent, and for vessels < 4 mm, the Palmaz-Schatz and MultiLink coronary stents are good choices. Third, coaxial guiding catheter alignment and extra-support guidewires are useful to ease stent delivery. Aggressive guiding catheter intubation should be avoided, since it will be necessary to retract the guiding catheter into the ascending aorta to achieve optimal stent position. Fourth, the stent must be deployed so that 1-2 mm of the proximal end of the stent is in the ascending aorta. Failure to position the stent in the ascending aorta may result in incomplete coverage of the ostial lesion. On the other hand, deployment of the stent too proximally in the aorta may result in placement of the stent articulation at the ostium (and inadequate coverage of the lesion) and/or damage to the stent from the tip of the guiding catheter. Since the guiding catheter must be retracted to allow ideal ostial stenting, adequate contrast opacification may be difficult. If possible, the operator should use auto-roadmapping, freeze frames, and other fluoroscopic landmarks (rib or lung markings, surgical clips, pulmonary artery catheters, pacemaker wires, etc) to ensure proper stent position. Fifth, final inflation with a full-size or slightly oversize balloon is recommended to flare the stent against the aortic wall. Finally, even in centers that do not routinely use IVUS for stenting, IVUS can be useful to ensure that the vessel ostium is completely covered by the stent, and that "optimal" stenting has been achieved. In the event the ostium is not completely covered, another stent should be implanted.

*****

STENT: OSTIAL DIAGONAL

Stent of an ostial lesion in the diagonal (reference diameter = 3.2 mm).

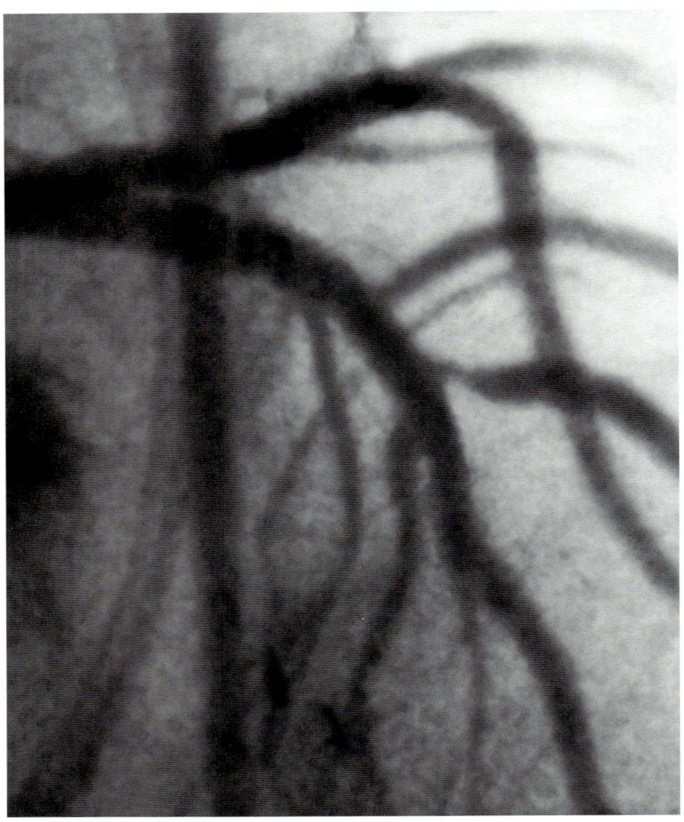

Is stenting reasonable for this lesion?

Paul Teirstein, MD, USA: This is an ostial diagonal branch stenosis; I do not recommend stenting. My preference is Rotablator atherectomy.

Masakiyo Nobuyoshi, MD, Japan: A stent is suitable.

Comment on device sizing and important technical tips.

Masakiyo Nobuyoshi, MD, Japan: I would predilate with a 3.0 x 20 mm balloon through an 8F JL4 guide using a 0.014-inch wire. Then I would place a 3.0 mm Palmaz-Schatz stent and postdilate with a 3.25 x 20 mm noncompliant balloon at 15 ATM. The important technical point is to place the proximal edge of the stent 1.0 mm in the LAD.

Editors' Perspective: Stenting this lesion may be more difficult than other techniques (e.g., PTCA, Rotablator, or directional atherectomy). It is essential that the stent completely cover the ostium. Since the diagonal has a right angle origin from the LAD, this is an ideal configuration for stenting because the proximal end of the stent can be deployed "flush" with the ostium. Balloon-expandable stents without an articulation are recommended, and stents with better radiopacity will be easier to deploy.

*****

STENT: OSTIAL LAD

Stent of an ostial lesion in the LAD (reference diameter = 3.8 mm).

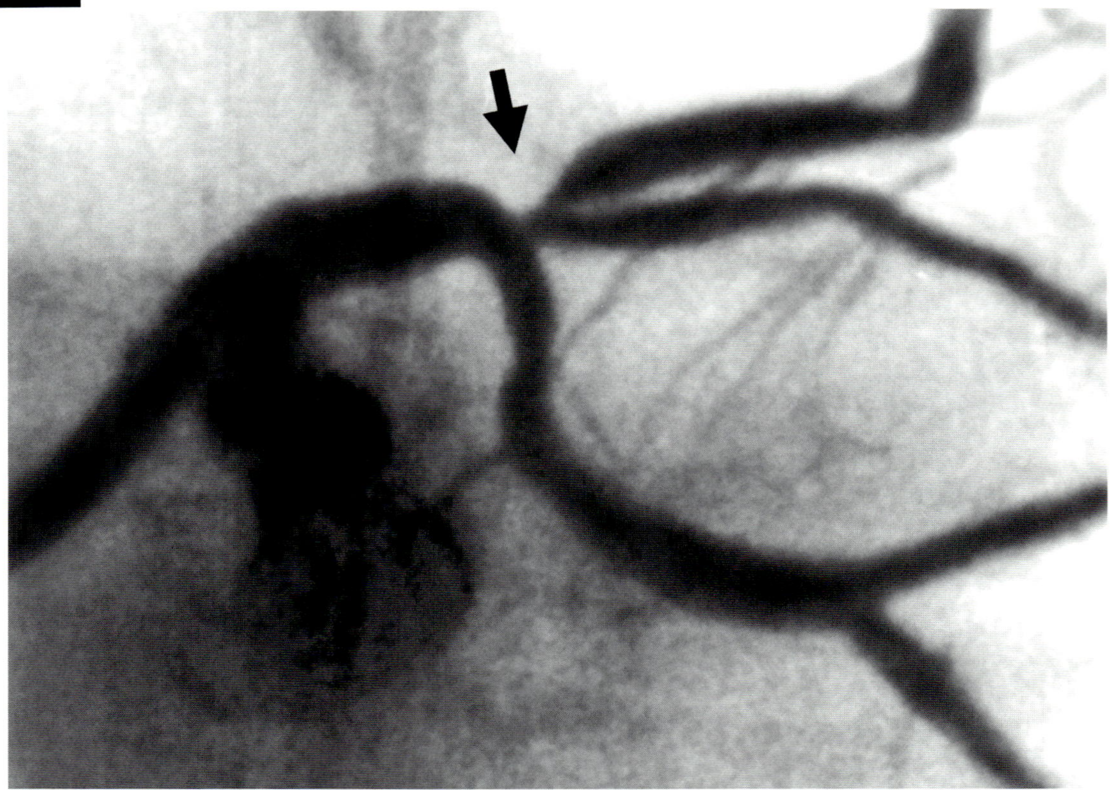

Is stenting reasonable for this lesion?

Paul Teirstein, MD, USA: This lesion is suitable for stenting.

Masakiyo Nobuyoshi, MD, Japan: Two treatment options include stenting and directional atherectomy.

Comment on device sizing and important technical tips.

Paul Teirstein, MD, USA: If this lesion is calcified by fluoroscopy, I would pretreat with rotational atherectomy. I would use an 8F Judkins left guide and a 1.5 mm followed by a 2.0 mm Rotablator burr. I would then use a 3.0 mm balloon to further predilate this lesion. While the balloon is across the target lesion, I would exchange the Rotablator-C wire for a 0.014-inch Extra-S'port wire, and deploy a 3.5 mm Palmaz-Schatz stent precisely at the ostium of the LAD. This necessitates a small portion of the stent "overhanging" the ostium of the LCX. This used to cause great concern when stent thrombosis was a more frequent complication. In 1996, the incidence of stent thrombosis is < 1%. I would use a 3.5-4.0 x 9-10 mm balloon at 20 ATM for final inflations, and I would use IVUS as part of an ongoing, randomized trial at Scripps Clinic.

Editors' Perspective: Lesions at the origin of the LAD create a number of concerns about stenting: First, proper stent deployment mandates that the proximal end of the stent be deployed in the distal left main coronary artery, which may partially impinge on the origin of the LCX. Second, there is considerable vessel tapering from the distal left main bifurcation to the proximal LAD, raising the question of balloon sizing (which can readily be addressed by IVUS). Third, marginal dissections following high-pressure balloon inflations, although relatively uncommon, could have dramatic impact on procedural safety and outcome if located in the left main coronary artery. Finally, stent restenosis at the proximal margin of the stent could result in significant stenosis of the left main coronary artery.

*****

STENT: OSTIAL LCX

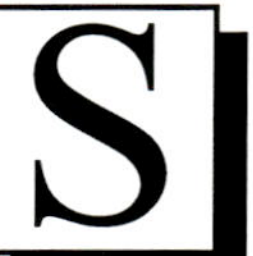tent of an ostial lesion in the LCX (reference diameters: left main = 4.2 mm; LCX = 3.8 mm).

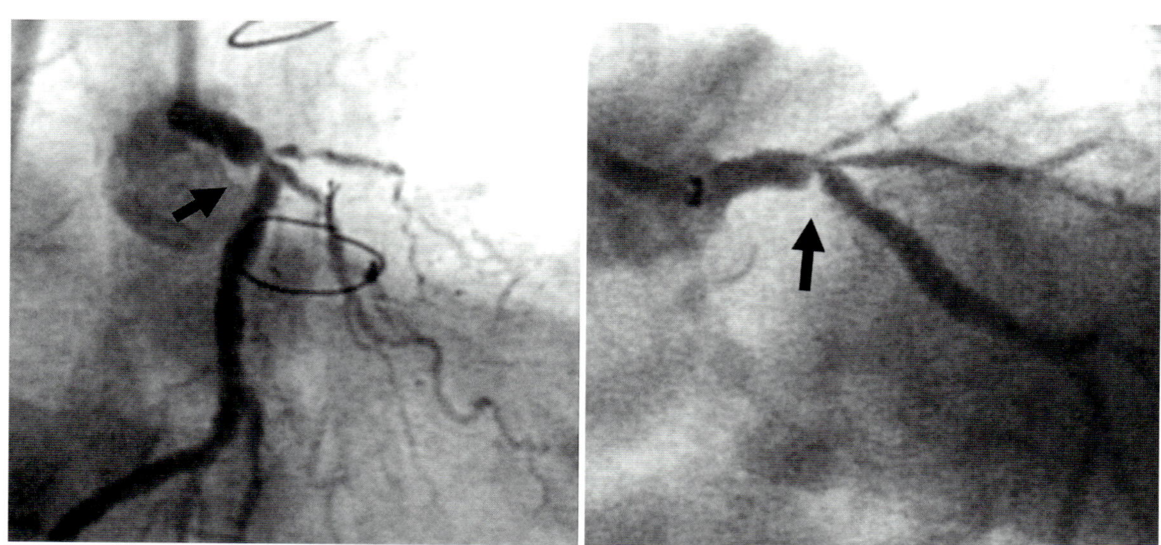

Is stenting reasonable for this lesion?

Paul Teirstein, MD, USA: The left main stenosis involves the ostium of the LCX; stenting is reasonable.

Masakiyo Nobuyoshi, MD, Japan: Stenting is the best choice.

Comment on device sizing and important technical tips.

Paul Teirstein, MD, USA: Distal left main stenoses such as this are usually highly calcified and, in my experience, are best treated with Rotablator atherectomy. I would use a Judkins left guide catheter, a Rotablator-C wire, start with a 1.5 mm burr, and follow with a 2.0 mm burr. I have found that the 1.5 mm burr often creates substantial debulking, probably because it abrades deeply into the vessel wall as it travels around the severe bend, and sometimes a larger burr is unnecessary. I would then use a 3.0 mm balloon to further dilate the vessel, and exchange for an Extra-S'port wire or a Platinum-Plus wire. I would then deploy a 3.5 mm Palmaz-Schatz coronary stent in the distal left main extending into the proximal LCX, and postdilate with a 3.75-4.0 mm high-pressure balloon at 18-20 ATM. I would use intravascular ultrasound as part of an ongoing randomized trial at Scripps Clinic.

Masakiyo Nobuyoshi, MD, Japan: I would predilate with a 4.0 x 20 mm balloon at 8-10 ATM, using an 8F JL4 guide and a flexible 0.014-inch guidewire. I would place a Palmaz-Schatz stent, and postdilate with a 4.0 mm noncompliant balloon at 18 ATM. The technical tip is not to place the stent articulation in the middle of the stenosis.

Editors' Perspective: This lesion is readily treated by any of a number of different types of stents. As mentioned by Dr. Nobuyoshi, care should be taken to avoid placing the articulation of the Palmaz-Schatz coronary stent at the left main bifurcation. Extra-support guidewires may be necessary to straighten the bend and ease stent insertion. Because of the large vessel caliber, a biliary stent may provide better radial support than a coronary stent. Since there is a significant step-down in vessel caliber after the left main bifurcation, the stent will need to be "molded" with balloons of different size or with a tapered balloon.

*****

STENT: DEGENERATED VEIN GRAFT

Stent of a degenerated vein graft to the OM (reference diameter = 3.9 mm).

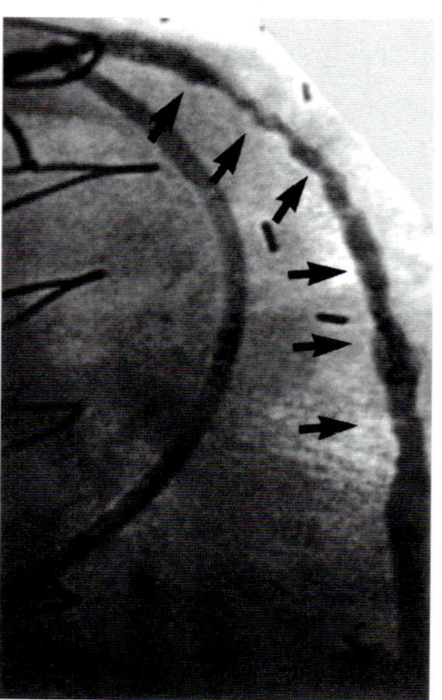

Is stenting reasonable for this lesion?

Masakiyo Nobuyoshi, MD, Japan: The angiogram shows a long, diffuse vein graft stenosis. Multiple stents or a long Wallstent are best.

Ulrich Sigwart, MD, England: Stent implantation has the greatest chance of long-term success in this situation.

Patrick Serruys, MD, PhD, The Netherlands: I have more than 7 years experience with Wallstents in bypass grafts, and consider them ideal for degenerated grafts.

Comment on device sizing and important technical tips.

Masakiyo Nobuyoshi, MD, Japan: I would use a 10F hockey stick guide, a TEC guidewire, and a 7F TEC device. I would follow with adjunctive PTCA with a 4.0 x 40 mm balloon at 8-10 ATM. After PTCA, I would place multiple stents from distal to proximal to cover the entire length of the lesion. A 6.0 x 38 mm Wallstent stent may also be used. In either case, I would postdilate with a 4.5 mm balloon at 15 ATM. Important technical tip: This lesion contains losts of thrombus and every effort must be made to avoid distal embolization, which might have severe consequences!

Ulrich Sigwart, MD, England: I would take a 70 mm long peripheral Wallstent which goes through a 9F guiding catheter over a 0.038-inch Wholey wire. It may protrude slightly into the aorta, but this is not of major significance. If it turns out to be too short, a balloon expandable stent can also be deployed. Predilatation is not recommended!

Patrick Serruys, MD, PhD, The Netherlands: I recommend a 6.0 x 60 mm Wallstent, an 8F El Gamal guiding catheter, and a Schneider 0.014-inch x 300 cm guidewire. I would not predilate this lesion because of the risk of distal embolization. However, if on-line QCA suggests a MLD < 1.5 mm, or if the Wallstent does not cross the lesion easily, predilation would be performed with a 3.5 x 40 mm Europass. The Wallstent would then be dilated with a 4.0 mm Speedy; a larger balloon would be used if necessary, depending on on-line QCA. IVUS is recommended if there is uncertainly about optimal stent deployment.

Editors' Perspective: Stents offer the best hope for palliation of symptoms associated with degenerated vein grafts. The best stent for this situation is unknown, but it is likely that the Wallstent will become the most widely employed. Advantages of the Wallstent are its ease of insertion, availability in multiple lengths, excellent conformability, and radial support. New designs will simplify delivery and increase radioopacity. Most operators who deploy Wallstents in degenerated vein grafts do not recommend predilation, although adjunctive PTCA is recommended after stent deployment.

*****

STENT: OSTIAL VEIN GRAFT

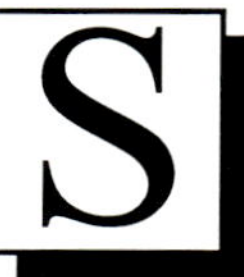tent of an ostial lesion in a vein graft to the LAD (reference diameter = 3.9 mm).

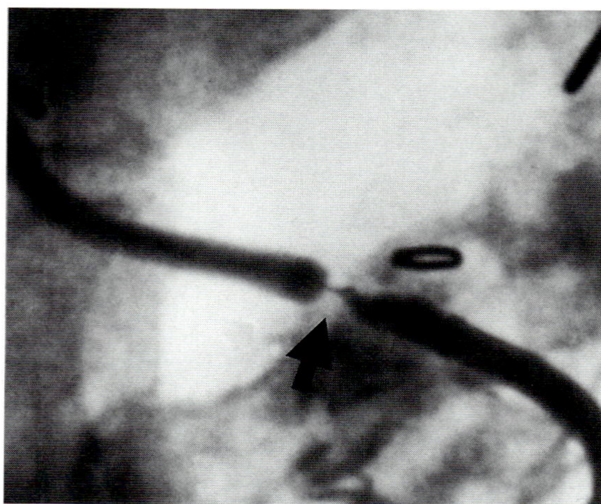

Is stenting reasonable for this lesion?

Masakiyo Nobuyoshi, MD, Japan: The angiogram shows a focal stenosis in a vein graft, which is well-suited for stenting.

David Foley, MD, The Netherlands: This problem will be treated by a Wallstent.

Comment on device sizing and important technical tips.

Masakiyo Nobuyoshi, MD, Japan: I would use an 8F JR4 guide, a 0.014-inch wire, predilate with a 4.0 x 20 mm balloon at 10 ATM, and implant a 4.0 mm Palmaz-Schatz stent. I would postdilate the stent with a 4.25 x 20 mm noncompliant balloon at 18 ATM. Important technical tip: The proximal part of the stent must be in the aorta; if the stent is inside the ostium, unrecognized residual ostial stenosis will remain.

David Foley, MD, The Netherlands: I recommend a 5.0 x 20 mm Wallstent. A 4.0 x 9 mm Microstent or a 4.0 x 10 mm Palmaz-Schatz stent are acceptable alternatives.

> Editors' Perspective: **The only important clinical issue in this case is not whether to stent, but which stent to use. Biliary stents have excellent radioopacity and radial strength, and are ideal for target lesions in the ostium of large saphenous vein grafts. Other balloon-expandable stainless steel stents, such as the Palmaz-Schatz coronary stent, the Microstent, the MultiLink stent, and the Nir stent may also be effective for this lesion. The Wallstent is a nice stent for most vein graft lesions, but may not be the best choice for ostial lesions; because of stent shortening, adequate stenting of the ostium is unpredictable, except in very experienced hands.**

*****

STENT: VEIN GRAFT

Stent of a vein graft to the RCA (reference diameter = 3.9 mm).

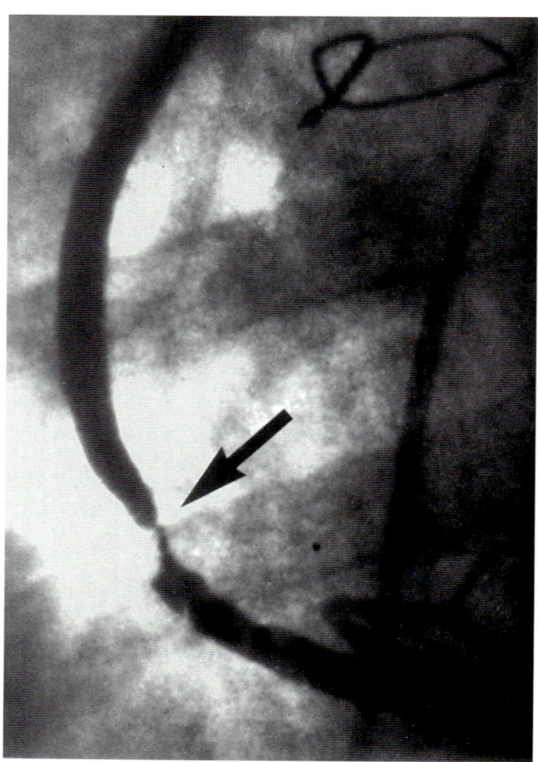

Is stenting reasonable for this lesion?

Masakiyo Nobuyoshi, MD, Japan: This stenosis is ideal for stenting, because the vessel is large, the lesion is short, and there is no tortuosity. Stenting results in a lower incidence of restenosis compared to PTCA.

Ulrich Sigwart, MD, England: This is an ideal case for a Wallstent.

Patrick Serruys, MD, PhD, The Netherlands: I have 7 years of experience with Wallstents in bypass grafts, and consider them ideal for degenerated grafts.

Comment on device sizing and important technical tips.

Masakiyo Nobuyoshi, MD, Japan: I would use an 8F JR4 guide, a flexible 0.014-inch wire, predilate with a 4.0 x 20 mm balloon, place a 4.0 mm Palmaz-Schatz coronary stent, and postdilate with a 4.0 mm noncompliant balloon at 18-20 ATM.

Ulrich Sigwart, MD, England: I would implant a 4.5 x 30 mm Wallstent. One might be surprised that the lesion is fibrous in nature and therefore I would always "palpate" the stenosis with a balloon; this does not mean that the lesion has to be fully dilated.

Patrick Serruys, MD, PhD, The Netherlands: Of course, distal embolization may be a problem, but will be a bigger problem if the vessel is predilated. My practice is to have adenosine and verapamil ready, in case of embolization. Regarding selection of Wallstents, I usually choose a diameter at least 1 mm larger than the QCA-measured diameter. I choose a length which is clearly ample to allow safe anchoring of the stent in healthy graft proximal and distal to the lesion. For this lesion, I recommend a 5.0 x 27 mm Wallstent. I use exclusively El Gamal guiding catheters for deep intubation. I generally use a Schneider 0.014-inch x 300 cm guidewire, which will provide adequate support for the Wallstent.

Editors' Perspective: Stenting has become the treatment of choice for vein graft lesions like this, so the only real issue is which stent to use. In grafts measuring 4.0 mm in diameter, the most commonly employed stents in the United States are biliary stents and the Palmaz-Schatz coronary stent. In our practice, we prefer biliary stents because of their superior radioopacity and excellent radial strength. The vertical downward origin of this graft favors use of a 9F multipurpose guiding catheter, through which a nonarticulated P204 biliary stent will easily pass. Extra-support guidewires are useful to ease passage of the biliary stent into the vessel origin. In Europe, there is a large experience with the Wallstent, which could be readily deployed in this lesion without difficulty. Although high-pressure inflations are recommended after stent deployment in native vessels, high-pressure inflations in vein grafts may increase the risk of distal embolization and no-reflow. Nevertheless, postdilation is recommended using a noncompliant balloon inflated to 8-12 ATM. IVUS may be useful to determine the adequacy of stent deployment and the need for higher inflation pressures. This patient was treated with a single nonarticulated P204 biliary stent, using a 0.014-inch TEC guidewire and a 10F multipurpose guide. The lesion was predilated with a 3.5 mm Cobra-18, and postdilated with a 4.0 x 20 mm NC Cobra at 18 ATM. After high-pressure inflations, there was transient slow-flow (TIMI-2), which resolved after intracoronary verapamil.

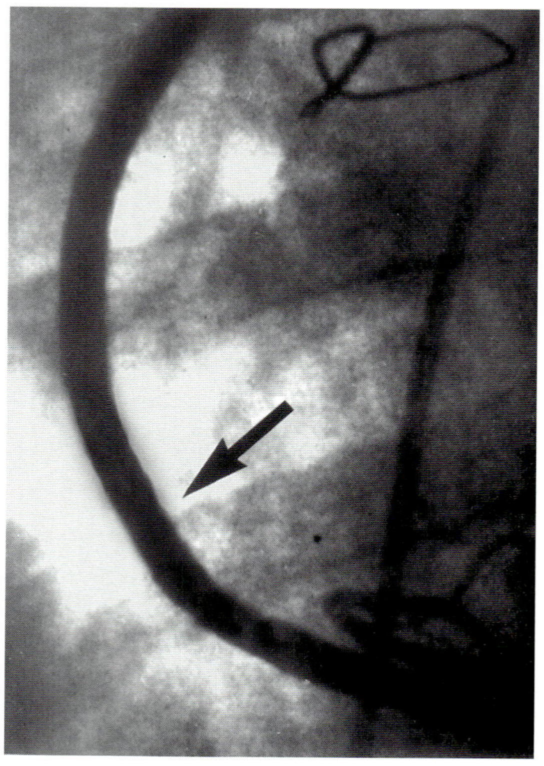

*****

STENT: LARGE THROMBUS

Stent of a large thrombus in a degenerated vein graft (reference diameter = 5.2 mm).

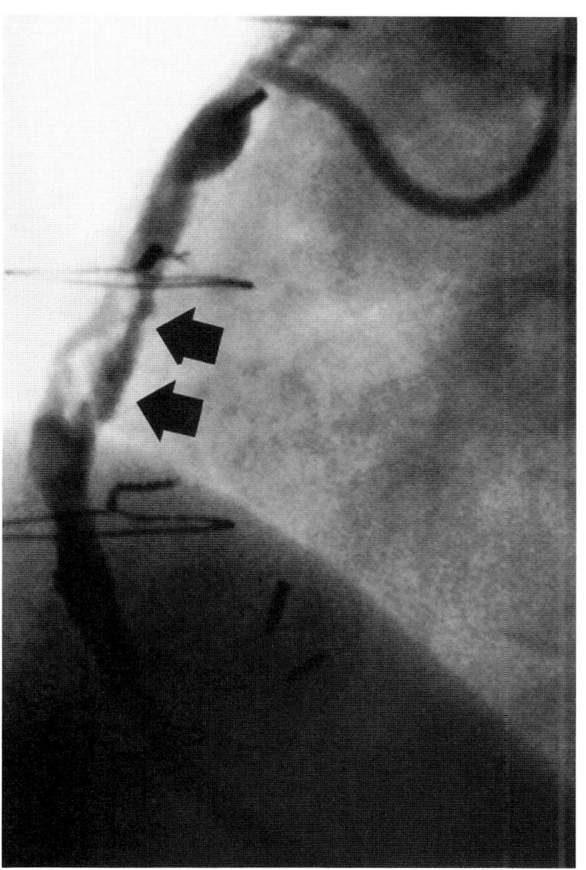

Is stenting reasonable for this lesion?

Richard Schatz, MD, USA: This lesion is ideally suited for coronary stenting once the thrombus is eliminated.

Ulrich Sigwart, MD, England: This is a terrible looking graft to the RCA, which could be treated by stenting.

Comment on device sizing and important technical tips.

Richard Schatz, MD, USA: Since the risk of distal embolization is high, every measure should be taken to prevent this potentially fatal complication. I would start with a Stabilizer wire and a 6F multipurpose guiding catheter, place a 6.0 cm Tracker catheter, and infuse tPA (20 mg) or urokinase (500,000 units over 18-24 hours). I would administer heparin (600-800 units per hour) through the guiding catheter, leaving it in the ostium unless it is occlusive. If the clot resolves after 18 hours, I would place two overlapping Palmaz-Schatz coronary stents and a Palmaz biliary stent in the ostium. I would postdilate all stents with a 5.0 mm Total Cross at 15 ATM. I would not use ReoPro in this setting, since there are relatively few data about its value. However, my early experience with the AngioJet is favorable, and this device may become the device of choice for lesions such as this.

Ulrich Sigwart, MD, England: I would intubate the graft with a 9F multipurpose guiding catheter, pass a Wholey wire into the distal graft, and immediately place a 7.0 x 60 mm Wallstent. If the stent is too short, I would place a 5.0 x 10 mm biliary stent in the ostium. There is no need for predilation of such a friable atheroma. The embolization rate with primary implantation of large self-expanding Wallstents is minimal.

Antonio Colombo, MD, Italy: I would administer intragraft urokinase (100,00 units per hours for 8-9 hours). If thrombus resolves, I would implant multiple biliary stents or a Wallstent. After stenting, I would give 12-24 hours of IV heparin prior to sheath removal. The best guiding catheter is a left Amplatz (8F for a Palmaz-Schatz stent, 10F for a Wallstent).

Editors' Perspective: Stenting offers the best hope for long-term palliation of symptoms associated with disease in vein grafts. However, implantation of stents in degenerated vein grafts with substantial thrombus should be avoided until the thrombus has been aggressively treated and the thrombus burden reduced. Potential adjuncts for decreasing thrombus include bolus intracoronary injection of thrombolytic agents (tPA 20 mg or urokinase 250,000-500,000 units), prolonged intracoronary infusion of thrombolytic agents (urokinase 50,000-200,000 units/hour for 6-24 hours), local delivery of urokinase or tPA through a Dispatch or Localmed catheter, TEC atherectomy, the Cordis Hydrolyzer, and the Possis AngioJet. If the thrombus burden can be substantially reduced, stenting can be performed immediately or within 2-4 weeks. The risk of distal embolization seems to be less if stenting is deferred, but there is a definite risk of graft occlusion prior to definitive therapy when this approach is used. The choice of stents is a matter of operator preference. Potential advantages of the Wallstent include its availability in multiple lengths and its self-expanding properties, which may obviate the need for high-pressure adjunctive PTCA. The ideal post-stent medical therapy is unknown, but recent data suggest that Coumadin may be deleterious; aspirin, ticlopidine, and subcutaneous heparin seem reasonable. Although ReoPro has not been specifically evaluated in degenerated vein grafts, anecdotal experience suggests potential benefit for reducing no-reflow.

*****

STENT: SMALL THROMBUS

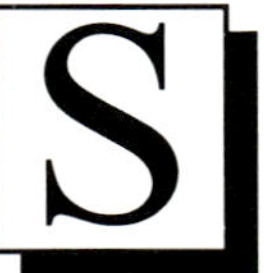

Stent of a small thrombus in the proximal RCA (reference diameter = 3.4 mm)

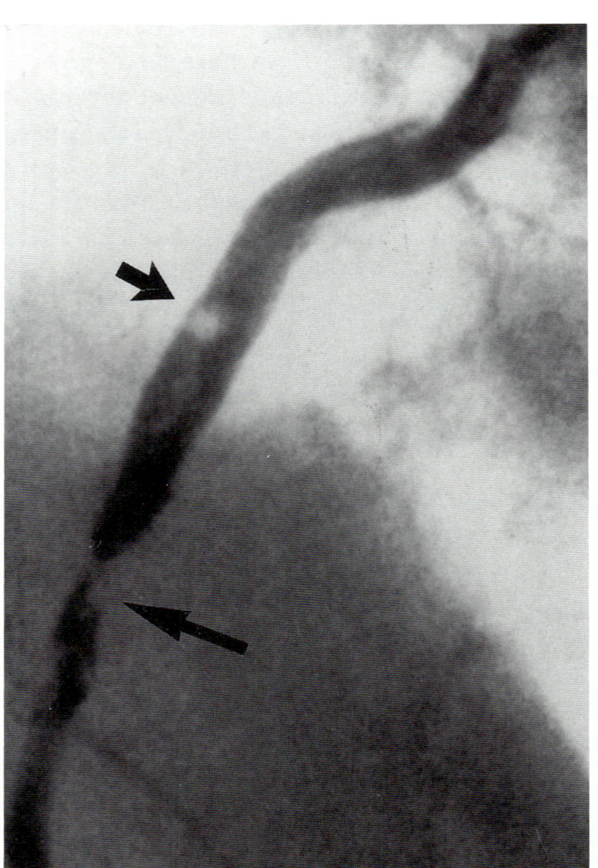

Is stenting reasonable for this lesion?

Richard Schatz, MD, USA: Coronary stenting is very appropriate for this lesion due to the presence of good inflow and good outflow, despite complex morphology characterized by ulceration and fresh thrombus. Once clot is removed, coronary stenting is ideal.

Ulrich Sigwart, MD, England: A long stent would cover the entire lesion in the RCA.

Comment on device sizing and important technical tips.

Richard Schatz, MD, USA: Although the clot burden is small, the risk of distal embolization is high. I recommend overnight lysis with tPA (20 mg) or urokinase (500,000 units IC). This case is more complex than the previous one, since a 3F Tracker may cause ischemia when placed across the target lesion. If this occurs, a brief inflation with a 1.5 mm balloon would solve the problem by creating a small channel for the Tracker. I would bring the patient back the next day and if the clot is gone, I would perform intracoronary stenting. If a single stent covers the lesion, I would predilate with a 3.5 mm NC Bandit, implant a 3.5 mm Palmaz-Schatz stent, and postdilate with same NC Bandit at 20 ATM. If there is some residual clot following overnight lysis, I would place a 4.0 mm Dispatch followed by intramural injection of urokinase (250,00 units) or tPA (10 mg). There is no indication for ReoPro.

Ulrich Sigwart, MD, England: I recommend a Wallstent to cover the entire lesion.

Antonio Colombo, MD, Italy: I would predilate with a 3.5 mm balloon, and perform multiple inflations until thrombus resolves. When the thrombus has cleared, I would deploy one or two stents on a 3.5 mm balloon; final IVUS evaluation is important. I would administer 12 hours of IV heparin prior to sheath removal. Discharge medications include aspirin and ticlopidine.

> **Editors' Perspective: This lesion is readily amenable to stenting, but the question is whether stenting can be performed without first removing the thrombus. In this case, the thrombus burden is small; predilating the lesion with a balloon may result in resolution of thrombus, which may have little or no impact on stenting. On the other hand, incomplete thrombus removal might predispose to stent thrombosis (we personally think this is quite unlikely). General options for thrombus removal include local delivery of thrombolytic agents or heparin using the Dispatch or Localmed catheter, bolus intracoronary infusion of urokinase (250,000-500,000 units) or tPA (20 mg), prolonged infusion of urokinase (50,000-100,000 units/hr for 6-24 hours), TEC atherectomy, the Cordis Hydrolyzer, and the Possis AngioJet.**

*****

PTCA
Techniques

PTCA: ECCENTRIC LESION (LAD)

PTCA of an eccentric lesion in the proximal LAD (reference diameter = 3.4 mm).

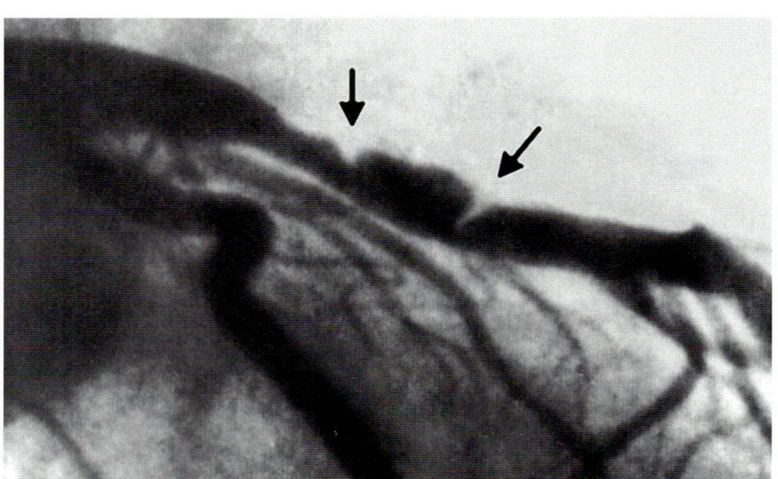

Is PTCA alone reasonable for this lesion?

Spencer King III, MD, USA: PTCA is a reasonable alternative for this lesion using a 3.5 x 20 mm perfusion balloon and prolonged inflations. It is likely that PTCA will be quite adequate, and PTCA might be as cost-effective over the long run as two stents.

David Foley, MD, The Netherlands: PTCA alone is not a reasonable alternative because the lesion is ulcerated and complex, and an optimal result is highly unlikely.

Barry George, MD, USA: Stand-alone PTCA can be undertaken, and in the hands of an operator with minimal experience with directional atherectomy, it is an appropriate intervention.

Cindy Grines, MD, USA: PTCA is an acceptable approach. I would use prolonged inflations with a 3.5 x 40 mm balloon.

Michael Cowley, MD, USA: While PTCA alone is reasonable, the likelihood of an excellent result is higher with directional atherectomy or stenting.

Nicolaus Reifart, MD, Germany: PTCA alone is a reasonable alternative if stents are not available. I would use an 8F JL 4 guiding catheter, a 0.014-inch Hi-torque floppy wire, and a 3.5 x 40 mm balloon (Europass or Speedy), and gradually increase the pressure from 2-8 ATM. In case of severe dissection or residual stenosis > 30%, I would place a stent.

Raimund Erbel, MD, Germany: I do not recommend PTCA because of an increased risk of restenosis and severe dissection.

John Bittl, MD, USA: The treatment of choice is PTCA and conditional stenting, using a 3.5 mm Lifestream at 3-6 ATM. If the residual stenosis is > 20%, I would place one or two overlapping Palmaz-Schatz stents and postdilate with the 3.5 mm Lifestream at 13.5 ATM.

Frank Litvack, MD, USA: PTCA alone is reasonable, but not the best way to approach this lesion. The results of PTCA will probably be suboptimal because of lesion eccentricity, proximal LAD location, and length, which predict a very high restenosis rate.

> **Editors' Perspective: Eccentric lesions such as this have been treated successfully by PTCA for many years, with good angiographic and clinical results. Nevertheless, the collective experience of many high-volume interventionalists suggests that results are more predictable with other techniques. For operators who prefer PTCA, a strategy of "conditional stenting" is reasonable, as described by Dr. Bittl. Using this strategy, PTCA is performed with guiding catheters and guidewires that are "stent-compatible." If suboptimal lumen enlargement (elastic recoil, dissection, etc) or abrupt closure occurs after PTCA, stenting can be readily accomplished without delay.**

*****

PTCA: ECCENTRIC LESION (RCA)

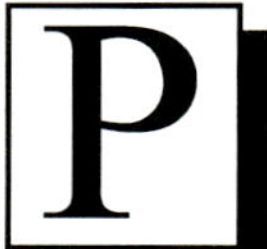

TCA of an eccentric lesion in the mid-RCA (reference diameter = 3.2 mm).

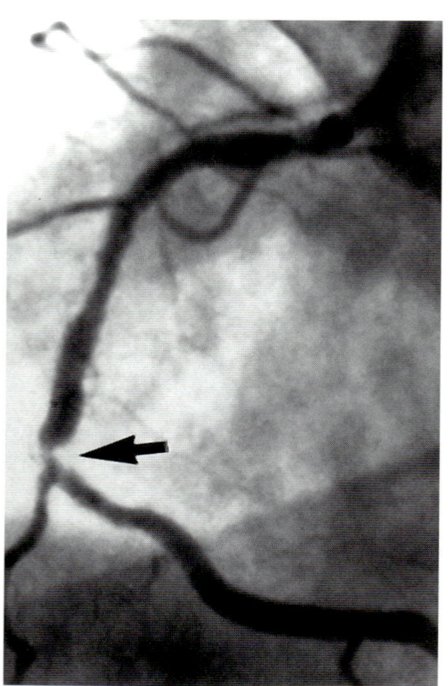

Is PTCA alone reasonable for this lesion?

David Holmes, MD, USA: I would use a 3.0 x 30 mm balloon to straighten the lesion.

Spencer King III, MD, USA: My first choice is PTCA because of diffuse disease and the risk of damage with bulky devices. I would place a 3.0 x 30 mm balloon with the proximal end in the ectatic segment of artery just before the lesion, and the distal end in the relatively normal artery. I would not dilate the remaining portion of the vessel. If a distal dissection occurs, then I would predilate the whole vessel, and place multiple bailout Gianturco-Roubin stents.

Patrick Serruys, MD, PhD, The Netherlands: PTCA will virtually always result in a long, extensive dissection in this type of lesion, which is why I prefer a primary Wallstent.

William O'Neill, MD, USA: I would perform PTCA with a 3.0 x 20 mm Edge and a 0.014-inch guidewire. If severe dissection occurs, I would place a Palmaz-Schatz coronary stent. I would use IVUS after stenting to identify the normal reference size.

Cindy Grines, MD, USA: I prefer PTCA with an 8F guiding catheter and a 3.0 x 40 mm compliant balloon (which could achieve a diameter of 3.5 mm).

Michael Cowley, MD, USA: PTCA alone is reasonable using an oversize 3.5 mm semicompliant balloon at 4 ATM for 2-3 minutes, if possible. If the result is suboptimal, I would implant a 3.0 mm Palmaz Schatz stent followed by a 3.25 mm balloon at 16-18 ATM.

Nicolaus Reifart, MD, Germany: PTCA alone is a reasonable alternative, but there is a high incidence of spiral dissection. I would use a 0.014-inch Extra-S'port wire, an 8F JR4 guiding catheter, and 60-second inflations to at least 6 ATM to avoid dissection.

Raimund Erbel, MD, Germany: PTCA alone is not a reasonable alternative, because this complex lesion is associated with a high incidence of severe dissection and restenosis.

John Bittl, MD, USA: The treatment of choice is PTCA and conditional stenting, using a 3.5 mm ACS Lifestream at 3-6 ATM. For a residual stenosis > 20%, I would place one or two Palmaz-Schatz stents and postdilate with the Lifestream at 13.5 ATM.

Timothy Sanborn, MD, USA: PTCA alone is reasonable using an 8F JL4 guide, a 0.014-inch Hi-torque floppy guidewire, and a 3.0 x 30 mm balloon. I would be prepared to place a 3.5 mm Gianturco-Roubin stent or two 3.5 mm Palmaz-Schatz stents if the result is suboptimal.

Frank Litvack, MD, USA: The lesion could be approached with conventional PTCA, with an expectation of an excellent immediate result and a restenosis rate of 20-35%.

Antonio Colombo, MD, Italy: I would first try to get a good result with PTCA alone, and place a stent in case of a poor result or large dissection. In the near future, the availability of long stents may change this consideration. I would use a 3.0 mm perfusion balloon. If stenting is necessary, I would exchange for a 0.014-inch Extra-Support guidewire and predilate with a 3.5 mm balloon. Up to four Palmaz-Schatz stents are likely to be needed, followed by high-pressure inflation with a 3.5 mm balloon. IVUS evaluation is important after stenting. I would then prescribe aspirin (ticlopidine for 2 weeks is optional).

Ian Penn, MD, Canada: PTCA is definitely reasonable. In this case, I would use a low-pressure inflation at 3-4 ATM with a 3.5 x 30 mm Duralyn balloon.

Marty Leon, MD, USA: My experience is that PTCA is relatively ineffective in this setting, due to significant residual stenosis and a high likelihood of dissection. If PTCA is attempted, I recommend 30-40 mm balloons to distribute the axial straightening forces over a longer length. I would avoid high pressures and excessive vessel straightening, regardless of balloon material.

Editors' Perspective: There is little consensus about the use of PTCA for this lesion. However, PTCA is certainly not contraindicated, and has been performed on lesions like this for many years with excellent results. Long (30-40 mm) balloons (to conform to the vessel contour without excessive straightening) and possibly perfusion balloons (to permit prolonged inflations) may improve PTCA results. As with all percutaneous interventions, operators should be comfortable with stenting if the PTCA result is suboptimal or complicated by abrupt closure. This lesion was treated with conventional PTCA, using a 3.0 x 40 mm compliant balloon at 6-8 ATM, without complications (below).

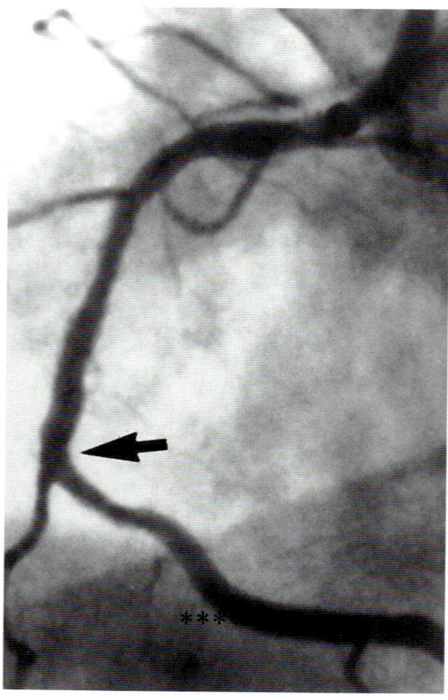

PTCA: ULCERATED LESION

PTCA of an ulcerated lesion in the mid-LAD (reference diameter = 3.2 mm).

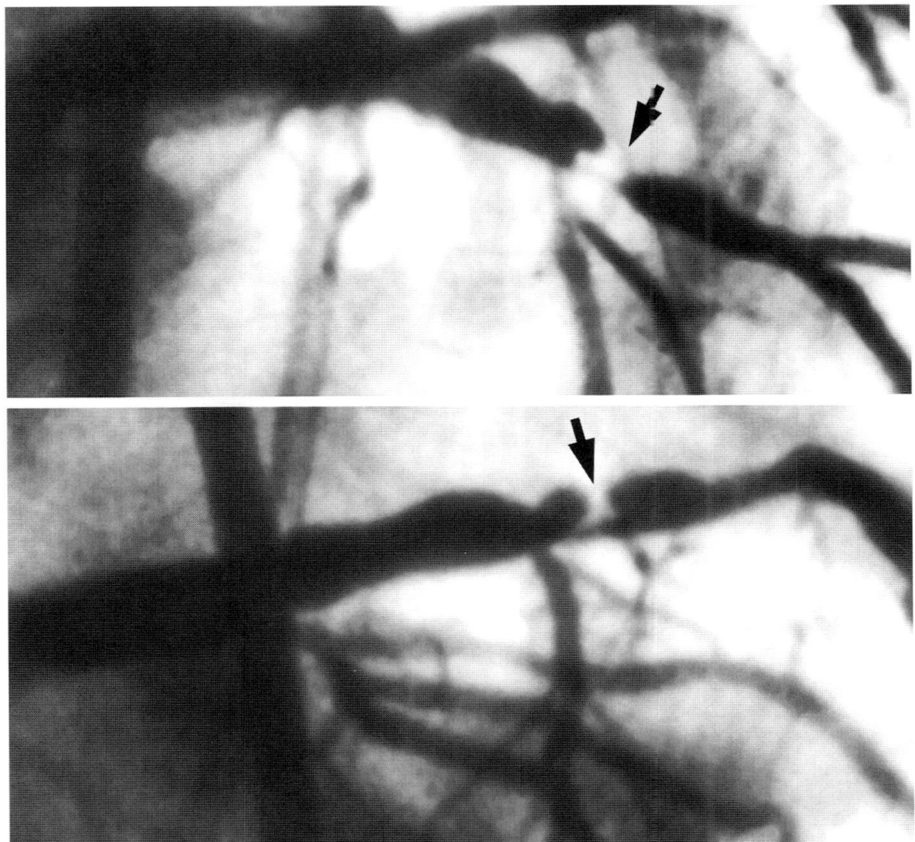

Is PTCA alone reasonable for this lesion?

David Williams, MD, USA: PTCA alone will not provide a satisfactory result for this lesion. Although PTCA is safe, the marked eccentricity and ulceration preclude significant improvement in lumen diameter without dissection. Ulcerated lesions are usually extremely elastic and do not respond well to PTCA.

Michael Cowley, MD, USA: I would not use PTCA alone for this lesion due to the high likelihood of suboptimal results and complications. Whether the lesion is soft or rigid, there is significant likelihood that stenting will be necessary following PTCA. While this is an acceptable strategy, this type of highly eccentric lesion is ideal for directional atherectomy.

David Foley, MD, The Netherlands: PTCA alone is not useful because of the high risk of embolization.

William O'Neill, MD, USA: PTCA alone should not be done.

Cindy Grines, MD, USA: Conventional PTCA will not achieve an acceptable result, due to recoil and residual stenosis. If other devices are not available, I would refer the patient elsewhere.

Barry George, MD, USA: PTCA with adjunctive ReoPro is reasonable.

Raimund Erbel, MD, Germany: PTCA alone is not a reasonable alternative because of the risk of dissection and distal embolization. Most important, PTCA may occlude the first septal branch.

Paul Teirstein, MD, USA: I do not believe that PTCA alone is a reasonable alternative for this lesion because of severe ulceration, leading to a suboptimal result with significant recoil and/or dissection. I favor stenting.

John Bittl, MD, USA: The treatment of choice is PTCA and conditional stenting. If inflation of a 3.5 mm perfusion balloon to 3-6 ATM fails to achieve a residual stenosis < 20%, I would place a Palmaz-Schatz stent and postdilate with a 3.5 mm noncompliant balloon at 18 ATM.

Frank Litvack, MD, USA: PTCA alone could be performed, but with a higher risk of acute complications.

Antonio Colombo, MD, Italy: If stents are not available, I would perform kissing balloon angioplasty with a 3.0 mm perfusion balloon in the LAD and a 2.0 mm ACE in the septal branch.

Gary Roubin, MD, PhD, USA: PTCA alone is unlikely to achieve a good late result in this long and complex lesion; much better immediate and long-term results are achieved after stenting.

Editors' Perspective: Because of the markedly abnormal lesion contour, there is more consensus (and less controversy) about the limited usefulness of PTCA for this lesion. In fact, PTCA was performed, and resulted in no change in the appearance of the stenosis; definitive lumen enlargement was achieved with laser balloon angioplasty. For operators who favor PTCA over other devices, our impression is that PTCA failure in lesions such as this is more often due to suboptimal lumen enlargement than severe complications (such as abrupt closure or distal embolization). Although ReoPro is a worthwhile consideration to decrease the risk of complications, it has no value in facilitating lumen enlargement. For this reason, PTCA operators should be prepared to implant a stent in case of a suboptimal result. If stenting is not an option, the patient should probably be referred to a center with stent experience.

*****

PTCA: TUBULAR LESION

PTCA of a tubular lesion in the mid-RCA (length = 15 mm; reference diameter = 2.5 mm).

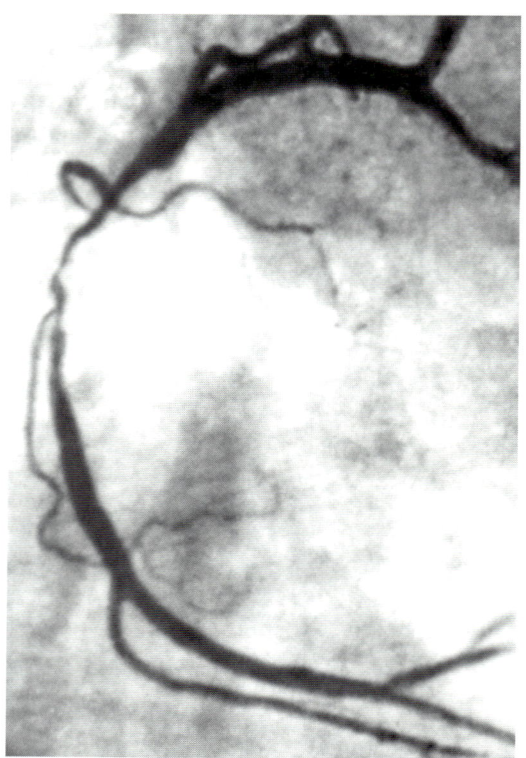

Is PTCA alone a reasonable alternative for this lesion?

Spencer King III, MD, USA: PTCA alone is a viable alternative for this lesion, using a 2.5 x 40 mm balloon for at least 2 minutes.

David Williams, MD, USA: PTCA alone is a poor choice for this lesion, since extensive dissection or suboptimal luminal improvement are likely. I prefer Rotablator atherectomy.

Cindy Grines, MD, USA: My first choice for this lesion is PTCA with a 2.5-3.0 x 40 mm balloon.

Michael Mooney, MD, USA: If rotational atherectomy is not available, referral to a tertiary center experienced in rotational atherectomy is appropriate. Angioplasty alone is not an acceptable strategy due to the length of the lesion and the risk of acute complications and subsequent restenosis.

Patrick Whitlow, MD, USA: PTCA is reasonable for 15 mm lesions in noncalcified, nontortuous vessels; a 3.0 x 30 mm balloon at 3-5 ATM will give a good result.

Richard Myler, MD, USA PTCA is a reasonable alternative for this lesion using a 2.5 x 20 mm PET balloon. I would inflate very slowly at 3-4 ATM for 2 minutes.

John Bittl, MD, USA: The treatment of choice is PTCA; a 3.0 Palmaz-Schatz stent should be placed for dissection or inadequate result.

Timothy Sanborn, MD, USA: I am impressed with the greater clinical success and fewer complications when tackling these lesions with long balloons. I would use a 2.5-3.0 x 30 mm balloon.

Frank Litvack, MD, USA: PTCA with a long balloon is reasonable in this patient, though I believe that prior debulking will yield a larger lumen diameter and potentially reduce the risk of acute and long-term complications.

Marie-Claude Morice, MD, France: My first choice is to dilate this artery with a 2.5 x 30 mm semicompliant balloon over a 0.014-inch Traverse wire through a 6F hockey stick guiding catheter. I would perform a single 3-4 minute inflation at 4-6 ATM.

Richard Schatz, MD, USA: PTCA is not an alternative for this lesion under any circumstances, due to its unpredictability. The risk of dissection, recoil, or acute closure is 5-10%, compared to almost 0% with coronary stenting. It is difficult to justify a 5-10% risk of acute closure in a patient requiring bail-out stenting, when an elective stent will achieve greater primary success, fewer complications and probably a lower restenosis rate in the long run. There is no downside to elective stenting in this patient.

Editors' Perspective: **Before the availability of lasers and Rotablator, long (30-40 mm) balloons were commonly applied to such lesions. In our practice, the use of PTCA for this type of lesion is more influenced by long-term outcome rather than concerns about immediate complications, since excellent immediate results are achieved with a low incidence of abrupt closure. The relative merits of PTCA, Rotablator, and stents for long lesions await definition. In our opinion, PTCA with a long balloon is a perfectly reasonable approach, with stenting for a suboptimal result or abrupt closure. This patient was treated with conventional PTCA using a 2.5 x 30 mm balloon without complications (below).**

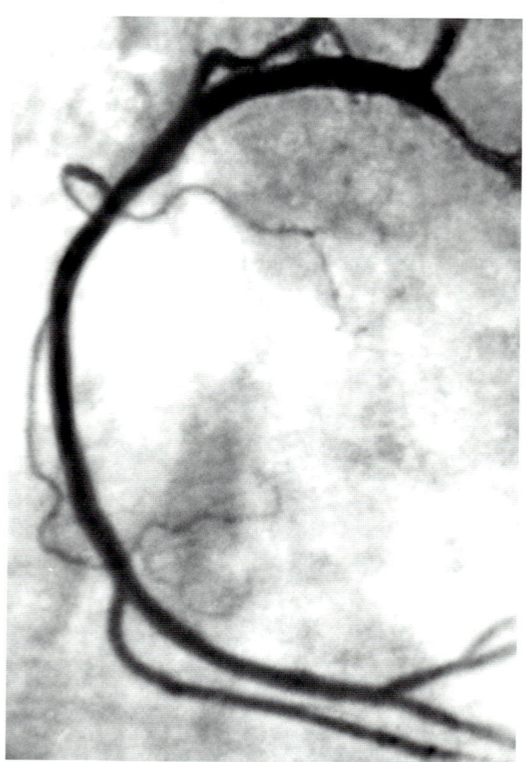

*****

PTCA: LONG LESION

PTCA of a long lesion in the mid-LAD (length = 25 mm; reference diameter = 3.3 mm).

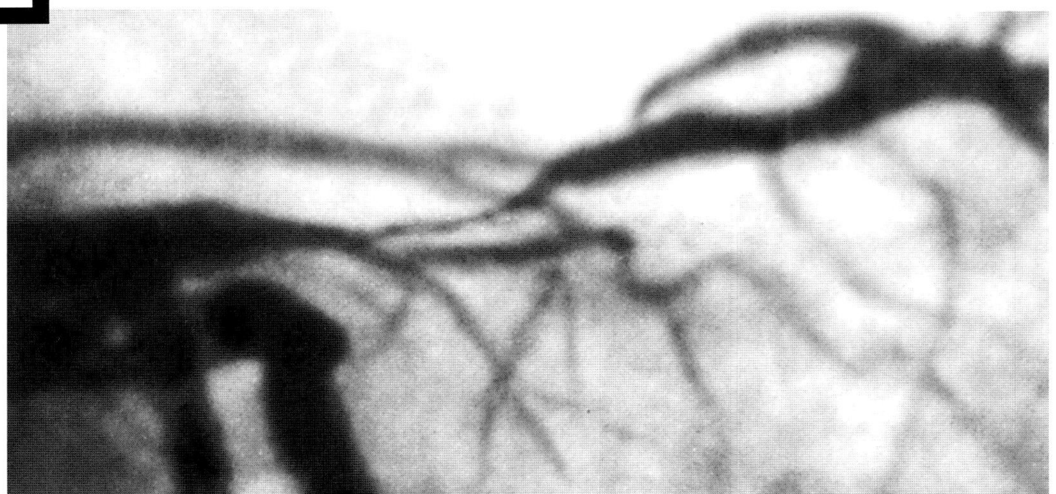

Is PTCA alone a reasonable alternative for this lesion?

Spencer King III, MD, USA: I would not select PTCA alone for this lesion because of the high risk of dissection and restenosis. Certainly, PTCA with an eye toward bailout stenting is reasonable.

David Williams, MD, USA: The LAD lesion is so long and severe that it may not be possible to advance the balloon across the lesion. I would expect substantial dissection after PTCA alone.

Barry George, MD, USA: PTCA alone with stent backup is a reasonable alternative approach. If left ventricular function is impaired, PTCA alone is my first choice.

Cindy Grines, MD, USA: If the patient has "hot" unstable angina or acute MI, a long balloon is appropriate to reduce the chance of distal embolization of thrombus.

Michael Mooney, MD, USA: Angioplasty alone is not appropriate. This long stenosis requires intravascular ultrasound, rotational atherectomy, and stenting to adequately treat this patient. If these resources are not available, referral to a highly experienced center is appropriate.

Patrick Whitlow, MD, USA: PTCA is a reasonable approach for this type of long lesion, which is in a straight segment without calcification. A 3.5 x 30 mm noncompliant balloon at 3-5 ATM is my initial choice. Having a stent for back-up is optimal in case of major dissection.

Richard Myler, MD, USA: PTCA alone is a reasonable alternative for this lesion, especially if calcification is absent by IVUS. I would use a slow inflation technique with a 3.5 x 30 mm PET balloon.

John Bittl, MD, USA: The treatment of choice is PTCA with a 3.5 x 30 mm Trakstar. If an inadequate result is obtained, I would implant a 3.5 mm Palmaz-Schatz stent.

Timothy Sanborn, MD, USA: I would use a 3.5/3.0 x 25 mm tapered balloon.

Frank Litvack, MD, USA: I would not perform conventional PTCA alone on this lesion because its length and morphology are associated with a higher risk of complications and restenosis. Depending on the age of the patient, status of the other coronary arteries, ventricular function, and general health of the patient, bypass surgery is reasonable using an internal mammary graft.

Marie-Claude Morice, MD, France: PTCA alone can be performed on this lesion. However, stenting must remain an option in case of a suboptimal result or dissection. It is unacceptable to treat this lesion without the availability of stents. In this case, good results (and low risk) are associated with internal mammary artery grafting.

Masakiyo Nobuyoshi, MD, Japan: PTCA of such a long lesion may lead to a large dissection; it is best to have stents available.

Richard Schatz, MD, USA: PTCA alone is not a good option for this long lesion, due to the high risk of acute occlusion and restenosis.

<u>Editors' Perspective</u>: The ideal treatment for long lesions in the proximal LAD is unknown. Certainly, a variety of devices could be employed safely, including PTCA, Rotablator, stents, lasers, and directional atherectomy. If PTCA is performed, the operator should be prepared for stenting should a suboptimal result or abrupt closure occur; operators without stent experience should probably refer this patient to another center. As suggested by Dr. Litvack, coronary artery bypass surgery with a left internal mammary artery graft might offer the best option: a recent randomized trial (MASS) of medical therapy, PTCA, and LIMA-CABG for single-vessel proximal LAD disease suggested fewer symptoms, antianginal medications, and repeat procedures for patients undergoing CABG. This patient was treated by Dr. Gregory Robertson with a 3.0 x 40 mm balloon, achieving a good angiographic result.

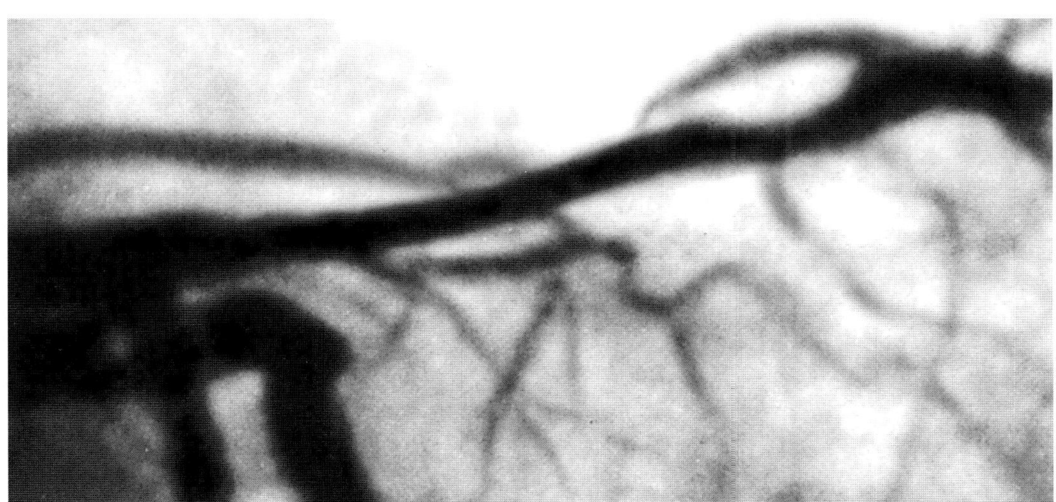

*****

PTCA: ANGULATED LESION (LAD)

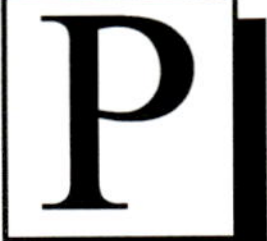

TCA of an angulated lesion in the proximal LAD (lesion on inner curve; reference diameter = 3.4 mm).

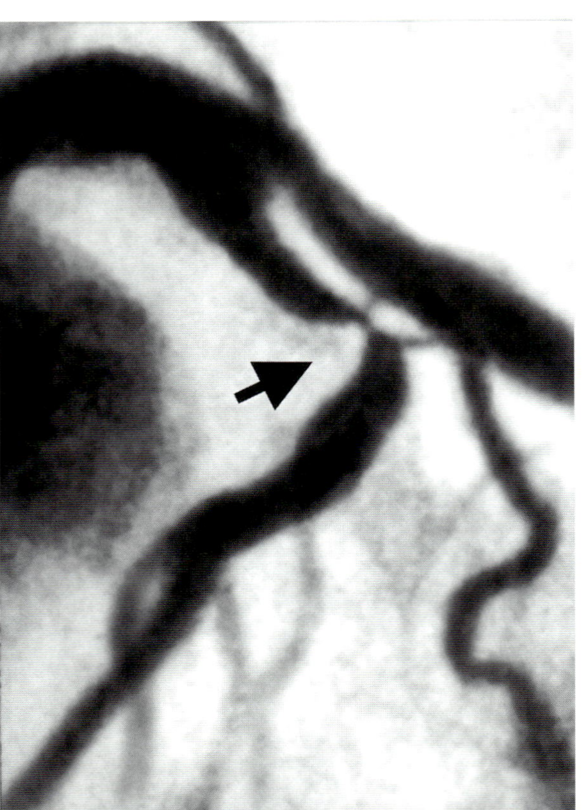

Is PTCA alone reasonable for this lesion?

David Williams, MD, USA: PTCA alone may be satisfactory for the LAD lesion, using a long balloon. Stenting is recommended if the result is suboptimal.

Michael Cowley, MD, USA: PTCA alone is a reasonable alternative for this lesion, but might be associated with a higher residual stenosis and restenosis rate than after an optimal atherectomy. I recommend a 3.5 x 30 mm noncompliant balloon.

Michael Mooney, MD, USA: PTCA is reasonable using a 3.5 mm x 30 mm compliant balloon.

William O'Neill, MD, USA: PTCA is reasonable with a 3.5 x 40 mm balloon and prolonged inflation.

Patrick Whitlow, MD, USA: I would not consider PTCA alone without backup stenting; lesion angulation and eccentricity make it highly likely that a suboptimal result or dissection would follow.

Nicolaus Reifart, MD, Germany: PTCA alone is a reasonable choice, but the likelihood of occlusive dissection is about 15 %.

Paul Teirstein, MD, USA: PTCA alone is not a reasonable alternative for this lesion because of the high risk of dissection. Furthermore, restenosis rates will be lower using the Palmaz-Schatz stent.

Ian Penn, MD, Canada: PTCA is reasonable in the LAD. I would use a perfusion balloon and aim for a 5-10 minute inflation at 4-5 ATM.

David Foley, MD, The Netherlands: PTCA could be attempted using kissing balloons. However, I do not anticipate a high success rate.

> **Editors' Perspective: PTCA of this angulated lesion is relatively straightforward, with stenting reserved for suboptimal results or acute closure. Long (30-40 mm) balloons are useful for minimizing straightening forces and enhancing conformability. Most available data suggest no advantage for one balloon material over another.**

*****

PTCA: ANGULATED LESION (RCA)

PTCA of an angulated lesion in the proximal RCA (lesion on outer curve; reference diameter = 3.1 mm).

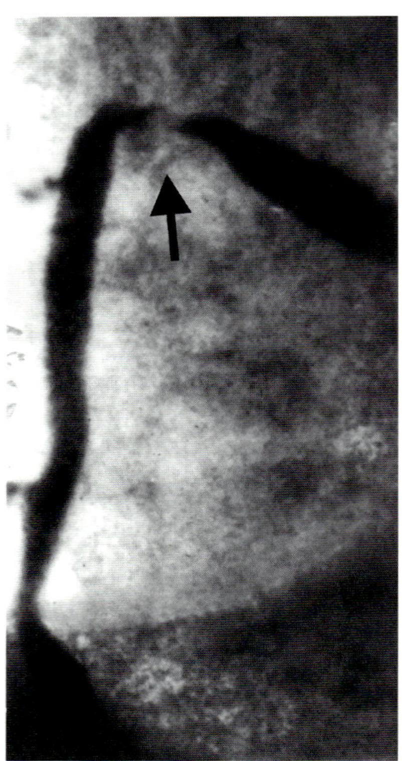

Is PTCA alone reasonable for this lesion?

Michael Cowley, MD, USA: PTCA alone is reasonable but would be associated with a significant likelihood of a suboptimal result, for which stenting might be necessary.

Nicolaus Reifart, MD, Germany: PTCA alone a reasonable alternative, since the vessel is not calcified and since the lesion is located in a bend. I recommend an 8F AR2, AL1, or right Voda guiding catheter to achieve adequate backup.

Barry George, MD, USA: Because of the upward takeoff and severe stenosis, I would choose a hockey stick guide with sideholes, an Extra-S'port guidewire, and a 3.5 x 20 mm Bandit inflated at 2-3 ATM. I would take special care to avoid positioning the heel or toe of the balloon on the sharp angle. A longer balloon might help distribute tangential forces. I would reserve stenting for suboptimal results.

Patrick Whitlow, MD, USA: PTCA alone is reasonable, but the extreme angle distal to the lesion may predispose to dissection, especially at moderately high inflation pressures.

Paul Teirstein, MD, USA: I do not believe that this is a good lesion for PTCA alone because of the risk of dissection. A better result will be achieved with coronary stenting.

John Bittl, MD, USA: Because the lesion abuts the "angle of death" (the sharply angulated shepherd's crook) this lesion should not be treated with conventional PTCA because of a high likelihood of dissection, closure, and refractory cardiogenic shock from right ventricular failure.

Ian Penn, MD, Canada: PTCA alone could be performed with a 30 mm balloon to decrease the risk of disk dissection. A short tip JR4 guide is adequate.

Editors' Perspective: PTCA with A long (30-40 mm) balloon followed by stenting for suboptimal results or acute closure is a reasonable approach to this lesion.

*****

PTCA: TORTUOUS LCX

PTCA of a focal lesion in a tortuous LCX (right angle takeoff; reference diameter = 2.6 mm).

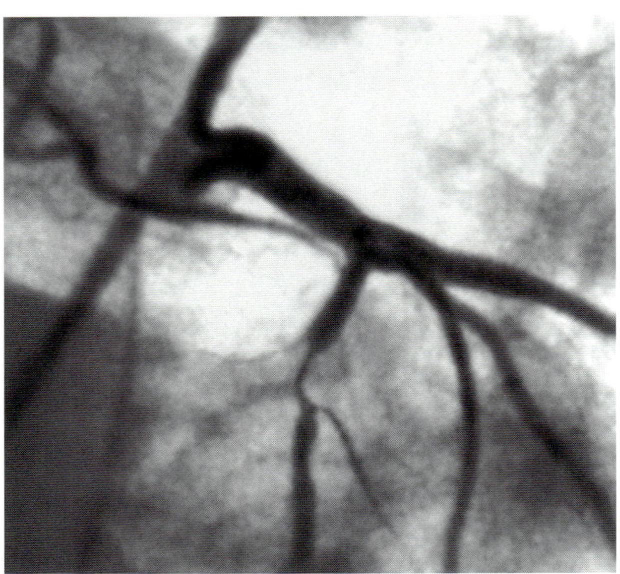

Is PTCA alone reasonable for this lesion?

William O'Neill, MD, USA: I would simply treat with a 5-minute inflation with a 2.5 mm balloon. This patient could be easily treated as an outpatient with a 6F AL3 guiding catheter via the right radial artery. The patient can be immediately ambulated and discharged twelve hours later.

Michael Cowley, MD, USA: PTCA alone is a reasonable treatment for this lesion. I would use a 2.75 mm noncompliant balloon or a 3.0 mm semicompliant balloon, a 0.014-inch Hi-torque floppy wire, and inflation pressures at 3-4 ATM.

Paul Teirstein, MD, USA: If there is no calcification, I favor conventional PTCA since the lesion is concentric and discrete. I would use a JL4 guide, but an Amplatz may be necessary given the difficult right angle takeoff of the LCX. A relatively "transitionless" guidewire will be helpful, such as the Cordis Reflex, the ACS Traverse, or the ACS Balance guidewire. Once guidewire access is obtained, if I have trouble tracking a balloon around this angle, I would exchange for a Platinum-Plus guidewire. When using the Platinum-Plus guidewire, it is important to keep in mind that the tip of this guidewire is relatively stiff; I have encountered coronary artery perforation and pericardial tamponade on two occasions.

Michael Mooney, MD, USA: I favor conventional PTCA.

Frank Litvack, MD, USA: This lesion is on the long and bulky side, but conventional PTCA is certainly reasonable using a JL4 or Voda guide, a 0.014-inch Hi-torque floppy guidewire, and a 2.5-3.0 mm balloon.

Timothy Sanborn, MD, USA: Conventional PTCA will yield a satisfactory result. I would use an 8F JL4 guide, a 0.014-inch Hi-torque floppy guidewire, and a 2.5 mm compliant balloon.

John Bittl, MD, USA: The treatment of choice is PTCA with 2.5 mm Cordis Trakstar. It is possible that the vessel diameter is 3.0 mm, so a 3.0 mm Palmaz-Schatz stent would be implanted if an inadequate result is obtained.

Ian Penn, MD, Canada: I recommend a low profile monorail system such as a 2.5 mm Europass, which tracks extremely well over the wire despite proximal angulation and tortuosity. Balloons work surprisingly well in most difficult situations, as this appears to be.

Patrick Whitlow, MD, USA: PTCA is a reasonable approach, because the lesion itself is in a relatively straight segment, and the artery is not calcified. I would utilize an Amplatz catheter to make sure that the balloon tracks into the LCX without difficulty. I prefer noncompliant or semicompliant balloons and attempt to achieve full balloon expansion utilizing oscillating inflations with a slightly oversized (2.75-3.0 mm) over-the-wire balloon at 3-4 ATM (approximately 300 seconds for the first inflation).

David Williams, MD, USA: PTCA alone could be performed and should give satisfactory angiographic results. I recommend an Amplatz guide for extra backup given the long left main, and a Cordis Stabilizer wire, in case stenting is required.

David Foley, MD, The Netherlands: PTCA alone is a reasonable alternative, but is best approached from the point of view of which stent will be needed if PTCA is unsatisfactory. Thus, trackability and support are of paramount importance, and the shortest stent necessary to cover the lesion should be chosen to minimize tracking difficulties.

Editors' Perspective: The simple lesion morphology favors use of conventional PTCA. Non-balloon devices may be used successfully, but the level of technical difficulty required to negotiate the right angle takeoff of the LCX will be substantially increased over that for simple PTCA. Access to the target lesion may be facilitated by power guides (Amplatz, Voda, XB, EBU, GL, etc), low-profile balloons, and extra-support or heavy-duty guidewires. This patient was referred to Dr. Gregory Robertson for possible directional atherectomy, but the takeoff of the LCX was felt to be too acute. Conventional PTCA was performed successfully using an 8F left Amplatz guide, a 0.014-inch Hi-torque floppy guidewire, and a 2.5 x 20 mm balloon.

*****

PTCA: TORTUOUS RCA

PTCA of a focal lesion in a tortuous RCA (reference diameter = 3.2 mm).

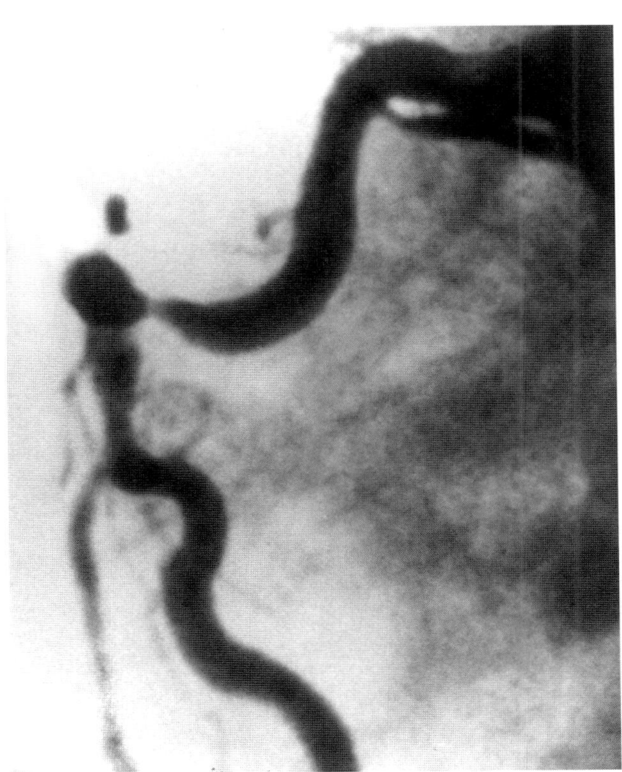

Is PTCA alone reasonable for this lesion?

David Williams, MD, USA: PTCA alone could be performed. Although the risk of dissection and abrupt closure is increased, a flexible (rather than extra-support) guidewire may enhance conformability of the balloon. I favor a slightly undersized 3.0 x 30 mm balloon, and I would accept a final residual stenosis of 20-30% if there is no dissection. If significant dissection occurs, I would exchange the flexible wire for an extra-support wire, to facilitate stent implantation.

Patrick Whitlow, MD, USA: If an Extra-Support wire does not straighten the artery, I would utilize PTCA alone. Although lesion angulation is a risk factor for coronary dissection, no other device is associated with a lower incidence of dissection. However, I would start with a guiding catheter with good support, and position a guidewire in stable position in the distal RCA; coronary stenting could be accomplished without changing equipment. I would utilize a noncompliant 3.5 mm balloon at 3-5 ATM (my usual approach).

William O'Neill, MD, USA: I would simply treat with a 3.0 x 10 mm balloon to avoid dissection. For a suboptimal result, I would deploy a half-stent. This can be accomplished by partially removing the articulated stent, cutting it in half, and placing it back into the delivery sheath. I would use a short stent to avoid placing the articulation of a 15 mm stent in the bend.

Paul Teirstein, MD, USA: Due to my concerns about dissection, I do not recommend PTCA alone for this lesion. I favor stenting.

Michael Cowley, MD, USA: PTCA alone is reasonable for this lesion. However, because of the marked proximal tortuosity and angulation distal to the lesion, the likelihood of dissection is higher. I would use a less aggressive inflation strategy with a 3.0 mm balloon at sufficient pressure to resolve any balloon indentation, for 3 minutes. If the angiographic result is suboptimal, I would use a perfusion balloon for 10 minutes. If the angiographic result is still suboptimal, stenting is appropriate.

Michael Mooney, MD, USA: My initial strategy is to utilize an Amplatz guiding catheter, a 0.014-inch floppy wire, and PTCA. If there is dissection, I would deploy a 3.0 mm stent and postdilate with a 3.5 x 10 mm balloon.

Frank Litvack, MD, USA: I favor conventional PTCA. To minimize the risk of dissection, I recommend a PET or 10 mm balloon, a 0.014-inch Hi-torque floppy guidewire, and a JR4 guide. I would position the tip of the balloon proximal to the bend, inflate slowly, and use nominal inflation pressure.

Ian Penn, MD, Canada: My advice is to perform PTCA with a 3.0 x 30-40 mm semicompliant balloon at 7-8 ATM. Excellent guiding support is essential for success.

Editors' Perspective: Conventional PTCA may be the most reasonable approach to such lesions, and could be performed with less technical difficulty compared to other devices. There are several suggestions for ensuring successful PTCA: First, begin the case with a guiding catheter that will offer excellent back-up support and coaxial alignment; Left Amplatz, hockey stick, and right Voda configurations will work nicely. Although double-loop Arani guides provide excellent support, they are difficult to engage, and their overall performance is generally inferior to that of right Voda guiding catheters. Second, a flexible wire, S'port wire, Stabilizer wire, or a Roadrunner wire may be best to access the target lesion and the distal vessel; the Platinum-Plus wire also provides excellent rail support, but its use is limited by its poor steerability. Third, low-profile over-the-wire or monorail balloons will perform best in this type of anatomy, but if unsuccessful, a fixed wire-balloon catheter could be employed. Fourth, the balloon length should be selected to avoid bends proximal and distal to the target lesion (such as a 9-10 mm balloon) or to conform to the these bends (such as a 30-40 mm balloon). "Standard" 20 mm balloons may result in dissection at the interface between plaque and normal wall, and balloon oversizing should also be avoided because of the risk of dissection. Balloon material is probably irrelevant, and should be based on operator preference and cost.

*****

PTCA: LARGE THROMBUS

PTCA of a large thrombus in a degenerated vein graft (reference diameter = 5.2 mm).

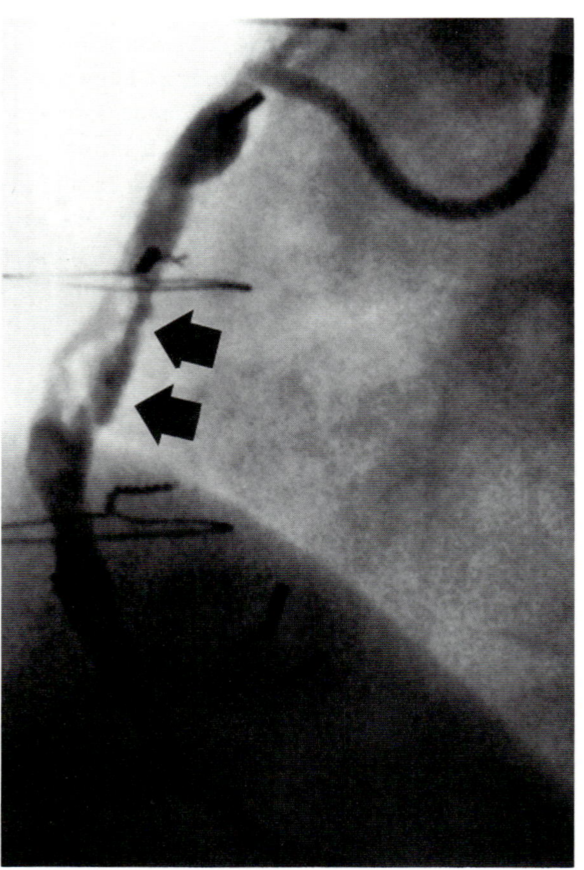

Is PTCA alone reasonable for this lesion?

Patrick Whitlow, MD, USA: PTCA alone is not a suitable alternative because of the high risk of distal embolization and restenosis.

Richard Myler, MD, USA: PTCA is not reasonable in view of diffuse disease and the risk of embolization. The long-term results of all interventional therapies on diffusely diseased grafts are problematic. I would consider elective CABG especially if there are other diseased grafts and native vessels.

Michael Cowley, MD, USA: PTCA alone is not a reasonable treatment alternative for this lesion due to the high likelihood of distal embolization and no-reflow.

Timothy Sanborn, MD, USA: PTCA alone is not a reasonable alternative in view of the large thrombus burden.

Richard Schatz, MD, USA: PTCA alone is not a reasonable alternative for this lesion due to the high likelihood of distal embolization, which I estimate at 30%.

Editors' Perspective: There is no role for PTCA, except as an adjunct to stenting.

*****

PTCA: SMALL THROMBUS

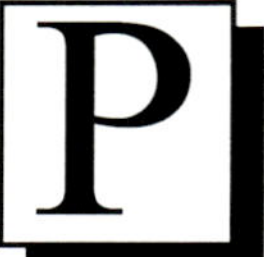

PTCA of a small thrombus in the proximal RCA (reference diameter = 3.4 mm).

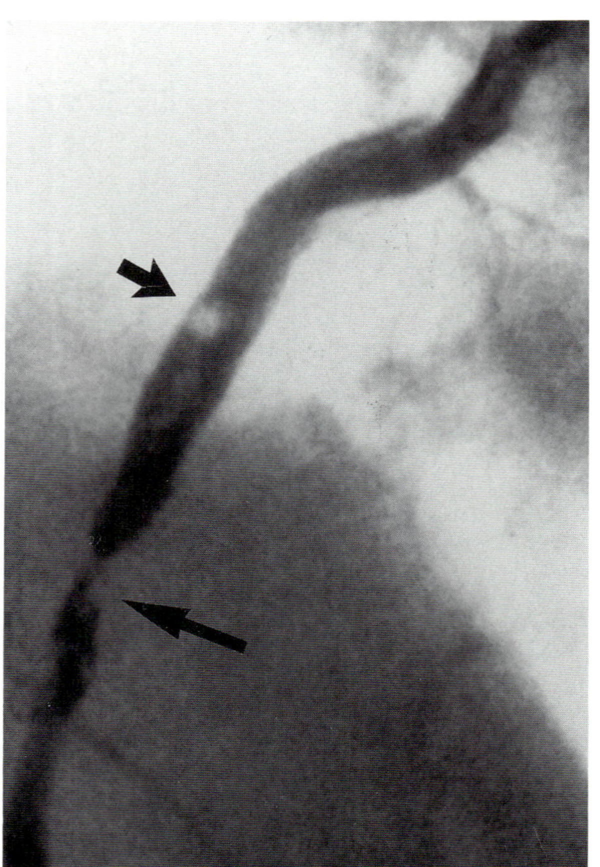

Is PTCA alone reasonable for this lesion?

Spencer King III, MD, USA: I recommend PTCA despite the risk of distal embolization of the small thrombus. I would approach the lesion with a 6F JR4 guide and a 3.0 mm compliant balloon. If I did not achieve a good angiographic appearance, I would increase the inflation pressure to try to enlarge the balloon. If the proximal thrombus remains stationary, I would not make any further attempt to dislodge or treat it. I would use a bolus plus infusion of ReoPro for 12 hours.

David Holmes, MD, USA: PTCA alone could be useful in this setting, although the chance of distal embolization is substantial. Local treatment with a Dispatch catheter or intravenous ReoPro may be very helpful.

Cindy Grines, MD, USA: I would consider PTCA alone, but I would achieve an ACT greater than 350 seconds and use ReoPro (0.25 mg/kg bolus and 0.125 mcg/kg/min infusion for 12 hours). I would avoid intracoronary thrombolytics, due to evidence from three trials showing a worse clinical outcome. If the patient is stable, an alternative approach is to pretreat with ticlopidine (250-500 mg BID for 3 days) prior to PTCA.

Patrick Whitlow, MD, USA: PTCA, ReoPro (0.25 mg/kg bolus and 10 mcg/min infusion for 12 hours), and weight adjusted heparin (70 units/kg) is my first choice for this lesion. I would utilize a 3.5 x 30 mm noncompliant balloon at 3-4 ATM for 3-5 minutes. Ulcerated plaques are frequently very soft, and tend to mold very well with prolonged low-pressure inflations.

Richard Myler, MD, USA: PTCA is reasonable; ReoPro is very helpful in these cases.

Michael Cowley, MD, USA: Immediate PTCA could be used to treat this lesion, using a 3.5 x 30 mm noncompliant balloon, ReoPro, and weight-adjusted heparin. I would continue heparin for 24-36 hours.

John Bittl, MD, USA: If the patient has unstable angina, I recommend heparin to achieve an ACT ~ 250 seconds. I recommend ReoPro bolus and infusion, PTCA with a 3.5 mm Lifestream at 3 ATM, and conditional stenting with a 3.5 mm Palmaz-Schatz stent for a suboptimal result.

Masakiyo Nobuyoshi, MD, Japan: Because of elastic recoil, PTCA alone is not suitable for this lesion. A Palmaz-Schatz stent or MultiLink stent is preferred.

Patrick Serruys, MD, PhD, The Netherlands: PTCA is extremely unlikely to provide good results.

Ulrich Sigwart, MD, England: I would try to aspirate the globular clot and then proceed with PTCA (with or without stenting). Urokinase has not been successful in my experience.

Richard Schatz, MD, USA: PTCA alone is contraindicated in this case due to the fresh thrombus. The unpredictability of PTCA creates a hazardous situation of potential dissection, abrupt closure and overwhelming thrombus, with or without embolization. It is imperative that fresh clot be removed before aggravating the lesion with any intervention.

Antonio Colombo, MD, Italy: Conventional PTCA with a 3.5 x 20-30 mm balloon is a good choice. For residual stenosis > 20% and/or dissection, stenting is reasonable.

Editors' Perspective: PTCA of thrombus-containing lesions is associated with an increased risk of complications. Adjunctive thrombolytic therapy is often considered for such lesions, but may have little impact on procedural success. Although bolus plus infusion ReoPro are often advocated for such lesions, ReoPro has not been specifically tested in thrombotic lesions. Nevertheless, it is widely used for this purpose and may be effective. This patient was treated with 3 days of continuous intravenous heparin, but at the time of intervention, the angiographic appearance was essentially unchanged. Conventional PTCA was performed using a 3.5 x 40 mm balloon, with a good result and without complications. After PTCA, an overnight heparin infusion was prescribed; ReoPro was not used. The patient presented 3 months later with restenosis, which was treated by stenting.

*****

PTCA: FUNCTIONAL TOTAL OCCLUSION

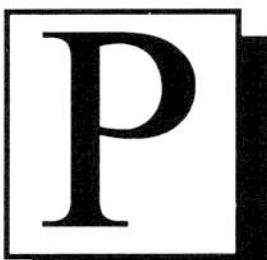

PTCA of a functional total occlusion in the proximal LAD (reference diameter = 2.7 mm). Assume the occlusion can be crossed with a guidewire.

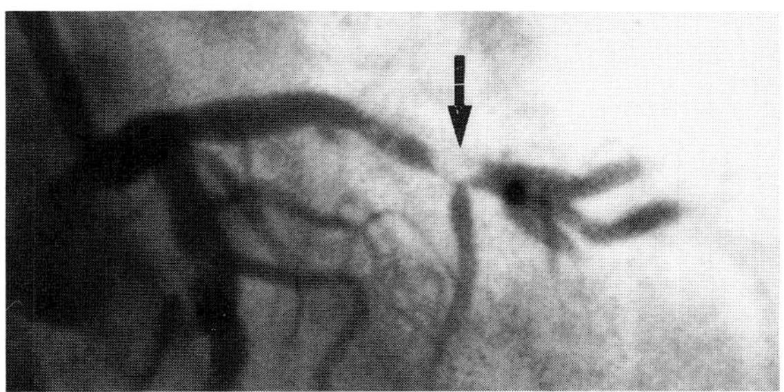

Is PTCA alone reasonable for this lesion?

David Holmes, MD, USA: My first choice for this lesion is conventional PTCA with a 2.5 mm balloon to allow me to decide whether PTCA is the definitive approach or whether another modality will be useful. Stent implantation often produces superb results in the setting of a total occlusion.

Spencer King III, MD, USA: My first choice for this lesion is PTCA with a 3.0 mm balloon. If the result is adequate, I would stop. If the lumen is < 2 mm or there is dissection, I would place a 3.0 mm Palmaz-Schatz stent and postdilate to high pressure. If the occlusion is recent, I would use ReoPro.

William O'Neill, MD, USA: This is not a good lesion for PTCA alone. If necessary, I would perform PTCA with a 24-hour ReoPro infusion and administer intracoronary heparin (5,000 units, diluted 50:50 with saline).

Patrick Whitlow, MD, USA: I would strongly recommend PTCA rather than TEC as my first choice for this lesion. Now that ReoPro is available, the results of PTCA in this setting are excellent, as documented in the EPIC trial. I would use a Traverse wire and a 3.0 x 30 mm Lifestream at low pressure for 5 minutes.

Richard Myler, MD, USA: PTCA has been used for years with good (but not excellent) success. Thrombus (associated with acute ischemic syndromes) is the only statistically significant predictor of untoward events, and late results are compromised in the presence of intracoronary thrombus.

Nicolaus Reifart, MD, Germany: My first choice is PTCA with a 3.0 x 35 mm Speedy with long inflations at low pressure to compress the thrombus. I would approach the lesion with a 6F JL4 guiding catheter and a 0.014-inch Hi-torque floppy guidewire.

Frank Litvack, MD, USA: Conventional PTCA alone is reasonable, especially if this is an acute thrombotic occlusion. I would use an SL4 guide and any 2.5 mm balloon. ReoPro is a good idea if thrombus is evident.

Timothy Sanborn, MD, USA: PTCA alone is unlikely to yield a good long term result.

John Bittl, MD, USA: I recommend low-dose heparin to achieve an ACT of 250 seconds, ReoPro bolus and infusion, and PTCA with a perfusion balloon.

Masakiyo Nobuyoshi, MD, Japan: PTCA is a better choice than a stent. I recommend a 3.0 x 20 mm balloon at 8-10 ATM. If a large dissection occurs, I would use a 3.0 mm Palmaz-Schatz stent.

Ulrich Sigwart, MD, England: I recommend a small amount of urokinase (selective infusion over 15 minutes into the LAD or via a drug delivery balloon). If this helps, I recommend PTCA with a 3.0 mm balloon at low pressure.

Marie-Claude Morice, MD, France: It is likely that a good result will not be achieved with PTCA for such an eccentric lesion. However, PTCA alone is indeed reasonable. It has not been proven that stenting prevents restenosis in total occlusions. I would select a 6F JL4 guiding catheter, a 0.014-inch Traverse wire, and a 3.0 mm Cobra balloon. Although I usually use Monorail catheters, total occlusions are better approached with coaxial systems; one can reshape or exchange the wire and the balloon can be positioned 1-2 cm proximal to the tip of the wire to provide support. The only technical difficulty in this case is crossing the occlusion with the guidewire.

Editors' Perspective: A reasonable approach to this lesion is conventional PTCA followed by stenting or directional atherectomy, depending on the appearance of the vessel and lesion after crossing the occlusion with the guidewire. Since the caliber of the distal vessel is uncertain, it is a good idea to "dotter" the occlusion with a deflated balloon or transfer catheter before dilating the occlusion with what is thought to be the proper size balloon. Failure to consider vessel tapering or placement of the guidewire in a smaller sidebranch before dilating with a balloon sized to match the the proximal reference diameter can lead to dissection, abrupt closure, or rarely coronary artery perforation. For these reasons, we recommend using an angioplasty wire through a 3.5F transfer catheter to provide support for the wire and to permit wire exchanges, if necessary. If adequate flow can be achieved, subsequent angiography will permit the operator to select a full size balloon or other device for definitive revascularization. Although ReoPro has been shown to decrease complications associated with PTCA, it has not been specifically tested in total occlusions (with or without thrombus). Nevertheless, off-label use of ReoPro for this type of lesion seems reasonable.

*****

PTCA: TOTAL OCCLUSION

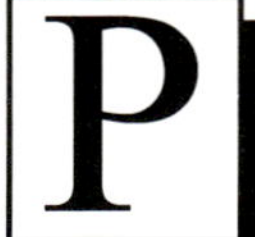

PTCA of a total occlusion in the proximal RCA (reference diameter = 4.5 mm). Assume the occlusion can be crossed with a guidewire.

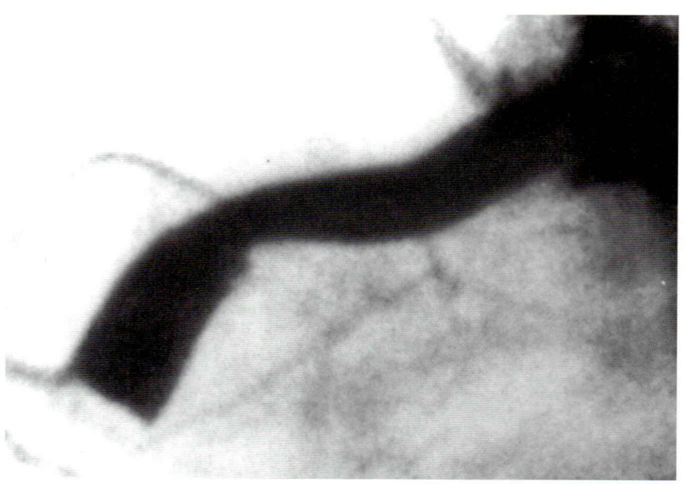

Is PTCA alone reasonable for this lesion?

Michael Mooney, MD, USA: The initial strategy I would use is PTCA with an Implants F1 guiding catheter and a 0.014-inch Hi-torque floppy wire. I like long balloons in this setting because thrombus can be approached with a longer dilating surface. If dissection occurs, I would use a Palmaz-Schatz stent.

David Holmes, MD, USA: I would use conventional PTCA with a small balloon and see what the distal bed looks like. If a large thrombus is present, I recommend ReoPro.

Spencer King III, MD, USA: My first choice for this lesion is PTCA with a 4.0 mm compliant balloon. I would withdraw the balloon without inflating it and perform angiography to assess distal flow, thrombus burden, and determine if any additional therapy is needed before definitive balloon inflations.

Patrick Whitlow, MD, USA: PTCA is my first choice for this type of thrombotic lesion that conceals the distal anatomy. I generally start with a Traverse wire or Hi-torque floppy wire, then intermediate and standard wires, and then a Meditech Gold Glidewire, if necessary. A stent can be utilized if excellent results are not obtained with PTCA alone.

Richard Myler, MD, USA: PTCA as sole device is reasonable. However initial and late outcome may be less than optimal. Adjunctive intracoronary urokinase or ReoPro may be helpful for persistent thrombus.

Nicolaus Reifart, MD, Germany: My first choice is PTCA with an 8F AR2 or multi-purpose guiding catheter, a 0.014-inch Hi-torque intermediate guidewire, and a 4.5 x 40 mm Europass or Speedy balloon for 6 minutes. For residual stenosis > 30%, I would implant a stent if there is no visible clot.

John Bittl, MD, USA: I recommend prolonged intravenous heparin and aspirin for 4-7 days, followed by PTCA with a 3.0 mm Lifestream. Adjunctive ReoPro can be given if large intracoronary filling defects persist after PTCA.

Frank Litvack, MD, USA: I would perform conventional PTCA using a JR4 guide, a 0.014-inch Hi-torque floppy guidewire, and any 4.0 mm balloon. I would implant a stent if the result is suboptimal.

Marie-Claude Morice, MD, France: PTCA alone is indeed a reasonable approach; PTCA may be preferable to multiple stents, since I am not sure if stents prevent restenosis in such lesions.

> **Editors' Perspective: For the last 17 years, PTCA has been the standard approach to this type of lesion. There are two major limitations to the use of PTCA in this case: First, the length of occlusion, diameter of the distal reference vessel, and extent of thrombus are unknown; and second, PTCA balloons (in the United States) are available in diameters ≤ 4 mm, mandating the use of peripheral balloons to achieve satisfactory lumen enlargement. When PTCA is performed, excellent guiding catheter support and coaxial alignment using a left Amplatz or hockey stick guide is essential. The choice of guidewires is largely a matter of personal preference; if floppy guidewires are unsuccessful, other options include intermediate or standard guidewires, the Glidewire, the Magnum wire, or Choice-PT wires. Personally, we feel that the choice-PT wire is the best wire for crossing chronic total occlusions.**

*****

PTCA: CALCIFIED LESION

PTCA of a calcified lesion in the mid-LAD (reference diameter = 2.9 mm).

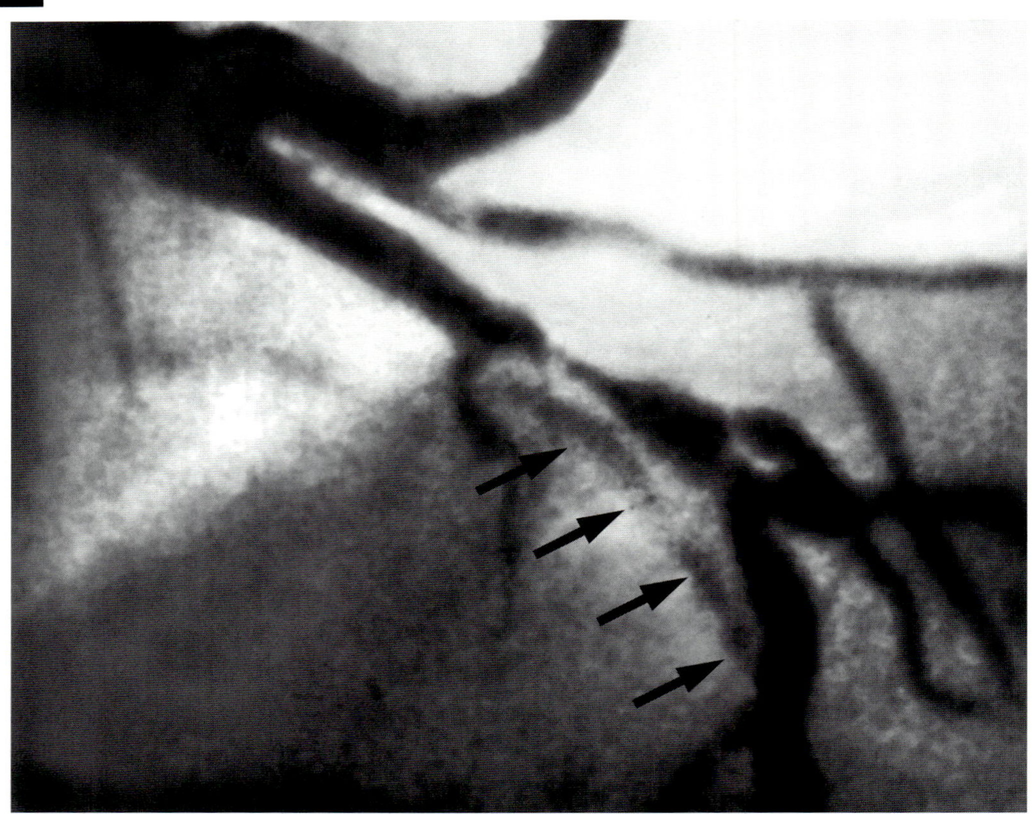

Is PTCA alone reasonable alternative for this lesion?

Michael Cowley, MD, USA: I do not consider PTCA alone a reasonable approach in current interventional practice, due to the high likelihood of a suboptimal result. If PTCA is done, a noncompliant balloon will allow high inflation pressures.

David Williams, MD, USA: PTCA alone could be attempted but will likely lead to suboptimal results. I prefer Rotablator atherectomy, PTCA, and possible stenting.

Patrick Serruys, MD, PhD, The Netherlands: PTCA alone could be performed, but with calcification, the risk of dissection and restenosis are high, and the chance of achieving an optimal result with a diameter stenosis < 35% is low. Be prepared for bailout stenting.

Patrick Whitlow, MD, USA: I would seriously consider sending the patient to a center where coronary stents and rotational atherectomy are available, rather than attempt PTCA alone. If the lesion is mildly calcified, PTCA is reasonable. I would use a 3.0 mm perfusion balloon and aim for a 5-10 minute inflation with progressive increases in pressure up to 4-6 ATM. If this strategy fails, I would use oscillating inflations up to 10 ATM. If this fails, I would change to a noncompliant 3.0 mm balloon; the complication rate goes up because major dissections are more common with inflation pressures >10 ATM.

Raimund Erbel, MD, Germany: PTCA alone is not a suitable technique.

Paul Teirstein, MD, USA: PTCA alone will probably result in dissection, and stenting will be required.

John Bittl, MD, USA: I recommend a strategy of PTCA with a perfusion balloon and conditional stenting with a 3.0 mm Palmaz-Schatz stent. Stenting is contraindicated if the balloon is incompletely expanded at high pressure.

Marie-Claude Morice, MD, France: PTCA alone is a good alternative, if stents are available for suboptimal results.

> **Editors' Perspective: The results of PTCA alone for calcified lesions are unpredictable for several reasons: First, compared to IVUS, fluoroscopy is insensitive to the presence, distribution, and extent of calcification, factors that influence procedural outcome. PTCA is reasonable if extensive superficial calcification is absent. Second, the risk of dissection is increased in the presence of superficial calcification, and usually occurs at the interface between calcified and noncalcified plaque. Rotablator is extremely useful for ablating superficial calcium, and can increase lesion compliance and decrease the risk of subsequent dissection after PTCA. Third, extensive calcification may cause marked lesion rigidity and impair full balloon expansion, resulting in suboptimal lumen enlargement. Again, Rotablator can improve lesion compliance and facilitate subsequent lumen enlargement by PTCA or stenting.**

*****

PTCA: CALCIFIED OSTIAL RCA

PTCA of a calcified ostial lesion in the RCA (reference diameter = 2.8 mm).

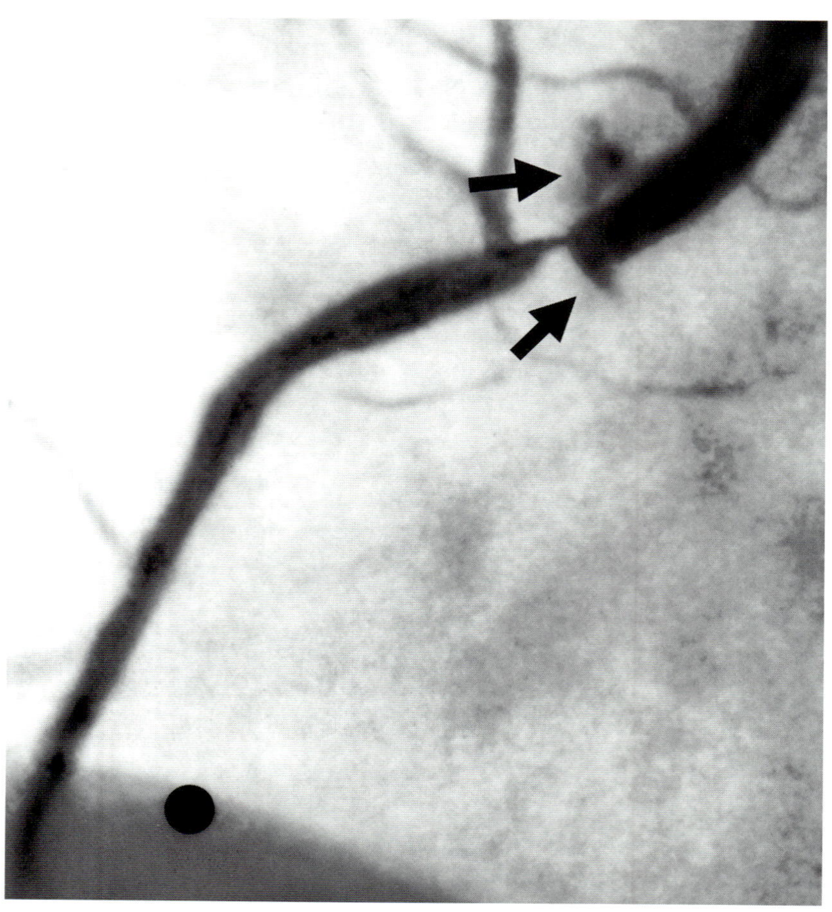

Is PTCA alone reasonable alternative for this lesion?

Michael Cowley, MD, USA: PTCA alone is not a reasonable treatment for a calcified ostial lesion. Such a patient should be referred to a center experienced in new devices, if these options are not available locally.

David Williams, MD, USA: PTCA alone could be attempted but will likely be suboptimal. Ostial lesions need some type of debulking or stenting to achieve an acceptable result.

Patrick Serruys, MD, PhD, The Netherlands: PTCA may be attempted in this type of lesion but is almost always associated with suboptimal results and frequent restenosis. Optimal results will be obtained with Rotablator, followed by adjunctive PTCA and stenting.

Barry George, MD, USA: If the operator does not have experience with rotational atherectomy or stenting, the patient should be referred to a center with such experience.

Patrick Whitlow, MD, USA: PTCA is not a reasonable approach for this type of heavily calcified ostial lesion. The primary success rate is 50-70%, and the recurrence rate exceeds 50%.

Raimund Erbel, MD, Germany: PTCA alone is not a suitable technique.

Michael Mooney, MD, USA: PTCA is not an acceptable approach in this case. Rotational atherectomy and stenting are necessary to achieve optimal results. This patient should be referred to another center, if appropriate resources are not available.

Timothy Sanborn, MD, USA: This type of calcified ostial lesion simply does not dilate well with conventional PTCA, due to dissection, abrupt closure, and a high incidence of restenosis.

Marie-Claude Morice, MD, France: PTCA could be performed in this lesion, but is not recommended because it entails two major risks: Acute occlusion and restenosis. Furthermore, such lesions are extremely resistant and cannot be adequately dilated by balloons.

> **Editors' Perspective: Conventional PTCA for calcified ostial lesions is limited by lesion rigidity, elastic recoil, and suboptimal lumen enlargement. Final residual stenoses < 50% are extremely unusual after PTCA alone, thus making restenosis a virtual certainty. The results of PTCA alone are so poor (even with high-pressure balloons) that patients with this type of lesion should be referred to centers with Rotablator, atherectomy, and stents.**

*****

PTCA: OSTIAL DIAGONAL

PTCA of an ostial lesion in the diagonal (reference diameter = 3.2 mm).

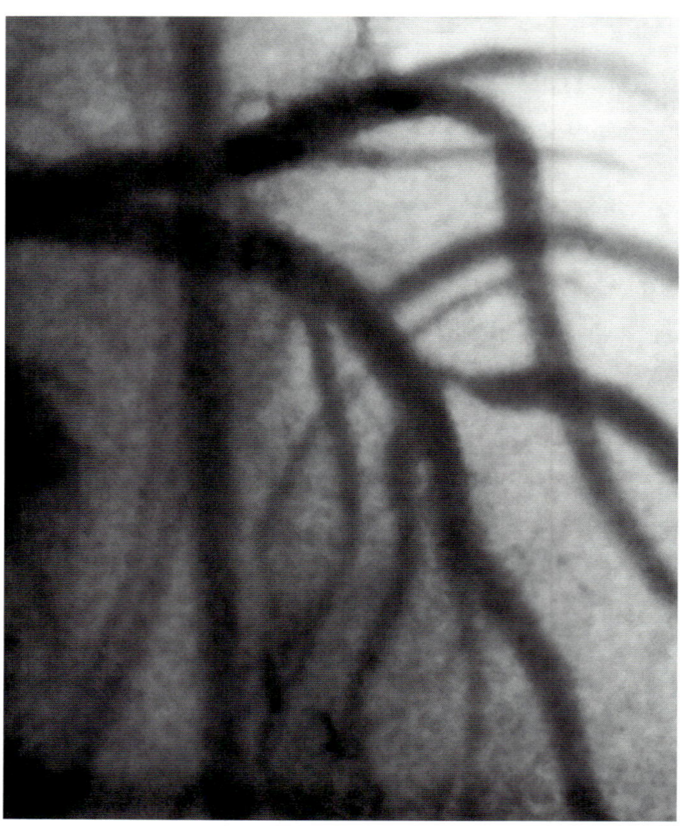

Is PTCA alone a reasonable alternative for this lesion?

Spencer King III, MD, USA: PTCA is reasonable for this lesion, although ostial lesions usually do not respond as well after PTCA compared to directional atherectomy. I would utilize a 3.5 mm balloon to slightly oversize the orifice. It is not necessary to position another wire in the LAD.

David Foley, MD, The Netherlands: PTCA in this type of lesion is associated with a high risk of dissection and restenosis, and is not recommended.

Donald Baim, MD, USA: I do not favor conventional PTCA due to marked elastic recoil in ostial lesions.

Cindy Grines, MD, USA: I would avoid conventional PTCA, due to significant elastic recoil.

Michael Mooney, MD, USA: I do not recommend PTCA alone, due to the high incidence of dissection and elastic recoil.

Patrick Whitlow, MD, USA: I personally would not utilize PTCA when I have debulking devices like the Rotablator, directional atherectomy, or laser, but PTCA is not unreasonable. If none of these devices are available, I would use a 3.25 x 20 mm PET balloon to permit high-pressure inflations.

Richard Myler, MD, USA: PTCA alone is reasonable, although recoil is common. Results with Rotablator, directional atherectomy, and stents are better.

John Bittl, MD, USA: I would perform PTCA with a 3.5 mm Lifestream at 3-4 ATM, and conditional stenting with a 3.0 mm Palmaz-Schatz stent for inadequate result.

Frank Litvack, MD, USA: Ostial diagonal lesions are notoriously prone to recoil; PTCA is not recommended.

Paul Teirstein, MD, USA: I do not recommend PTCA for this lesion because of significant elastic recoil.

> <u>Editors' Perspective</u>: **PTCA alone is often associated with significant elastic recoil and suboptimal lumen enlargement; residual stenoses ≥ 50% are common. Although slightly oversized balloons were commonly used to enhance lumen enlargement, such a strategy merely increases the risk of dissection. Patients with such lesions should be referred to another center with Rotablator, atherectomy, and stents.**

*****

PTCA: OSTIAL LAD

PTCA of an ostial lesion in the LAD (reference diameter = 3.8 mm).

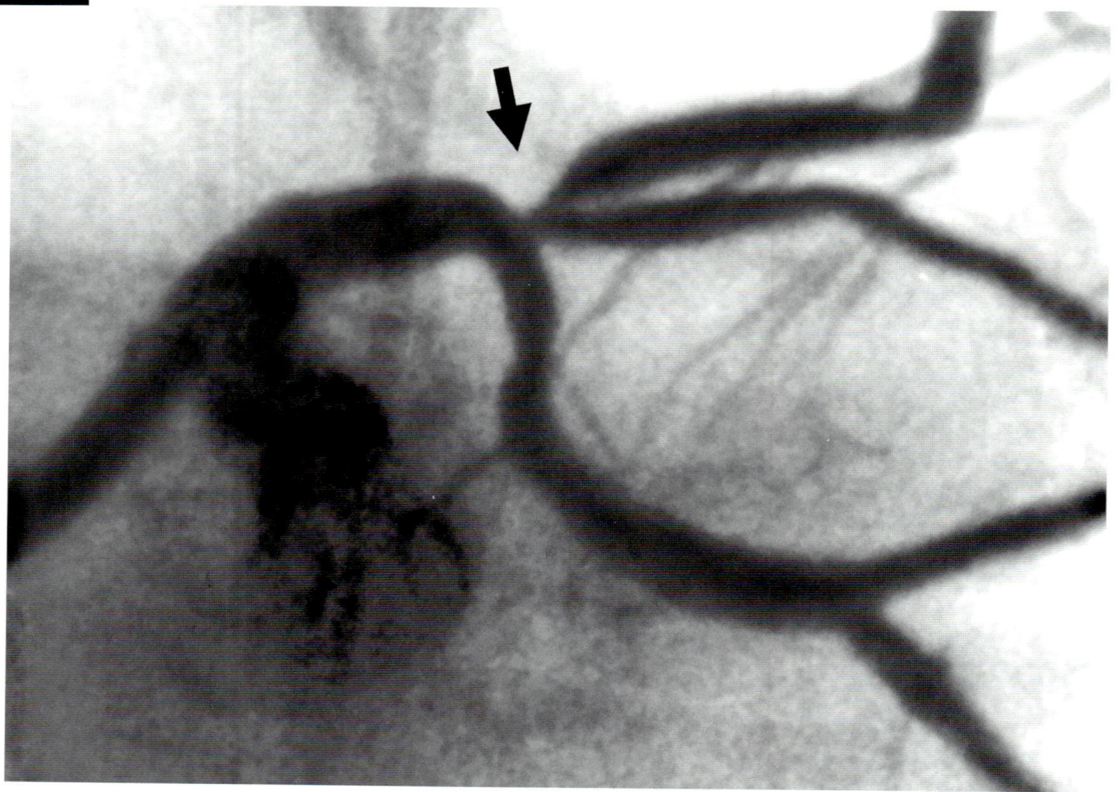

Is PTCA alone a reasonable alternative for this lesion?

Donald Baim, MD, USA: I would not favor conventional PTCA due to marked elastic recoil in ostial lesions.

Spencer King III, MD, USA: I would not consider PTCA in this case, since it would simply shift the plaque burden.

Cindy Grines, MD, USA: I do not expect a good result with conventional PTCA due to the ostial location and eccentricity of the lesion.

Michael Mooney, MD, USA: PTCA alone is often complicated by significant recoil, and is not recommended.

Patrick Whitlow, MD, USA: PTCA alone is not reasonable for this lesion, because of the risk of left main dissection, prolonged ischemia, and a suboptimal result.

Richard Myler, MD, USA: PTCA is not reasonable; Rotablator, directional atherectomy and stents offer better results.

John Bittl, MD, USA: Conventional PTCA alone is inadequate for this type of lesion because a residual stenosis > 50% and a hazy appearance usually persist after treatment.

> **Editors' Perspective: Conventional PTCA in this location has several problems, including significant elastic recoil, suboptimal lumen enlargement, and left main dissection.**

*****

PTCA: OSTIAL LCX

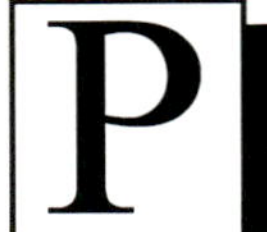
PTCA of an ostial lesion in the LCX (reference diameters: left main = 4.2 mm; LCX = 3.8 mm).

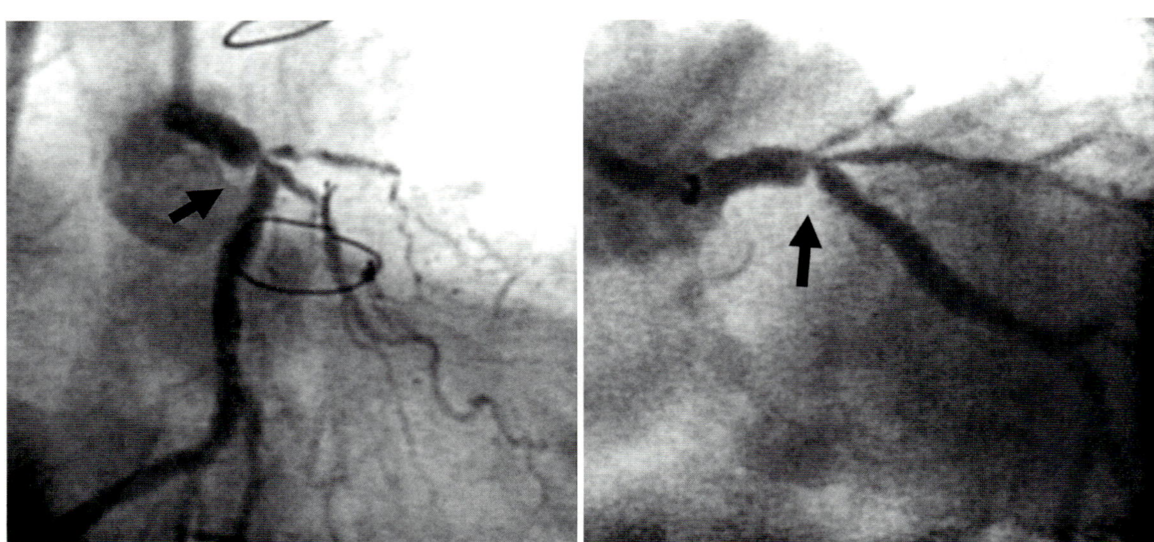

Is PTCA alone a reasonable alternative for this lesion?

Donald Baim, MD, USA: I do not favor conventional PTCA due to marked elastic recoil in ostial lesions.

Spencer King III, MD, USA: PTCA with a 4.0 mm balloon could be performed in this lesion.

Michael Mooney, MD, USA: These lesions respond poorly to PTCA alone, due to recoil, lesion rigidity, and calcification.

Patrick Whitlow, MD, USA: PTCA alone is reasonable, though I would expect a much better result with other devices. One of the difficulties in dilating such a lesion is the discrepancy in size between the left main and the LCX. I would choose a USCI 4.0/3.5 x 25 mm tapered balloon.

Richard Myler, MD, USA: PTCA can be used if there is no calcium. However, Rotablator and stents offer better results.

Frank Litvack, MD, USA: I would approach this lesion with conventional PTCA; occasionally, excellent angiographic results can be achieved.

Paul Teirstein, MD, USA: PTCA alone is not a reasonable alternative for this lesion, which is usually noncompliant due to fibrous tissue or calcium. I favor Rotablator atherectomy.

> **Editors' Perspective: PTCA is certainly feasible and can be readily performed with standard equipment and techniques. However, because of the high likelihood of elastic recoil and suboptimal lumen enlargement, stents should be available.**

*****

PTCA: VEIN GRAFT

PTCA of a vein graft to the RCA (reference diameter = 3.9 mm).

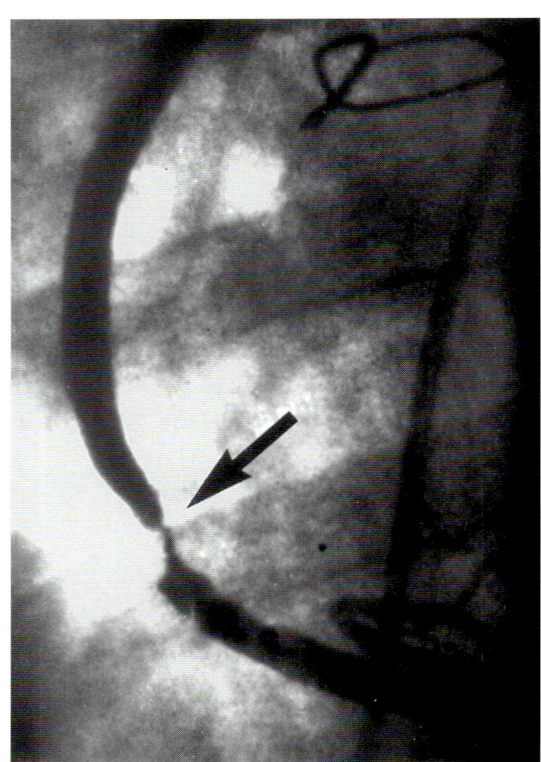

Is PTCA alone reasonable for this lesion?

Michael Mooney, MD, USA: PTCA is not an acceptable strategy given the high rate of restenosis.

Patrick Whitlow, MD, USA: PTCA alone would likely be successful, but I expect a restenosis rate of at least 45-50%. Since stenting and directional atherectomy have higher restenosis rates when used in restenotic lesions, I believe that stenting should be performed as the primary procedure.

Richard Myler, MD, USA: PTCA alone can be used, but stenting is better.

Michael Cowley, MD, USA: PTCA is reasonable, but the high likelihood of restenosis makes it unattractive.

John Bittl, MD, USA: PTCA alone can be attempted for this lesion, but the risk of embolization and restenosis is extremely high.

Patrick Serruys, MD, PhD, The Netherlands: PTCA is certainly a reasonable alternative, but there is a high risk of distal embolization. Wallstent implantation is better and safer.

> Editors' Perspective: **PTCA alone is technically feasible, and can be readily accomplished with any contemporary PTCA hardware. However, the high rate of restenosis limits the long-term effectiveness of PTCA in vein grafts, and virtually all operators recommend PTCA only as an adjunct to stenting.**

*****

PTCA: DEGENERATED VEIN GRAFT

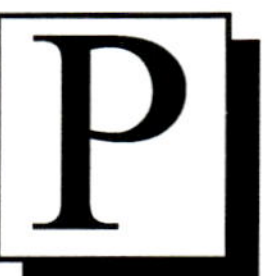TCA of a degenerated vein graft to the OM (reference diameter = 3.9 mm).

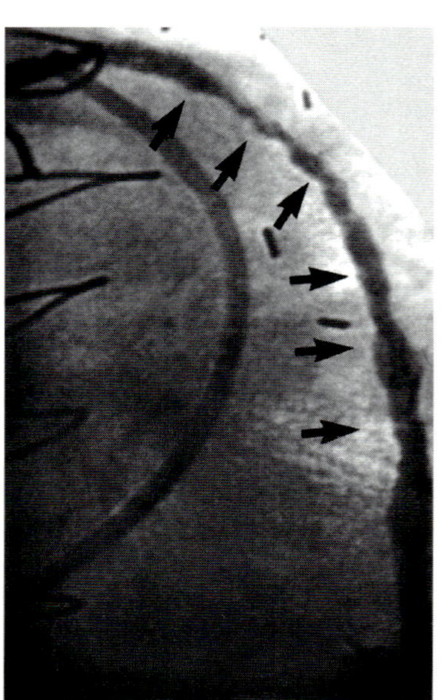

Is PTCA alone reasonable for this lesion?

David Holmes, MD, USA: PTCA with a long balloon could be performed but would increase the potential for distal embolization and a suboptimal result. I would use ReoPro at the start of the procedure to decease the risk of distal embolization.

Patrick Whitlow, MD, USA: PTCA alone is not a reasonable choice for this lesion because of the extremely high recurrence rate and the initial risk of distal embolization.

Richard Myler, MD, USA: PTCA is associated with unfavorable outcomes due to distal embolization, and should be avoided.

Michael Cowley, MD, USA: PTCA alone is occasionally successful in this setting, but the likelihood of major complications is high. PTCA alone should be reserved for urgent situations, when other options are not available.

John Bittl, MD, USA: PTCA alone is not recommended for this lesion because of the risk of embolization and restenosis.

Masakiyo Nobuyoshi, MD, Japan: Because this lesion has old thrombus, PTCA alone is not suitable.

David Foley, MD, The Netherlands: PTCA is dangerous, with a high likelihood of distal embolization of friable material.

> Editors' Perspective: **PTCA alone has no advantage over medical therapy for degenerated vein grafts such as this. The extremely high risk of distal embolization, no-reflow, and restenosis mitigate against PTCA, except as an adjunct to stenting.**

*****

PTCA: OSTIAL VEIN GRAFT

PTCA of an ostial lesion in a vein graft to the LAD (reference diameter = 3.9 mm).

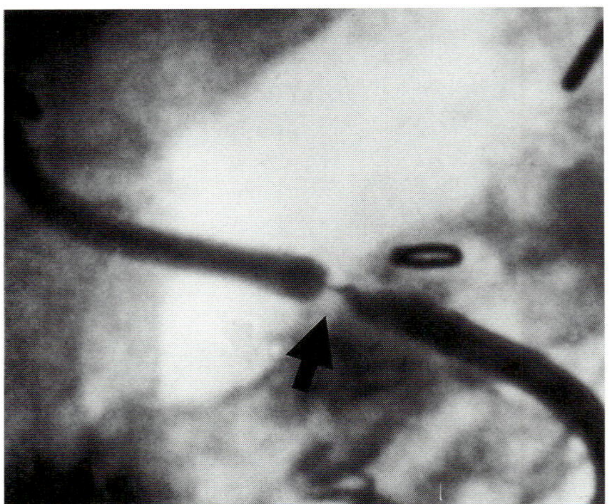

Is PTCA alone reasonable for this lesion?

David Holmes, MD, USA: PTCA is not a reasonable option given the high incidence of recoil and restenosis. Aortoostial vein graft lesions remain among the most difficult lesions to treat.

Patrick Whitlow, MD, USA: PTCA is not a reasonable choice for this lesion because of elastic recoil. A suboptimal result is certain, and restenosis approaches 100%.

Richard Myler, MD, USA: PTCA is not suitable; stenting is best.

Michael Cowley, MD, USA: PTCA alone is not appropriate for this lesion due to consistently poor results.

John Bittl, MD, USA: PTCA alone is not recommended because of the high likelihood of elastic recoil.

Timothy Sanborn, MD, USA: In general, aortoostial lesions like this one do not respond well to conventional PTCA.

Masakiyo Nobuyoshi, MD, Japan: Because of elastic recoil, PTCA alone is not suitable for this lesion and a stent is preferred.

Patrick Serruys, MD, PhD, The Netherlands: PTCA is extremely unlikely to provide good results.

<u>Editors' Perspective</u>: **PTCA is certainly safe and easy, but rigidity and elasticity of the aortoostial junction limit the immediate and long-term effectiveness of balloon dilation. Patients with ostial vein graft lesions should be referred to centers with atherectomy or stents, and should not be treated with PTCA alone.**

*****

PTCA: TRIFURCATION LESION

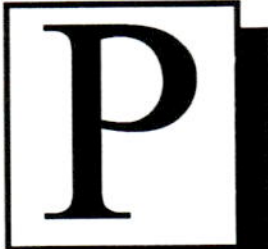TCA of a trifurcation lesion in the proximal LCX (reference diameter of proximal LCX = 3.4 mm).

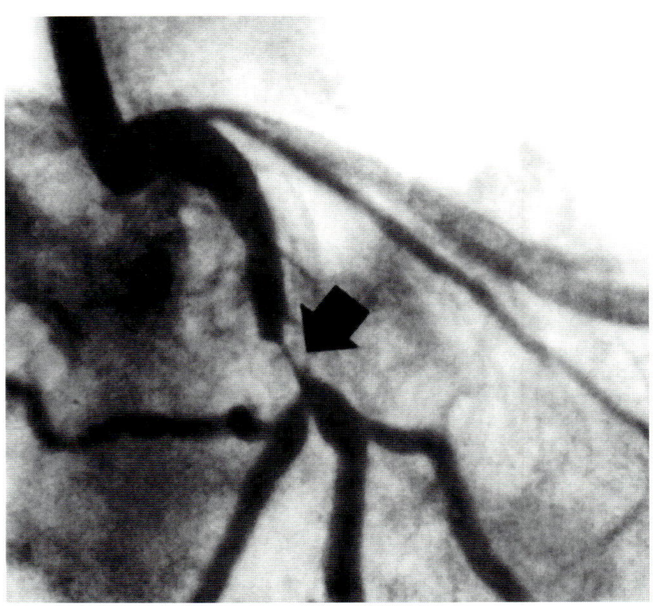

Is PTCA alone reasonable alternative for this lesion?

Michael Mooney, MD, USA: PTCA is reasonable for this lesion. I would only use coronary stenting if the PTCA result is suboptimal.

William O'Neill, MD, USA: PTCA with a 3.5 mm balloon could be easily performed.

Patrick Whitlow, MD, USA: PTCA alone is a reasonable approach. I would place one wire down the middle branch and try to dilate at low pressure with a 3.5/3.0 x 25 mm tapered balloon. I would then place the wire down the continuation of the AV groove, and perform PTCA with same balloon.

Michael Cowley, MD, USA: PTCA alone is reasonable for this lesion. I would use a 3.75 noncompliant balloon at low pressure, an 8F JL4 large lumen guide, and a 0.014-inch Hi-torque floppy wire.

Nicolaus Reifart, MD, Germany: PTCA alone is reasonable, using a 0.014-inch Hi-torque floppy wire and a long monorail balloon at 4-6 ATM.

John Bittl, MD, USA: The treatment of choice is "kissing" balloon angioplasty with a 2.5 mm Edge in the LCX, a 3.0 mm ACE in the obtuse marginal branch, and an 8F giant-lumen guide.

Frank Litvack, MD, USA: Conventional PTCA alone will yield an excellent angiographic and clinical result, using a single guidewire in the main marginal branch, and any 3.5 mm balloon.

Timothy Sanborn, MD, USA: I would treat the proximal LCX lesion with conventional PTCA using a single wire technique. I would use a Voda guide, a 0.014-inch Hi-torque floppy guidewire, and a 3.5/3.0 mm tapered balloon to decrease the risk of dissection in the distal vessel.

Richard Schatz, MD, USA: PTCA alone is not a great alternative due to the high likelihood of spasm, recoil, and restenosis.

> **Editors' Perspective: PTCA is readily accomplished; there are no features of the target vessel or lesion that preclude safe PTCA. Adjunctive stenting is reasonable if the result is suboptimal.**

*****

PTCA: BIFURCATION LESION

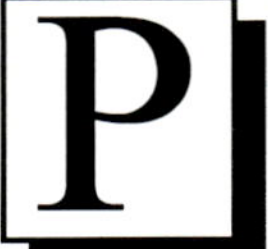TCA of a bifurcation lesion in the distal RCA (reference diameters: RCA = 3.6 mm; PDA= 2.7 mm; PLV = 2.2 mm).

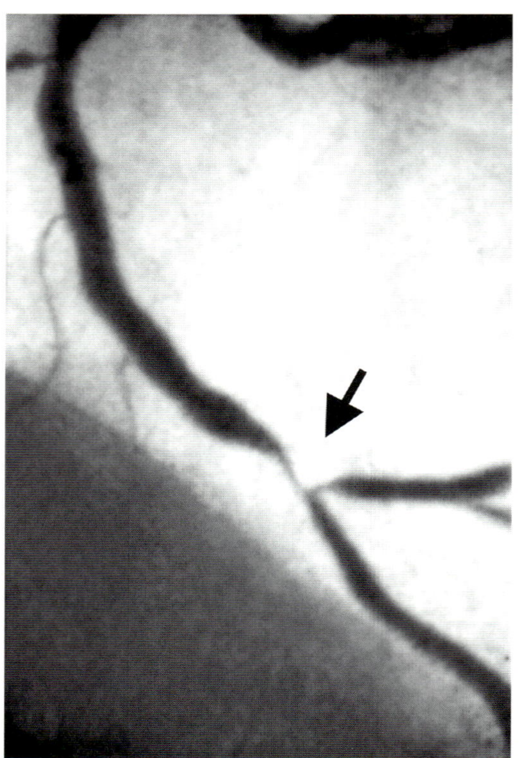

Is PTCA alone reasonable alternative for this lesion?

David Holmes, MD, USA: I do not think that PTCA is reasonable because of the potential for sidebranch occlusion, even using a double-balloon, double-wire technique.

Donald Baim, MD, USA: I do not believe that conventional PTCA would yield satisfactory results as a primary modality, because of shifting plaque and dissection.

William O'Neill, MD, USA: If PTCA is done, I would place two 2.0 x 40 mm balloons across each branch and do "kissing" balloon inflations. The risk of PTCA is increased in this case.

Patrick Whitlow, MD, USA: PTCA is certainly reasonable. The combination of a Probe and an over-the-wire balloon works quite nicely for this approach. I would use one wire in the AV continuation of the RCA and a 2.25 mm balloon inflated at low pressure. I would pull the balloon back into the guiding catheter and advance a 3.0 mm Probe into the PDA. I would reposition the 2.25 mm balloon in the distal RCA so the tip of the balloon is just in the AV continuation. I would inflate both balloons simultaneously (kissing balloons). This approach is effective when the proximal lesion is in a large artery, and each bifurcation vessel is considerably smaller.

Michael Cowley, MD, USA: PTCA alone is not an appropriate choice for a bifurcation lesion of this type, because of the high likelihood of an unsatisfactory result.

Nicolaus Reifart, MD, Germany: I recommend PTCA with a 0.014-inch ACS Traverse in the posterolateral branch (more difficult to wire), a 0.014-inch floppy wire in the PDA, and a 2.5 x 20 mm Europass to dilate each branch sequentially. If the result is unsatisfactory, I would perform kissing balloon inflations with another 2.5 x 20 mm Europass.

John Bittl, MD, USA: The treatment of choice is "kissing" balloon angioplasty with a 3.0 mm Edge in the PDA, a 2.0 mm ACE in the posterior left ventricular branch, and an 8F giant-lumen guide.

Frank Litvack, MD, USA: I recommend conventional PTCA with a double-wire technique, and sequential PTCA of the posterolateral branch and PDA. Unfortunately, branch point lesions tend to have a lot of recoil, and PTCA may not yield an adequate result.

Timothy Sanborn, MD, USA: The distal RCA lesion involves the posterolateral branch and is best treated with double-wire, sequential PTCA, or the "kissing balloon" technique, if necessary.

Ulrich Sigwart, MD, England: My preference is to place Extra-Support wires in the PLV branch and PDA, and do kissing balloon inflations with two 2.0 mm balloons.

Editors' Perspective: **Conventional PTCA has been performed for many years on this type of bifurcation lesion, and the advantages, disadvantages, and limitations of PTCA are well known. Although atherectomy, laser, and stent devices can be used to treat bifurcation lesions, these procedures are technically demanding and may not provide better results than conventional PTCA. To achieve the best results and minimize complications, a kissing balloon approach is recommended. Contemporary 8F guiding catheters (internal diameter ≥ 0.084 inches) can accommodate a variety of fixed wire-balloon catheters and low-profile over-the-wire or monorail systems.**

*****

— Section 3 —

Ischemic Syndromes

ANTERIOR MI: PRIMARY PTCA

A 50-year-old Democratic congressman presents with an acute anterior myocardial infarction of 4 hours duration, which began immediately after learning that his new nextdoor neighbor is Rush Limbaugh. Angiography reveals total occlusion of the LAD (reference diameter = 3.2 mm). No other significant disease is present, and the patient is hemodynamically stable.

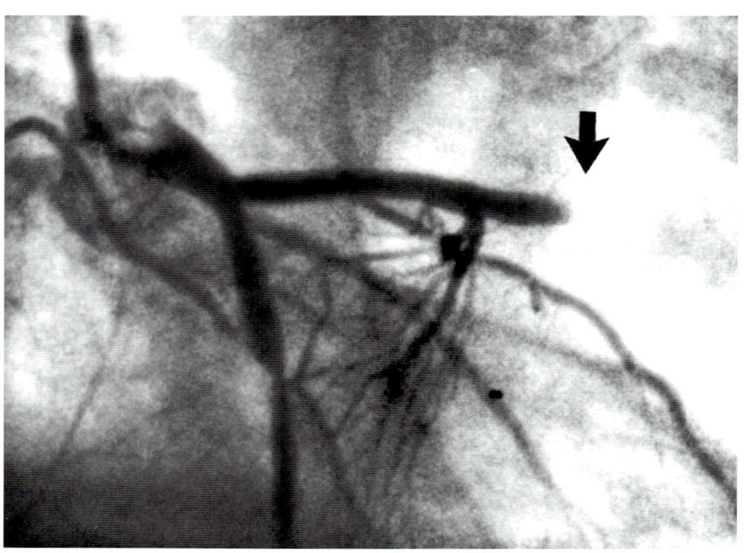

Is reperfusion therapy indicated?

Cindy Grines, MD, USA: This case demonstrates total occlusion of the mid-LAD. The patient clearly has indications for reperfusion therapy, given the fact that he has a large infarction of short duration.

David Williams, MD, USA: The mid-LAD is occluded. Of importance, there is some tapering of the LAD just proximal to the total occlusion. This patient is already in the catheterization laboratory, instrumented, and the pathology has been well demonstrated. It is appropriate to proceed with PTCA; the goal being to establish perfusion to the region of infarction. Typically a lesion like this should respond nicely to PTCA with a success rate of 90%. Delivering a wire and balloon to the lesion should be simple and straightforward. The tapering of the lesion suggests that a relatively small amount of thrombus is located at the target site. Although flow may be restored to the anterior wall, the patient may or may not experience any clinical improvement. It is common to see little change in ST segments or left ventricular function 4 hours into infarction. Had the patient been experiencing ongoing chest pain, I would expect to observe relief of symptoms.

Describe your technical approach.

Cindy Grines, MD, USA: I would use an 8F JL4 guiding catheter, and start with an 0.014-inch Hi-torque floppy wire and a 3.0 mm compliant balloon. If the lesion could not be easily crossed with a Hi-torque floppy wire, I would exchange for a Hyperflex or Reflex wire. After crossing the occlusion with the wire, I would wait a minute to see if the patient develops reperfusion arrhythmias. After a minute or so, I would cross the lesion with the balloon. I would inflate it to nominal pressure for 2-3 minutes, deflate the balloon, and obtain a repeat angiogram. If the result is suboptimal due to dissection or residual stenosis > 30%, recurrent ischemia is likely and stenting should be performed.

David Williams, MD, USA: I would perform PTCA with a 3.0 mm balloon, since it is likely that the mid-LAD beyond the lesion is smaller than the proximal LAD. (It is also possible that a large diagonal branch may arise shortly after this occlusion, which would result in a smaller mid-LAD.) I would start with a 0.014-inch Hi-torque floppy wire, which should readily cross the lesion, and then "dotter" the lesion with the balloon catheter. Next, I would inject contrast to ensure that the wire is in the proper location, and to assess the amount of thrombus distal to the occlusion. After this assessment, I would dilate for 3-5 minutes. If the lesion recurs despite prolonged inflations, I would deploy a Palmaz-Schatz stent.

Eric Topol, MD, USA: I would perform PTCA on the mid-LAD with a 3.0 mm balloon.

What problems do you anticipate?

Cindy Grines, MD, USA: Clinical experience and animal studies suggest that slow reperfusion will prevent reperfusion arrhythmias, which are commonly observed in this setting.

David Williams, MD, USA: Several complications can occur in association with intracoronary thrombus. In the presence of total occlusion, it is impossible to judge the extent of thrombus, but in the setting of acute myocardial infarction involving native arteries, the amount of thrombus is usually small. However, if thrombus burden is large, PTCA may result in embolization of collaterals. Second, thrombus can be inadvertently withdrawn into the proximal left coronary artery and cause additional flow impairment. Third, PTCA can result in retrograde dissection. Finally, slow-flow can occur secondary to edema and necrosis, microembolization, or microvascular spasm, but usually responds to intracoronary verapamil (100-900 mcg). The chance of these adverse events is small, and should certainly not preclude PTCA in this patient.

Describe your recommendations for adjunctive medical therapy and radiographic contrast.

Cindy Grines, MD, USA: The patient should receive chewable aspirin (5-10 grains) and ticlopidine (500 mg) in the Emergency Center. I would administer heparin (13,000 units) and maintain the ACT ≥ 350 seconds throughout the procedure. Since patients with unstable angina and acute myocardial infarction tend to be refractory to heparin, I would recheck the ACT every 20-30 minutes. I would use ionic contrast (high or low osmolar) and avoid nonionic contrast, due to the increased risk of thromboembolic complications. I would also use beta-blockers, but not calcium-blockers, dextran, or lidocaine.

David Williams, MD, USA: I would use low-osmolar ionic contrast (Hexabrix), because of its favorable hemodynamic profile and reduced likelihood of stimulating thrombus formation. I would not administer intracoronary or intravenous thrombolytic agents unless refractory thrombus was observed. ReoPro may be useful to decrease the risk of abrupt closure and reinfarction.

Eric Topol, MD, USA: ReoPro may have value during primary PTCA for acute MI; the results of the RAPPORT trial are pending.

Editors' Perspective: Primary PTCA for acute myocardial infarction is common practice for most interventional cardiologists. Advantages of primary PTCA over intravenous lytic therapy include improved survival in high-risk patients, higher

immediate vessel patency and less reocclusion, less recurrent ischemia and reinfarction, immediate definition coronary anatomy, early risk stratification, application to lytic-ineligible patients, reduced risk of myocardial rupture and intracranial hemorrhage, lower cost, and shorter hospital stay. Potential disadvantages of primary PTCA include the need for a skilled interventional cardiologist and ancillary staff, and logistical delays in mobilizing the cath lab. The results of primary PTCA are excellent, with acute patency of the infarct vessel in 83-97% and in-hospital mortality in 1.5-9.3% (Table 37). Nevertheless, these patients remain at risk for complications related to PTCA (dissection, abrupt closure, emergency bypass surgery, distal embolization, no-reflow, thrombotic occlusion) and myocardial infarction itself (heart failure, cardiogenic shock, mechanical complications, arrhythmia, death). Dr. Grines and Dr. Williams point out a number of technical considerations that may improve outcome during primary PTCA: First, nonionic contrast should not be used routinely in this setting because of its prothrombotic potential. Ionic contrast is recommended, and the ionic low osmolar

Table 37. Primary PTCA: Results of Nonrandomized Studies

		In-hospital Outcome (%)		
	N	Patency	Mortality	Reocclusion
Stone[23]	47	86	6.3	13
O'Keefe[12]	1000	94	7.7	13
Nakagawa[15]	190	90	4	-
O'Neill[4]	63	92	6.3	-
Brodie[13]	383	91	9	-
Beauchamp[14]	214	92	7.9	-
Rothbaum[16]	151	87	9	9
Miller[17]	127	92	8.6	8
Dageford[18]	65	97	1.5	9
Marco[20]	43	95	9.3	-
Kimura[19]	58	88	-	2
O'Neill[21]	29	83	6.8	8
Pooled Results	**2370**	**93**	**7.4**	**10**

agent Hexabrix may be especially useful in patients with hemodynamic dysfunction. Second, although crossing the occlusion with a guidewire is usually accomplished with little difficulty, "rapid" reperfusion may increase the chance of reperfusion arrhythmias, particularly in the RCA. Waiting a minute or so after crossing with the wire before inflating the balloon may attenuate reperfusion arrhythmias. Third, if the infarct vessel is occluded so that the distal vessel cannot be sized, it is reasonable to reestablish some antegrade flow before sizing the balloon for definitive lumen enlargement, either by using a small (2.0 mm) balloon to "predilate" the occlusion, or a deflated balloon or transfer catheter to "dotter" the occlusion. Failure to accurately size the vessel distal to the occlusion and confirm that the guidewire is in the main vessel (and not a small branch) can result in advertent dissection and/or perforation. Fourth, all patients must receive aspirin and heparin before intervention, and careful monitoring of the ACT throughout the case, since patients with acute myocardial infarction may be resistant to heparin.

*****

If, in addition to total occlusion of the LAD, this acute anterior MI patient also had high-grade lesions in the LCX and RCA, but was hemodynamically stable at the time of presentation, would you recommend immediate PTCA of the LAD or CABG?

Cindy Grines, MD, USA: During acute myocardial infarction, PTCA is performed only on the infarct-related artery.

David Williams, MD, USA: The primary role of PTCA in this setting is to achieve reperfusion to the zone of infarction, not to dilate other vessels.

If the high-grade lesions in the LCX and RCA were amenable to PTCA, would you recommend immediate- or staged-intervention on these other vessels?

Cindy Grines, MD, USA: Multivessel PTCA has been performed in patients with profound cardiogenic shock as a last ditch effort, but is not recommended in other cases of acute myocardial infarction, and may be harmful. I would stage PTCA depending on the severity and location of the other lesions.

David Williams, MD, USA: If the patient has high-grade lesions in two other vessels, I would certainly not try to revascularize those vessels at this time. Should additional revascularization be required, the procedure is much safer once the patient has stabilized after infarction.

Eric Topol, MD, USA: Further intervention would be staged at some point after the initial hospitalization. Ideally, these lesions can be confronted if reversible ischemia is objectively defined 3-6 weeks after acute myocardial infarction.

What factors influence your judgement about the timing of staged intervention?

Cindy Grines, MD, USA: The timing of intervention depends on the presence, severity, and timing of recurrent ischemia. If unstable ischemia occurs during the hospital stay, the staged procedure should be performed early. If there are no signs of ischemia, I would stage PTCA at one month.

What factors influence your choice of PTCA or CABG for the LCX and RCA?

Cindy Grines, MD, USA: If the lesions are very proximal and severe, I would consider bypass surgery in 1-2 weeks. If the lesions are mid or distal, I would consider staged PTCA in 2-4 weeks. Regardless of the type of revascularization, I would expect the anterior wall to have limited recovery, especially since reperfusion occurred during the fifth hour.

David Williams, MD, USA: The choice between bypass surgery and PTCA depends on characteristics of the lesions and the status of the left ventricle. If PTCA does not salvage myocardium and the patient has a large area of anterior akinesis and a low ejection fraction, I favor bypass surgery, since patients with 3-vessel disease and impaired left ventricular function have better survival following bypass surgery, but not following PTCA.

If this patient has 3-vessel disease and cardiogenic shock, what would you recommend?

Cindy Grines, MD, USA: Patients with 3-vessel disease and cardiogenic shock have a very poor prognosis. I would quickly place an intraaortic balloon pump, and perform PTCA on the occluded LAD. Following reperfusion, I would perform left ventriculography (unless the pulmonary capillary wedge pressure is ≥ 30 mmHg) to identify mechanical defects, which can be easily missed or underestimated by echocardiography. I would then convince the surgeons to take the patient for emergency revascularization.

David Williams, MD, USA: If the patient is in cardiogenic shock, I would initially place an intraaortic balloon pump, intubate the patient, and initiate assisted ventilation and appropriate pharmacologic therapy. I would then proceed with PTCA of the LAD.

Eric Topol, MD, USA: PTCA of the LAD is still indicated. If bypass surgery can be done very quickly, it could be considered. For a young patient with cardiogenic shock, an intraaortic balloon pump with reperfusion of the infarct vessel would be a good start, and bypass surgery could still be considered, if necessary.

Editors' Perspective: The ideal approach to acute myocardial infarction in patients with left ventricular dysfunction and multivessel disease is unknown. In most centers (including our own), emergency bypass surgery is not considered primary therapy because of the delays in mobilizing the operating room and ancillary staff, uncertainties about the viability of myocardium in the infarct zone, and excellent results of PTCA. Although multivessel PTCA is safe and feasible in highly selected patients with acute myocardial infarction, most operators prefer to initially treat the culprit vessel (to reestablish normal blood flow and salvage myocardium in the infarct zone) and stage further interventions 2-8 weeks later, depending on the clinical setting. Acute multivessel revascularization should be considered when severe hemodynamic instability and ongoing ischemia persist despite successful PTCA of the infarct-related artery.

*****

ANTERIOR MI: SUBOPTIMAL PTCA

PTCA is performed for acute anterior myocardial infarction and the angiogram reveals a residual stenosis < 30%, TIMI-2 flow, and mild haziness. The patient's chest pain, which was 8 out of 10 on presentation, is now 3 out of 10.

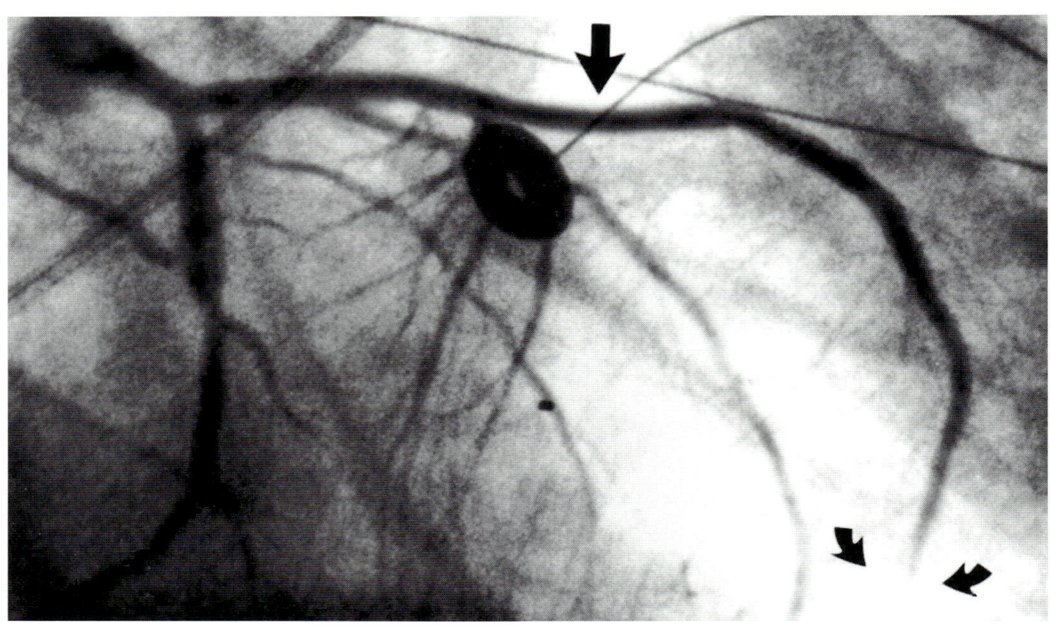

How do you explain persistent flow impairment and mild residual stenosis?

David Williams, MD, USA: The angiogram shows an excellent result at the site of initial occlusion, but there is cutoff of the distal LAD, suggesting embolization of a large amount of thrombus. Although the patient has experienced clinical improvement, the effectiveness of the procedure has been limited by distal embolization.

Eric Topol, MD, USA: The residual stenosis < 30% and TIMI-2 flow can be explained by embolization to the distal LAD.

How would you manage this patient now?

Cindy Grines, MD, USA: I would give intracoronary nitroglycerin and verapamil (in an attempt to increase flow), recheck the ACT to make sure it is > 350 seconds, and obtain several angiographic views to make sure that the lesion has been adequately dilated. For residual stenosis > 30% or dissection, additional balloon inflations or upsizing is indicated. It is not unusual to see persistent ST elevation and mild lingering chest pain following primary PTCA for acute MI, even with excellent results.

David Williams, MD, USA: I would advance the floppy wire through the new obstruction into the distal LAD, and then simply "dotter" the lesion with the balloon catheter. This may result in complete dislodgment of the obstructive thrombus, precluding the need for additional balloon inflations. It will also allow visualization of the distal vessel for optimal balloon sizing in the event PTCA is required. Should thrombotic occlusion recur at that site, I would administer intracoronary urokinase (500,000 units over 30 minutes) or intracoronary tPA (20 mg bolus, followed by a 40-60 mg intravenous infusion). ReoPro may decrease the risk of thrombosis.

Eric Topol, MD, USA: If there is evidence of thrombus, bolus (0.25 mg/Kg) and infusion (10 mcg/min for 12 hours) of ReoPro is appropriate. Heparin should be given as a bolus (70 units/Kg) to achieve an ACT of 250 seconds. Additional heparin is not necessary, and sheaths should be removed as soon as possible.

Do you recommend insertion of an IABP?

Cindy Grines, MD, USA: I do not believe that there is a definite need for an intraaortic balloon pump if the patient is hemodynamically stable. In the PAMI studies, TIMI-2 flow was not predictive of reocclusion, and although a prophylactic balloon pump did alleviate chest pain, it did not prevent reocclusion.

Eric Topol, MD, USA: An intraaortic balloon pump is indicated only if there is hemodynamic instability or a suboptimal result after repeat inflations.

Would you restudy the patient?

Cindy Grines, MD, USA: Followup angiography is not routinely performed in patients who have an acceptable result.

Eric Topol, MD, USA: Repeat angiography is not indicated unless the patient has recurrent ischemia or reinfarction.

Editors' Perspective: Persistent flow impairment after primary PTCA for acute myocardial infarction may be due to residual stenosis, dissection, thrombus or spasm at the original target lesion, and should be evaluated in multiple angiographic projections. Even if a residual stenosis is not identified, contrast "pooling" in the target lesion suggests the presence of dissection and/or thrombus. Prolonged balloon inflations (with or without a perfusion balloon) are recommended if such a finding is present; stenting (and rarely directional atherectomy) may be employed if necessary. If thorough angiographic evaluation of the target lesion fails to identify an explanation for impaired flow, angioscopy (to identify residual plaque, dissection, or thrombus) and IVUS (to identify residual plaque or dissection) should be considered. Other possible explanations for impaired flow despite minimal residual stenosis include distal embolization of thrombus and no-reflow. Distal embolization is usually due to thromboembolism of an epicardial vessel, and is identified angiographically as abrupt vessel cutoff. In most cases, the embolus can be disrupted by guidewire manipulation, "dottering" with a deflated balloon or transfer catheter, or local delivery of thrombolytic therapy. No-reflow is usually due to microvascular thromboembolism and/or spasm, and is identified angiographically as a stagnant column of contrast in the absence of dissection, thrombus, spasm, residual stenosis, or distal embolization to an epicardial vessel. Treatment options for no-reflow include intracoronary calcium channel blockers and/or adenosine.

*****

POSTERIOR MI

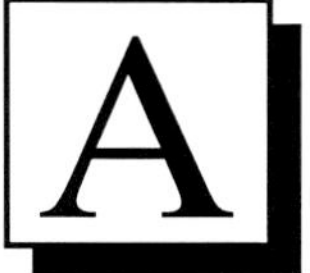

A 63-year-old cardiologist is 4 hours into an acute posterolateral myocardial infarction. Angiography shows an ulcerated 80% stenosis in the proximal LCX (reference diameter = 3.2 mm) with TIMI-3 flow. Other coronary arteries are normal and the patient is hemodynamically stable.

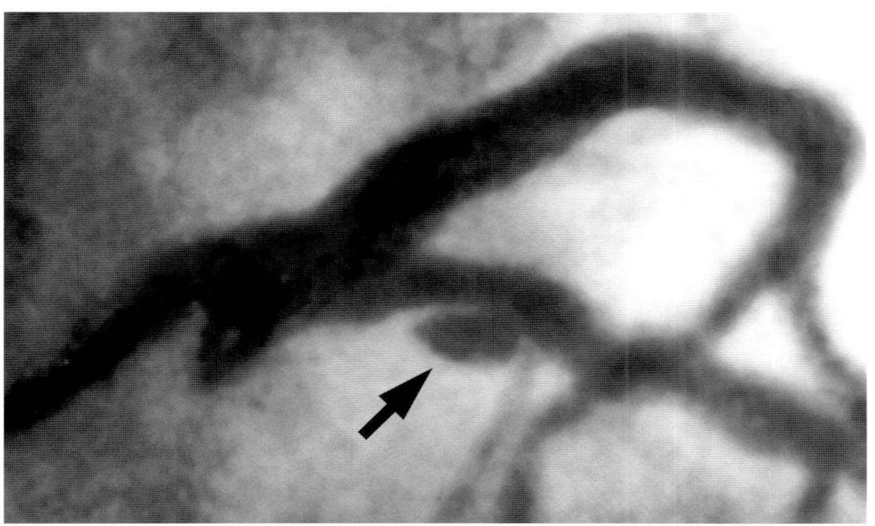

During the angiogram, chest pain and ST elevation resolve. How would you manage this patient?

Cindy Grines, MD, USA: I would administer chewable aspirin, ticlopidine, high-dose intravenous heparin, and beta blockers. Due to the ruptured plaque lesion morphology, this vessel may clean up substantially and leave a borderline residual stenosis.

David Williams, MD, USA: This case is quite unusual. The patient has experienced spontaneous improvement, and although reperfusion is common after thrombolytic therapy, it is uncommon in the absence of lytic therapy or heparin. One potential mechanism of infarction in this patient is that the site of ulceration is not the site of infarction. Thrombus may have originated in the ulcerated segment and embolized to the distal circulation. It is possible that the ulcerated lesion contains more thrombus than is evident from the angiogram. Accordingly, thrombolytic therapy and heparin are most appropriate to "clean up" the culprit segment.

Eric Topol, MD, USA: With TIMI-3 flow, there is no indication for PTCA. The 80% lesion in the proximal LCX can be treated 5-7 days later. When the lesion is dilated, bolus and infusion of ReoPro should be administered to reduce the risk of abrupt thrombotic closure. Stenting is reasonable if there is a suboptimal result after PTCA; I would use a 3.0 mm Palmaz-Schatz stent and postdilate with a 3.25 mm noncompliant balloon at high pressure.

During the angiogram, chest pain resolves completely, but ST elevation persists. How would you manage this patient?

Cindy Grines, MD, USA: I would treat the patient conservatively, as above. It is not unusual to see persistent ST elevation after reperfusion therapy. Since the patient is completely free of pain and has TIMI-3 flow, I would not perform PTCA now.

David Williams, MD, USA: ST elevation is a poor indicator of reperfusion, and many patients achieve TIMI-3 flow but have persistent ST elevation. Clinical outcome correlates with achieving TIMI-3 flow, not relief of ST elevation. ST segment elevation should not be a trigger for mechanical intervention, especially if TIMI-3 flow has already been achieved.

During the angiogram, ST elevation resolves, but chest pain persists. How would you manage this patient?

Cindy Grines, MD, USA: Continued chest pain makes me worry that a high-grade stenosis persists, causing ongoing ischemia. I would perform PTCA with prolonged inflations using a 3.5 mm balloon at 2 ATM. I expect the result to look hazy. Stenting is indicated if there is a flow-limiting dissection or residual ulceration. For PTCA in this setting, I use ionic contrast and maintain the ACT > 350 seconds throughout the procedure.

David Williams, MD, USA: If chest pain persists but ST elevation resolves, I would consider other explanations for persistent chest pain if TIMI flow is normal. Certainly, pericarditis should be considered. Another possible cause is distal embolization. Again, chest pain with TIMI-3 flow should not trigger mechanical intervention.

Editors' Perspective: This case illustrates one of several management dilemmas when treating patients with acute myocardial infarction, namely, the presence of a high-grade stenosis but normal flow at the time of emergency angiography. In the setting of acute MI and TIMI-3 flow, clinical markers of ongoing ischemia (e.g., chest pain, ST elevation) are not very reliable. Microbubble studies have shown that coronary microvascular flow may be impaired despite TIMI-3 epicardial flow, which may explain some cases of persistent chest pain and/or ECG changes following "successful" PTCA. In the present case, since the goal of normal antegrade flow has already been achieved before PTCA (heparin alone can restore patency in 10-20% of lesions), the risk of delayed reocclusion must be weighed against the risk of immediate PTCA. In the absence of published data, it may be reasonable to treat the patient with aspirin and heparin, and defer intervention for a few days. Bolus plus infusion of ReoPro is reasonable if PTCA is performed at that time.

*****

ACUTE MI: CARDIOGENIC SHOCK

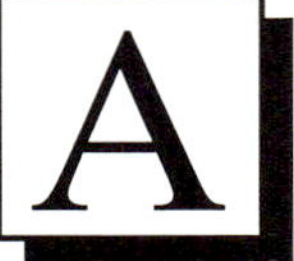

A 50-year-old man presents 1 hour into an extensive anterior myocardial infarction with cardiogenic shock. Angiography reveals subtotal occlusion of the distal left main and a severe stenosis in the RCA.

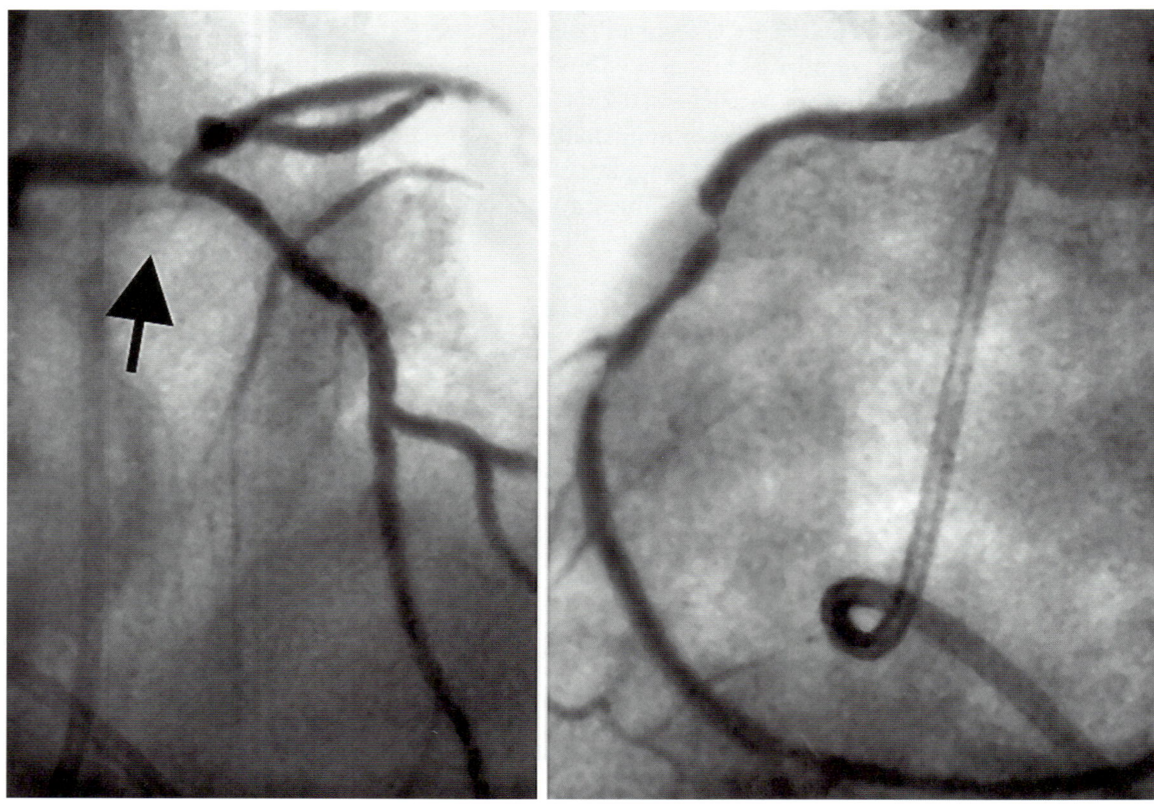

How would you manage this patient?

Cindy Grines, MD, USA: After angiography with Hexabrix, I would insert an intraaortic balloon pump and a Swan-Ganz catheter, and consult our cardiovascular surgeon for immediate bypass surgery.

David Williams, MD, USA: This young man develops extensive myocardial infarction and cardiogenic shock, due to significant stenoses of the distal left main coronary and RCA. The best treatment for this patient is immediate coronary bypass surgery. If an operating room is available, the patient should be taken directly to surgery, where he will be promptly intubated and placed on cardiopulmonary bypass — this is the most effective and quickest way to manage the patient. The patient should not be rejected for emergency bypass surgery. If clinical improvement is required before surgery, the patient should be intubated and supported with intraaortic balloon counterpulsation. Although percutaneous cardiopulmonary bypass may be more effective in improving hemodynamics, this temporizing maneuver takes longer to initiate than intraaortic balloon counterpulsation and does not protect the myocardium.

Eric Topol, MD, USA: The patient should have emergency bypass surgery. Rescue PTCA would only be considered as a temporizing measure in such a complex patient.

The patient is turned down for emergency CABG, but the surgeons will reconsider surgery if the patient improves. An echocardiogram shows extensive anterolateral wall motion abnormalities, moderate MR, and EF = 25%. How would you proceed at this point?

Cindy Grines, MD, USA: If death was imminent (persistent shock despite intra-aortic balloon pump, vasopressors and intubation), I would perform PTCA of the left main coronary artery. I would also position a wire in the LCX in case of abrupt closure, and use a kissing balloon technique, if possible. I would use Hexabrix and ReoPro, limit the number of contrast injections, use brief balloon inflations, and maintain the ACT ≥ 350 seconds. I would avoid intracoronary thrombolytics. In the absence of persistent shock and imminent death, I would send the patient to the Coronary Care Unit on high-dose heparin.

David Williams, MD, USA: It is likely that the left main stenosis is responsible for the infarction. Fortunately, flow has been reestablished so it is not essential to attempt intervention at this time. Should the patient deteriorate or reocclude the left main, then every effort should be made to restore flow with PTCA and possibly stenting.

Eric Topol, MD, USA: If surgery is not available, PTCA and stenting could be used as a temporizing measure.

You perform PTCA on the distal left main and reduce the stenosis to 30%. Hemodynamic performance improves and the patient is stable. What do you recommend now? If you send the patient to surgery, are you concerned about competitive flow adversely affecting graft patency?

Cindy Grines, MD, USA: If the patient stabilizes, I would push the surgeons to perform bypass surgery. This young man obviously does not tolerate partial left main occlusion. The left main and ostial LAD are at extremely high risk for restenosis. In addition, 10-13% of infarct vessels reocclude after primary PTCA, and an additional 40% develop restenosis within 6 months. If I send the patient to surgery, competitive flow may be an issue. However, I would leave it to the surgeons to determine the appropriate course of action. Generally, they would place vein grafts to provide greater flow.

David Williams, MD, USA: PTCA of the left main results in luminal enlargement and clinical improvement. The patient should still have coronary bypass surgery since abrupt closure or restenosis could be fatal. I am not concerned about the lesion potentially affecting the longevity of the bypass graft; this is a small theoretical issue.

Eric Topol, MD, USA: Even though PTCA is successful, coronary artery bypass surgery should still be performed.

> **Editors' Perspective: In-hospital survival for cardiogenic shock is 10% when treated medically, 30% after thrombolytic therapy, and 40-80% after successful PTCA. In the present case of severe left main stenosis causing acute myocardial infarction and cardiogenic shock, acute revascularization is the only hope for extended survival. Since some of these patients may be denied surgical intervention, percutaneous therapy may be required. In our opinion, stents offer the best option, since stenting offers the most reliable and predictable result. Coil stents offer the theoretical advantages of preserved access to the LCX if the stent is placed in the LAD (and vice versa). If stenting is**

considered, the ideal anticoagulation regimen is unknown. Given the potentially fatal consequences of stent thrombosis, reasonable (but unproven) pharmacologic adjuncts include ReoPro (during and after the procedure) and subcutaneous heparin (for 2 weeks), in addition to aspirin and ticlopidine. This patient was successfully treated with PTCA and stenting of the distal left main and LAD using 2 overlapping Palmaz-Schatz stents. Recurrent chest pain developed several days later and was managed with PTCA of the RCA using a 2.5 x 40 mm balloon (below). The patient remains asymptomatic, now 2 years after intervention.

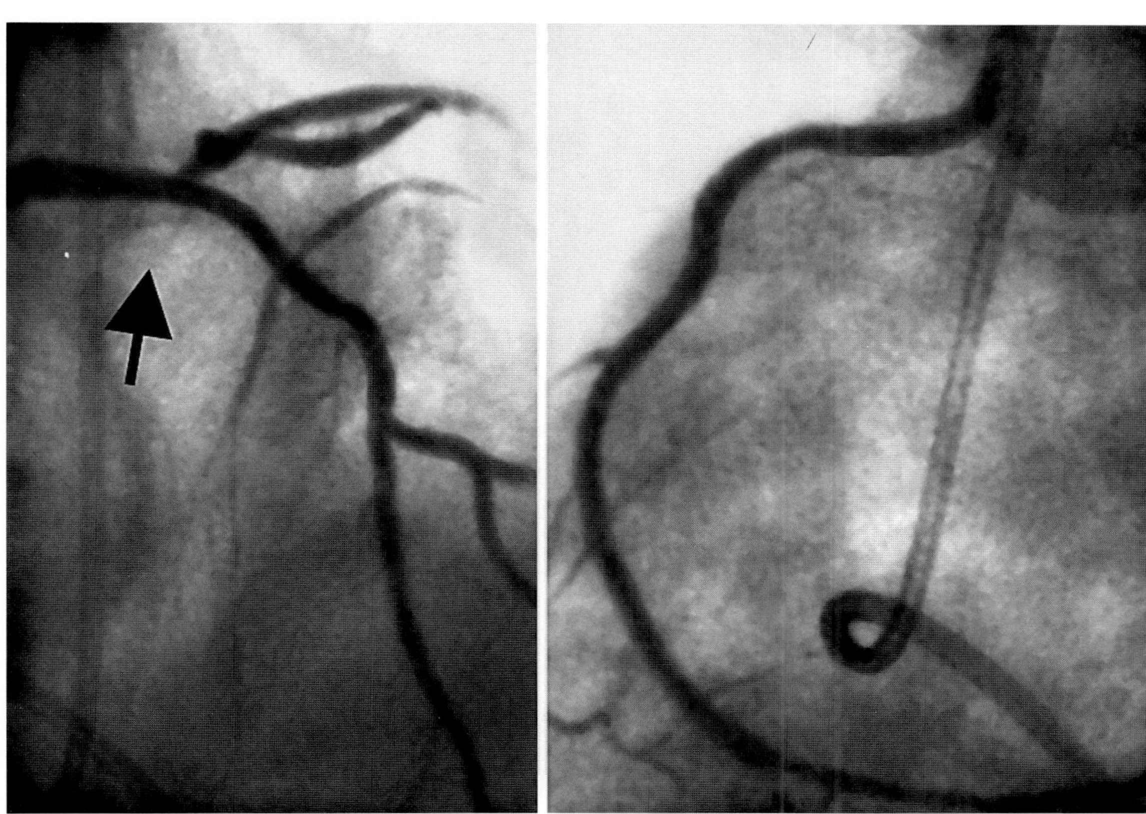

*****

ACUTE MI: RESCUE PTCA

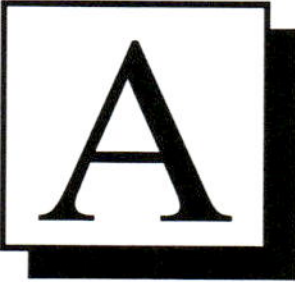
67-year-old woman presents to an outside hospital within 3 hours of acute inferior myocardial infarction. Front-loaded tPA is given and the patient is transported to your center.

How would you manage the patient if she is hemodynamically stable and chest pain and ST elevation have resolved 90 minutes after thrombolytic therapy?

Cindy Grines, MD, USA: I would make sure that chewable aspirin and heparin have been administered. If chest pain and ST elevation resolve, I would admit the patient to the Coronary Care Unit and treat her medically. In the absence of recurrent ischemia or hemodynamic problems, she falls into a low risk category. Routine catheterization or exercise testing may be performed in this patient, but due to her low risk it is unlikely that either will have a substantial impact on her prognosis.

David Williams, MD, USA: Since the patient is clinically improved after thrombolytic therapy, there is no need for catheterization or intervention at this time.

Eric Topol, MD, USA: If chest pain and ST-segment elevation completely resolve, the patient should not undergo emergency coronary angiography.

How would you manage the patient if she is hemodynamically stable but chest pain and ST elevation are present 90 minutes after thrombolytic therapy?

Cindy Grines, MD, USA: Since chest pain and ST-elevation persist in a patient with myocardial infarction < 12 hours duration, I would perform emergency PTCA of the infarct-related vessel. I would reperfuse the vessel slowly with the wire, since rescue PTCA of the RCA is associated with a higher incidence of reperfusion arrhythmias.

David Williams, MD, USA: Despite thrombolytic therapy, the patient continues to have chest pain and ST elevation. In this situation it is likely that reperfusion has not occurred, although chest pain and ST elevation are more predictive of failed reperfusion if each had improved and then recurred. In this situation, catheterization and PTCA are appropriate. However, the results of PTCA after failed thrombolytic therapy are not as good as the results of primary PTCA. The reasons for this are not clear but may relate to the selection of patients with refractory thrombosis. If this patient had initially responded to lytics but chest pain and ST elevation recurred, then repeat treatment with thrombolytics would be a legitimate option; in this situation, a single dose of intravenous tPA (20 mg) has a 50 percent chance of causing immediate and sustained relief.

Eric Topol, MD, USA: Chest pain and ST-elevation are still present, so angiography should be performed.

How would you manage the patient if she is hemodynamically stable and chest pain has resolved, but ST segments remain elevated 90 minutes after thrombolytic therapy?

Cindy Grines, MD, USA: Patients with persistent ST elevation and resolution of chest pain present a diagnostic and therapeutic dilemma. It is uncertain whether reperfusion has occurred. I recommend immediate angiography if she has any other high-risk features, such as tachycardia, heart failure, poor left ventricular function, mitral regurgitation, or right ventricular infarction.

David Williams, MD, USA: Chest pain has resolved but ST segments remain elevated; there is no indication for catheterization.

Eric Topol, MD, USA: Persistent ST-segment elevation in the absence of chest pain 90 minutes after lytic therapy is not an indication for rescue PTCA.

How would you manage the patient if she is hemodynamically stable and chest pain persists but ST elevation has resolved 90 minutes after thrombolytic therapy?

Cindy Grines, MD, USA: Persistent chest pain with resolution of ECG changes also represents a diagnostic and therapeutic dilemma. I would perform emergency angiography to identify a collateralized total or subtotal occlusion.

David Williams, MD, USA: Persistent chest pain in the absence of ECG changes raises the possibility of other etiologies for chest pain, such as pericarditis or aortic dissection. If unexplained severe chest pain persists, catheterization should be strongly considered.

Editors' Perspective: In the setting of acute myocardial infarction and intravenous thrombolytic therapy, clinical markers of reperfusion are relatively unreliable. Since current data suggest that resolution of ischemic chest pain and ECG changes is predictive of successful reperfusion, emergency angiography and PTCA are not indicated. However, if either chest pain or ECG changes persist (and the other resolves), there is less certainty about the patency of the infarct vessel, and emergency angiography can be used to identify persistent occlusion (TIMI flow $\leq$ 2) of the infarct vessel. Available data suggest that rescue PTCA is indicated for failed thrombolytic therapy, with the goal of achieving TIMI-3 flow. Rescue PTCA restores vessel patency in approximately 85% of vessels; however, among these patients, reocclusion occurs in 18% and in-hospital mortality in 10% (compared to 30-40% mortality rates when rescue PTCA is unsuccessful). Compared to patients with persistent occlusion, those with successful rescue PTCA have less heart failure, less shock, and better left ventricular function. If the infarct vessel is patent with TIMI-3 flow, PTCA should be deferred, even if a high-grade residual stenosis is present — routine PTCA fails to improve LV function, and is associated with more transfusions and emergency bypass surgery compared to a more conservative stategy (i.e., PTCA for spontaneous or provokable ischemia).

*****

ACUTE MI: RESCUE PTCA

A 67-year-old woman presents to an outside hospital within 3 hours of acute inferior myocardial infarction. Front-loaded tPA is given and the patient is transported to your center, where coronary angiography is performed for persistent chest pain and ST elevation. The angiogram shows a 90% stenosis in the mid-RCA and TIMI-2 flow (reference vessel diameter = 3.3 mm). No other disease is evident.

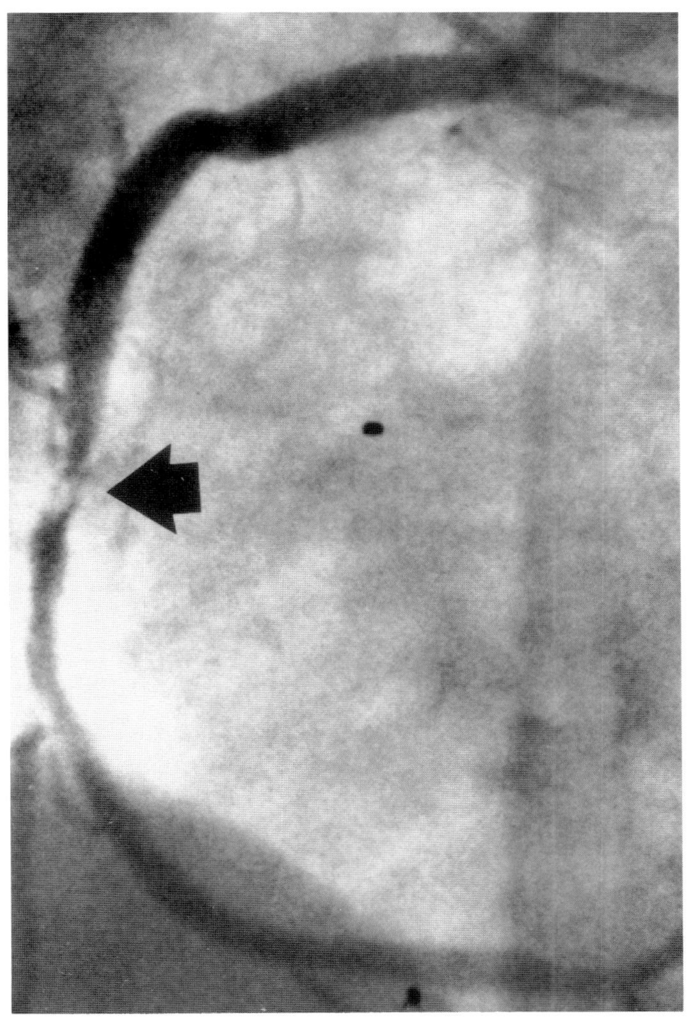

How would you manage this patient?

Cindy Grines, MD, USA: If the patient continues to have chest pain and ECG changes, I would perform PTCA with a 3.5 mm balloon at 2-3 ATM. I would use chewable aspirin, ticlopidine, low-dose intracoronary nitroglycerin, ionic contrast, and maintain the ACT ≥ 350 seconds. I would avoid ReoPro due to the increased risk of intracranial hemorrhage after recent thrombolytic therapy.

David Williams, MD, USA: The patient has TIMI-2 flow with a complex irregular lesion in the RCA. This lesion was the site of total occlusion and partial lysis has occurred. I would perform PTCA with a 3.0 mm balloon, and use a larger balloon if necessary. The objectives of PTCA in this setting are to relieve chest pain and ST elevation, and to restore TIMI-3 flow. ReoPro may be useful in this setting.

Eric Topol, MD, USA: Persistent chest pain and ST elevation justify a decision to perform emergency cardiac catheterization and PTCA. The data for ReoPro after thrombolysis are quite sparse; at this time, I do not recommend it. Ultimately, it is highly likely that a stent will be required in this complex lesion if the result is suboptimal.

How would you manage this patient if chest pain and ST elevation resolve during angiography?

Cindy Grines, MD, USA: If chest pain and ST elevation resolve during cardiac catheterization, I would treat the patient medically, given the poor outcome of PTCA immediately after lytic therapy (presumably due to platelet aggregation). However, the APRICOT study demonstrated that 90% stenoses are more likely to reocclude than other lesions, which suggests that severe, nontotal occlusions should also be treated.

David Williams, MD, USA: If chest pain and ST elevation resolve, I would reassess epicardial blood flow. These favorable changes should not occur unless flow improves. I would proceed with PTCA only if TIMI flow remains ≤ 2.

How would your approach differ if chest pain and ST elevation resolve and TIMI-3 flow is present?

Cindy Grines, MD, USA: If the patient has TIMI-3 flow during the diagnostic angiogram, I would not perform PTCA. However, it is difficult to correlate TIMI flow with the risk of reocclusion.

David Williams, MD, USA: If the patient improves clinically and flow improves to TIMI-3, there is no justification for PTCA.

> **Editors' Perspective: If chest pain and ECG changes persist despite lytic therapy, emergency angiography is indicated. Angiographic findings of impaired flow and high-grade residual stenosis justify percutaneous intervention. If the results of PTCA are suboptimal, stenting should be performed. In the setting of acute MI and a high-grade residual stenosis, the temptation to perform an acute intervention ("oculostenotic reflex") after lytic therapy should be resisted when normal (TIMI-3) flow is present.**

*****

ACUTE MI: MILD LESION

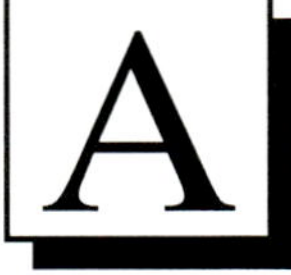

67-year-old woman presents to an outside hospital within 3 hours of acute inferior myocardial infarction. Front-loaded tPA is given and the patient is transported to your center. Coronary angiography reveals a 40% stenosis in the mid-RCA and TIMI-3 flow.

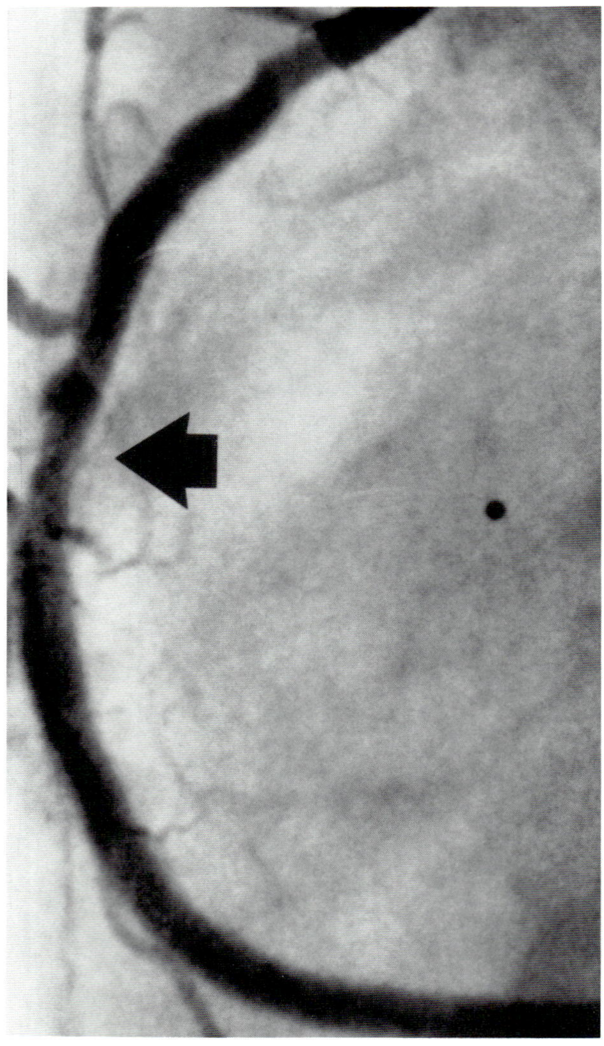

How would you manage this patient if chest pain and ST elevation have resolved?

Cindy Grines, MD, USA: I recommend chewable aspirin and intravenous heparin for 5 days.

David Williams, MD, USA: This patient has a noncritical stenosis of the RCA and brisk flow. I would maintain heparin for at least 24 hours (PTT 50-70 seconds) and daily aspirin.

Eric Topol, MD, USA: If there is TIMI-3 flow, the patient is stable, and there is no evidence for intracoronary thrombus, I would not do anything else at this time.

How would you manage this patient if chest pain persists but ST elevation has resolved?

Cindy Grines, MD, USA: I would administer intracoronary nitroglycerin and intracoronary verapamil, and obtain multiple angiographic projections to be sure that I did not miss a lesion. If the vessel is patent with TIMI-3 flow and there is minimal residual stenosis, persistent pain may be due to pericarditis or myocardial infarction.

David Williams, MD, USA: I would treat the patient with medical therapy, as above.

Eric Topol, MD, USA: I would maintain heparin for at least 24 hours (PTT 50-70 seconds) and daily aspirin.

How would you manage this patient if ST elevation persists but chest pain has resolved?

Cindy Grines, MD, USA: I recommend medical therapy, as above.

David Williams, MD, USA: I recommend medical therapy, as above.

Eric Topol, MD, USA: I would maintain heparin for at least 24 hours (PTT 50-70 seconds) and daily aspirin.

How would you manage this patient if chest pain and ST elevation persist?

Cindy Grines, MD, USA: I am worried about distal embolization, and I would place an intraaortic balloon pump.

David Williams, MD, USA: If chest pain and ST elevation persist, I would look for other causes. It is important to perform left coronary angiography to exclude other lesions, and aortography to exclude aortic dissection. There is no reason to believe that PTCA of the culprit lesion will have any benefit, since a noncritical stenosis is present with normal antegrade flow.

Eric Topol, MD, USA: I would maintain heparin for at least 24 hours (PTT 50-70 seconds) and daily aspirin.

How would you approach differ (if at all) if the angiogram revealed TIMI-2 flow in the RCA?

Cindy Grines, MD, USA: I would use higher doses of nitroglycerin.

David Williams, MD, USA: I would consider IVUS to further evaluate the stenosis. If a significant stenosis is not identified, I favor ReoPro and possibly verapamil to treat small vessel obstruction.

Eric Topol, MD, USA: I would maintain heparin for at least 24 hours (PTT 50-70 seconds) and daily aspirin.

Editors' Perspective: In some instances, emergency angiography after successful thrombolytic therapy reveals normal antegrade flow and only a moderate residual stenosis. In the absence of clinical signs of ischemia, medical therapy is indicated. If clinical signs of ischemia persist, the operator should search for other causes of ischemia, such as distal embolization, and consider causes of non-ischemic chest pain that can mimic ischemia (such as pericarditis or aortic dissection). If the target lesion appears moderate in severity but antegrade flow is impaired, multiple angiographic projections should be performed to evaluate and exclude a persistent severe stenosis. If absent, treatment for no-reflow is indicated, using intracoronary calcium channel antagonists and possibly adenosine.

*****

ACUTE MI: DELAYED PTCA OF TOTAL OCCLUSION

A 51-year-old man has an uneventful recovery after receiving thrombolytic therapy for an acute anterior myocardial infarction. Noninvasive evaluation reveals an akinetic anterior wall and apex, with a left ventricular ejection fraction of 35%. Your partner performs cardiac catheterization on day 6, revealing total occlusion of the LAD (reference diameter = 3.2 mm).

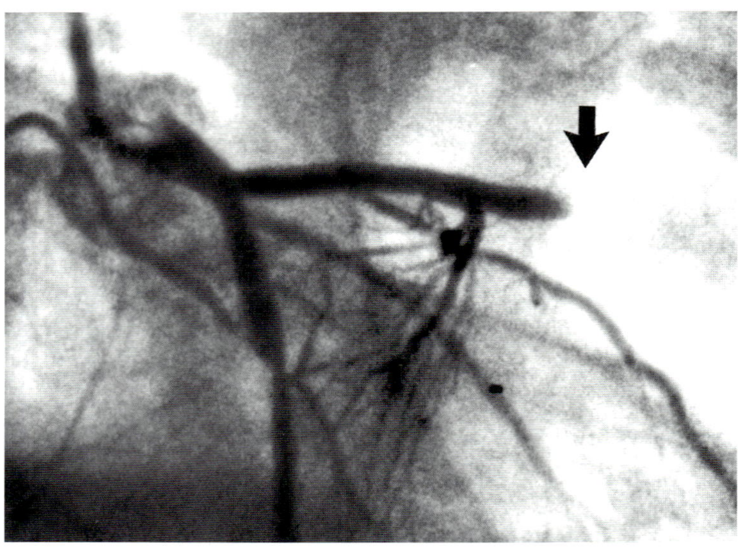

How would you manage this patient if a stress test had not been performed.

Cindy Grines, MD, USA: I would perform PTCA since this is a large LAD in a young patient. The presence of an akinetic anterior wall is extremely common following acute anterior myocardial infarction, and does not necessarily indicate nonviable myocardium; minimal (if any) recovery in regional wall motion is observed during the first week after infarction. I believe that

PTCA is indicated to restore flow, improve long-term healing, reduce aneurysm formation, and prevent ventricular arrhythmia. If the PTCA result is anything but perfect, I recommend stenting.

David Williams, MD, USA: This is a middle-aged male with recent myocardial infarction and total occlusion of the infarct-related vessel on day six. If a stress test had not been performed or failed to show ischemia, there are no strong data to indicate that this artery should be revascularized. Nevertheless, this is a relatively young man and the risks of an untoward event after PTCA are small. Since there may be long-term benefit after achieving a "patent infarct artery," I would share these thoughts with the patient and recommend PTCA.

Eric Topol, MD, USA: If a stress test had not been performed, PTCA is not indicated.

How would you manage this patient if a stress test fails to show reversible ischemia.

Cindy Grines, MD, USA: Failure to demonstrate reversible ischemia does not necessarily mitigate against PTCA in this situation. Total and subtotal occlusions may require a 24-hour redistribution scan to identify ischemia. I would still perform PTCA.

David Williams, MD, USA: If a stress test fails to show ischemia, there are no strong data to indicate that this artery should be revascularized. Nevertheless, this is a relatively young man and the risks of PTCA are small. I would share these thoughts with the patient and recommend PTCA. If significant lesions are present in the RCA, there is greater justification for revascularization of the LAD.

How would you manage this patient if a stress test demonstrates reversible anterior ischemia.

Cindy Grines, MD, USA: Reversible anterior ischemia is clearly an indication for PTCA and possibly stenting. These patients are at increased risk for abrupt closure and clinical complications. For that reason, I use ionic contrast, maintain the ACT $\geq$ 350 seconds, and continue heparin for 24 hours after PTCA.

David Williams, MD, USA: I recommend PTCA.

Eric Topol, MD, USA: I would perform PTCA and implant a Palmaz-Schatz coronary stent if the result is suboptimal.

Editors' Perspective: Spontaneous or provokable ischemia soon after thrombolytic therapy for acute myocardial infarction is a clear indication for coronary angiography and revascularization. Data are less compelling for intervention when persistent total occlusion is present 1 week after thrombolytic therapy in a patient with a fixed myocardial perfusion defect, or in whom a stress test was not performed. Nevertheless, successful delayed PTCA of a persistent total occlusion may improve left ventricular function and remodeling, and enhance survival. Antegrade flow into the infarct zone may also serve as a source of collaterals for other vessels. Since the risk of PTCA of an occluded vessel is small, and since there may be some derived benefit (particularly in a young patient), some operators recommend delayed PTCA in this setting. Clinical and angiographic factors suggesting viable myocardium in the infarct zone include preservation of R-waves on the ECG, retained wall motion by echo or ventriculography, collaterals to the infarct-related vessel, ischemic chest pain, viability on PET scan, and reversible ischemia by myocardial perfusion imaging.

*****

ACUTE MI: DELAYED PTCA OF SUBTOTAL OCCLUSION

A 51-year-old man has an uneventful recovery after receiving thrombolytic therapy for an acute anterior myocardial infarction. Noninvasive evaluation reveals an akinetic anterior wall and apex, with a left ventricular ejection fraction of 35%. The patient is submitted for cardiac catheterization on day 6, and angiography reveals an 80% stenosis in the LAD with TIMI-3 flow (reference diameter = 3.2 mm).

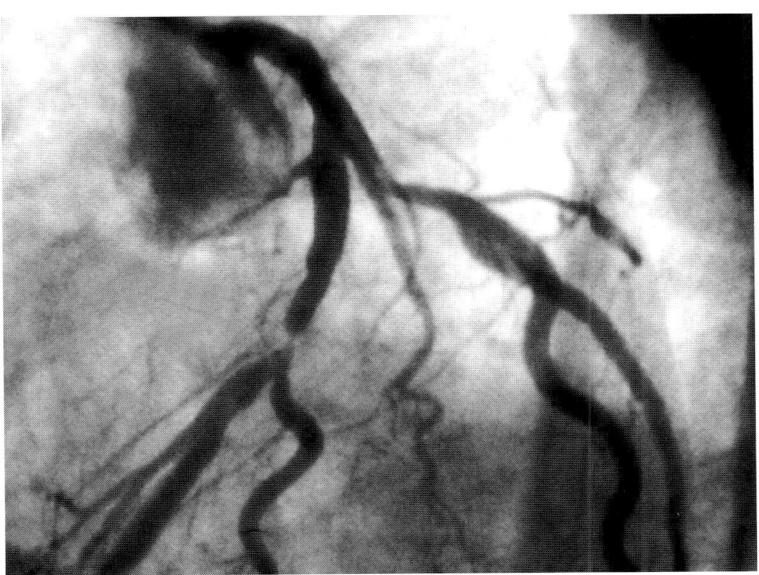

How would you manage this patient if a stress test had not been performed.

Cindy Grines, MD, USA: Based on the severity of the stenosis, I would perform PTCA and possibly stenting (if the diagonal is not involved) to prevent late occlusion. Following thrombolytic therapy, 30-40% of initially patent vessels may reocclude within the first 6 months.

David Williams, MD, USA: This patient has a patent artery with a severe stenosis and TIMI-3 flow. I recommend PTCA since this patient may have achieved some degree of myocardial salvage and has the potential for ischemia.

Eric Topol, MD, USA: If a stress test has not been performed, no intervention would be done.

How would you manage this patient if a stress test fails to show reversible ischemia.

Cindy Grines, MD, USA: If there is no evidence for reversible ischemia, I would obtain a 24 hour redistribution scan.

David Williams, MD, USA: If this artery serves a totally necrotic myocardium, there is no value in performing PTCA.

Eric Topol, MD, USA: If the stress test fails to show reversible ischemia, no intervention would be done.

How would you manage this patient if a stress test demonstrates reversible anterior ischemia.

Cindy Grines, MD, USA: Reversible anterior ischemia is a clear indication for PTCA. I would give ticlopidine, ionic contrast, and maintain the ACT at 350 seconds during the procedure. I would maintain heparin for 24 hours following PTCA, and taper to half-dose heparin for 12 hours before complete discontinuation, to reduce rebound thrombosis. I would not use ReoPro since the lesion is not thrombotic, and I would not protect the diagonal branch with another guidewire.

David Williams, MD, USA: If the stress test is positive, PTCA should be performed.

Eric Topol, MD, USA: If there is reversible anterior ischemia, kissing balloon angioplasty is indicated with a 3.0 mm balloon in the LAD and a 2.5 mm balloon in the diagonal. I would also use ReoPro. Intravascular ultrasound is quite helpful in this case and would be used sequentially in both the LAD and diagonal. Directional atherectomy might be necessary to remove plaque. This is not a good case for stenting.

How would you manage this patient if coronary angiography was performed on day 2 instead of day 6? (The patient has been pain-free since receiving lytic therapy).

Cindy Grines, MD, USA: My management does not differ; I would perform PTCA.

David Williams, MD, USA: If catheterization is performed on day 2, I would defer PTCA, giving thrombolytic and anticoagulant therapy an opportunity to work. I would perform repeat angiography on day 6.

> **Editors' Perspective: The considerations about delayed PTCA of a severely stenotic (but not occluded) lesion are similar to those for an occluded vessel (p. 466).**

*****

CHEST PAIN: SIMPLE LESION

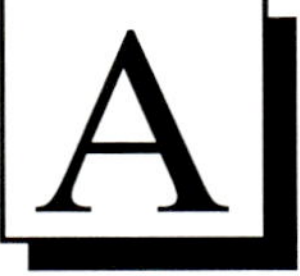

A 51-year-old man develops a chest pain syndrome. The patient is not on any medical therapy except aspirin and has not had a stress test. Another cardiologist performs cardiac catheterization, which shows a severe stenosis in the mid-RCA, and mild disease in the distal RCA (reference diameter = 3.7 mm).

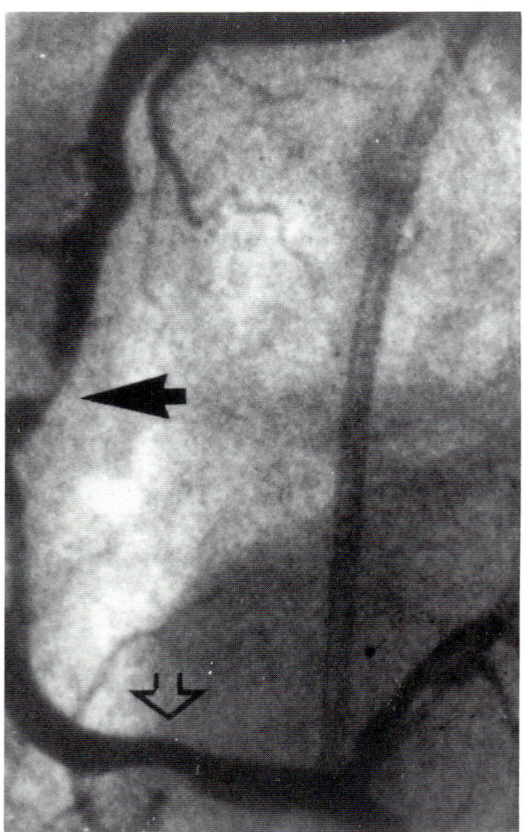

What would you recommend if the patient has atypical chest pain and a normal resting EKG.

Cindy Grines, MD, USA: If the patient has atypical chest pain, I would inform the patient that PTCA may not relieve his chest pain syndrome. However, many patients wish to have the lesion treated once they know they have coronary artery disease. If the patient prefers PTCA, I would perform the procedure.

David Williams, MD, USA: I would certainly expect that a lesion of this severity would have the potential of causing ischemia in an artery of this size and distribution. Since the patient is symptomatic, I would offer the patient percutaneous intervention.

Eric Topol, MD, USA: It is important to verify that the patient has ischemia due to this lesion, before intervention is performed.

What do you recommend if the patient has angina and a normal resting EKG.

Cindy Grines, MD, USA: I recommend PTCA with a 3.5 x 40 mm balloon to reduce the risk of dissection. If a suboptimal result is obtained, I would place a Palmaz-Schatz stent.

David Williams, MD, USA: PTCA is recommended since it is more effective in relieving angina than medical therapy.

Eric Topol, MD, USA: Stenting the mid-RCA is indicated, with intravascular ultrasound first to characterize the lesion. I would predilate with a 3.0 mm balloon followed by a 3.5 mm Palmaz-Schatz stent.

Editors' Perspective: See p 501.

*****

CHEST PAIN: COMPLEX LESION

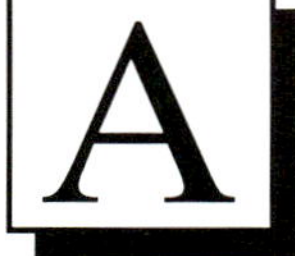

A 51-year-old man develops a chest pain syndrome. The patient is not on any medical therapy except aspirin and has not had a stress test. Another cardiologist performs cardiac catheterization which shows a severe stenosis in the LAD (reference diameter = 3.3 mm). Other vessels and LV function are normal.

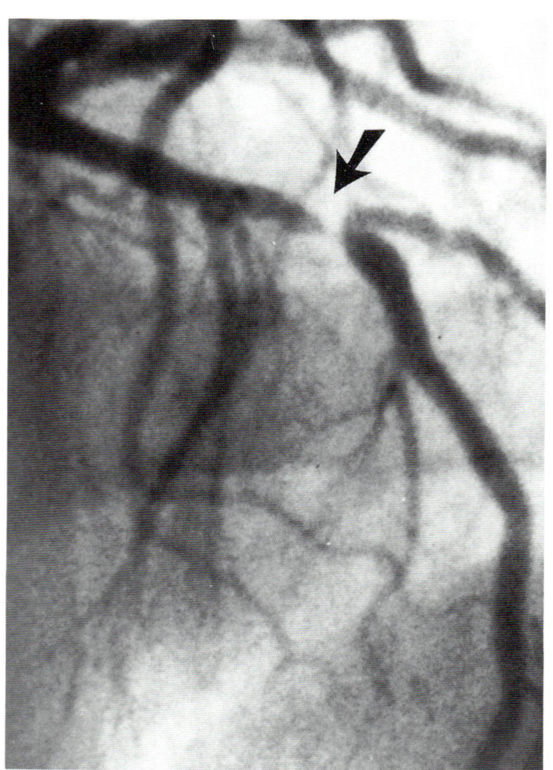

What would you recommend if the patient has atypical chest pain and a normal resting EKG.

Cindy Grines, MD, USA: If the patient has atypical chest pain, I still recommend PTCA because of the stenosis severity and large amount of jeopardized myocardium. Stenosis severity can be further evaluated with IVUS or a Doppler FloWire.

David Williams, MD, USA: This patient has an atypical chest pain syndrome and a very complex lesion (rather than a simple lesion as in the previous patient). This lesion is just proximal to a large diagonal branch arising from the LAD, and it is severe and extremely eccentric. It is quite unlikely that a lesion of this severity would not result in myocardial ischemia. I would perform directional atherectomy.

Eric Topol, MD, USA: The stenosis just prior to bifurcation of the LAD and diagonal would be approached only if the patient has rest angina, an abnormal stress test, or spontaneous ECG changes.

What would you recommend if the patient has angina and a normal resting EKG.

Cindy Grines, MD, USA: I would place a wire in the LAD, and perform PTCA with a 3.5 mm balloon. Since the diagonal branch is not involved, I would not protect this vessel with a wire. Coronary stenting with a 3.5 mm stent is an option, but I am concerned about jailing the diagonal branch.

David Williams, MD, USA: The procedure of choice for this lesion is directional atherectomy, since the lesion is eccentric and located near the origin of a major branch. Alternative treatments include Rotablator atherectomy (using a 2.5 mm burr), PTCA alone, and stenting with a Cordis or Gianturco-Roubin stent to preserve access to the diagonal.

Eric Topol, MD, USA: If intervention is indicated, a double wire is necessary. Intravascular ultrasound would be performed on the LAD prior to PTCA or directional atherectomy.

Editors' Perspective: In general, the two major reasons to recommend revascularization are to improve event-free survival (e.g., severe 3-vessel disease with LV dysfunction, acute MI, cardiogenic shock) and to improve angina or anginal-equivalent symptoms. The decision to perform PTCA on patients with coronary artery disease depends on several factors: First, the operator must assess the likelihood that PTCA will relieve ischemia. If the patient does not have symptomatic ischemia, it seems reasonable to us that objective evidence of ischemia should be demonstrated. Second, the operator should weigh the risk of intervention against the potential benefit. Third, the operator should weigh the risk of restenosis against the risk of spontaneous disease progression; in many instances, the risk of restenosis outweighs the risk of disease

progression, particularly for lesions of moderate severity. Fourth, the risk/benefit ratio of percutaneous intervention must be weighed against that of CABG and medical therapy. Finally, these issues should be communicated to the patient and family to ensure that they have realistic expectations and a reasonable understanding of what they're getting into. Lesions of borderline significance can be assessed while in the cath lab with the Doppler FloWire; coronary flow reserve > 2 suggests that critical ischemia is not present and that intervention can be safely deferred.

*****

— Section 4 —

High-Risk Patients

MULTIVESSEL DISEASE: SIMPLE

A 70-year-old female presents with a 10-year history of chronic stable angina that has progressed over the last month to Class-3 angina despite medical therapy. Angiography reveals high-grade focal lesions in the LAD, RCA, and LCX. LV ejection fraction = 45%. (Reference vessel diameters: LAD = 3.6 mm, RCA = 3.8 mm, LCX = 3.2 mm).

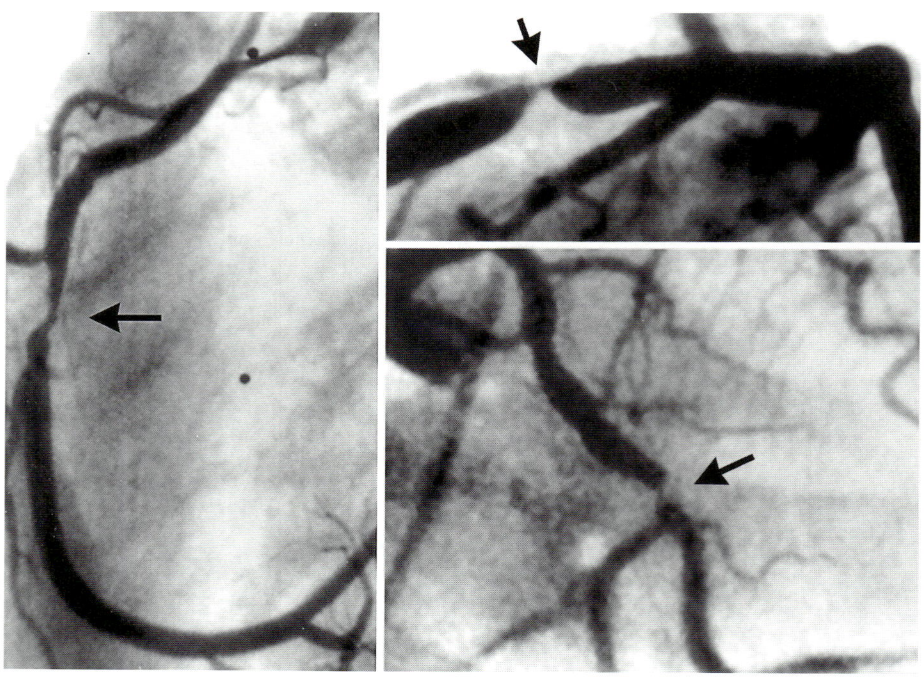

Do you recommend percutaneous or surgical revascularization?

John Douglas Jr., MD, USA: This patient has 3-vessel disease with three discrete lesions in mid and distal vessels. Since all lesions are suitable, I recommend percutaneous revascularization as a less invasive option than CABG. The EAST results indicate similar mortality at 3 years, but more repeat revascularization and less complete angina relief in patients treated with PTCA.

Dean Kereiakes, MD, USA: Although this woman has 3-vessel disease, the disease is focal and involves large caliber vessels. The longest stenosis is in the dominant RCA, but the most severe stenoses are in the LAD and LCX. Because the lesions are relatively focal and not calcified, I recommend percutaneous revascularization.

Describe your technical approach.

John Douglas Jr., MD, USA: The RCA lesion is about 15 mm long without apparent calcification, but given the chronicity of symptoms, I expect this stenosis to be rigid. The mid-LAD lesion is eccentric but the distal LCX stenosis is concentric; both do not have apparent calcification. If there is fluoroscopic calcium in the RCA, I would perform rotational atherectomy (1.5, 2.0, and 2.5 mm burrs followed by adjunctive PTCA with a 3.75 mm noncompliant balloon at 3 ATM). If there is no apparent calcification on fluoroscopy, I would use conventional PTCA with a low-profile 3.5 mm compliant balloon capable of high-pressure inflation. If results of several balloon inflations are not excellent, I would place a 4.0 mm Palmaz-Schatz stent and postdilate with a 4.0 x 15 mm NC Bandit at 15-20 ATM. If the RCA intervention is successful and less than 250 cc of contrast have been used, I would dilate the LCX. I would approach the LAD the next day, probably with a 3.5 mm compliant balloon (although the lesion is fine for directional atherectomy or a Palmaz-Schatz stent).

Dean Kereiakes, MD, USA: I would perform primary stent placement in the LAD utilizing an 8F JL4 short tip guiding catheter, a 0.014-inch Extra-Support guidewire, and predilation with a 2.5 mm MC Rail balloon. I would then place a 4.0 mm Palmaz-Schatz stent and postdilate with a 4.0 x 9.0 mm Titan at 16 ATM. I would perform intravascular ultrasound to identify optimal stent deployment. I would then place a 0.014-inch Traverse guidewire in the LCX and perform PTCA with a 3.5 mm Flowtrack perfusion balloon, using gradual (1 ATM every 30-60 seconds) inflations for > 10 minutes. For the RCA, I recommend an 8F multipurpose guide with sideholes, a 0.014-inch Extra-Support wire, predilation with a 2.5 mm MC Rail balloon, and implantation of a 4.0 mm MultiLink or Palmaz-Schatz stent. If lesion length is ≥ 15 mm, the GR-II stent will provide excellent results since it is available in 20 mm lengths. I would postdilate with a 4.0 x 9.0 mm Titan at 18 ATM.

If you perform percutaneous revascularization, which lesion would you approach first?

John Douglas Jr., MD, USA: If evident, I would first treat the vessel that receives collaterals. If no collaterals are present, I would first treat the RCA because of the lesion length, followed by the LCX. I would treat the LAD on the following day. Although a single procedure is more cost-effective, I prefer to treat three major vessels with staging.

Dean Kereiakes, MD, USA: The presence of collaterals influences my staging sequence; I would first revascularize the vessel receiving collaterals, since collaterals offer some protection if an occlusive complication occurs. Otherwise, I would treat the LAD first because it is the most severe stenosis in the largest vessel. I would treat the LCX next to allow use of the same guiding catheter and continued observation of the LAD. The RCA would be the third target because it has the least severe obstruction and requires a separate guiding catheter. If optimal results are obtained in the LAD and LCX, the RCA would be treated at the same sitting. Otherwise, I recommend deferring PTCA of the RCA for 4-6 weeks.

Is "complete" revascularization necessary or desirable?

John Douglas Jr., MD, USA: Complete revascularization should be attempted since all lesions are severe and each vessel is large.

Dean Kereiakes, MD, USA: Complete revascularization is desirable because of the severity of the lesions. Complete revascularization may not be necessary for other cases, particularly in the context of smaller sidebranch stenoses with normal left ventricular function or target stenoses < 70%.

How would your approach differ if left ventricular ejection fraction was 20%?

John Douglas Jr., MD, USA: I recommend bypass surgery, since abrupt closure of any one of the three vessels would be poorly tolerated.

Dean Kereiakes, MD, USA: My approach would be different if the left ventricular ejection fraction is 20% and the patient has signs of congestive heart failure. In this patient population, I use PET scans to identify myocardial viability. If this patient has residual viability > 50%, I recommend surgical revascularization. Large nonrandomized studies in patients with severe 3-vessel disease and left ventricular ejection fraction < 40% suggest improved 1-year outcome following surgical revascularization. This patient population requires a more "durable" procedure in the context of limited myocardial reserve.

How would your approach differ if the patient is 50 years old, extremely active, and angina began 6 months ago? LV function is normal.

John Douglas Jr., MD, USA: For the young patient with recent symptoms, I would offer PTCA with a bit more encouragement than CABG, attempting to postpone CABG as long as possible. I would perform PTCA on the RCA and LCX, and directional atherectomy or PTCA on the LAD. If the results are suboptimal, I would implant Palmaz-Schatz stents.

Dean Kereiakes, MD, USA: I recommend percutaneous revascularization. In particular, my utilization of intracoronary stents is more aggressive in this patient population. I would stent the LAD, stent or PTCA the LCX, and stent the RCA.

How would your approach differ if the patient presents with prolonged rest angina and reversible ST depression in the anterior leads?

John Douglas Jr., MD, USA: Since the LAD is the culprit vessel, I would treat it first. I would use ReoPro, and directional atherectomy or PTCA. I would reserve stenting for suboptimal results.

Dean Kereiakes, MD, USA: This syndrome identifies the LAD as the "culprit" lesion, and would dissuade me from utilizing Rotablator atherectomy because of a higher risk of no-reflow. I would still place a stent in the LAD and dilate the LCX at the same sitting. Patients with rest pain and fluctuating ST-T abnormalities are ideal for ReoPro and at least 48 hours of heparin before intervention. The benefit of antecedent heparin is additive to ReoPro. I also recommend ReoPro during stent implantation in the LAD. With this antecedent unstable syndrome, I would treat the patient with Coumadin for one month, even after optimal stent deployment.

Editors' Perspective: The decision to perform percutaneous vs. surgical revascularization for patients with multivessel disease depends on anatomical suitability, left ventricular function, patient and physician preference, and comorbid medical conditions, as discussed in the cases to follow. As shown in Tables 38-40, results from randomized trials suggest similar overall and infarct-free survival. In general, patients treated by PTCA have more angina, and require more antianginal medications and revascularization procedures in the first 5 years, while patients treated by CABG have a longer convalescence and often develop saphenous vein graft disease. Important limitations of these trials include the frequent exclusion of new devices, which were not widely available when these studies were performed, and the short duration of patient follow-up, which preceded the peak incidence of vein graft failure. These factors and their nuances should be shared with the patient and family before making final recommendations about treatment.

In addition to device selection, important technical considerations for percutaneous therapy include the completeness of revascularization, and the timing and sequence of intervention. Complete "anatomical" revascularization refers to successful revascularization of all lesions with diameter stenoses > 50%, and is distinguished from complete "functional" revascularization, which refers to successful revascularization of only those lesions causing ischemia (i.e., "culprit" lesions). Available data suggest that patients with multivessel disease and *normal* LV function have similar long-term survivals regardless of whether complete anatomical or functional revascularization is achieved (this may explain the lack of differences in survival between PTCA and bypass surgery in current randomzied trials). In contrast, patients with multivessel disease and *poor* LV function appear to do better with complete anatomical revascularization, which may explain the survival advantage for CABG over PTCA in this high-risk patient population. Since late outcome is most influenced by the completeness (rather than the mode) of revascularization, CABG may be preferred if PTCA cannot achieve complete anatomical revascularization in patients with multivessel disease and left ventricular dysfunction.

With regard to the timing and sequence of intervention, potential approaches include complete revascularization during one sitting, complete revascularization during separate sittings (days or weeks apart), or revascularization of the "culprit" lesion and reassessment of ischemia in the distribution of other vessels before further intervention. In general, total occlusions or severely stenotic lesions that supply large areas of viable myocardium or receive collaterals from other vessels are dilated first. If a suboptimal

result is obtained in one vessel, further intervention on remaining vessel(s) should be deferred. The time interval between staged procedures is a matter of operator discretion, and can vary from 1 day to 4 weeks after the initial intervention, depending on anginal stability, lesion morphology, left ventricular function, and comorbid medical conditions.

Table 38. Randomized Trials of PTCA vs. CABG: In-Hospital Results

Trial	Group	Complications (%)			Other (PTCA vs CABG)
		D	MI	CABG	
RITA[34]	PTCA	0.7	3.5	4.5	Length of stay (4 vs. 12 days)
	CABG	1.2	2.4	-	
ERACI[35]	PTCA	1.5	6.3	1.5	Stroke (1.5% vs. 3.1%)
	CABG	4.6	6.2	-	
GABI[36]	PTCA	1.1	2.3	2.8	Stroke (0% vs. 1.2%); post-op pneumonia (1.1% vs. 10.6%, p < 0.001); length of stay (5 vs. 19 days); angina (18% vs. 7%, p < 0.005)
	CABG	2.5	8.1*	-	
CABRI[37]	PTCA	1.3	-	3.3	-
	CABG	1.3	-	-	
EAST[38]	PTCA	1	3	10.1	Stroke (0.5% vs. 1.5%)
	CABG	1	10.3*	-	
BARI[39]	PTCA	1.2	2.1	6.3	Stroke (0.2% vs. 0.8%), respiratory failure (1% vs. 2.2%, p < 0.05)
	CABG	1.3	4.6*	-	

CONCLUSIONS:

- **In-hospital mortality was similar between PTCA and CABG groups.**
- **In-hospital MI was more frequent in CABG group.**
- **Emergency CABG for failed PTCA was required in 1.5-10%.**
- **Length of hospital stay was 2-3 fold higher in CABG group.**

Abbreviations: D = death; Q-MI = Q-wave myocardial infarction; CABG = emergency coronary artery bypass grafting; - = Not reported

* p < 0.01

Table 39. Randomized Trials of PTCA vs. CABG: Late Outcome

Trial	F/U (yrs)	Modality	D / MI / TLR / ASX (%)	Other
RITA[34]	2.5	PTCA	3.1 / 6.1 / 35 / 69	See 1, below
		CABG	3.6 / 3.9 / 3.8^{+} / 79^{+}	
ERACI[65]	3	PTCA	9.5 / 7.8 / $37^{\#}$ / $57^{\#}$	PTCA less expensive at 1- and 3-year follow-up
		CABG	4.7 / 7.8 / 6.3 / 79	
GABI[36]	3	PTCA	- / - / 37 / 60	
		CABG	- / - / 3.2^{+} / 80^{+}	
	1	PTCA	2.6 / 4.5 / 44 / 71	See 2, below
		CABG	6.5 / 9.4 / 6 / 74	
CABRI[37]	1	PTCA	3.9 / 4.9 / 35.6 / 67	Need for antianginals (84% vs. 65%)
		CABG	2.7 / 3.5 / 2.1 / 75^{+}	
EAST[38]	3	PTCA	7.1 / 14.6 / 54 / $80^{\dagger}$	See 3, below
		CABG	6.2 / 19.6 / 13^{+} / $88^{\dagger+}$	
BARI[39]	5	Overall		See 4, below
		PTCA	14 / 8 / 54 / -	
		CABG	11 / 9 / 8^{+} / -	
		Diabetic^{++}		
		PTCA	35 / - / 62 / -	
		CABG	19 / - / 8^{+} / -	

CONCLUSIONS:

- **Infarct-free survival at 1-year was similar between PTCA and CABG groups, but diabetics treated with PTCA had higher late mortality.**
- **PTCA resulted in more angina, antianginal therapy, and repeat revascularization (3-10 fold) compared to CABG; ~ 20% of PTCA patients required CABG at 1-3 years.**

Abbreviations: ASX = asymptomatic; D = death; MI = myocardial infarction; TLR = target lesion revascularization; CABG = emergency coronary artery bypass grafting; EF = ejection fraction; - = not reported

Other results:

1. PTCA vs. CABG: Death, MI, or reintervention (38% vs. 11%);$^{+}$ severe angina 6% in both groups; PTCA less expensive. Pre vs. post-revascularization: 40% of those not working at baseline had returned to work at 6 months; revascularization had no effect on ejection fraction
2. PTCA vs. CABG: Death or MI (5% vs. 11%) $^{+}$ *, antianginals (88% vs 78%)$^{+}$
3. PTCA vs. CABG: Abnormal thallium stress (9.6% vs. 5.7%); use of antianginals (66% vs. 51%)$^{+}$; costs equal; no difference in LVEF
4. PTCA vs. CABG: Infarct-free survival (79% vs. 80%); 70% of PTCA patients survived 5 years without CABG and at most one repeat PTCA procedure; severe angina present in only 3% of PTCA & CABG groups, but PTCA patients more likely to have angina of all grades

+ $p < 0.05$,
# $p < 0.001$
++ Patients receiving oral hypoglycemics or insulin at study entry

Table 40. Randomized PTCA vs. CABG Trials: Summary of Conclusions

Trial	In-hospital (%)		Late (%)				Other
	D	MI	D	MI	TLR	Angina	
RITA[34]	ND	ND	ND	ND	↑	↑	Severe angina (ND), cost (↓), exercise capacity (ND)
ERACI[35]	ND	ND	ND	ND	↑	↑	Cost (↓)
GABI[36]	ND	↓	ND	ND	↑	ND	Death or MI (↓), need for antianginals (↑)
CABRI[37]			ND	ND	↑	ND	Need for antianginals (↑)
EAST[38]	ND	↓	ND	ND	↑	↑	Abnormal thallium (ND), need for antianginals (ND), cost (ND), exercise capacity (ND)
BARI[39]		ND	ND*	-	↑	↑	

CONCLUSIONS:

- **For patients with multivessel disease and significant ischemia who are candidates for either PTCA or CABG and meet the entry criteria for the randomized trials (i.e., no previous PTCA or CABG; well-preserved LV function; and no left main stenosis, evolving or very recent MI, or severe noncardiac illness):**
  - **PTCA and CABG result in similar acute and longterm (1-5 yr) infarct-free survival. However, diabetic patients treated by PTCA have higher mortality than CABG patients.**
  - **Patients treated by PTCA have more angina, require more antianginal therapy, and need more revascularization procedures in the first 1-5 years, including CABG in 20%.**
  - **Patients initially treated with CABG have a longer convalescence. Longterm follow-up will determine whether more revascularization is needed after 5 years in CABG patients (i.e., to treat vein graft disease).**
- **For patients with multivessel disease and either left main stenosis, single stenosis supplying > 50% of viable myocardium, severe LV dysfunction, diffusely diseased vessels, or undilatable occlusions supplying viable myocardium, CABG may be preferred over PTCA.**

Abbreviations: D = death; MI = in-hospital myocardial infarction; CABG = emergency coronary artery bypass grafting: TLR = target lesion revascularization; - not reported
ND = No difference between PTCA and CABG groups
↑ Incidence higher in PTCA group
↓ Incidence lower in PTCA group
* Diabetics treated by PTCA had higher late mortality compared to those treated by CABG

*****

MULTIVESSEL DISEASE: COMPLEX

A 70-year-old female presents with a 10-year history of chronic stable angina, which has progressed over the last month to Class-3 angina despite optimal medical therapy. Angiography reveals high-grade complex lesions in the LAD (long, calcified), RCA (eccentric, angulated), and LCX (eccentric, ulcerated). LV ejection fraction = 45%. (Reference vessel diameters: LAD = 2.9 mm, RCA = 3.1 mm, LCX = 3.2 mm.)

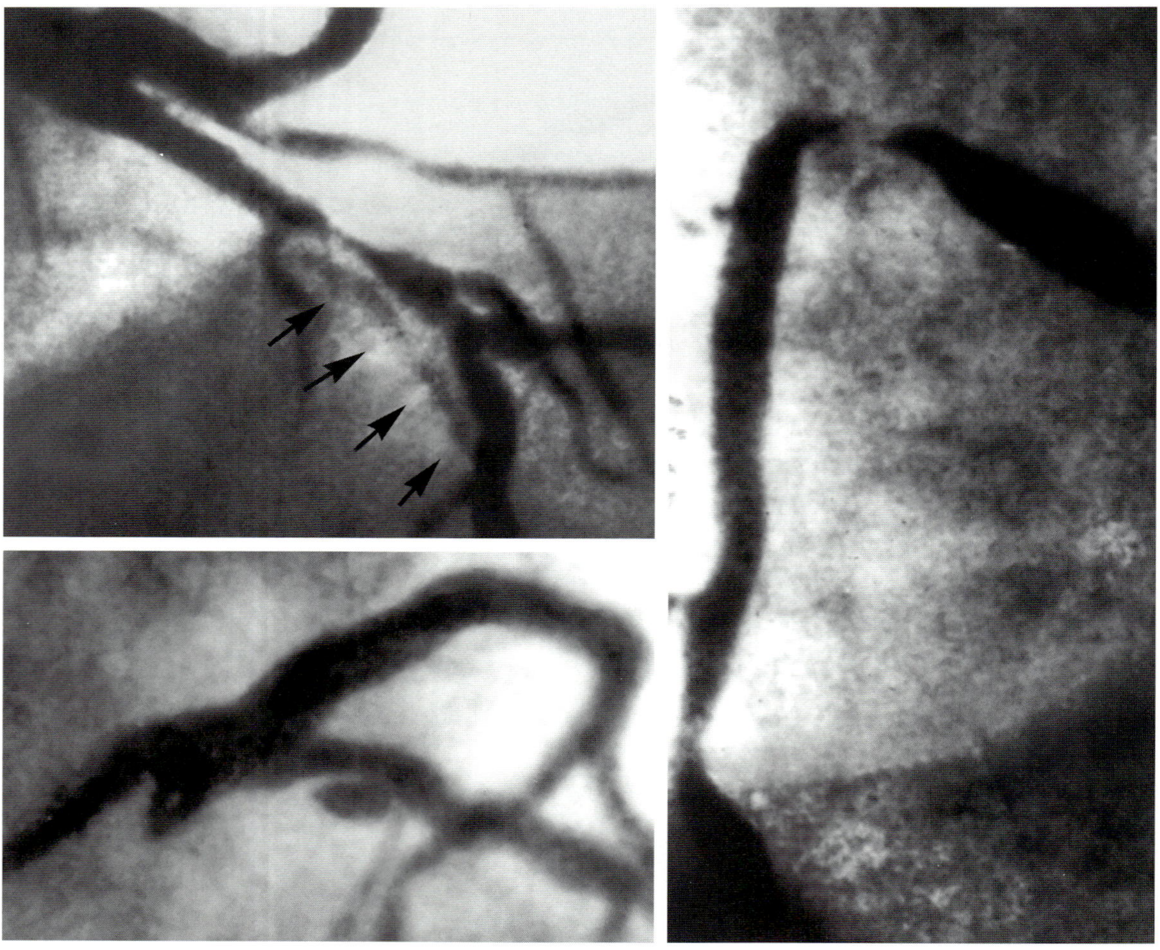

Do you recommend percutaneous or surgical revascularization?

David Faxon, MD, USA: Each of the target lesions is complex and is associated with an increased risk of complications. For this reason, I favor bypass surgery, unless there are other factors that increase the risk of bypass surgery. While PTCA can be done, the overall duration of hospitalization, the likelihood of complications, and ultimately, the high cost of interventional therapy (given the high probability of restenosis) make percutaneous revascularization less desirable than surgical revascularization.

Spencer King III, MD, USA: I recommend surgical revascularization because of the good quality of the distal vessels, impaired left ventricular function, and the complexity of each lesion, which increases the risk of acute complications and restenosis.

Ferdinand Kiemeneij, MD, The Netherlands: I recommend coronary bypass surgery. All lesions are type C lesions, with increased risk of suboptimal results and acute closure after PTCA.

If you perform percutaneous revascularization, which lesion would you approach first?

David Faxon, MD, USA: If percutaneous intervention is indicated, I would revascularize the most severe lesion first, which appears to be the RCA. Because of the risk of dissection, I recommend a 2.75 x 30 mm balloon, upsizing to a 3.0 mm balloon, if necessary. If a significant dissection occurs, I would place a Gianturco-Roubin stent, and bring her back at another setting. If the RCA is successfully treated without complications, I would dilate the LAD next. But the approach to the LAD, given the heavy calcification, is problematic. I might perform intravascular ultrasound to assess whether the calcium is in the media and intima, or whether it is purely localized to the adventitia. In any case, it is better to treat this diffuse disease with Rotablator than with PTCA. I would use a 9F JL4 guide with sideholes, a Rotablator-C wire, a 1.5 mm burr, and then upsize to a 2.0 mm or 2.25 mm burr. Following Rotablator, I would place a 3.25 x 20-30 mm balloon inflated at 1-1.5 ATM. I would avoid high-pressure inflation unless absolutely necessary to achieve an adequate angiographic result. The LCX lesion is also problematic; I would leave it alone unless there is objective evidence of ischemia.

Spencer King III, MD, USA: If surgical revascularization is high risk, I would dilate the RCA, which seems to be the culprit lesion. Following PTCA, I would reassess the patient's symptomatic condition; if she performs a modest level of exercise without symptoms, I would not treat the LAD or LCX. On the other hand, if she remains symptomatic or has a strongly positive exercise test suggesting anterior ischemia, I would approach the LAD in a staged procedure. I would examine the LAD with intravascular ultrasound to judge the extent and location of calcium. If there is extensive superficial calcium, I would choose Rotablator as the initial strategy, using a step-burr approach followed by adjunctive PTCA. I would avoid dilating the LCX.

On what basis would you decide to revascularize all 3 lesions at the same time or stage the procedure?

Spencer King III, MD, USA: I would not revascularize all three lesions at the same time.

Is "complete" revascularization necessary or desirable?

David Faxon, MD, USA: Complete revascularization is my goal, since many studies demonstrate that incomplete revascularization is associated with greater likelihood of recurrent angina and the need for further revascularization. The only setting in which incomplete revascularization is acceptable is when a vessel is too small to be bypassed or the vessel serves nonviable territory.

Spencer King III, MD, USA: Complete revascularization may not be necessary since the patient was adequately treated for 10 years with chronic stable angina, and is now suffering from progressive disease in the RCA. In any case, after stabilization of the RCA, I would perform exercise stress testing to determine whether there is evidence to warrant revascularization of the LAD or LCX.

How would your approach differ if left ventricular ejection fraction was 20%?

David Faxon, MD, USA: The surgical option is better than the percutaneous one.

Spencer King III, MD, USA: It would strengthen my recommendation for surgery.

How would your approach differ if the patient is 50 years old, extremely active, and angina began 6 months ago? LV function is normal.

David Faxon, MD, USA: If the patient is young, extremely active, and has new onset angina, I favor PTCA, particularly if one lesion can be identified as the culprit.

Spencer King III, MD, USA: If the patient is 50 years old and extremely active, I would have more enthusiasm for surgery, to achieve maximum functional benefit.

Ferdinand Kiemeneij, MD, The Netherlands: I would refer this patient for coronary bypass surgery.

How would your approach differ if the patient presents with prolonged rest angina and reversible ST depression in the anterior leads?

David Faxon, MD, USA: If there is reversible ST depression in the anterior leads, I would approach the LAD first, and bring the patient back for treatment of the other lesions at another setting.

Spencer King III, MD, USA: I would stabilize the patient on heparin for several days, and use ReoPro at the time of PTCA to decrease the risk of acute thrombotic complications.

Ferdinand Kiemeneij, MD, The Netherlands: I would still refer this patient for coronary bypass surgery.

Editors' Perspective: Unlike the previous patient, this patient has very complex 3-vessel disease, for which conventional PTCA is not ideally suited. For operators who perform only PTCA, bypass surgery may be preferred given the risk of restenosis and repeat intervention associated complete anatomical revascularization. Rotablator and stents may improve the safety of percutaneous therapy for complex lesions, and may be a reasonable alternative to bypass surgery if left ventricular function is normal, although bypass surgery is more likely to provide sustained clinical benefit.

*****

MULTIVESSEL DISEASE: PROXIMAL LAD & OSTIAL RCA

A 49-year-old malpractice attorney develops progressive angina. A recent stress test shows extensive anterior and inferior ischemia. Angiography shows a high-grade angulated lesion in the proximal LAD, and a high-grade calcified lesion in the ostium of the RCA. Left ventricular ejection fraction = 55%. (Reference vessel diameters: LAD = 3.4 mm, RCA = 2.8 mm).

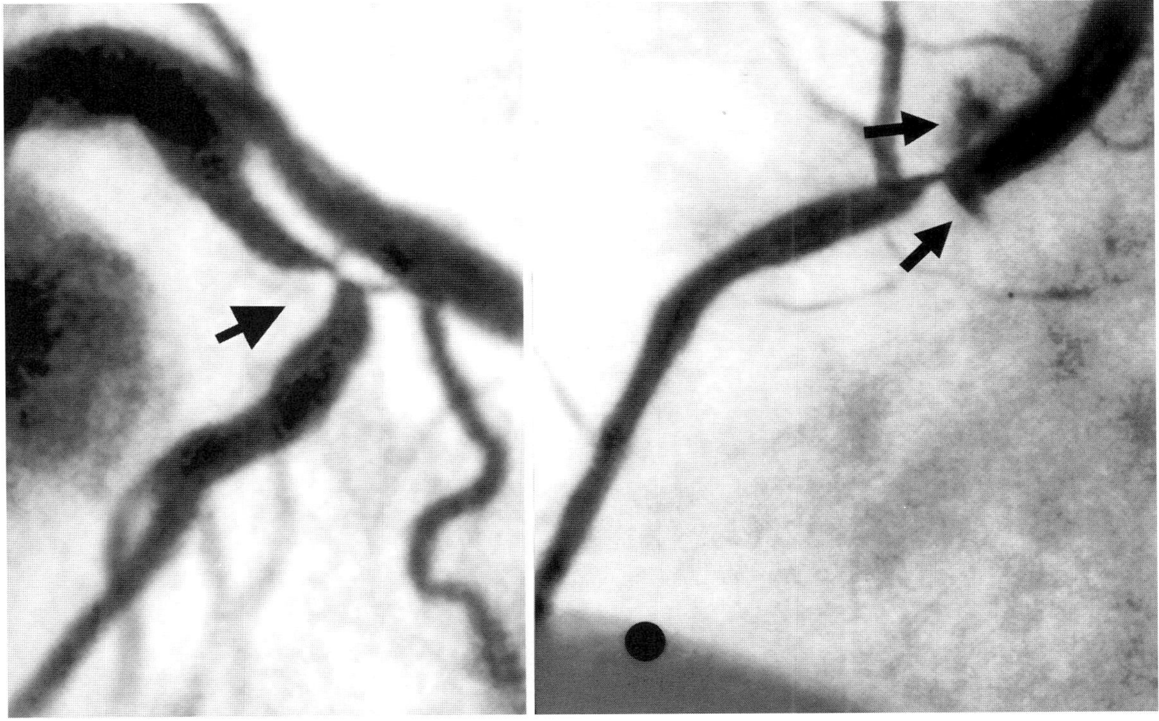

How would you manage this patient?

Dean Kereiakes, MD, USA: This attorney has high-grade proximal disease in two large vessels. These are complex lesions, and the risk of percutaneous intervention is slightly increased.

Nevertheless, I prefer a percutaneous strategy for either vessel if the patient presented with "single vessel disease." For this reason, I would offer this patient staged percutaneous intervention or bilateral internal mammary artery bypass surgery.

Bernhard Meier, MD, Switzerland: There is no doubt that this malpractice attorney needs coronary revascularization if he intends to continue to make the lives of cardiologists miserable. There are 2 discrete lesions: One is concentric but in a tortuous segment of the LAD and the other involves the origin of the RCA. The availability of stents will allow me to do both lesions in one setting. Bypass surgery is recommended if you feel that you have a score to settle with this particular lawyer or with lawyers in general.

Morton Kern, MD, USA: This young patient has progressive angina and 2-vessel disease involving the proximal LAD and ostial RCA. Both lesions are associated with a higher risk of complications and restenosis. Treatment options include 2-vessel coronary bypass surgery or complex multivessel intervention. In favor of bypass surgery are the severe nature of the ostial RCA lesion and the acute bend in the LAD, both predisposing to more difficult PTCA with increased complications. However, in view of the patient's young age, postponement of surgery is desirable since progressive coronary artery disease is likely. My approach is to discuss with the patient and family the options, risks of PTCA and restenosis, and recommend a stent in the LAD and Rotablator plus stenting of the RCA.

If you and the patient prefer percutaneous intervention, what is your approach to the 1st lesion?

Dean Kereiakes, MD, USA: If the patient is willing to undergo staged intervention, I would first perform PTCA of the LAD using an 8F JLR guiding catheter, a 0.014 Traverse wire, and a 3.5 mm perfusion balloon. Because of the acute angulation (approximately 90°), I would not utilize atherectomy or a stent as the primary therapy. Although stent deployment may work in this vessel, the acute angulation may result in a less-than-optimal stent result due to prolapse of plaque through the stent (using designs currently available in the United States); this may require placement of a superimposed stent to achieve definitive lumen enlargement. In my experience, the optimal stent for this lesion is the ACS MultiLink stent, because of its flexibility, conformability, and lack of a central articulation. I would image the LAD in 2-3 weeks and perform intervention on the RCA at that time.

Bernhard Meier, MD, Switzerland: First I would insert a 6F AL2 guiding catheter into the left coronary artery. The LAD lesion can easily be negotiated with any coronary guidewire. I would predilate with a 3.0 mm balloon at 10 ATM for 1 minute, and implant an 8 mm Palmaz-Schatz stent in the LAD.

Morton Kern, MD, USA: The more difficult of these two procedures is the Rotablator and stent in the RCA, which I would perform first, followed by PTCA and stent in the LAD, which I would perform the following day. For the RCA, I would use a 9F JR4 large-lumen guide, a 1.75 mm burr, and a Rotablator-C wire. I would increase to a 2.25 burr if the angiographic appearance is unsatisfactory, and finish with a 3.0 mm balloon at nominal pressures to obtain an adequate lumen. At this point, I would implant a 3.0 x 15 mm stent or a 10 mm biliary stent. I would give ReoPro for a suboptimal result.

What is your approach to the 2nd lesion?

Dean Kereiakes, MD, USA: Two weeks after successful PTCA of the LAD, I would perform intervention on the RCA using an 8F JR4 short-tip guiding catheter, a Rotablator-C wire, and rotational atherectomy with 1.5 mm and 2.0 mm burrs at 180,000 RPM. My choice of rotational atherectomy is guided by the presence of dense ostial calcification and the desire to facilitate stent deployment. I believe the best result in this type of lesion is obtained with rotational atherectomy and stenting. My own bias is to place a 3.0 mm Palmaz-Schatz stent and postdilate with a 3.0 x 9 mm balloon at 14 ATM.

Bernhard Meier, MD, Switzerland: The RCA can be tackled during the same session unless there is a long dissection in the LAD that cannot be covered completely by stents. It is very likely that the ostial RCA lesion will require a short stent (e.g. the saved half stent from the LAD), which should be implanted by crimping it on the balloon before the second inflation. With a little luck, these two lesions can be successfully dilated using only one 6F guiding catheter, one 3.0 mm balloon, one coronary guidewire, and one Palmaz-Schatz stent. Aspirin with or without ticlopidine is sufficient.

Morton Kern, MD, USA: After 24 hours, the patient would return to the cath lab for PTCA and stent placement in the LAD. I would use a 0.086-inch large-lumen JL4 guide, a 0.014-inch x 300 cm extra-support wire, a 3.0 x 20 mm balloon, and a 3.5 x 15 mm Palmaz-Schatz stent positioned so the articulation is not over the plaque. I would follow with intravascular ultrasound to ensure adequate stent deployment, and discontinue heparin after 4 hours. The patient would be discharged on aspirin (325 mg QD), ticlopidine (250 mg BID), and a calcium channel blocker for 6 weeks.

Intervention on the LAD results in a residual stenosis of 40% and a non-flow-limiting dissection. The patient is asymptomatic and the ECG is normal. What would you do now?

Dean Kereiakes, MD, USA: This is a suboptimal result in a large vessel and further intervention is indicated. I recommend directional atherectomy if a localized or eccentric plaque can be identified, using a 7F GTO or EX device. If a suboptimal result persists, I would implant a GR-II stent or MultiLink stent, and defer intervention on the RCA.

Bernhard Meier, MD, Switzerland: I would try to optimize the result in the LAD using one or more stents. If more than 2 cm of the LAD had to be stented to achieve a good result, I would postpone intervention on the RCA for at least 4 months, to get an idea about restenosis in the LAD. I would use heparin or ReoPro infusion for 12 hours and leave the sheath in place until the next morning.

Morton Kern, MD, USA: I would place a 3.5 mm Palmaz-Schatz stent in the LAD and then proceed with the RCA after a 2-day interval between procedures (off heparin).

Editors' Perspective: This type of patient may not have been enrolled in any randomized study of PTCA vs. CABG because of the unsuitability of the calcified ostial RCA stenosis for PTCA. For operators who perform only PTCA, it is unlikely that complete revascularization could be achieved. For operators experienced with new devices, this type of lesion could be readily treated by Rotablator (with adjunctive PTCA), directional atherectomy, or stenting. However, even with the availability of Rotablator and stents, the potential advantages and disadvantages of surgery should be frankly discussed with the patient before proceeding with percutaneous revascularization.

*****

COMPLEX PATIENT: SIMPLE LESION

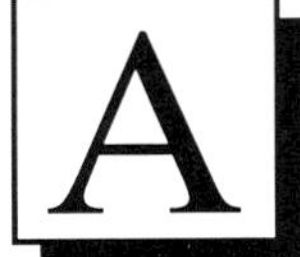

78-year-old man develops refractory angina. Past medical history is significant for chronic renal failure and peripheral vascular disease. Angiography shows a single, tubular stenosis in the mid-RCA (reference diameter = 3.0 mm). Ejection fraction = 25%.

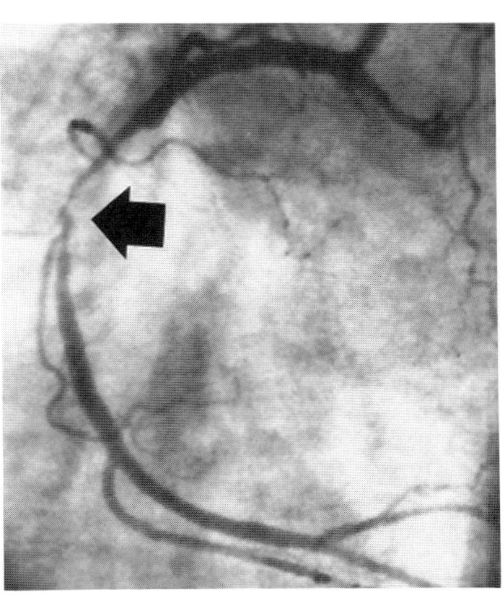

What is your overall assessment of the risk of revascularization?

David Faxon, MD, USA: This patient has chronic renal failure, peripheral vascular disease, and a long, tubular lesion in the RCA. The patient is at increased risk for acute complications and restenosis. Nevertheless, renal failure patients are more difficult to manage with surgical therapy, and I prefer PTCA over CABG in a patient with single vessel disease.

Bernhard Meier, MD, Switzerland: This elderly man is a high-risk candidate for any type of intervention, due to chronic renal failure and poor left ventricular function. It can be assumed that the poor left ventricular ejection fraction is at least partially due to a previous occlusion of the

RCA, which reduces the risk of PTCA of this artery. If, however, the RCA subtends the only viable myocardium, PTCA of the RCA is equivalent to PTCA of an unprotected left main. Bypass surgery is associated with a high risk of mortality, and is not a perfect alternative either.

What approach would you recommend?

David Faxon, MD, USA: I prefer Rotablator and low-pressure balloon inflation, since this will result in a better outcome than PTCA alone. I would use a 9F guiding catheter with sideholes, a Rotablator-C wire, and a 1.25 mm burr. Depending on the result, I would upsize to a 1.75 mm and perhaps a 2.0 mm burr. I would follow with a 3.25 x 30 mm balloon inflated at 1-1.5 ATM. For dissection or suboptimal result, I recommend ReoPro.

Bernhard Meier, MD, Switzerland: I recommend a 6F JR4 guide and a 3.0 x 40 mm balloon over a 0.014-inch guidewire, and 1 inflation for only 20 seconds. Stent implantation is indicated unless the result is absolutely pristine. The ideal stent for this lesion is a 3.5 x 40 mm GR-II stent, which can pass easily through a 6F guiding catheter. After deployment at 8 ATM, I would withdraw the balloon a little to prevent the distal end from extending beyond the stent, and inflate at 14 ATM. Coumadin is indicated because of poor left ventricular function.

Is supported angioplasty indicated?

Bernhard Meier, MD, Switzerland: I do not recommend percutaneous cardiopulmonary bypass or intraaortic balloon pumping, but recommend brief balloon inflations. If the vessel occludes due to a long dissection, mechanical support may be necessary.

<u>Editors' Perspective</u>: The overall risk of intervention is dependent on angiographic characteristics, clinical factors, and left ventricular function (Table 41). The risk of abrupt closure for focal, uncomplicated lesions as displayed in this angiogram is low (2-4% for PTCA; < 1% for stents). Nevertheless, this patient is at increased risk of death if abrupt closure occurs because of advanced age, left ventricular dysfunction, and a jeopardy score > 2.5 (Figure 1, p. 112).

In this type of patient, supported angioplasty (intraaortic balloon pump or percutaneous cardiopulmonary bypass) is often considered (p. 113-114). "Standby" support (access to contralateral femoral artery before intervention; support initiated only if needed) is often considered for patients with left ventricular ejection fractions < 30%, complex lesions (bifurcation, thrombus, severe angulation), and stable hemodynamics (systolic blood pressure > 100 mmHg and mean pulmonary wedge pressure < 20 mmHg). Prophylactic IABP (support initiated at start of case) is often recommended for patients with left ventricular ejection fractions < 30%, abnormal hemodynamics (systolic blood pressure < 100 mmHg or mean pulmonary wedge pressure > 20 mmHg), or a jeopardy score ≥ 3. Prophylactic CPS, the most aggressive level of support, is generally reserved for patients with a single patent vessel, unprotected left main intervention, or a jeopardy score ≥ 5.

Table 41. Estimation of Procedural Mortality

Lesion Closure Risk*	+	Patient Mortality Risk**	∝	Procedural Risk
High		High		Highest
Low		High		High
High		Low		Intermediate
Low		Low		Low

Lesion Closure Factors::
- Unstable angina
- Thrombus
- Multilesion/multivessel CAD
- Angulation > 45-60°
- Long lesion (> 20 mm)
- Branch point stenosis
- No aspirin
- Suboptimal ACT
- Balloon-to-artery ratio > 1
- Residual stenosis > 30%
- Dissection: long, spiral, cap

Patient Mortality Factors:
- LVEF < 35%
- Age > 65 years
- Three-vessel or left main CAD
- Recent MI
- No prior CABG
- Jeopardy score ≥2.5
- Female gender

Abbreviations: ACT = activated clotting time; CABG = coronary artery bypass graft; CAD = coronary artery disease; LVEF = left ventricular ejection fraction

* The risk of developing acute closure; estimated from the number of lesion closure factors.

** The risk of death following acute closure; estimated from the number of patient mortality factors.

*****

COMPLEX PATIENT: COMPLEX LESION

A 78 year-old man develops refractory angian. Past medical history is significant for chronic renal failure and peripheral vascular disease. Angiography shows complex 3-vessel disease including a severe LAD bifurcation lesion (proximal LAD = 3.4 mm, diagonal = 2.9 mm); a tortuous LCX with a severe distal stenosis (reference diameter = 3.2 mm); and a tortuous RCA with a severe, eccentric, ulcerated stenosis in a bend (reference diameter = 3.2 mm). Left ventricular ejection fraction = 25%.

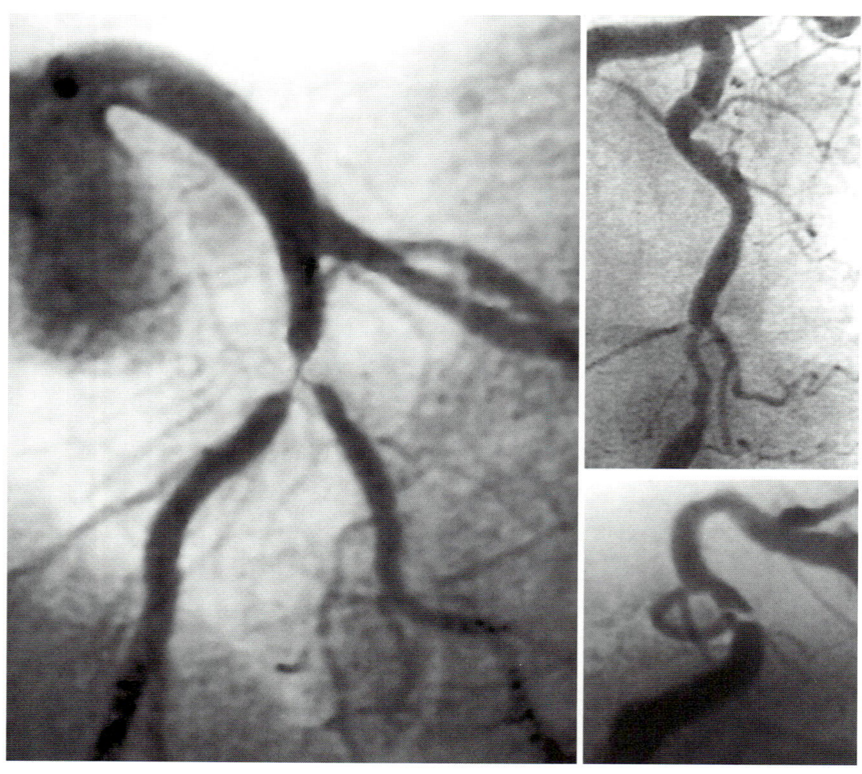

What is your overall assessment of the risk of revascularization?

David Faxon, MD, USA: This patient has 3-vessel disease with three complex lesions that are at increased risk for acute complications and restenosis. I recommend bypass surgery.

Bernard Meier, MD, Switzerland: PTCA is not a viable option. Each of the individual lesions has a high risk of complications and restenosis. The patient should be referred for coronary artery bypass surgery or treated medically if the surgeons refuse.

Editors' Perspective: Unlike the previous case, the risk of ischemic complications in this patient is extremely high. Complex lesion morphology imparts a high risk of abrupt closure, and advanced age, left ventricular dysfunction, multivessel disease, and jeopardy score > 2.5 impart a high risk of procedural mortality in the event abrupt closure occurs. In this complicated and high-risk patient, CABG may offer a survival advantage over PTCA. If percutaneous intervention is performed, standby support or prophylactic insertion of an intraaortic balloon pump is recommended.

*****

RISK STRATIFICATION: LEFT VENTRICULAR FUNCTION

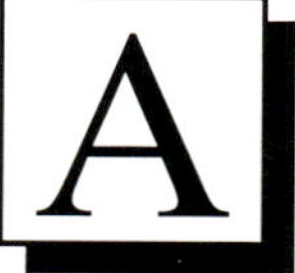 57-year-old woman develops unstable angina. Angiography reveals a high-grade stenosis in the mid-LAD (reference diameter = 3.1 mm). No other coronary disease is evident.

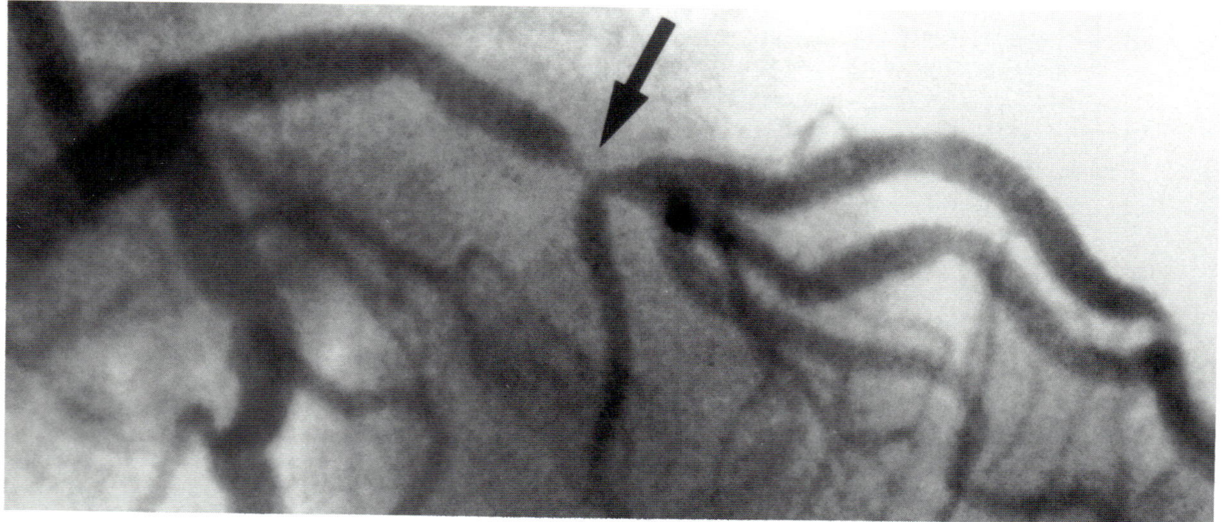

How would manage this patient if left ventricular ejection fraction = 60%.

Ferdinand Kiemeneij, MD, The Netherlands: This patient has a severe, short, eccentric lesion in the mid-LAD. PTCA may result in occlusion of the septal branch and there is some risk of diagonal occlusion. I would approach this patient from the right radial artery with GR-II stent implantation. The rationale for stenting is to obtain a safe and predictable result and to prevent restenosis; the new Gianturco-Roubin stent is associated with reduced risk of sidebranch occlusion.

David Faxon, MD, USA: This mid-LAD lesion is optimal for PTCA. Since stenting will jeopardize the septal and diagonal, it would not be an ideal choice, except as bailout. Directional atherectomy is reasonable, but the distal LAD has some disease and tortuosity, raising concerns about nosecone injury. Since the lesion is concentric and non-calcified, PTCA is my first choice, regardless of left ventricular function.

Spencer King III, MD, USA: Since the lesion is short and dissection is infrequent (although it could jeopardize a large amount of myocardium), I would perform PTCA with a 3.0 mm balloon. Directional atherectomy is also reasonable, but I would avoid stenting.

How would manage this patient if left ventricular ejection fraction = 30%.

Spencer King III, MD, USA: I would proceed with PTCA, as long as the anterior wall is viable.

David Faxon, MD, USA: I would proceed with PTCA, as above.

How would manage this patient if left ventricular ejection fraction = 10%?

Ferdinand Kiemeneij, MD, The Netherlands: I would approach the LAD via the right femoral artery, with a prophylactic intraaortic balloon pump in the left femoral artery. I would use a 6F Scimed Voda left guiding catheter, allowing optimal support, coaxial alignment, and selective cannulation of the LAD. I would work fast ("hit and run") with short inflations and few contrast (Omnipaque) injections, to reduce ischemia. I would implant a GR-II stent as described previously. I recommend Coumadin (INR 2.5-3.0) because of poor left ventricular function.

This procedure can be performed by interventionalists without access to percutaneous cardiopulmonary bypass, if they can implant coronary stents.

David Faxon, MD, USA: An intraaortic balloon pump prior to PTCA and a perfusion balloon will reduce the risk of the procedure. I would not place the patient on percutaneous cardiopulmonary bypass, but would have it on standby.

Spencer King III, MD, USA: With an ejection fraction of 10%, there must be a cardiomyopathy with generalized left ventricular dysfunction. If the patient has severe angina related to the LAD lesion, I would consider PTCA (but only in that case). The role of cardiopulmonary support would not enter my thinking here since my defense would be ready availability of a stent if dissection occurs. However, I would place a prophylactic intraaortic balloon pump.

Editors' Perspective: Procedural risk of percutaneous intervention is dependent on lesion morphology, clinical characteristics, and left ventricular dysfunction. This lesion is associated with a low risk of abrupt closure, particularly with stenting. However, the risk of patient mortality increases with decreasing ejection fraction. For operators who perform only PTCA, standby support should generally be considered when left ventricular ejection fraction is < 30%, and prophylactic support when the ejection fraction is ≤ 15% (or < 30% when hypotension or decompensated heart failure is present). The availability of stents may decrease the need for supported angioplasty.

*****

SINGLE PATENT VESSEL

A 72-year-old man with a history of CABG in 1984 develops unstable angina despite optimal medical management. Angiography reveals a high-grade stenosis in the saphenous vein graft to the LAD (reference diameter = 4.5 mm), total occlusion of the vein graft to the obtuse marginal branch, and total occlusion of the vein graft to the RCA. Collaterals from the LAD supply two large obtuse marginal branches. The native circulation is not amenable to percutaneous revascularization.

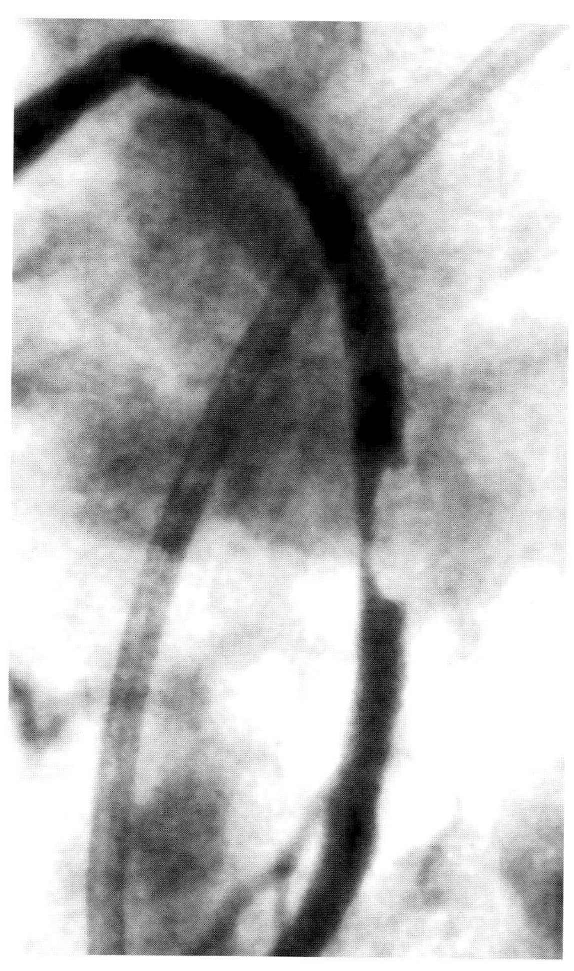

How does left ventricular ejection fraction influence your decision to perform percutaneous intervention?

David Faxon, MD, USA: This case illustrates a high-grade, irregular lesion in the middle of a large saphenous vein graft to the LAD, which also supplies collaterals to large obtuse marginals. Thus, the lesion supplies a large amount of myocardium. Since the risk of the procedure is largely related to the percentage of viable myocardium, this needs to be carefully assessed prior to the procedure. A number of studies demonstrate that the extent of viable myocardium is the best predictor of hemodynamic collapse: The worse the ejection fraction, and more importantly, the greater the amount of viable myocardium served by this lesion, the greater the need for support techniques. Thus, if the ejection fraction is 30% and this lesion serves most of the viable territory, I would place an intraaortic balloon pump. If the ejection fraction is 15% and the lesion serves a large area of viable myocardium, I would place an intraaortic balloon pump and have percutaneous cardiopulmonary bypass on standby.

Spencer King III, MD, USA: I recommend bypass surgery to all distal vessels, regardless of ejection fraction, since the patient is surviving on an LAD graft that is severely diseased. The likelihood of maintaining long-term graft patency might be improved by stenting, but data to support this are weak. Restenosis within a stent may produce a fatal outcome, and a percutaneous approach is risky in this patient.

Ferdinand Kiemeneij, MD, The Netherlands: This patient is living on a severely diseased graft to the LAD, equivalent to an unprotected left main stenosis. Procedural failure and occlusion is not compatible with life. Temporary occlusion has a high risk of cardiogenic shock. If the ejection fraction is > 30%, I recommend a second bypass operation. If an operable patient absolutely refuses surgery and has an ejection fraction of 15%, I would stent the LAD graft with an intraaortic balloon pump in place.

Describe your percutaneous approach.

David Faxon, MD, USA: My major concern is the severity and irregularity of the lesion. Old degenerated vein grafts are predisposed to distal embolization; directional atherectomy or TEC might be associated with a higher risk of complications. Therefore, I would approach this lesion with a 3.0-4.0 mm balloon, then place a 4.5 mm biliary stent, and follow with a high-pressure inflation with a 4.5 mm balloon. Optimum deployment should be checked with intravascular ultrasound, given the large size of the vein graft, to ensure proper apposition to the vessel wall. If distal embolization occurs, intracoronary nitroglycerin or verapamil is helpful. If stents are not available, a 4.0 mm perfusion balloon is an alternative.

Spencer King III, MD, USA: If the patient absolutely refuses surgery, I would predilate the lesion with a 3.0 mm balloon, implant a 4.0 mm Palmaz-Schatz stent, and postdilate with a 4.5 mm balloon at high pressure to achieve 0% residual stenosis. I would not utilize cardiopulmonary support but would depend on rapid stent placement; an intraaortic balloon pump might be useful.

Ferdinand Kiemeneij, MD, The Netherlands: I would insert an intraaortic balloon pump. I would use a 6F multipurpose guiding catheter to cannulate the graft, an ACS 0.014-inch Extra-Support guidewire, a 3.5 x 40 mm Flowtrack at 6-8 ATM to allow distal perfusion, an 18 mm Palmaz-Schatz stent on a 4.0 x 20 mm balloon, and Hexabrix or Omnipaque. At the start of the procedure, I would administer aspirin (500 mg IV) and heparin (10,000 units IV). To prevent no-reflow, I would give verapamil (100-200 mcg IC). I would discharge the patient on aspirin and Coumadin because of poor left ventricular function. This procedure can be performed by interventionalists without access to percutaneous cardiopulmonary bypass, provided they can implant coronary stents and an intraaortic balloon pump is available.

Editors' Perspective: This patient is at high risk for ischemic complications with percutaneous intervention. Both the risk of vessel closure and patient mortality are high because of complex lesion morphology (possible thrombus-laden lesion in a vein graft) and a large territory at risk (single patent vessel). For operators who perform only PTCA, this patient should be referred for CABG or to a center experienced with stents and support devices. Even with stenting (and adjunctive TEC), the risk of no-reflow is 5-15%, which could be potentially fatal. If otherwise reasonable, redo bypass surgery is recommended.

*****

— Section 5 —

Suboptimal Results

RIGID LESION: LAD

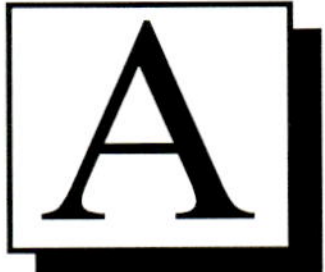

60-year-old cardiologist has unstable angina. Coronary angiography demonstrates a mildly calcified tubular stenosis in the mid-LAD (reference vessel = 3.0 mm). Your partner performs conventional PTCA and states that despite inflation pressures of 10 ATM, there is a persistent waist in the PET balloon ("dog-boning").

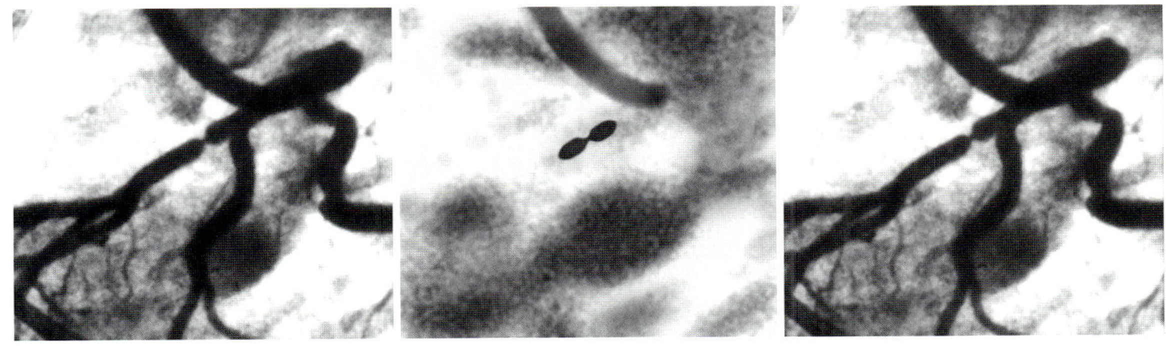

What would you do now?

Patrick Whitlow, MD, USA: This unfortunate cardiologist has an "undilatable" lesion that has just been assaulted with a balloon at 10 ATM. In my experience, the worst complications with PTCA occur at high inflation pressures. Therefore, I would not persist with PTCA, since more effective alternatives are now available. As long as no major lesion disruption is apparent, I would exchange the PTCA guidewire for a Rotablator C-wire. The Rotablator is uniformly successful in resolving "undilatable" lesions. I would utilize a 1.5 mm burr, which fits through a 7F or 8F guiding catheter. If an 8F large-lumen catheter has been used, a 2.15 mm burr can be utilized, which would likely give adequate debulking and allow successful PTCA with a 3.0 mm balloon at 2-4 ATM.

Spencer King III, MD, USA: This lesion is resistant to balloon inflation. Since the patient has unstable angina, I think further therapy is needed at this time. The severe constriction on the balloon suggests that it is a very fibrotic and calcified, and although high-pressure balloon inflation might break this lesion, it would respond better to rotational ablation.

Bernhard Meier, MD, Switzerland: I would certainly go to 20 ATM. If this pressure fails, a Rotablator wire should be inserted. If a 6F guiding catheter has been used, the burr size is limited to 1.25 mm but this may suffice to split the rigid plaque and allow successful PTCA. If a larger guiding catheter is used, a larger burr can be employed. However, the burr should not be larger than 1.75 mm. After just one passage of the burr, I would reinsert the balloon and inflate at high pressure.

If Rotablator is desirable, do you have concerns about using it immediately after PTCA?

Patrick Whitlow, MD, USA: In 1992, I was very concerned about using the Rotablator immediately after PTCA. However, my current philosophy is to abandon PTCA if the waist is not resolved at 10 ATM, and switch immediately to rotational atherectomy. As long as there is no apparent intimal disruption, I would proceed immediately with Rotablator. I have never seen the Rotablator extend or cause a tear in such cases, as long as very slow passes are made with a step-burr approach. It is not necessary to pass the initial Rotablator burr all the way through a lesion before stopping the run; the run should be limited to 15-30 seconds, since longer runs are associated with a higher incidence of no-reflow. The major lesson we learned over the last few years is never allow the rotational speed to drop more than 5,000 RPM, to avoid generation of heat and dissection.

Spencer King III, MD, USA: Although delaying the procedure until the vessel has healed may sound desirable, leaving this severe lesion (especially after endothelial denudation after PTCA) poses a greater risk for acute thrombotic closure. I would start with a 1.5 mm burr and pass it very slowly into the lesion, being certain that the rotational speed does not drop more than 5,000 RPM, and then exchange for a 2.0 mm burr. I would inspect the artery with intravascular ultrasound to determine the degree of residual plaque, and decide whether to move up to a 2.15 mm burr or use a balloon.

Bernhard Meier, MD, Switzerland: The use of a Rotablator after an initial attempt at PTCA is not commonly recommended. However, if the balloon cannot be passed or fully expanded, a small burr is the only alternative. It should not create a problem, as long as there is no significant dissection after PTCA.

Editors' Perspective: Occasionally, conventional PTCA fails because lesion rigidity prevents full balloon expansion. Although this scenario creates considerable frustration and anxiety for the operator, there are a number of approaches that can be used to salvage these "nondilatable" lesions. One approach is to deliver higher pressures using one of several balloons capable of > 20 ATM without rupture. A second approach is to use "force-focused" angioplasty. This technique requires placement of a second 0.012-0.018-inch guidewire parallel to the original wire, followed by balloon inflation over the original wire using a noncompliant balloon. The parallel wire outside the inflated balloon can "score" the plaque, increasing lesion compliance and facilitating balloon inflation. A third technique relies on the cutting (Barath) balloon, which uses razor-sharp microtomes on a conventional balloon to score the plaque and facilitate balloon expansion. A fourth approach is to use the Rotablator, which is extremely effective and virtually always successful in nondilatable lesions. However, the risk of extending an inapparent dissection after PTCA must be weighed against the advantage of successful revascularization. It is reassuring that all 3 experts have experience with immediate Rotablator after failed PTCA, and the risks appear to be low. However, if gross angiographic dissection is apparent after PTCA, Rotablator is contraindicated.

*****

RIGID LESION: VEIN GRAFT

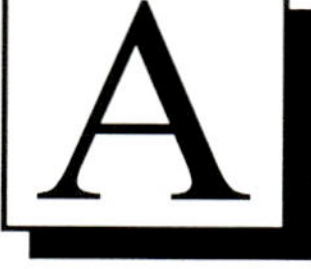

A saphenous vein graft to the LAD is treated with a 4.5 mm high-pressure balloon (reference vessel = 4.5 mm). Despite inflation pressures up to 16 ATM, the waist in the balloon persists and the lesion is unchanged. All other grafts and left ventricular function are normal.

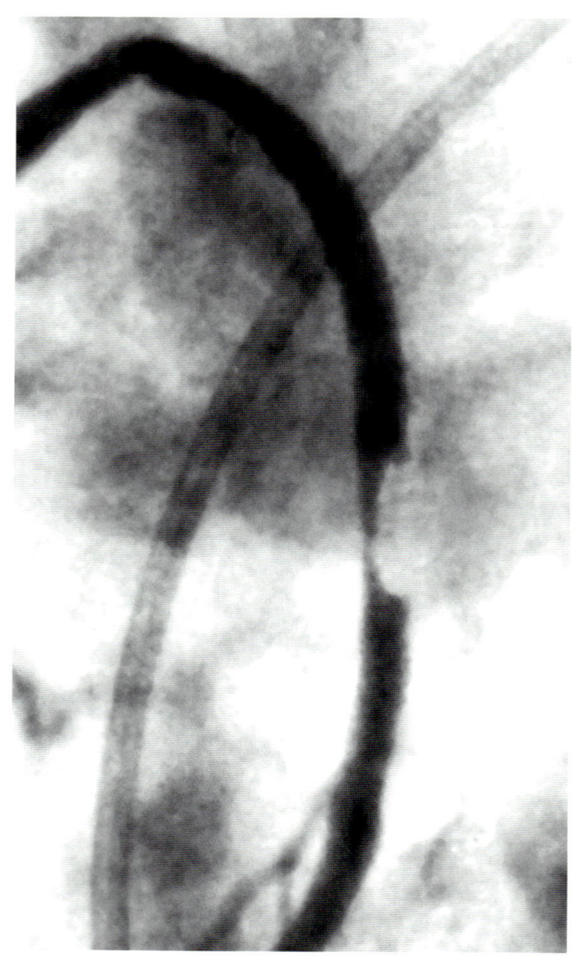

How would you approach this lesion now?

Richard Schatz, MD, USA: We do not know the age of this vein graft, but if we assume it is greater than 5 years, I would assume that it is extremely fragile. Therefore, although inflation pressures >16 ATM are possible, one has to consider the potential hazards of vessel rupture and distal embolization. If intravascular ultrasound reveals heavy calcification, procedural failure, restenosis, and complications are likely; the patient should be treated with bypass surgery. If the patient is not a candidate for repeat bypass surgery and is unstable, one must accept the attendant risks of more aggressive strategies. If there is no calcium, the lesion is ideal for directional atherectomy due to its eccentricity and accessibility, despite an increased risk of distal embolization. I would use a 7F AtheroCath and do multiple passes guided by ultrasound.

Richard Heuser, MD, USA: This patient has a rigid stenosis in a saphenous vein graft. Directional atherectomy is reasonable, using a 7F AtheroCath and a DVI guide. I would use a 0.014-inch x 300 cm Extra-S'port or Hi-torque floppy wire. I would predilate with a 3.0 mm high-pressure balloon. Because sole therapy with directional atherectomy does not reduce restenosis, I would also implant a biliary stent.

Ulrich Sigwart, MD, England: Direction atherectomy is the preferred approach, followed by PTCA and stenting. Directional laser angioplasty could also be used to "precondition" the lesion for stenting.

Are adjunctive imaging modalities useful? Should specific techniques or devices be avoided?

Richard Schatz, MD, USA: Rotational atherectomy of vein grafts is not recommended, but might be considered if there is heavy calcification by intravascular ultrasound.

Richard Heuser, MD, USA: This can be a difficult scenario because you do not want to place a stent if you can't expand the lesion before intervention. I don't think IVUS is going to help before intervention, but I would definitely use angioscopy to be sure that thrombus and friable plaque are absent.

Ulrich Sigwart, MD, England: A TEC device does not seem the right thing here, nor would I use the Rotablator, primarily because of lesion eccentricity.

Editors' Perspective: The general considerations and approaches to nondilatable lesions in vein grafts are similar to those in native coronary arteries (see p. 535). An important exception is the use of Rotablator in the body of vein grafts, which has been considered an absolute contraindication because of the risk of distal embolization and no-reflow. Personally, we have no experience with Rotablator in the body of vein grafts, but if performed, it is probably best to use the smallest burr possible to unroof the plaque while minimizing distal embolization. In many cases such as this, even slight unroofing of the rigid cap can favorably impact lesion compliance; directional atherectomy can be used for this purpose, followed by stenting, if necessary.

*****

ELASTIC RECOIL

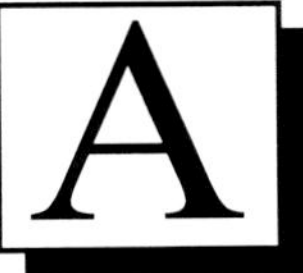

An eccentric lesion in the distal RCA is treated with a 3.5 x 20 mm balloon (reference vessel = 3.5 mm). Despite full balloon expansion at low pressure, the lesion is unchanged. Other vessels and left ventricular function are normal.

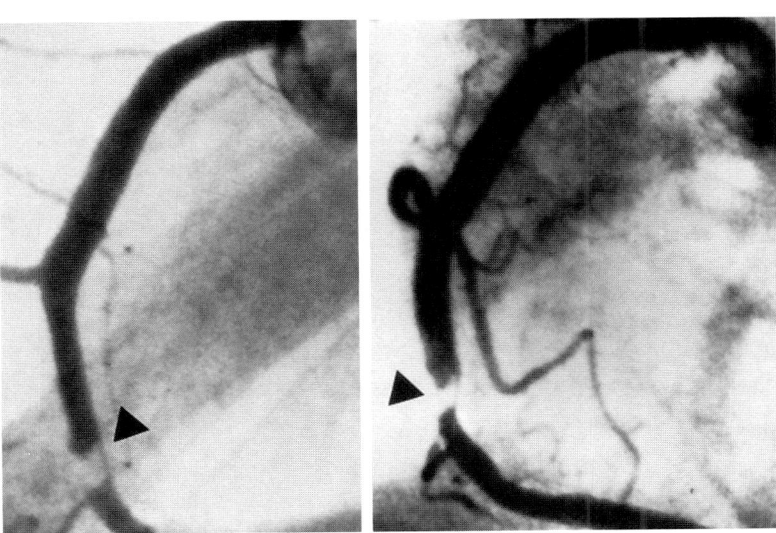

What causes this type of suboptimal PTCA result?

John Douglas Jr., MD, USA: The patient has an eccentric RCA stenosis with a very unusual angiographic appearance There is no response to PTCA. The lesion does not have the appearance of a simple atherosclerotic plaque, since it is extremely eccentric and has a sharp leading edge. The most likely explanation is plaque rupture and superimposed thrombus, but other possibilities include localized dissection or eccentric plaque.

Takeshi Kimura, MD, Japan: This patient has a highly eccentric lesion unresponsive to PTCA.

Three possible explanations are thrombus, rigid plaque, and a highly elastic lesion. Since full balloon expansion was obtained at low pressure, rigid plaque can be excluded.

Ian Penn, MD, Canada: This patient has failed PTCA. I would assume there is an area of plaque prolapsing into the vessel that does not remodel with PTCA. The lesion morphology is that of a bulky filling defect without staining or embolization to suggest clot.

How would you approach this lesion now?

John Douglas Jr., MD, USA: The two strategies that appeal to me are stenting and directional atherectomy. My first choice is implantation of a 3.5 mm Palmaz-Schatz stent, but if considerable thrombus is present, I would perform directional atherectomy with a 7F Graft AtheroCath over a 0.014-inch Platinum-Plus wire (avoiding cuts toward the normal wall). I would use ReoPro and a 3.5 x 20 mm perfusion balloon to optimize the result.

Takeshi Kimura, MD, Japan: I would perform stent implantation without angioscopy. Although directional atherectomy is reasonable for elastic recoil, stent implantation is more predictable and user-friendly, and guiding catheter exchange is not required. I would use an 8F JR4 large-lumen guiding catheter without sideholes and a 0.014-inch x 300 cm guidewire. I would implant a 3.5 x 15 mm Palmaz-Schatz stent with a spiral articulation and postdilate at 16-18 ATM with a 3.5-4.0 x 20 mm balloon. Anticoagulation consists of aspirin (243 mg QD) and ticlopidine (200 mg QD).

Ian Penn, MD, Canada: I recommend stenting with a 3.5 x 18 mm Palmaz-Schatz stent with a spiral articulation. A JR4 guide, a 0.014-inch Extra-Support wire, and a 4.0 x 9 mm Titan or High-energy balloon are reasonable. Although directional atherectomy could debulk this lesion, the restenosis rate is similar to PTCA. I would prescribe aspirin alone; the only indication for additional antiplatelet therapy is an inadequate result based on QCA and ultrasound.

Are adjunctive imaging modalities useful or indicated?

John Douglas Jr., MD, USA: The most helpful modality is angioscopy, to clarify whether thrombus is a major component of the lesion. This important issue is not easily resolved by other imaging methods. Intravascular ultrasound will not provide conclusive information.

Takeshi Kimura, MD, Japan: Although angioscopy is helpful to evaluate the presence or absence of thrombus, no significant angiographic change after PTCA suggests that the lesion is highly elastic, not thrombotic.

Ian Penn, MD, Canada: I may perform intravascular ultrasound to determine the reference vessel size and optimize stenting. I do not routinely use angioscopy in this setting.

If lasers, atherectomy devices, and stents are not available at your institution, how would you approach this lesion?

John Douglas Jr., MD, USA: In a center without devices, I recommend prolonged redilation with a 3.5 x 20 mm perfusion balloon, and subsequent referral for directional atherectomy or stenting if the result is inadequate.

Takeshi Kimura, MD, Japan: If atherectomy devices and stents are not available, this patient should be referred to another center where stents are available.

Ian Penn, MD, Canada: I would use a 4.0 mm x 20 mm perfusion balloon, removing the wire and retracting the guide to maintain perfusion for 15-20 minutes. However, perfusion balloon angioplasty is time-consuming and unpredictable. Based on randomized data from TASC-II, I favor stent deployment.

> **Editors' Perspective: This case represents an example of a nondilatable lesion due to elastic recoil (as opposed to lesion rigidity or calcification). Prolonged balloon inflations (with or without a perfusion balloon), higher inflation pressures, and oversize balloons may be of value, but the results are unpredictable and often associated with complications. Directional atherectomy is particularly well-suited for elastic, eccentric lesions in large vessels; other atherectomy devices are less useful unless there is associated thrombus (TEC) or calcification (Rotablator). Finally, stenting is a reasonable approach to such lesions, because of its predictability and reliability in eliminating elastic recoil.**

*****

WATERMELON SEEDING

PTCA of the LAD with a 3.25 x 20 mm balloon is unsuccessful because of "watermelon seeding." There is no apparent lesion calcification by fluoroscopy (reference vessel diameter = 3.2 mm). Other coronary arteries and left ventricular function are normal.

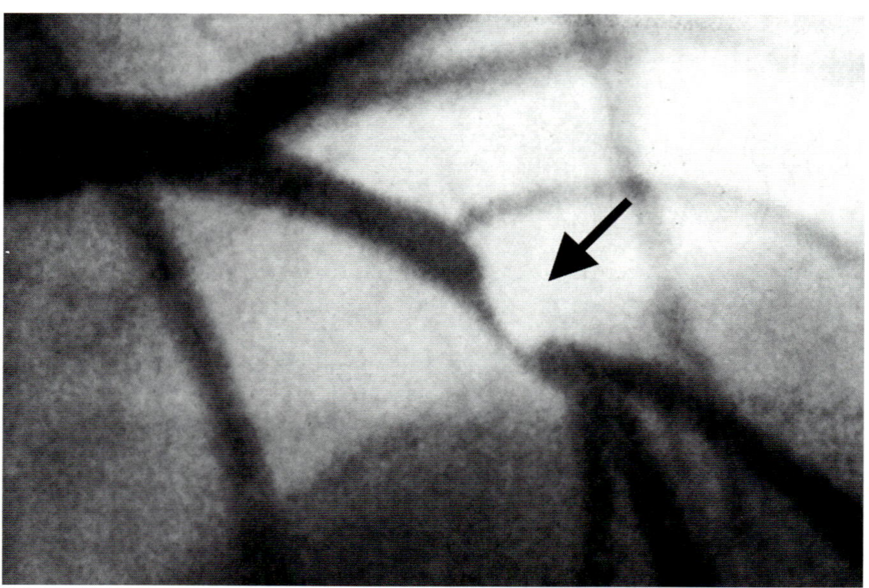

Are there specific "tricks-of-the-trade" to eliminate watermelon seeding?

John Douglas Jr., MD, USA: So called "watermelon seeding" is common, especially if the balloon has a slick coating and/or there is arterial tapering resulting in oversizing of one end of the balloon relative to the lumen it occupies. This can virtually always be managed by extremely slow balloon inflation. If this is not effective, I would try a tapered balloon (3.0-2.5 x 25 mm) or a slightly smaller long balloon without a slick coating (e.g. a 3.0 x 30 mm balloon).

Ferdinand Kiemeneij, MD, The Netherlands: The patient has an eccentric lesion in the LAD. If watermelon seeding occurs, I would try a slow inflation first, trying to keep the balloon centered in the stenosis by a "push-and-pull" technique.

If "watermelon seeding" persists, how would you approach this lesion?

John Douglas Jr., MD, USA: If "watermelon seeding" persists, I would implant a 3.5 mm Palmaz-Schatz stent or perform directional atherectomy using a 7F GTO Atherocath over a 0.014-inch Platinum-Plus guidewire, avoiding cuts along the normal wall. Adjunctive PTCA would be performed if necessary to achieve a residual stenosis < 20%. If chronicity of symptoms or advanced age suggest lesion calcification, IVUS might be useful to clarify the need for Rotablator atherectomy.

Ferdinand Kiemeneij, MD, The Netherlands: I would use a 30 mm balloon, which usually solves the problem. If this phenomenon persists, I would try a 3.25 mm cutting balloon. For an unsatisfactory result, I would implant a 14 mm Palmaz-Schatz stent. Other options are to perform Rotablator atherectomy with a 1.5 mm burr or directional atherectomy. Adjunctive imaging techniques are not necessary.

Editors' Perspective: "Watermelon-seeding" is a fairly common source of operator frustration. Generally, this problem arises when low-profile coated balloons are used to dilate rigid lesions. There are several approaches to this problem: One approach is to gently retract the balloon during slow inflation, to see if the balloon will "seat" across the lesion. Unfortunately, this maneuver often results in "watermelon-seeding" proximal to the stenosis. Another approach is to redilate the lesion with a long (30-40 mm) balloon, which generally works nicely. Since these lesions are frequently rigid, it is a good idea to use a noncompliant balloon, in case higher pressures are needed to achieve full balloon expansion. A third approach is to use Rotablator or directional atherectomy to "unroof" the rigid cap on the lesion and facilitate subsequent lumen enlargement. Although stenting has been suggested, we would be concerned about the ability to seat the stent in the lesion, and would not recommend stenting until the lesion can be fully expanded with a balloon.

*****

RESIDUAL STENOSIS: RCA

PTCA is performed using a 3.25 mm balloon (reference diameter = 3.1 mm), leaving a residual stenosis of 40% without dissection, thrombus, or impaired flow. Other vessels and left ventricular function are normal. The patient is pain-free.

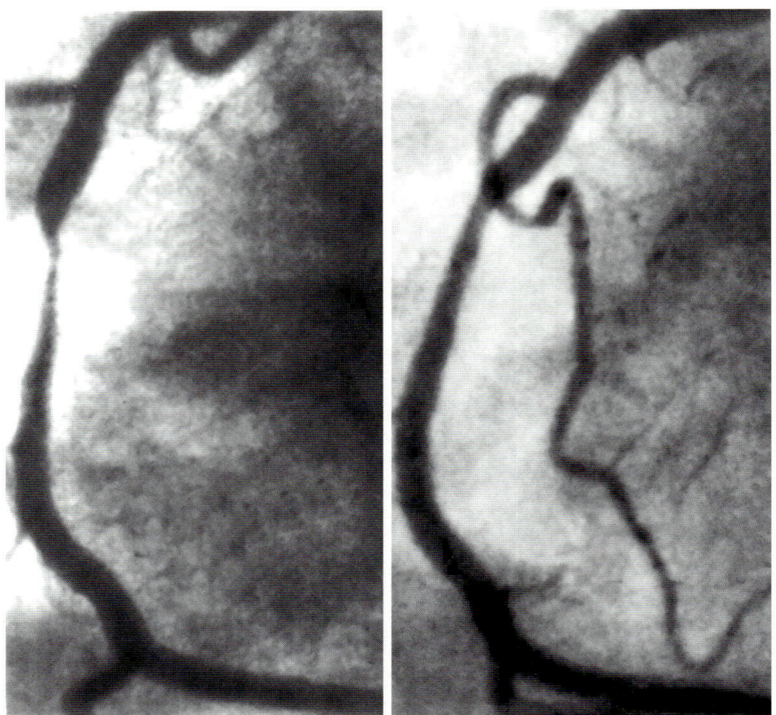

Following this "typical" PTCA outcome, would you do anything else to further assess your results?

Morton Kern, MD, USA: A 40% stenosis by angiography falls inside an intermediate range (40-70%), which may or may not be flow-limiting when measured directly with intracoronary flow velocity. There is a 50-50 chance that the residual stenosis will lead to early restenosis.

Richard Heuser, MD, USA: This stenosis has not been adequately dilated. With a 40% residual stenosis, restenosis is very likely. The entire lesion is perhaps 3 cm in length, so a 3.5 x 40 mm Wallstent is an excellent choice, using a 0.014-inch Extra-S'port wire and an 8F JR4 guide. Other options are the GR-II stent or multiple Palmaz-Schatz stents.

Takeshi Kimura, MD, Japan: This patient underwent "successful" PTCA, and will do well acutely. However, the final lumen diameter is suboptimal in the "new device era". The probability of restenosis is 40-50%.

If further assessment is warranted, what would you do?

Morton Kern, MD, USA: This typical PTCA result is satisfactory for many operators. A decision to proceed with further intervention is based on clinical features and restoration of normal coronary blood flow. An elderly individual may not require further intervention, but a younger patient might need a better result. IVUS at this point will tell me what I already know: There is residual plaque in the lumen. There are no criteria to determine whether the lumen is physiologically adequate, to assess the potential for restenosis or complications. The only way to identify a satisfactory physiologic result is to use a 0.014-inch FloWire and intracoronary adenosine (12 mcg), and stent the artery if coronary flow reserve is < 2.0.

Takeshi Kimura, MD, Japan: Although intravascular ultrasound might give us a little more information, clear guidelines have not been established for suboptimal PTCA. I would implant a 3.5 x 20 mm Palmaz-Schatz stent with a spiral articulation to reduce the risk of restenosis. I recommend an 8F JR4 guiding catheter (ID > 0.084-inch) without sideholes, and a 0.014-inch x 300 cm Extra-Support wire.

What do you recommend to operators who perform only PTCA?

Morton Kern, MD, USA: If in doubt and in-lab assessment is unavailable, STOP. If restenosis occurs, deal with it later as a stable problem. The use of stents has resulted in an "optical recalibration" of previously acceptable PTCA results. Operators now using stents have a hard time accepting residual lumen narrowing which they previously would have identified as satisfactory. Nonetheless, all should recognize the limitations of angiography and employ some objective data (such as flow reserve) to help guide decisions beyond the "calibrated eyeball."

Takeshi Kimura, MD, Japan: If the operator performs only conventional PTCA, a 3.5 mm balloon is acceptable to improve the suboptimal result. If the patient undergoes a second intervention for restenosis, referral to centers where stents are available is clearly indicated.

Editors' Perspective: Before the availability of stents, this type of angiographic result would have been considered a "success," even though the risk of angiographic restenosis (diameter stenosis > 50% at 6-months) is ~ 50% and the need for repeat intervention is ~ 30%. For operators who perform only PTCA, one option is to terminate the procedure and follow the patient clinically. A second option is to insert a perfusion balloon and perform a 5-30 minute inflation, with the hope that a better result will be achieved. A third option is to use higher pressures or larger balloons, but neither has been shown to improve results. In fact, oversize balloons (balloon/artery ratio > 1.1) may increase the risk of dissection and major complications. Finally, this patient could be referred to a center where stents are available. Unfortunately, the "right" answer is unknown. In most contemporary interventional practices, this lesion would be treated by stenting, because of the predictability of this approach and the expectation of a lower restenosis rate. If the Doppler guidewire is available, this is a perfect case for its use, since coronary flow reserve ≥ 2.0 predicts an excellent clinical outcome without further intervention.

*****

RESIDUAL STENOSIS: VEIN GRAFT

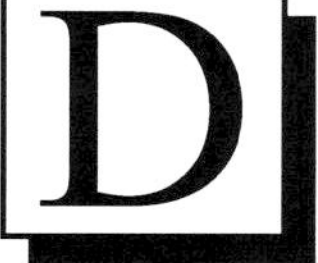

Directional atherectomy is performed on this focal vein graft lesion with a 7F AtheroCath (reference diameter = 4.0 mm). After 16 cuts, there is a mild residual stenosis.

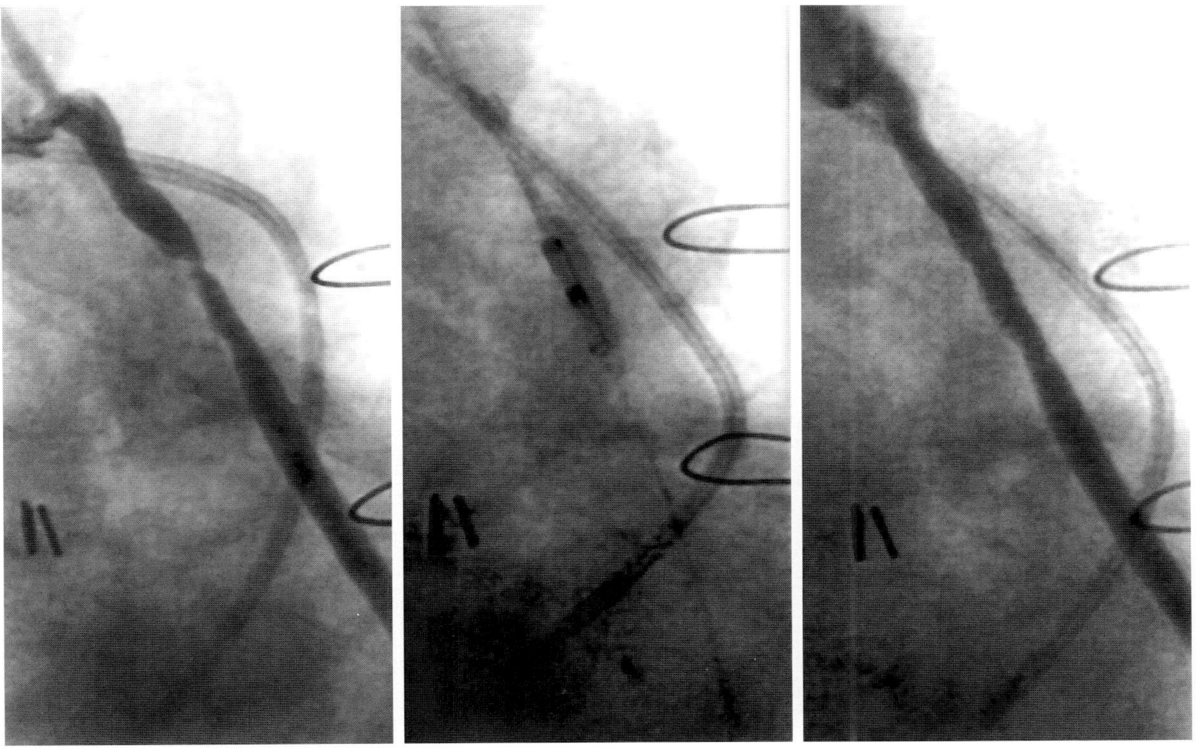

Is this result acceptable or suboptimal?

Richard Heuser, MD, USA: This is a suboptimal result with a significant residual lesion in a vein graft.

Morton Kern, MD, USA: This is an excellent result with mild luminal irregularities. By IVUS, however, atherectomy results are usually suboptimal; the long-term result is similar to PTCA.

If suboptimal, how would you optimize the result?

Richard Heuser, MD, USA: I would place a stent. Another option is to postdilate aggressively with a balloon, to achieve a superb angiographic and ultrasound result.

Morton Kern, MD, USA: The treatment of choice for residual stenosis in a vein graft is stent placement, to reduce restenosis. I would use a 4.0 x 20 mm biliary stent over a 0.014-inch Extra-Support wire, followed by high-pressure balloon expansion with 4.0 x 20 mm Titan at 15-20 ATM. After stenting, I recommend aspirin and ticlopidine, without Coumadin.

Are adjunctive imaging modalities useful?

Richard Heuser, MD, USA: If ultrasound confirms that the residual cross-sectional area is not significant, I would not perform further intervention.

Morton Kern, MD, USA: Before stenting, IVUS imaging might demonstrate residual plaque which could be addressed by further atherectomy and/or stenting.

Is conventional PTCA alone reasonable for this lesion?

Richard Heuser, MD, USA: I would never perform PTCA as sole therapy in vein grafts. A center that only does PTCA for such lesions should not be treating patients with vein graft stenoses.

Morton Kern, MD, USA: PTCA for vein graft lesions is generally unacceptable, due to high restenosis rates. Skip PTCA and refer the patient for directional atherectomy or primary stenting.

> **Editors' Perspective: In situations where atherectomy results in a mild persistent residual stenosis, the next course of action is to either perform additional atherectomy with the same AtheroCath at higher pressures, increase the size of the AtheroCath, or use adjunctive PTCA with a balloon/artery ratio ~ 1.0-1.1. Stenting is certainly feasible, and could have been employed as the original intervention without antecedent atherectomy.**

*****

INTRALUMINAL HAZINESS

A 58-year-old man with progressive angina and a severe stenosis in the RCA (left panel, reference diameter = 3.5 mm) is treated by PTCA with a 3.5 mm balloon (middle panel). In the orthogonal view, there is a moderate residual stenosis with intraluminal haziness (right panel). The patient is pain-free and has no ECG changes. Other vessels and left ventricular function are normal.

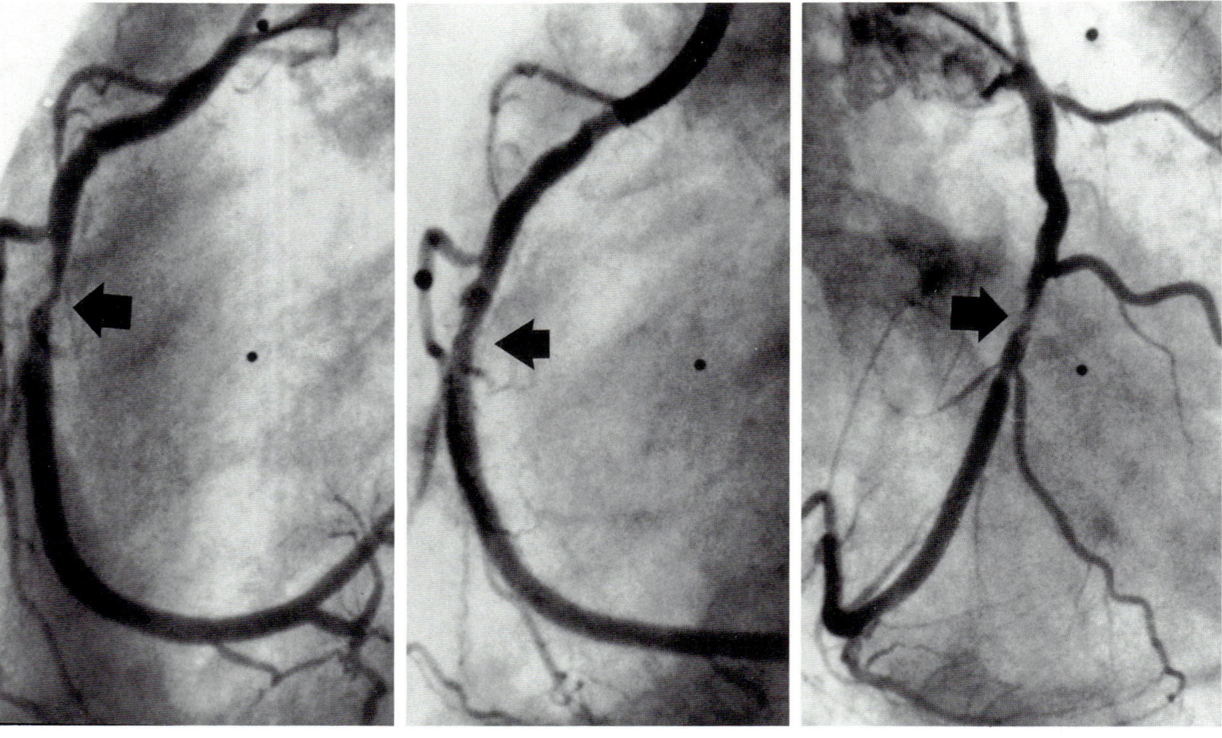

If you decide to terminate the procedure at this point, describe your post-PTCA management strategy.

Dean Kereiakes, MD, USA: This patient has a suboptimal result after PTCA, with moderate residual stenosis and intraluminal haziness. I would not terminate the procedure at this point because the risk of abrupt closure and late restenosis are clearly increased with this kind of suboptimal result.

Morton Kern, MD, USA: This patient has a severe irregular stenosis in the proximal RCA, with dissection and possible thrombus after PTCA. The LAO projection appears satisfactory, but the RAO projection is unacceptable. A suboptimal PTCA result has a high likelihood of abrupt closure; lesion stabilization should be assured prior to discharge from the lab.

Marty Leon, MD, USA: This is a suboptimal result after aggressive PTCA with a 3.5 mm balloon. There is moderate residual stenosis with haziness, plaque disruption, intimal irregularity, and possible dissection. I would definitely not leave this vessel in its current state without further therapy.

Is further assessment and/or intervention warranted?

Dean Kereiakes, MD, USA: I recommend further intervention with directional atherectomy or intracoronary stent placement. My first choice is to place a 3.5 mm Palmaz-Schatz stent. I would also administer a bolus and infusion of ReoPro, but no heparin after the procedure. I recommend aspirin and ticlopidine (250 mg BID for 1 month); I do not use Lovenox.

Morton Kern, MD, USA: I would continue with a prolonged balloon inflation using a 3.5 x 20 mm perfusion balloon (a Flowtrack-40 or RX-perfusion balloon), withdrawing the guidewire and guiding catheter to permit perfusion. After 5-10 minutes, I would reassess the stenosis by angiography. If haziness persists, I would administer intravenous ReoPro and place a 3.5 mm Palmaz-Schatz stent over a 0.014-inch Extra-S'port wire. Had I started the procedure with a Doppler FloWire, I would check coronary flow reserve prior to stent placement. If flow reserve is < 2.0, I would place a stent. Following stent placement, heparin would be discontinued and aspirin and ticlopidine would be prescribed.

Marty Leon, MD, USA: I would proceed immediately with stent placement using a 9F JL4 guiding catheter with sideholes, an ACS Extra-Support wire, a single 3.5 mm Palmaz-Schatz stent, and adjunctive PTCA with a high-pressure balloon guided by intravascular ultrasound. This vessel may be somewhat larger than it appears on the angiogram, and adjunctive PTCA with a 4.0 mm balloon may be necessary. I would not be satisfied with a residual stenosis > 0%. After an excellent angiographic result, my anticoagulation regimen would include aspirin and ticlopidine. If the result is suboptimal (residual dissection or stenosis), I would use ReoPro and/or 36-hours of intravenous heparin followed by 2 weeks of Lovenox. The dose of ReoPro for a suboptimal result (residual dissection, intraluminal thrombus, or residual stenosis) is the same dose used in the EPILOG study, which includes weight adjusted Heparin (70-100 units/kg) followed by a ReoPro bolus (0.25 mg/kg) and infusion (10 mcg/kg) for 12 hours.

Editors' Perspective: Intraluminal haziness is a common, relatively nonspecific angiographic finding after conventional PTCA. Although some operators equate intraluminal haziness with thrombus, the most common causes are intimal dissection and residual plaque. The following approach to the hazy result may be useful: First, confirm that the ACT is ≥ 300 seconds. Because of the lack of specificity of intraluminal haziness for thrombus, intracoronary lytic therapy is not recommended. Second, attempt to achieve optimal PTCA results using a full-size balloon (balloon/artery ratio ~ 1.0) for at least 2 minutes at nominal inflation pressure. If inflations are not tolerated or if longer inflations are desired, a perfusion balloon can be used. Third, consider use of IVUS (to help identify residual plaque and dissection) or angioscopy (the most sensitive tool for distinguishing thrombus, dissection, and residual plaque). Although these techniques are not mandatory, they can be useful in individual cases to help assess the results and guide further intervention, if necessary. Finally, as described by each of our experts, a practical solution to this problem is to simply implant a stent, because of the reliability and predictability of this approach.

*****

NEW FILLING DEFECTS

A tubular lesion in the vein graft to the LCX (reference diameter = 4.8 mm) is treated with a 4.5 mm balloon, leaving a moderate residual stenosis with considerable intraluminal filling defects and normal antegrade flow. The patient has mild chest pain and no ECG changes.

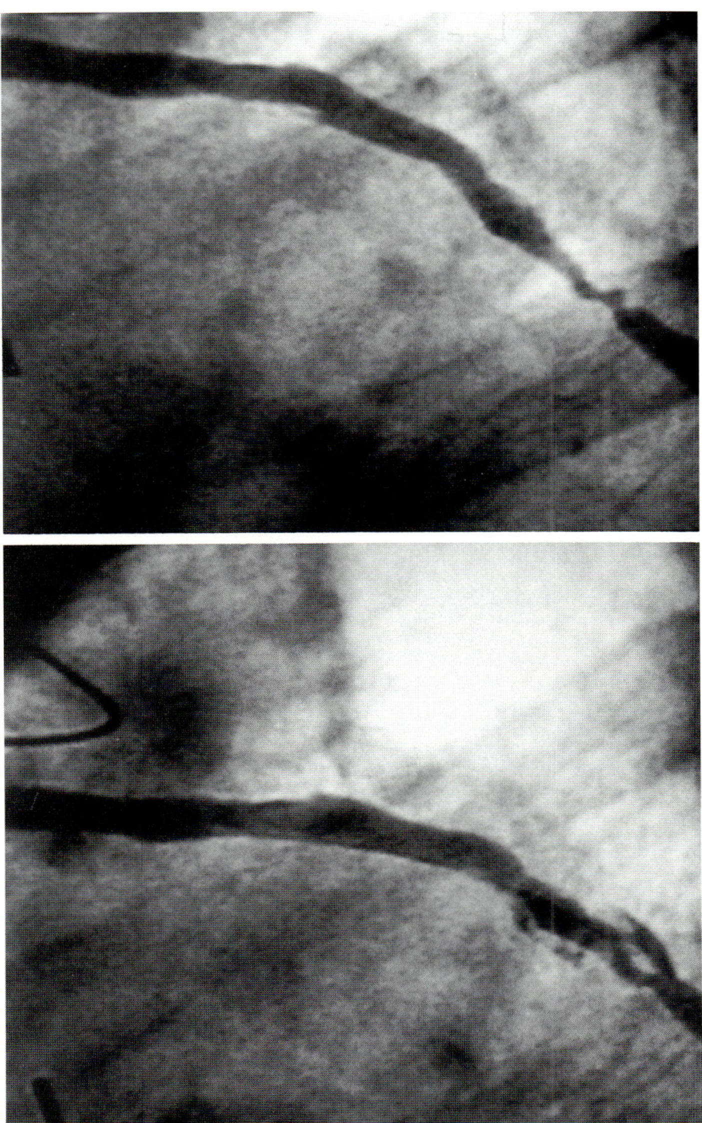

What is your impression of this angiographic result?

Masakiyo Nobuyoshi, MD, Japan: The angiograms show a tubular lesion in the vein graft with a large dissection and considerable intraluminal filling defects. If therapy is not added, abrupt closure may occur.

Richard Heuser, MD, USA: This patient had a tubular lesion with intraluminal filling defects, which could lead to abrupt closure.

Marie-Claude Morice, MD, France: This is a very suboptimal result after PTCA in a large graft with significant filling defects. This is a difficult situation with a high risk of complications, especially distal embolization, no-reflow, and myocardial infarction. Furthermore, there is a very high risk of restenosis.

How would you manage this lesion now?

Masakiyo Nobuyoshi, MD, Japan: I would implant a stent to obtain a well defined lumen; stenting is safer than directional atherectomy. I would use an 8F Judkins guide, a 0.014-inch guidewire, a 4.0 mm Palmaz-Schatz stent, and adjunctive PTCA with a 4.5 mm x 20 mm balloon at 10 ATM.

Richard Heuser, MD, USA: I would deploy a nonarticulated biliary stent on a 4.5 x 20 mm Schwarten peripheral balloon at 8 ATM, and postdilate with a 5.0 x 20 mm peripheral balloon.

Marie-Claude Morice, MD, France: In this situation, my primary choice is a Wallstent. I would select a 5.0 mm x 30 mm Wallstent to cover the whole lesion. The Wallstent is self-expanding, has good trackability, and can be used with a large-lumen 9F guiding catheter. I would smoothe the result with a 5.0 mm balloon. If no-reflow occurs, I would use verapamil.

Are other imaging modalities useful or necessary?

Masakiyo Nobuyoshi, MD, Japan: IVUS is necessary for evaluating the residual stenosis and the true lumen. If the dissection is not circumferential and residual stenosis is present, higher pressure is required. If the dissection is circumferential, higher pressures may result in rupture.

Richard Heuser, MD, USA: I wonder if this lesion is due to thrombus or dissection. Angioscopy is helpful to resolve this issue. If intraluminal thrombus is present, I would not proceed with a biliary stent.

Marie-Claude Morice, MD, France: I would not use angioscopy or ultrasound.

What adjunctive medical therapy would you recommend?

Masakiyo Nobuyoshi, MD, Japan: Medical therapy includes heparin, aspirin, and ticlopidine, as with any other stent implantation.

Richard Heuser, MD, USA: ReoPro might be useful.

Marie-Claude Morice, MD, France: Following a good angiographic result, this patient would receive the same treatment as all stented patients: ticlopidine and aspirin.

Editors' Perspective: This lesion has a disturbing angiographic appearance after PTCA, and angiography alone cannot accurately distinguish the relative contributions of dissection, thrombus, and plaque separation. Although angioscopy can be used to make these distinctions, most operators do not use it, and the future of angioscopy is questionable (at least from a marketing standpoint). The most important aspect of treating this patient is to stabilize the lesion and prevent abrupt closure; this is best accomplished by intracoronary stenting. The choice of stents is wide, but virtually all balloon-expandable (e.g., Palmaz biliary stent and all coronary stents) and self-expanding (e.g., as the Wallstent) stents would work nicely. Directional atherectomy is a reasonable technique, but would require exchange of vascular sheaths and guiding catheters, and could add considerable complexity to the procedure. Although ReoPro might be a useful adjunct, it is doubtful that ReoPro alone would have much impact on stabilizing this awful result.

*****

PERSISTENT FILLING DEFECTS

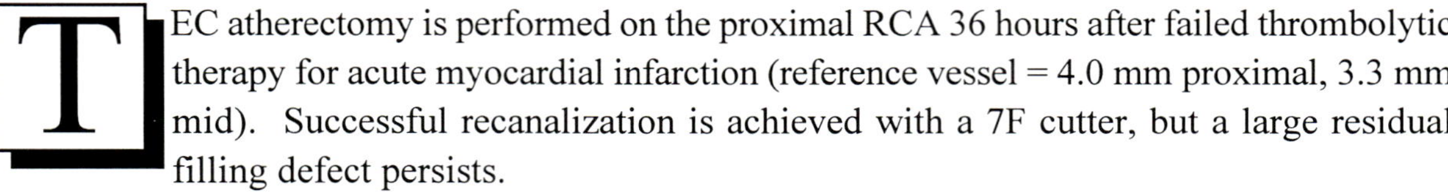

TEC atherectomy is performed on the proximal RCA 36 hours after failed thrombolytic therapy for acute myocardial infarction (reference vessel = 4.0 mm proximal, 3.3 mm mid). Successful recanalization is achieved with a 7F cutter, but a large residual filling defect persists.

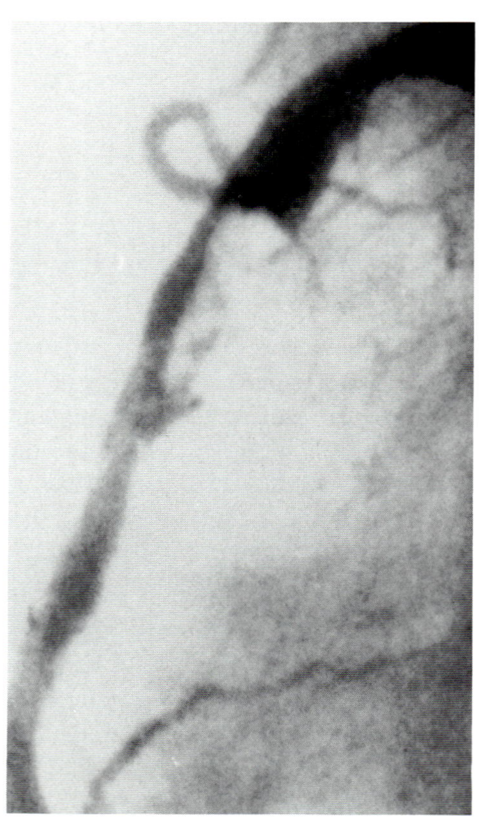

What do you recommend now?

Ferdinand Kiemeneij, MD, The Netherlands: I would insert a Tracker infusion catheter and infuse intracoronary streptokinase (50,000-100,000 units/hr for 24 hours). If the defect persists, I would perform PTCA on the RCA 2 weeks later, and pretreat with ReoPro.

Dean Kereiakes, MD, USA: There is a persistent large intraluminal filling defect following successful recanalization of the RCA with a 7F TEC cutter, consistent with residual organized thrombus 36-48 hours old. I look at this case largely as a mechanical problem. Although some interventionists would place a Dispatch catheter and delivery local urokinase (150,000 units over 30 minutes), the likelihood of achieving significant dissolution of organized thrombus and a good angiographic result is low. If available, I recommend a rheolytic thrombectomy catheter, such as the Possis AngioJet, which may be more effective at thrombus extraction. An alternative is to administer a bolus and infusion of ReoPro, followed by stenting to compress the thrombus.

Eric Topol, MD, USA: A Dispatch catheter can be deployed for local delivery of urokinase (250,00 units), followed by repeat angiography. Then I would consider conventional PTCA or stenting. An alternative strategy is to administer ReoPro (intravenous bolus and infusion), followed by PTCA or stenting.

Describe your anticoagulation regimen.

Ferdinand Kiemeneij, MD, The Netherlands: Medications consists of aspirin (500 mg IV) just before the procedure, bolus and 12-hour infusion of ReoPro, and weight-adjusted heparin at the start of intervention. I would continue heparin for 5 days (PTT 60-80 seconds), aspirin forever, and Coumadin for 1 month.

Dean Kereiakes, MD, USA: I would administer intravenous ReoPro in the standard intravenous weight-adjusted bolus and 12-hour infusion. Intravenous heparin would not be administered after the procedure until femoral hemostasis is achieved and the femstop device is applied. Following application of the femstop device, I would start intravenous heparin (10 units/kg) and monitor PTT every 6 hours with a target range of 50-70 seconds. I would discharge the patient on aspirin and Coumadin (INR of 2-3) for at least 1 month, at which time I recommend an outpatient angiogram.

Editors' Perspective: The presence of intracoronary thrombus substantially increases the risk of distal embolization, no-reflow, and myocardial infarction associated with percutaneous therapy. In the present case, persistent thrombus after TEC suggests the presence of a large clot burden or residual organized thrombus. Several mechanical and pharmacological approaches to residual thrombus exist: First, since there is normal antegrade flow and only a moderate residual stenosis, the patient could be treated with 2-4 weeks of oral Coumadin or subcutaneous heparin to "clean-up" the vessel. Repeat angiography could be performed with more definitive revascularization at that point, if needed. A second approach is to dissolve residual thrombus immediately after TEC, using intracoronary (bolus, prolonged infusion, or local delivery) or intravenous thrombolytic agents (tPA, urokinase, streptokinase). A third approach is to mechanically remove thrombus with directional atherectomy or direct aspiration via a supraselective catheter. Although devices such as the Hydrolyzer and AngioJet are very effective at removing fresh thrombus, they are not yet widely available. Finally, bolus plus infusion of ReoPro with PTCA or directional atherectomy could be utilized, although the value of ReoPro in this setting has not been adequately tested. While a larger (7.5F) TEC cutter may be able to aspirate additional clot, cutter/artery ratios > 0.7 increase the risk of vessel injury.

*****

FOCAL DISSECTION

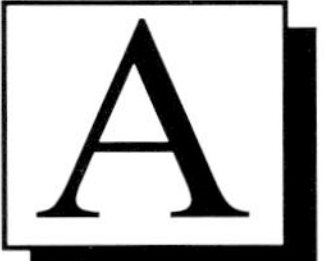

A 58-year-old man undergoes conventional PTCA of a focal stenosis in the proximal LCX, resulting in a non-flow-limiting dissection with an extraluminal "cap."

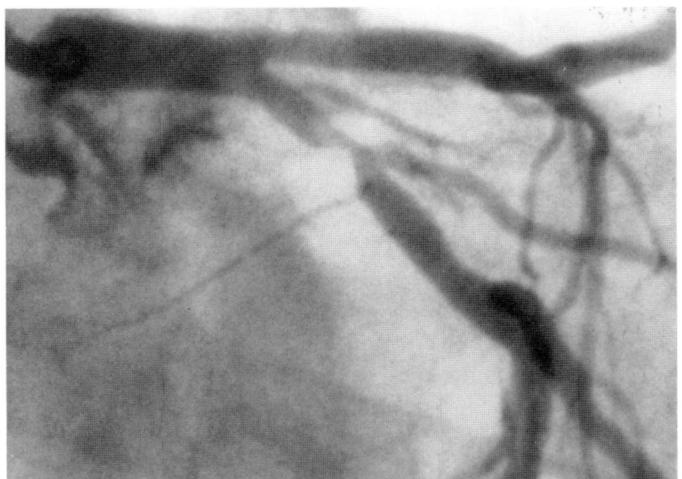

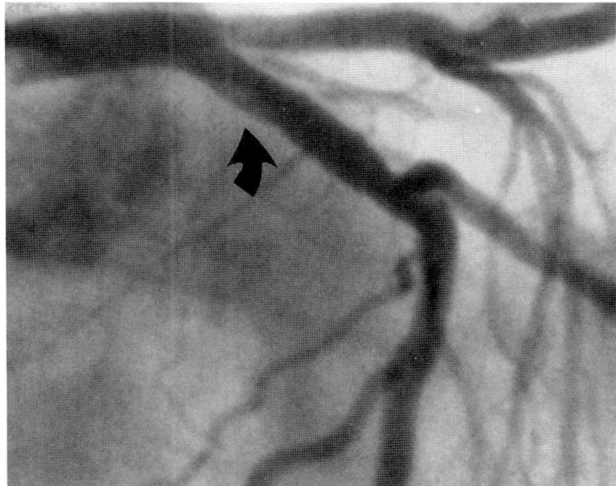

How would you manage this patient?

Donald Baim, MD, USA: Given the wide array of devices available, this is not a lesion that I would have treated with PTCA, given its marked eccentricity. Either directional atherectomy or coronary stent placement would have been better choices. The fact that PTCA was performed means that the operator should not be surprised by the presence of a residual stenosis and intimal defect. In that regard, this is a "typical" PTCA result, and should be managed with conventional care. The dissection is not sufficiently large or threatening to warrant bailout stent placement, but ReoPro (bolus and infusion) is reasonable to decrease the risk of abrupt closure.

Patrick Serruys, MD, PhD, The Netherlands: I would accept this result. The patient would receive aspirin (100 mg QD) and nifedipine (20 mg TID for 48 hours).

Ulrich Sigwart, MD, England: The chance of restenosis after such an unsatisfactory result is very high. I would not have the slightest hesitation in placing a Palmaz-Schatz stent in this lesion; it can be safely dilated to 4.0 mm. I would discharge the patient the next day on aspirin.

Marty Leon, MD, USA: This patient has an extraluminal "cap" dissection in the proximal LCX. At this time, I would make several additional assessments: First, it is important to wait 10-15 minutes to be certain that this is a stable focal dissection without further lumen compromise or ischemic sequelae. Second, I would definitely perform multiple angiographic views and intravascular ultrasound. If there is progressive lumen compromise, extension of the dissection, worsening of contrast retention, or diameter stenosis > 30% (by online QCA or ultrasound), I favor immediate stent placement. In the absence of these findings, I would simply observe the lesion. Previously, I recommended prolonged heparin infusion for patients with residual dissection. However, at the present time, I recommend ReoPro, removal of sheaths, and reinstitution of low-dose heparin for 12-24 hours. I predict that there is a 33% chance that stent placement will be required.

Editors' Perspective: This is a fairly typical result after conventional PTCA. If the operator has little experience with new devices, there are a number of alternatives to treat this fairly typical result after PTCA. First, in spite of the minor dissection (which is how PTCA works), this result may remain stable, and the procedure could be terminated at this point. If the operator is reluctant to pursue further intervention, it would be prudent to observe the patient in the catheterization laboratory for 15 minutes, and repeat the angiogram in multiple projections to be certain the result is stable. A second approach is to gather additional information about the lesion, using any one of a number of different techniques. The easiest technique is to advance the balloon catheter into the distal vessel and measure a translesional gradient. Although routine pressure gradient measurements have fallen out of favor, identification of a pressure gradient < 15 mmHg may be reassuring, whereas a gradient > 30 mmHg suggests that the result is unsatisfactory (a gradient of 15-30 mmHg is in the "gray zone"). Intravascular ultrasound can provide additional information about the nature and extent of dissection and more precise quantitation of lumen geometry. Measurement of coronary flow reserve with the Doppler FloWire is quick and easy, and offers important physiologic information that correlates with outcome; coronary flow reserve > 2 would argue against the need for further intervention. Another advantage of the Doppler FloWire is the potential for following trends in blood flow velocity over 15 minutes, which can be used to predict complications. Of all imaging modalities, angioscopy is probably the least useful, since it will simply corroborate the presence of dissection, but offers no quantitative or physiologic data. A third approach is to perform a prolonged inflation with a perfusion balloon, which could potentially "tack-up" the dissection flap and improve the angiographic result; before the availability of stents, this would have been considered "standard fare" for this lesion. Any of the above recommendations could be employed with ReoPro, although further studies using

this potent antiplatelet agent are required before firm recommendations can be offered. Data suggest that prolonged postprocedural heparin not only fails to prevent ischemic complications, but may increase bleeding and vascular injury. Finally, this lesion could be easily and successfully treated with virtually any stent. Directional atherectomy should be avoided since the presence of an extraluminal cap suggests medial dissection, which is associated with a higher risk of vessel perforation.

*****

FOCAL DISSECTION DURING ACUTE MI

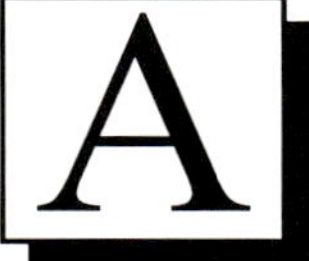

58-year-old man undergoes conventional PTCA of the proximal LCX (reference vessel = 3.5 mm) for acute myocardial infarction, resulting in restoration of TIMI-3 flow. There is a moderate residual stenosis with a focal "cap" and dye stain (arrow). The patient is asymptomatic and other vessels are normal.

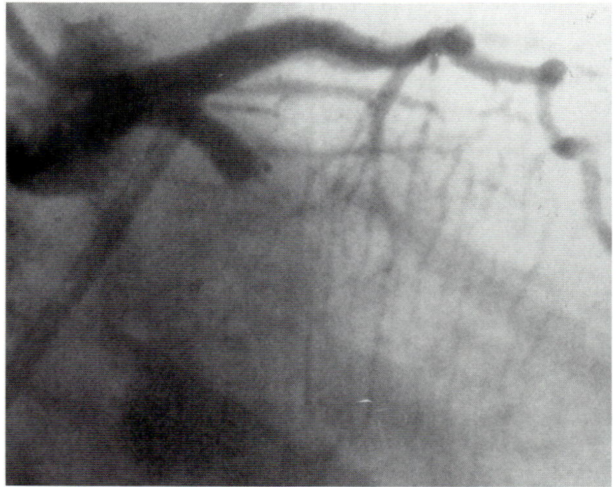

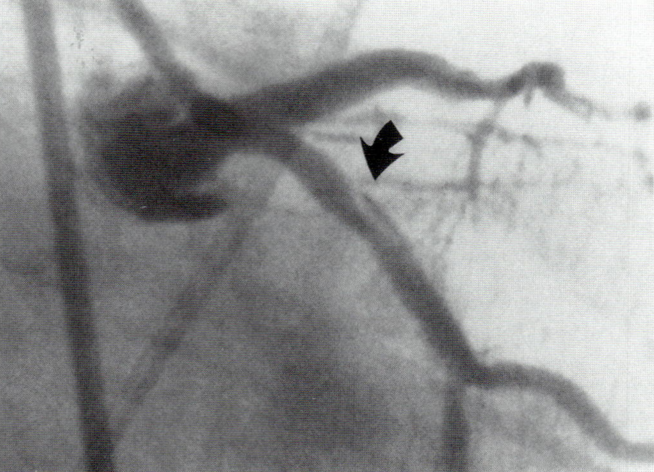

How would you manage this patient now?

Donald Baim, MD, USA: This patient has just undergone primary PTCA for acute myocardial infarction, producing a sizeable dissection in the mid-LCX. Although stent placement has been avoided in the peri-infarction period, I have had quite favorable results providing that good antegrade flow can be restored. I would place a 3.5 mm Palmaz-Schatz stent in this dissection and postdilate with a high-pressure balloon. The medical regimen would include aspirin, ticlopidine and low-molecular weight heparin (Lovenox 30 mg BID for 10 days).

Patrick Serruys, MD, PhD, The Netherlands: This is an unsatisfactory angiographic result in a reasonably large vessel in the setting of acute myocardial infarction. My current practice is to implant a 15 mm Palmaz-Schatz stent and postdilate using a noncompliant balloon at ≥ 16 ATM. Using quantitative angiography I would ensure a diameter stenosis < 10% after stent implantation, with a satisfactory step-up and step-down. I would perform intravascular ultrasound. My current practice is to give ReoPro for 12 hours, as well as aspirin and ticlopidine in the cath lab. I would leave the sheath in for 24 hours, and continue heparin.

Ulrich Sigwart, MD, England: My approach to this lesion is implantation of a Palmaz-Schatz or MultiLink stent. There is mounting evidence that stenting is not contraindicated in acute myocardial infarction. I recommend ReoPro, aspirin, and ticlopidine. The sheath should be taken out the same day, and if the result is perfect after stenting, there is no reason to prescribe Coumadin.

Marty Leon, MD, USA: Direct PTCA for acute MI is complicated by severe dissection and residual stenosis; stent implantation is appropriate. I would use an 8F transitionless left coronary guiding catheter (such as Cordis XB 3.5) and an Extra-support guidewire (the ACS Extra-Support wire, the Extra-S'port wire, or the Cordis Stabilizer-Plus). I would choose a 3.5 mm Palmaz-Schatz stent and use intravascular ultrasound to guide further adjunctive PTCA. I anticipate an excellent angiographic result without complications. The interesting question is adjunctive pharmacology. I would treat this patient with aspirin, ticlopidine (250 mg BID for 2 weeks), and ReoPro. It is my recent practice to use intravenous ReoPro for suboptimal results after bailout stenting for acute myocardial infarction, characterized by residual dissection at the stent margins, in-stent residual stenosis, or intraluminal haziness suggesting thrombus. I believe that ReoPro is the best choice for preventing stent thrombosis in this situation. After removal of the sheaths when the ACT reaches 150 seconds, I would continue ReoPro for 12 hours. Assuming the groin is stable, I would continue intravenous heparin for 24-36 hours (PTT 40-70 seconds). I would not use extended heparin therapy, outpatient subcutaneous heparin, or oral Coumadin.

Editors' Perspective: After primary PTCA, the risk of recurrent ischemia before discharge is approximately 10-15%; it is likely that many of these events are associated with the type of angiographic result observed in this patient. All of the considerations discussed in the previous case also apply to this patient, with the exception of the utility of the Doppler FloWire, since abnormal coronary flow reserve is difficult to interpret during acute myocardial infarction. The main issue surrounding this case is whether stents can be safely implanted during acute myocardial infarction. Data from our own institution and others suggest that stents should not be withheld from patients with failed primary PTCA, since the risk of stent thrombosis in this setting is no higher than for bailout stenting without acute myocardial infarction. When stenting is performed, contemporary studies suggest that Coumadin may be associated with a higher incidence of bleeding and ischemic complications than combined antiplatelet therapy with aspirin and ticlopidine. The use of ReoPro is unproven, but not unreasonable.

*****

FOCAL DISSECTION: ABRUPT CLOSURE

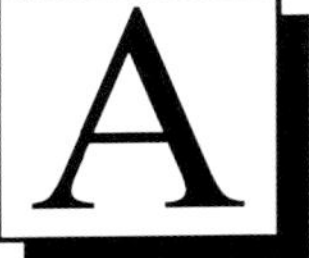

A 58-year-old man undergoes conventional PTCA of the proximal RCA, which is complicated by a focal dissection and TIMI-2 flow. The patient develops hypotension and bradycardia.

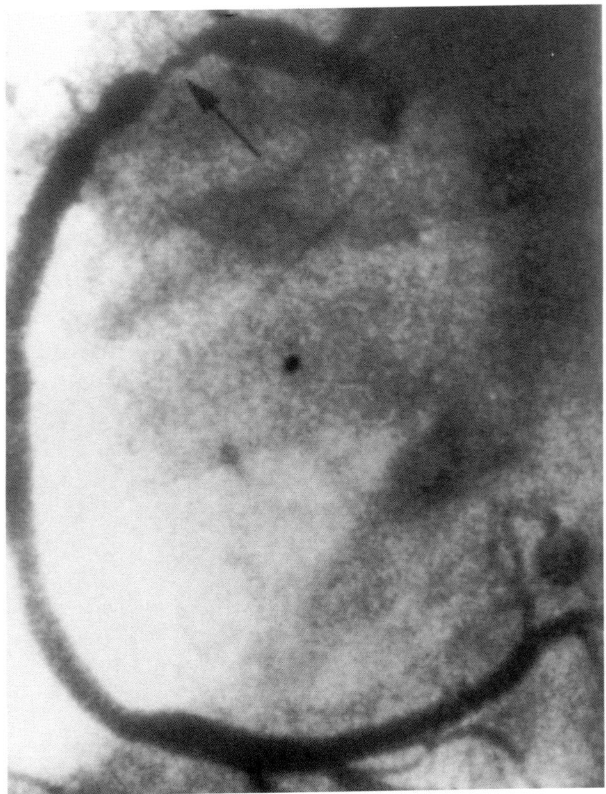

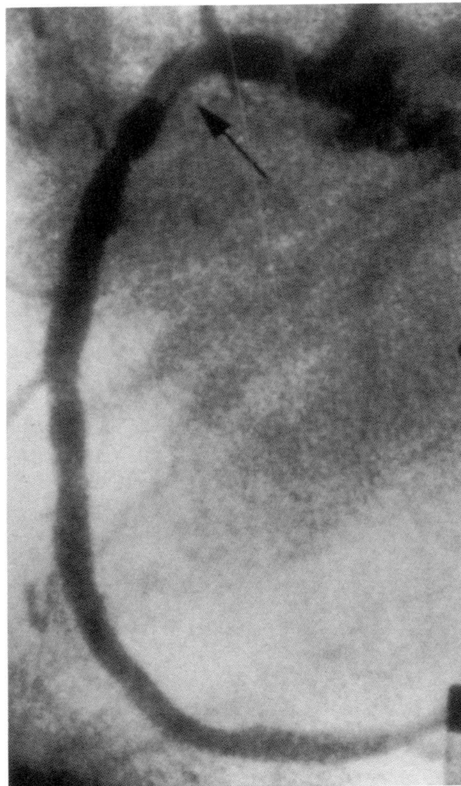

How would you manage this patient now?

Donald Baim, MD, USA: This is obviously a threatening dissection with hypotension, bradycardia, and reduced flow. When John Simpson and I did this case in 1980, there was no alternative but emergency surgery. Through the late 1980's, I would have attempted repeat PTCA, probably with prolonged inflations with a perfusion balloon. In the 1990's, the treatment for such a dissection is stenting using a Palmaz-Schatz or GR-II stent.

David Foley, MD, The Netherlands: The patient has a focal dissection with TIMI-2 flow, associated with hypotension and bradycardia. I would administer intravenous atropine, insert a temporary pacemaker, and deploy a 20 mm Gianturco-Roubin stent without further delay. A 15 mm Palmaz-Schatz stent would also be eminently suitable. Other considerations include a 15 mm ACS MultiLink stent, a 15 mm Cordis stent, a 16 mm Nir stent, a 20 mm Wallstent, or a 20 mm Freedom stent. The choice of stent depends on operator preference. Assuming an optimal angiographic result with residual stenosis < 10%, the patient would be discharged the following day on ticlopidine, aspirin, and nifedipine.

Ulrich Sigwart, MD, England: I would have no hesitation in putting a stent into this lesion. The quicker the better! An Extra-Support wire would help to advance the stent. A Wallstent is ideal if available; any other stent can be used as well. Aspirin alone is sufficient.

> **Editors' Perspective: This focal but severe dissection is best treated by stenting — virtually any stent would work nicely. Directional atherectomy is a reasonable alternative, since the dissection is focal and does not involve the deep layers of the arterial wall. For operators who perform only PTCA, prolonged balloon inflations with a perfusion balloon may reverse abrupt closure. Since flow impairment appears to be caused by dissection and/or plaque separation, rather than thrombus, it is doubtful that ReoPro alone would be beneficial.**

*****

DISSECTION & ABRUPT CLOSURE DURING ACUTE MI

Baseline angiography during acute anterior myocardial infarction reveals subtotal occlusion of the mid-LAD (reference vessel = 3.0 mm, open arrowhead) and TIMI-2 flow (closed arrowhead). After PTCA with a 3.0 x 20 mm balloon, there is a severe residual stenosis (open arrowhead) and TIMI-2 flow (closed arrowhead). Chest pain and ST elevation persist despite prolonged balloon inflations.

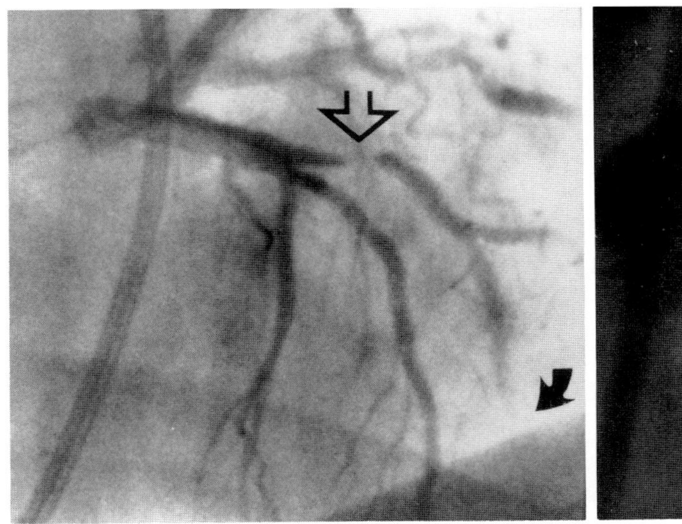

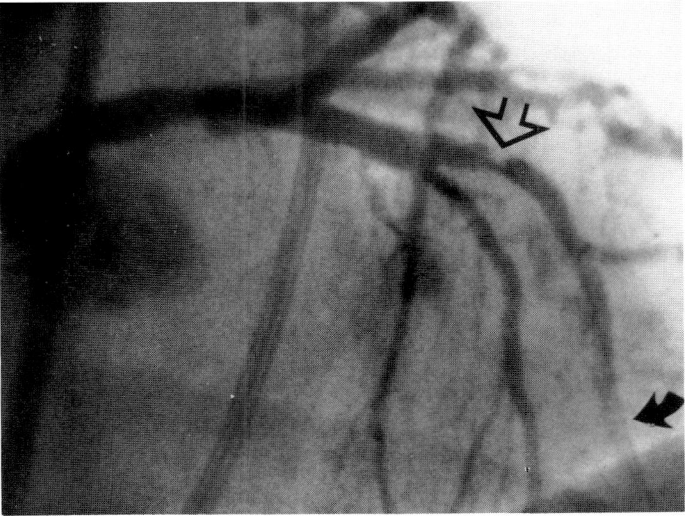

How would you manage this patient now?

Marie-Claude Morice, MD, France: In this case there is severe residual stenosis and delayed flow due to dissection, although the dissection is not very visible. I would immediately implant a Palmaz-Schatz 154 stent and postdilate with a 3.0 x 10 mm balloon at 16-18 ATM. In case of persistent flow impairment despite a good angiographic result, I would use intracoronary nitrates, verapamil, and ReoPro until TIMI-3 flow is obtained. I hardly ever use intracoronary lytics. The patient will receive heparin (for 72 hours), ticlopidine, and aspirin.

Dean Kereiakes, MD, USA: This is a focal, high-grade obstruction with well-defined margins. These defects are usually not thrombotic and do not respond well to coil stent placement. My approach is to place a 3.0 mm Palmaz-Schatz stent, and postdilate at ≥ 18 ATM. Adjunctive ReoPro is beneficial to reduce the incidence of embolization, subendocardial infarction and "slow flow," particularly in the setting of myocardial infarction. I would maintain the patient on aspirin and ticlopidine (250 mg BID for 1 month) following the procedure. I would not use Coumadin, intracoronary lytic therapy, or prolonged heparin.

Masakiyo Nobuyoshi, MD, Japan: I would implant a Palmaz-Schatz stent. In my experience, a high success rate is achieved by stenting, even during acute myocardial infarction. The likelihood of distal embolization is small. Post-interventional therapy includes heparin, aspirin, ticlopidine, and urokinase (96,000 units IV over 12 hours).

> **Editors' Perspective: Emergency bypass surgery is rarely undertaken in the setting of failed PTCA for acute myocardial infarction. Treatment options include repeat PTCA with a perfusion balloon for 15-30 minutes, directional atherectomy to resect the intimal flap, and stenting. As with most other dissections, the most reliable method for treating abrupt closure is stent implantation.**

*****

VEIN GRAFT DISSECTION

In preparation for stent implantation in this tubular vein graft stenosis (reference diameter = 3.7 mm, straight arrow, left panel), PTCA is performed with a 3.5 x 40 mm balloon (middle panel). After PTCA, the original lesion improves, but there is a focal dissection at the distal end of the balloon (curved arrow, right panel). The patient is asymptomatic.

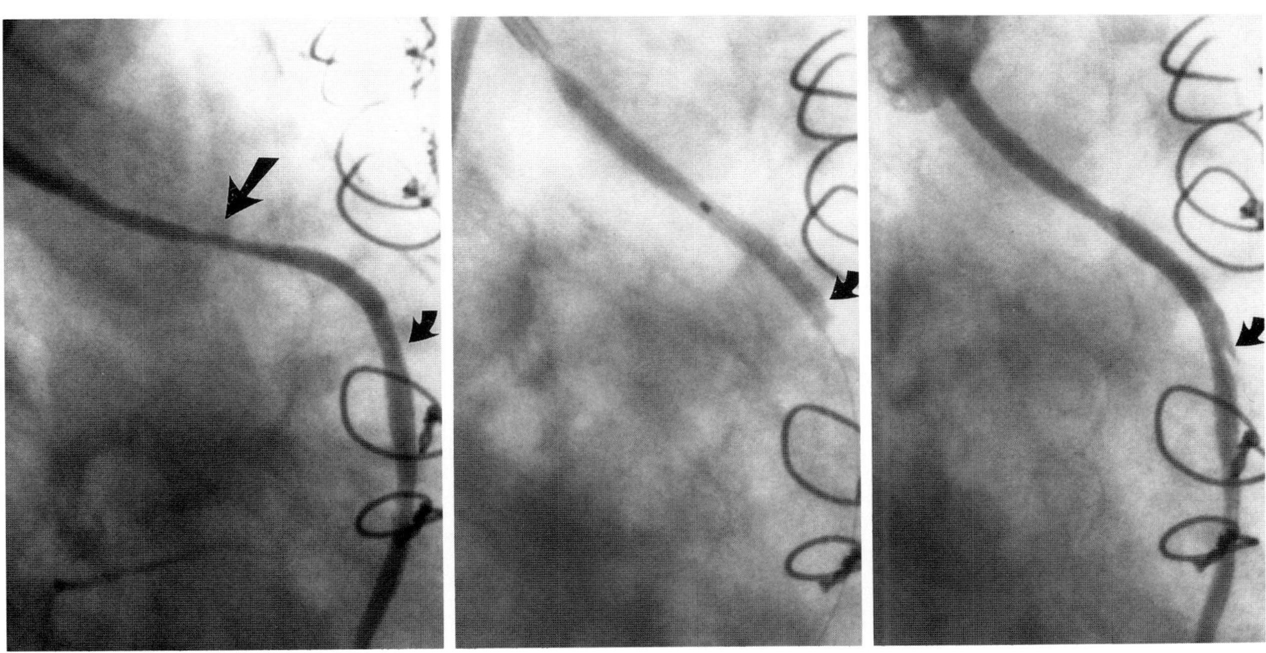

Please describe how you would have approached the original lesion, and what you recommend now.

Antonio Colombo, MD, Italy: Dissection at the time of PTCA prior to stenting is not a rare complication. It is rarely a problem, provided the operator meticulously stents the entire segment. In this particular situation the only problem is the lack of a stent of appropriate length. The lesion can be treated with multiple 4.0 mm Palmaz-Schatz or biliary stents, or ideally, a 4-6 cm

Wallstent. Following high-pressure dilation, IVUS should be performed.

Paul Teirstein, MD, USA: This is a long stenosis in the body of a vein graft. I believe the data are overwhelming to support the use of stents to treat vein graft stenoses. I would place 2-3 Palmaz-Schatz coronary stents, deploying the first stent just distal to the dissection, where the sternal wire intersects the vein graft. I would then work back to the ostium so that the entire lesion would be covered with coronary stents. I would then use a 3.75-4.0 mm high-pressure balloon at 16-20 ATM. I would use intravascular ultrasound as part of an ongoing randomized trial at Scripps Clinic. Assuming I achieve a pristine result, I would discharge the patient the next morning on aspirin and ticlopidine (250 mg BID).

Ulrich Sigwart, MD, England: The first balloon looks slightly long and oversized; I would have used a 3.0 x 30 mm balloon. Now, after the dissection occurs, I would implant multiple stents. I prefer two PS204 stents at high pressure, or a Wallstent.

> **Editors' Perspective: When PTCA is used to treat a lesion before stent implantation, the dilation strategy is different than for definitive PTCA. When preparing such a lesion for stenting, PTCA should be performed at nominal pressure (unless higher pressures are needed to fully expand the lesion) using a slightly undersized balloon (0.5 mm less than the reference diameter); this will preserve the "shoulders" of the lesion to facilitate proper stent position, and minimize the risk of dissection. When long balloons are used to predilate focal or tubular lesions, there is risk of dissection at the end of the balloon, which would then require multiple stents to cover the original lesion and distal dissection; balloon length should be selected just to cover the diseased segment.**

*****

LEFT MAIN DISSECTION

The mid-LAD (top left; reference vessel = 3.0 mm) is dilated with a 3.5 x 40 mm balloon (top right); abrupt closure ensues (middle left), and during deployment of a 3.0 mm Gianturco-Roubin stent, a contrast stain is noted (middle right, large arrowhead). Subsequent angiography (bottom) reveals a complex dissection involving the distal left main, proximal LCX, and LAD. Chest pain and ECG changes persist.

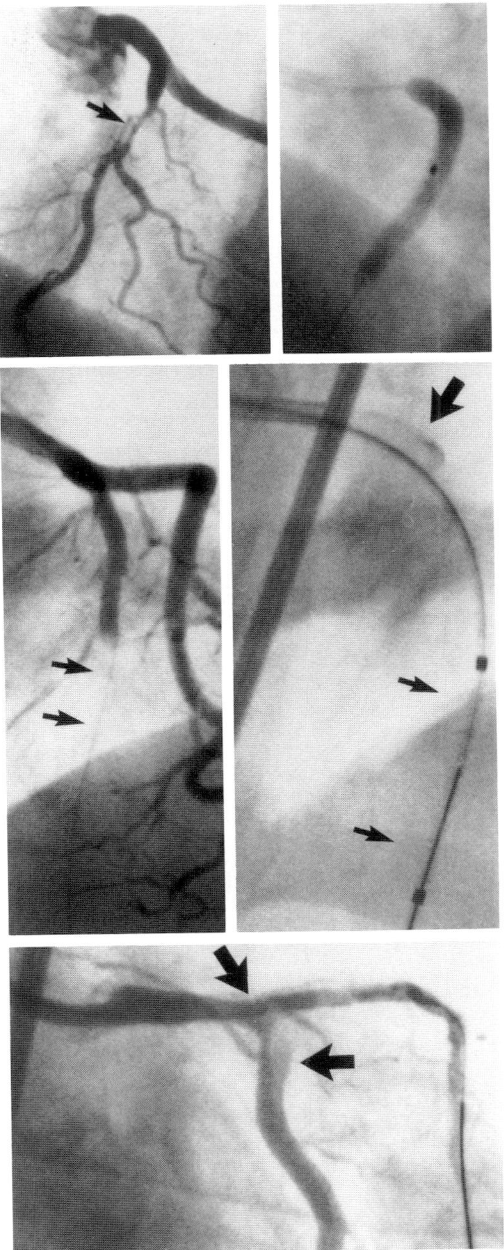

What do you recommend now?

Gary Roubin, MD, PhD, USA: In this case, left main dissection was probably caused by the guiding catheter. Left main dissection can be avoided by using guiding catheters that give you good support without requiring deep intubation into the left main stem. For this purpose, I use the Cook Lumax guiding catheter. I would insert an intraaortic balloon pump and immediately send the patient to surgery. If the patient is not a surgical candidate, I would leave a wire in the LAD and wire the LCX. I would place an additional Gianturco-Roubin stent in the proximal LAD and then remove the LAD wire prior to placing a stent in the LCX. I would not be concerned about leaving some coils in the distal left main I would do kissing balloons in the stents in the LAD and LCX. In this situation, I would also have percutaneous cardiopulmonary support on stand-by. In a high risk patient with stents in the left main bifurcation, LAD, and LCX, I would leave the intraaortic balloon pump in place for 24 hours, then manage the patient in-hospital for 10 days on aspirin, ticlopidine and low molecular weight heparin (30 mg BID).

Antonio Colombo, MD, Italy: This complication is likely due to the compliant balloon used to deliver the Gianturco-Roubin stent. One important point is not to inflate the Cook balloon over 5 ATM. Unfortunately, sometimes a higher inflation pressure may be necessary to deliver the stent. Whatever the cause of this complication, prompt surgical revascularization is appropriate. I would leave the wire in the LAD and insert an intraaortic balloon pump.

Ulrich Sigwart, MD, England: The dimensions of this case are difficult to understand. If the artery was dilated with a 3.5 mm balloon, why was a 3 mm stent implanted? I assume that the 3.5 mm balloon is oversized, and this was the cause of the problem. In a competent environment this could be solved by stenting the left main, the LAD, and the origin of the LCX. Perfusion balloons are helpful for stent delivery in this case.

> **Editors' Perspective: When dealing with dissections and failed PTCA, it is important for the operator to assess the length and extent of dissection in multiple views, before proceeding with stent implantation. In this particular case, the operator failed to recognize the dissection in the left main, which probably arose from the guiding catheter and/or oversized balloon before stent implantation. In general, it is not a good idea to proceed with stenting if the entire length of the dissection cannot be elucidated. In this patient, emergency bypass surgery was performed without complication.**

*****

LONG DISSECTION: ABRUPT CLOSURE

A 58-year-old man undergoes conventional PTCA of the mid-RCA (left panel), resulting in retrograde spiral dissection, subtotal occlusion, TIMI-2 flow, and a deep periadventitial dye stain (right panel).

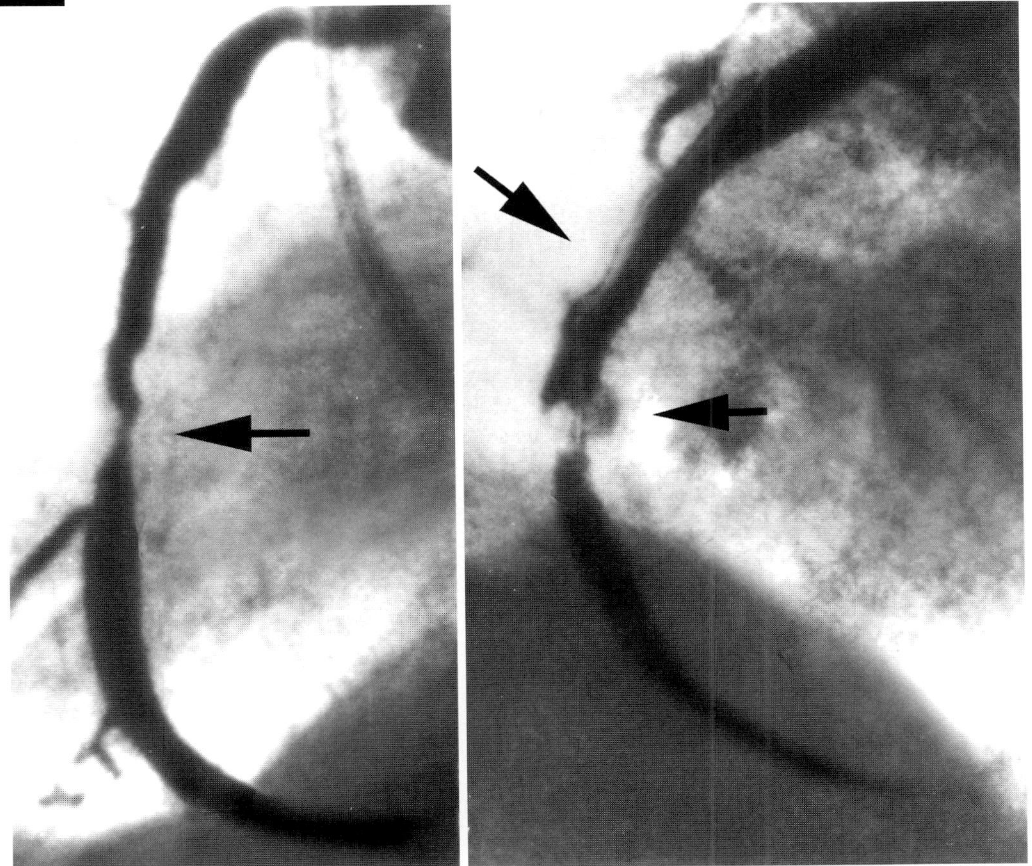

How would you manage this patient?

Donald Baim, MD, USA: This patient has unstable angina and it is not clear whether the linear defect after PTCA represents dissection or delamination of adherent thrombus. My first choice is repeat PTCA using a full-size balloon, with secondary stenting using a PS 204 biliary stent mounted on a 4.0 mm Schwarten balloon. Given the uncertainty of the integrity of the vessel wall, I would avoid directional atherectomy.

Patrick Serruys, MD, PhD, The Netherlands: PTCA has resulted in a horrible spiral dissection with probable local perforation. My first choice is to implant a 60 mm Wallstent (diameter should be 1 mm greater than the normal vessel diameter), covering the entire dissection; in my experience, this is the only treatment I would consider for this type of problem. The Gianturco-Roubin stent is also acceptable, but the Wallstent offers superior support for this vessel, since it can be safely postdilated to excellent dimensions (the Gianturco-Roubin stent can lose its shape). Having implanted the Wallstent and stabilized the situation, I would use online QCA to optimize the result and intravascular ultrasound to ensure adequate coverage of the dissection and to examine the perforated area. The localized perforation should not be a problem after Wallstent implantation. I would only prescribe aspirin and ticlopidine.

Ulrich Sigwart, MD, England: In this large RCA with a rather terrible looking dissection, a long stent is preferred. Speed is important here. A 5.0 x 40 mm Wallstent is perfectly adequate. If unavailable, I would deploy two 4.0 mm Palmaz-Schatz stents.

> **Editors' Perspective: This severe dissection may represent a contained perforation, and there is a real question as to the integrity of the vascular wall. Although prolonged inflations with a long (40 mm) balloon may stabilize the dissection, it is more likely that stent implantation would be required, using multiple balloon-expandable stents or a long Wallstent. Directional atherectomy is contraindicated due to the risk of perforation.**

*****

SPIRAL DISSECTION: ABRUPT CLOSURE

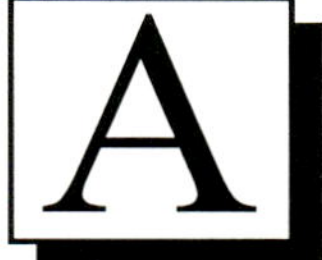

A 58-year-old man undergoes conventional PTCA of the mid-RCA with a 3.5 x 20 mm balloon, resulting in a long, spiral dissection and subtotal occlusion of the distal RCA.

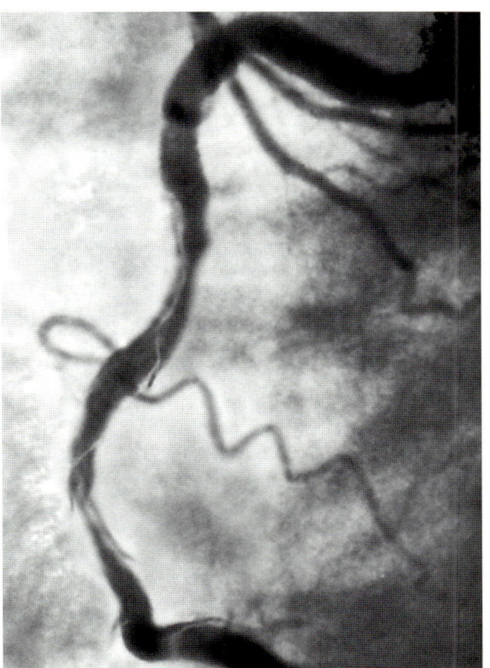

How do you manage this patient?

Patrick Serruys, MD, PhD, The Netherlands: If the last dissection was bad, this one is even worse! A long Wallstent is eminently suitable for this type of dissection. The singular advantage of the Wallstent above all others is the capacity to cover extremely long segments of disease with a single stent. I would redilate the distal lesion to facilitate passage of the Wallstent, using a long balloon. Fortunately the RCA is not particularly tortuous and I do not anticipate any difficulty placing a Wallstent. I would postdilate with balloons 0.5 mm larger than the QCA-measured reference diameter, at 16 ATM. Post-procedural therapy includes heparin (for 24 hours), aspirin, ticlopidine, nifedipine, and ReoPro (for 12 hours).

Donald Baim, MD, USA: Long spiral dissections are particularly problematic in the RCA where dissection may extend from the ostium to the crux. Although this vessel has moderate tortuosity, it should be possible to deliver a Gianturco-Roubin stent or multiple Palmaz-Schatz coronary stents to completely cover the dissection. I would begin distally, and work proximally, using an Extra-Support guidewire. Attention should be paid to covering the entire extent of the dissection and postdilating to achieve a perfect result. A "high-risk" anticoagulation protocol (including ReoPro) should be followed after stent deployment. If Gianturco-Roubin stents are used, special care should be taken to avoid the troublesome tendency of this stent to telescope when it is bumped by the nose of the delivery balloon of a second, more proximal stent. This tendency will be reduced with the second generation GR-II stent or Wallstent.

Ulrich Sigwart, MD, England: Perhaps the 3.5 mm balloon was oversized for this vessel. The trick is to seal the entry site with a stent, and then wait. I would put a rather solid stent into the original lesion and carefully compress the intramural hematoma at the most severe obstruction. This dissipates the blood within the wall and reduces the luminal narrowing. If the patient is stable, I would wait for 20 minutes and decide whether further stenting is necessary. Only if it is absolutely necessary would I put a stent into the distal lesion. A very long Wallstent would cover everything. My threshold for surgery would be rather low in this situation.

Despite your efforts, the distal RCA remains occluded. What factors do you consider when triaging between CABG or medical therapy for refractory acute closure?

Patrick Serruys, MD, PhD, The Netherlands: Unless there is a contraindication, this patient should be sent to emergency surgery with a long perfusion balloon to maintain distal perfusion. Of course, the presence of reasonable collaterals to the RCA would mitigate in favor of conservative therapy, as would prior inferior infarction. Other coronary disease, absence of collaterals, or a large area of myocardium at risk also favor emergency CABG.

Editors' Perspective: Long, complex spiral dissections with deep periadventitial dye staining represents a difficult problem for the interventional cardiologist and patient. Early surgical therapy is recommended if the dissection cannot be rapidly stabilized. For the operator who only performs PTCA, there are relatively few options. Because of the length of dissection, it is unlikely that a perfusion balloon will be useful, since removal of the guidewire to facilitate passive perfusion could potentially jeopardize subsequent guidewire access to the distal vessel. Overlapping inflations with a long (40 mm) balloon can occasionally stabilize the dissection and avoid the need for emergency bypass surgery. Directional atherectomy is absolutely contraindicated due to extensive disruption of the vessel wall and the risk of perforation. The GR-II stent and Wallstent have simplified the approach to such long dissections, but patient morbidity is still significant.

*****

LONG DISSECTION

A 58-year-old man undergoes conventional PTCA of a mid-LAD stenosis (left panel, reference diameter = 3.2 mm), resulting in abrupt closure of the diagonal branch with ST-segment elevation and chest pain. Salvage PTCA of the diagonal branch results in abrupt closure of the LAD (middle panel), which is managed by prolonged balloon inflation. After re-PTCA, the patient is pain-free and the ECG is normal. Angiography reveals a long, non-flow-limiting dissection (black arrows).

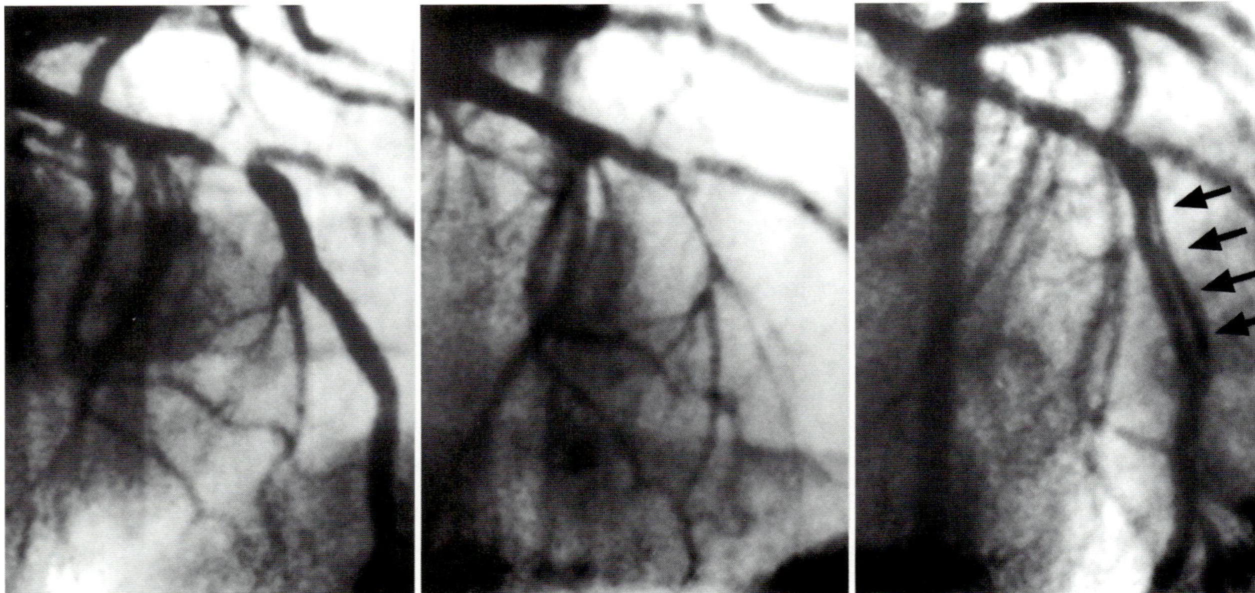

How would you manage this patient now?

Donald Baim, MD, USA: This long dissection in the LAD would qualify as threatened abrupt closure. Given the concerns about the diagonal sidebranch and the length of the dissection, I would place a 3.5 mm Gianturco-Roubin coil stent in the LAD to span the entire dissection. Having done so, it should not be difficult to regain access to the diagonal branch and redilate through the stent. Given the higher incidence of subacute thrombosis in emergency stenting such as this, I recommend ReoPro, aspirin, ticlopidine, and low-molecular weight heparin (Lovenox 30 mg BID for 10 days).

Patrick Serruys, MD, PhD, The Netherlands: The key decision in this case is not how to treat the dissection in the LAD (which I would stent), but rather whether to also stent the diagonal. Therefore, if the diagonal is more than 2.5 mm in diameter by QCA, I would also stent the diagonal. I would place two 300 cm guidewires in the diagonal and LAD, and stent the LAD using a 3.5 x 40 mm Gianturco-Roubin stent. After satisfactory postdilation with a 3.5 mm noncompliant balloon at 16 ATM, I would implant a 3.0 x 8 mm Microstent in the ostium of the diagonal, and postdilate with a short 3.0 mm Chubby balloon at 8-10 ATM. A more recent approach is deployment of a "half" Palmaz-Schatz stent or a 9 mm-long Nir stent in the LAD, leaving a wire in the diagonal. Another wire is positioned in the diagonal, after which time the original wire is removed. The diagonal can then be stented with a Nir stent. The post-procedure medical therapy is aspirin, ticlopidine, and nifedipine. If the angiographic result is not perfect, I recommend ReoPro for 12-18 hours.

Ulrich Sigwart, MD, England: Fifteen years ago I would have left this non-flow-limiting dissection alone. Nowadays I would not hesitate to put a stent into the bifurcation. The dissection must have started at this point and sealing the entry site is normally enough. On the other hand, one must use a stent with sufficient radial strength to achieve perfect sealing. These stents have limited side branch accessability. The 3.0 mm Palmaz-Schatz stent can easily be placed to allow access to the diagonal via the articulation between the two stent segments. If the entry site is not perfectly sealed after stent placement, another stent should be placed more distally. Anticoagulation is not required in these circumstances.

<u>Editors' Perspective</u>: This complex dissection involves the proximal and mid-LAD, as well as the origin of the diagonal branch. For interventionalists who do not implant stents, one option at this point is to observe the patient in the catheterization laboratory for 15-20 minutes to confirm that the angiographic appearance and clinical status remain stable. Another option is to send the patient to surgery for grafts to the LAD and diagonal branch. A third option is to administer ReoPro with the hope that this will stabilize the lesion and prevent further ischemic complications. A fourth option is to insert a perfusion balloon in the LAD (with or without a "kissing" balloon in the diagonal) and try a prolonged balloon inflation, hoping to "tack-up" the dissection.

Because of the length of the dissection, it may be difficult to achieve adequate antegrade perfusion without sacrificing guidewire position, which could jeopardize access to the distal LAD.

For operators experienced with new devices, other interventional strategies might be considered. Stenting is feasible but technically challenging. One stent approach is to use one or more coil stents in the LAD, and retrieve the diagonal branch if it becomes narrowed or occluded. Another approach is to implant a Palmaz-Schatz stent in the LAD with the articulation facing the origin of the diagonal branch, to facilitate access. Finally, depending on the caliber of the diagonal branch, it is possible to stent the origin of the diagonal and then stent the LAD in an end-to-side fashion ("T-stent"). Directional atherectomy, which can be used to resect focal flaps, is contraindicated in this type of long, spiral dissection due to the risk of perforation.

*****

COMPLEX DISSECTION

PTCA of the mid-LAD (reference vessel = 3.1 mm) is complicated by recurrent angina and ECG changes 48 hours later. Repeat angiography shows a patent vessel (left panel, RAO cranial) with significant dissection involving the diagonal branch (right panel, LAO cranial). Other vessels and left ventricular function are normal.

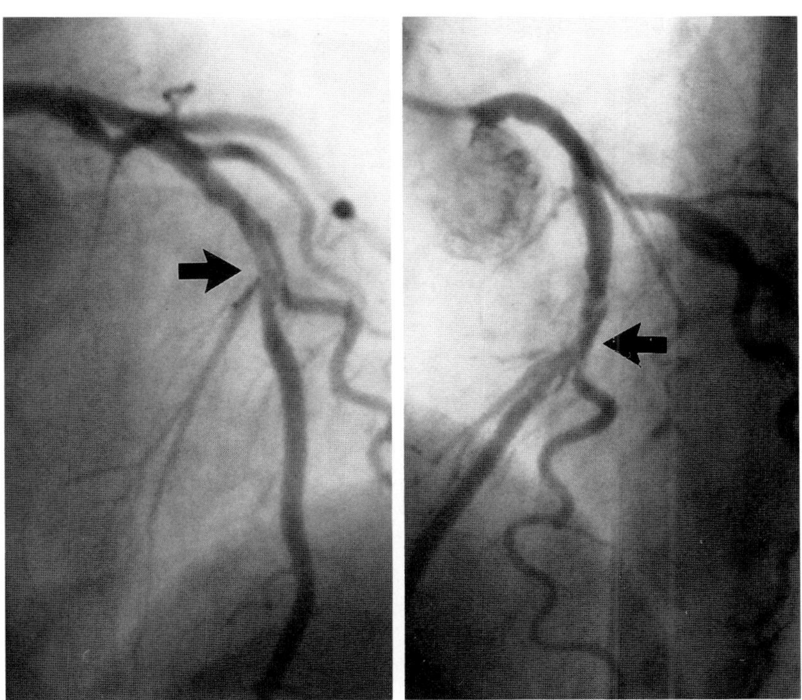

What do you recommend now?

Gary Roubin, MD, PhD, USA: I would use a Lumax JL 3.5 guiding catheter, recross the lesion with a 0.014-inch Traverse wire, place a 3.0 mm Bandit balloon in the distal LAD, and exchange the flexible wire for a 0.014-inch Platinum-Plus wire. I would then implant a Gianturco-Roubin stent at 4-5 ATM to cover the entire dissection. Then, I would withdraw the balloon 2-3 mm so the distal end of the delivery balloon is inside the stent, and repeat the inflation at 8 ATM for 2-3 minutes. I would then remove the delivery balloon, place a 0.014-inch wire through the stent coils into the diagonal branch, and perform kissing balloon angioplasty with a 3.0 mm Bandit in the LAD (16-18 ATM) and a 2.0 mm Bandit in the diagonal (16-18 ATM). The 3.0 mm Bandit balloon will give good expansion of the 3.5 mm stent. Having established good apposition of the Cook stent, I would deflate both balloons simultaneously and remove them. I would discharge the patient on aspirin, ticlopidine and subcutaneous low molecular weight heparin (for 10 days).

David Holmes, MD, USA: This is a difficult situation, with significant dissection involving the diagonal branch and LAD. Stent placement in the proximal LAD is the most ideal approach, but I would not stent the diagonal since it is small. My approach is to implant a 3.0 mm Gianturco-Roubin stent (use a GR-II, if available) in the LAD across the origin of the diagonal, and postdilate at high pressure. Then I would inflate a 2.0-2.5 mm balloon in the diagonal for a prolonged inflation. I would treat with aspirin, ticlopidine, and low molecular weight heparin or Coumadin. Another potential approach is directional atherectomy, although this is a relatively large dissection. I do not think conventional PTCA would work very well. I would not use a Palmaz-Schatz stent because of the potential for stent "jail."

Michael Cowley, MD, USA: PTCA is complicated by recurrent angina and ECG changes 48 hours later, and repeat angiography shows a patent vessel with severe dissection in the LAD extending across the diagonal branch, with high-grade narrowing in both vessels. Coronary stenting has a reasonable likelihood of successfully treating this occlusive dissection and avoiding urgent bypass surgery. I would recross the dissection using a 0.014-inch Hi-torque floppy wire. I would redilate with a 3.0 x 20 mm balloon at low pressure, and assess the length of the dissection by comparison with the inflated balloon (the dissection appears to be 20 mm in length). I would initially use a 3.5 mm Gianturco-Roubin stent at 4-5 ATM to cover the entire dissection (if the dissection is longer, multiple stents are required), followed by a 3.0 mm balloon at 12-16 ATM. If the diagonal branch is significantly narrowed or occluded, I would advance a wire into the diagonal branch and dilate with a 2.5 mm balloon. If the diagonal branch has residual narrowing or causes ischemia, stenting the diagonal branch is recommended with a 2.5 mm Gianturco-Roubin stent, positioned so most of the stent is in the diagonal and just covering the ostium. Further balloon inflation can be done in the LAD to treat any residual irregularity or narrowing after stenting the diagonal branch. If stenting achieves a good initial result, management includes Coumadin for 6 weeks.

<u>Editors' Perspective</u>: The constellation of moderately severe dissection, significant residual stenosis, normal antegrade flow, and recurrent ischemia is consistent with the diagnosis of "threatened" abrupt closure. When present, further intervention is required, either by repeat PTCA, stenting, or bypass surgery. Repeat PTCA is certainly reasonable as long as complete coverage of the dissection and optimal balloon sizing are assured. However, compared to PTCA, stenting results in better lumen enlargement and a more reliable angiographic outcome. The operator should be aware that multiple stents may be required to completely cover the dissection, and that stenting may jeopardize the diagonal branch ("stent jail"). Fortunately, stent jail is only a "minimum security prison," since sidebranch narrowing or abrupt closure can often be treated by PTCA (and sometimes stenting) through the coils or struts of previously implanted stents. Bypass surgery is certainly a reasonable approach, particularly if stenting is unsuccessful.

*****

BAILOUT STENT: RIGID LESION

A 3.0 mm Gianturco-Roubin stent is implanted (see original lesion on p. 583). There is a mild waist in the balloon (left panel, arrow) that persists after further inflations up to 20 ATM (middle panel, arrow). There is mild intraluminal haziness (right panel, arrow) and a severe stenosis in the diagonal branch (right panel, curved arrow). The patient is asymptomatic.

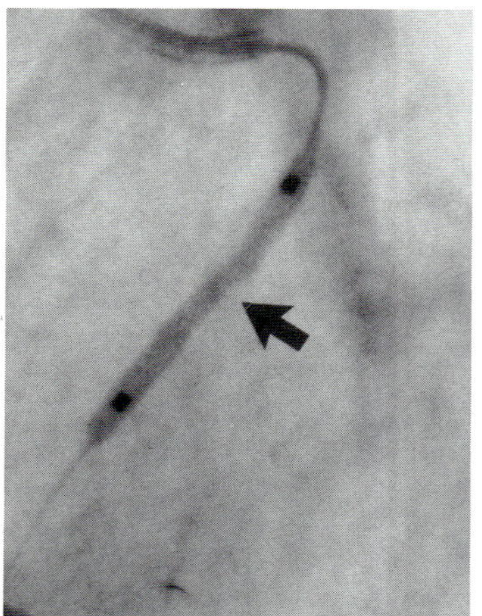
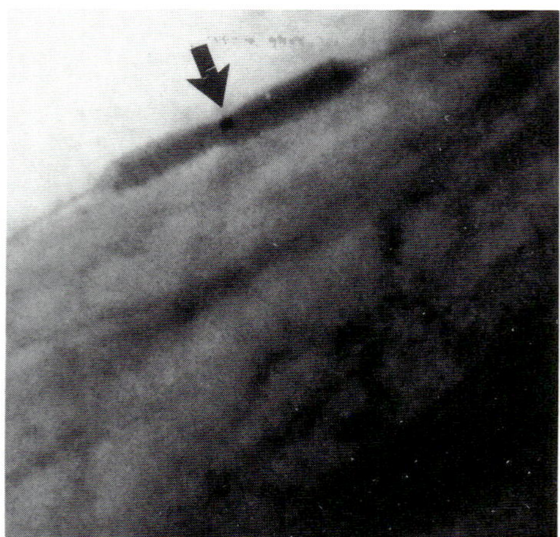
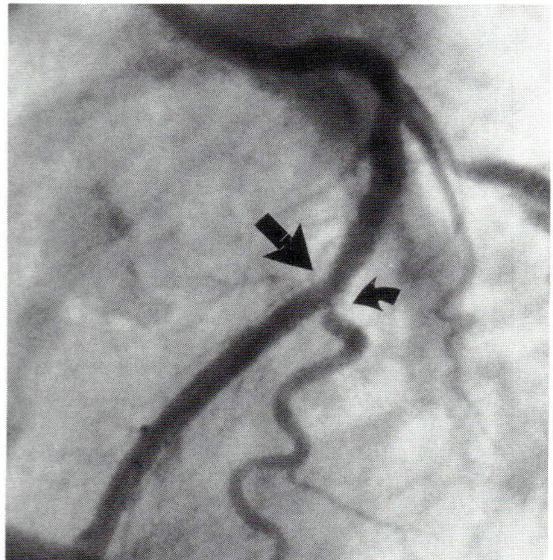

What do you recommend now?

Gary Roubin, MD, PhD, USA: This problem can be avoided by making sure that the lesion is fully released before advancing the stent. If a 3.0 mm balloon does not fully expand the lesion, the tip of a 3.5 mm balloon should be placed across the lesion and inflated to 20 ATM prior to stent placement. In the current situation, I would place the tip of a 3.5 mm high-pressure balloon just distal to the offending segment, inflated to at least 20 ATM. If the lesion does not yield, I would terminate the procedure, remove the sheaths the same day, and manage the patient with aspirin, ticlopidine and subcutaneous low molecular weight heparin (for 10 days).

David Holmes, MD, USA: This is a suboptimal result following implantation of a 3.0 mm Gianturco-Roubin stent. In this specific patient who is asymptomatic with a small diagonal side branch stenosis, I would consider medical management. I do not think other imaging techniques are useful. To further expand the lesion, I would use a 3.25 x 10 mm balloon at high pressure. If a stent deploys nicely and there is no residual stenosis, then I would use a high-pressure balloon to dilate the origin of the diagonal, realizing that if a downstream dissection occurs, I would not treat it. If the results improves, I would prescribe aspirin, ticlopidine and low molecular weight heparin (for one week). I recommend low-molecular weight heparin any time stent implantation is suboptimal.

Michael Cowley, MD, USA: After stenting, there is mild residual indentation on the balloon which persists despite inflation pressures to 20 ATM. Intravascular ultrasound imaging of the LAD is useful to assess the residual indentation and intraluminal haziness. If there is a good overall lumen for the LAD and the stent is well deployed, then further treatment to resolve the mild balloon indentation may not be necessary. In this setting of complicated stent placement, postprocedure medical therapy should include intravenous heparin and Coumadin (INR 2.5-3.0 for 4 weeks).

If the patient is symptomatic from the diagonal branch, describe your revascularization approach.

Gary Roubin, MD, PhD, USA: At this point, I am not concerned about occlusion of the diagonal branch. If the patient is symptomatic from the diagonal branch and there is reduced flow, I would proceed with kissing balloon angioplasty, as described above.

David Holmes, MD, USA: This is a small vessel. I would not sacrifice the LAD to try to save this small diagonal branch.

Michael Cowley, MD, USA: The diagonal branch should be dilated whether the narrowing is due to untreated lesion or dissection. I recommend a Hi-torque floppy wire to cross the ostium, and a proper size balloon to dilate the ostium. If PTCA of the diagonal branch disturbs the LAD, simultaneous balloon inflations are recommended ("kissing balloon") to eliminate shifting plaque.

Editors' Perspective: This lesion is characterized by mild residual narrowing inside the stent, consistent with suboptimal stent deployment. In this case, it is likely that residual narrowing was due to incomplete expansion of the rigid portion of the lesion, as opposed to stent recoil. The best way to deal with stent recoil is to implant another stent. The best way to deal with incomplete stent expansion due to lesion rigidity is to avoid stenting such lesions. This case illustrates the importance of ensuring that a lesion can be fully expanded with a balloon before stent implantation. Unfortunately, treatment options at this point are limited.

The ideal medical regimen after suboptimal stenting is unknown, since it is unclear whether anticoagulation per se will prevent stent thrombosis in this setting. Aspirin and ticlopidine are probably useful, and ReoPro may be helpful to disable the platelets as much as possible. Subcutaneous heparin and/or oral Coumadin are commonly prescribed after suboptimal stenting, but there are no data to confirm any benefit.

*****

STENT: SUBOPTIMAL DEPLOYMENT

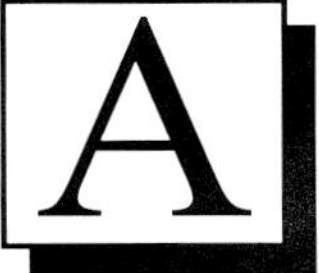

A focal lesion in the mid-RCA (reference = 2.6 mm) is treated by a single 3.0 mm Palmaz-Schatz stent after multiple episodes of restenosis. After stent deployment at 8 ATM there is no residual stenosis. Other vessels and LV function are normal.

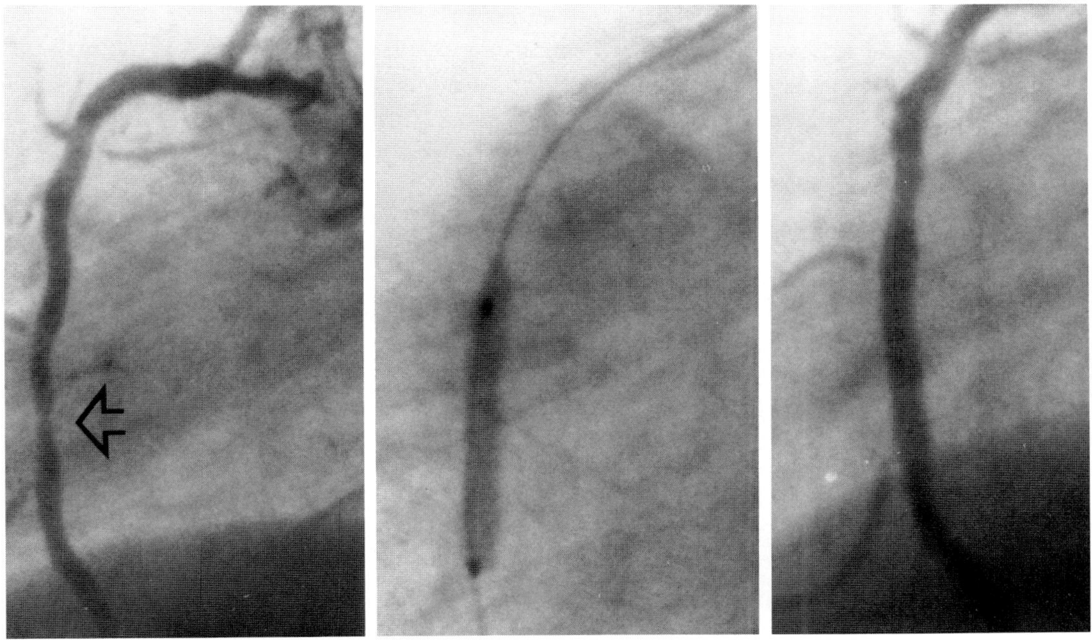

At this point, would you recommend adjunctive PTCA?

Richard Schatz, MD, USA: Although the immediate angiographic result is good, stent deployment took place at only 8 ATM. It is essential to postdilate every stent with a high-pressure balloon, regardless of the angiographic outcome. Intravascular ultrasound will always show that the stent is deformed, despite the excellent angiographic appearance. The stent achieves good wall contact and symmetric expansion only after high-pressure inflation.

Therefore, I would use a 3.0 mm NC Bandit at 20 ATM, and accept the risk of proximal or distal dissection. In this vessel, the risk of stent thrombosis is high without high-pressure inflations.

Antonio Colombo, MD, Italy: The angiographic result appears very satisfactory. Despite this fact, we know that after low-pressure stent deployment the cross sectional area inside the stent (by IVUS) is not optimal. I would proceed with an 18-20 ATM inflation with a 3.0-3.5 x 9-10 mm balloon. The vessel has mild diffuse disease, and for this reason I would use a short balloon. IVUS evaluation will determine the final balloon size and confirm optimal stent implantation. I urge IVUS evaluation to increase the level of confidence and patient safety.

> **Editors' Perspective: From an angiographic standpoint, this stent result is perfect. However, it is important to resist the temptation to do nothing. At this point, the operator should either perform IVUS to confirm optimal stent deployment, or dilate the stent at high-pressure (16-20 ATM) with or without IVUS guidance. This patient underwent adjunctive PTCA with a 3.0 x 20 mm high-pressure balloon at 16 ATM, which resulted in extensive distal dissection requiring emergency bypass surgery. It is important to limit high-pressure inflations to the stented segment; a 3.0 x 9-15 mm balloon would have been a better choice.**

*****

STENT: ARTICULATION DEFECT

A target lesion in the proximal vein graft to the LAD (reference diameter = 3.2 mm, left panel) is treated by implantation of a 4.0 mm PS204 biliary stent, and dilated at 18 ATM. After adjunctive PTCA, there is moderate disease just distal to the stent (right panel, higher magnification, curved arrows) and a prominent articulation defect (arrowhead). The patient is asymptomatic.

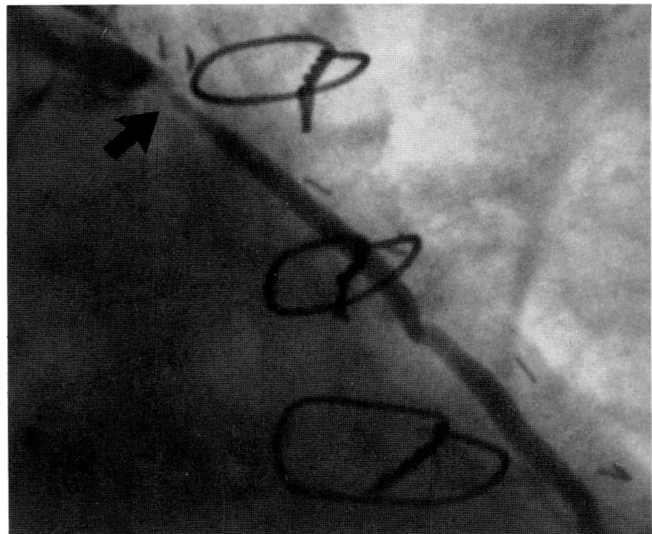

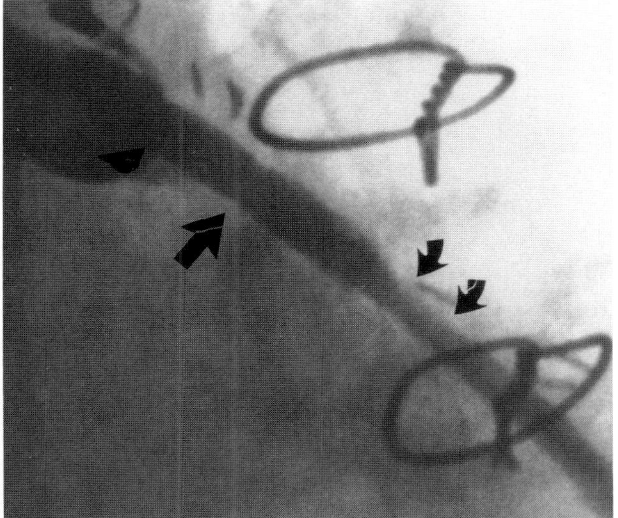

How would you approach this now?

Paul Teirstein, MD, USA: This vein graft has been treated with a PS204 biliary stent. A limitation of this type of stent is its large articulation. I would have used a Palmaz-Schatz coronary stent or a P154 biliary stent to treat this artery. At this point, I would use intravascular ultrasound to assess the degree of narrowing at the articulation and at the distal stent margin. If intravascular ultrasound does not show significant stenosis, I would discharge the patient the following day on aspirin and ticlopidine (250 mg BID). If significant narrowing is present at the distal stent margin, I would place a 3.5 mm Palmaz-Schatz coronary stent. If significant narrowing is present at the articulation, I would cut a 4.0 mm Palmaz-Schatz coronary stent in half, and place the "half" stent in the articulation defect.

Masakiyo Nobuyoshi, MD, USA: I would evaluate the distal stenosis with IVUS and if dissection or flap is evident, I would deploy a 3.5 mm Palmaz-Schatz stent at 8-10 ATM distally and 18 ATM proximally.

Ian Penn, MD, Canada: There is a hazy filling defect beyond the stent, due to atheroma and distal disease. I would perform intravascular ultrasound to determine the nature of the articulation defect, the reference size, and the nature and extent of distal disease. I assume the articulation defect is due to oversizing, and the distal disease is due to dissection at the interface between the stent and distal vessel. I would implant an 18 mm Palmaz-Schatz stent with spiral articulation to cover the distal lesion.

Editors' Perspective: Angiographic "irregularities" are occasionally observed after coronary stenting, which may be due to artifacts or significant lesions. IVUS may be superior to angiography in its ability to delineate the nature of these "irregularities." If IVUS is not available, these "irregularities" are best stented.

*****

STENT: INCOMPLETE EXPANSION

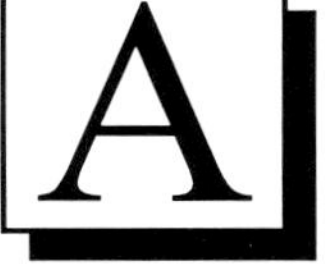

A lesion in a vein graft to the OM is predilated (left panel, arrow). A 5.0 mm P104 biliary stent is implanted (middle panel), and postdilated with a 5.5 mm balloon at 14 ATM. A small waist in the balloon persists, and there is mild tapering of the vessel within the stented segment (right panel).

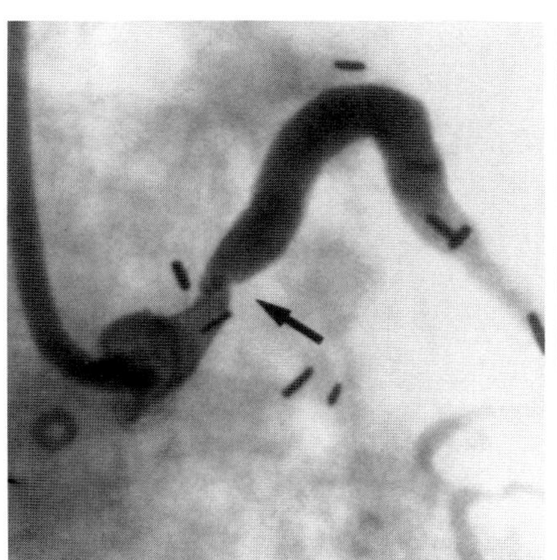

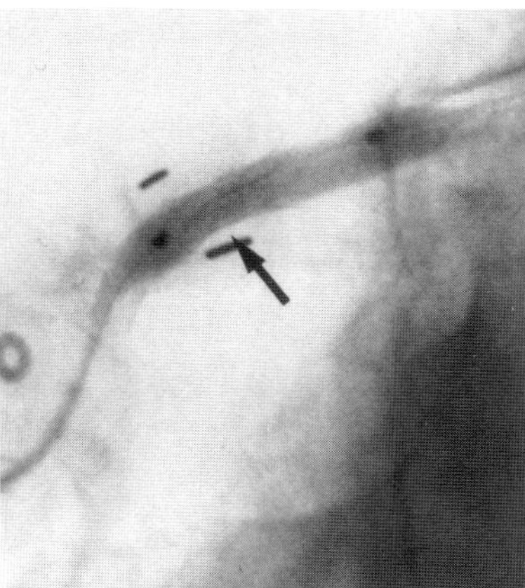

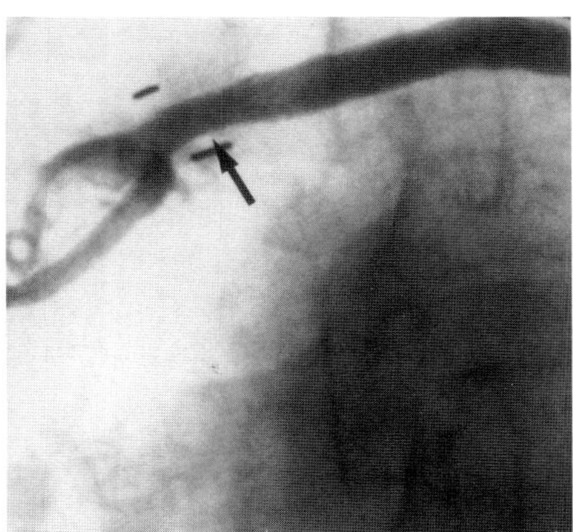

How would you approach this lesion now?

Richard Schatz, MD, USA: The final result is suboptimal with clear narrowing inside the stent. This represents a very difficult problem without a solution. The risk of restenosis and stent thrombosis is high. I would try a 6.0 mm Total Cross balloon, being sure that the majority of the balloon is in the aorta and only the distal marker is at the end of the stent. I would inflate to 15 ATM and hope that I get additional expansion of the stent, realizing that this approach may be associated with a risk of vessel perforation. If this is unsuccessful, there are no options other than to treat the patient expectantly. If the final result shows angiographic expansion of the stent, the patient can be discharged on aspirin and ticlopidine. If the stent remains underdilated and the patient has significant "muscle at risk", then the patient should stay in the hospital for 5-7 days on full anticoagulation, including aspirin, ticlopidine, intravenous heparin and Coumadin. The patient could then be discharged on this regimen for 30 days (including subcutaneous heparin).

Donald Baim, MD, USA: Vein graft lesions such as this one frequently require high pressures for full stent expansion, probably reflecting extensive peri-graft mediastinal fibrosis. Incomplete stent expansion increases the risk of thrombosis and restenosis, and I would make every effort to more fully expand this stent. I would use a 5.5 mm peripheral balloon capable of delivering 18-20 ATM, in an effort to achieve full stent expansion.

Masakiyo Nobuyoshi, MD, Japan: This lesion is resistant to the high-pressure inflation with the 5.5 mm balloon. I would use a short 5.5 mm high-pressure balloon (inflated to 20 ATM). The post-procedural anticoagulation includes heparin, ticlopidine, and aspirin (as with any other stent).

> **Editors' Perspective: The issues concerning incomplete stent expansion and rigid lesions in vein grafts are similar to those in native coronary arteries (p. 586). It is best to avoid this situation by ensuring full balloon expansion prior to stent deployment. On the other hand, mild residual in-stent narrowing in a large vein graft may have fewer implications than in a smaller native coronary artery. Meditech Symmetry balloons are excellent for high-pressure adjunctive PTCA in large vessels and vein grafts.**

*****

STENT MIGRATION

PTCA of the mid-RCA (top left, reference vessel = 4.0 mm) is complicated by severe dissection (top middle, short arrow). A 4.0 mm Gianturco-Roubin stent is implanted (top right), but there is persistent dissection (bottom left, short arrow) at the proximal end of the stent. A second 4.0 mm Gianturco-Roubin stent is inserted (bottom, middle), resulting in distal migration of the first stent (small arrowheads) and "telescoping" of the second stent (open arrowheads). Subsequent angiography (bottom right) reveals persistent dissection at the original site, which is not covered by stent coils (short arrow). The patient is asymptomatic.

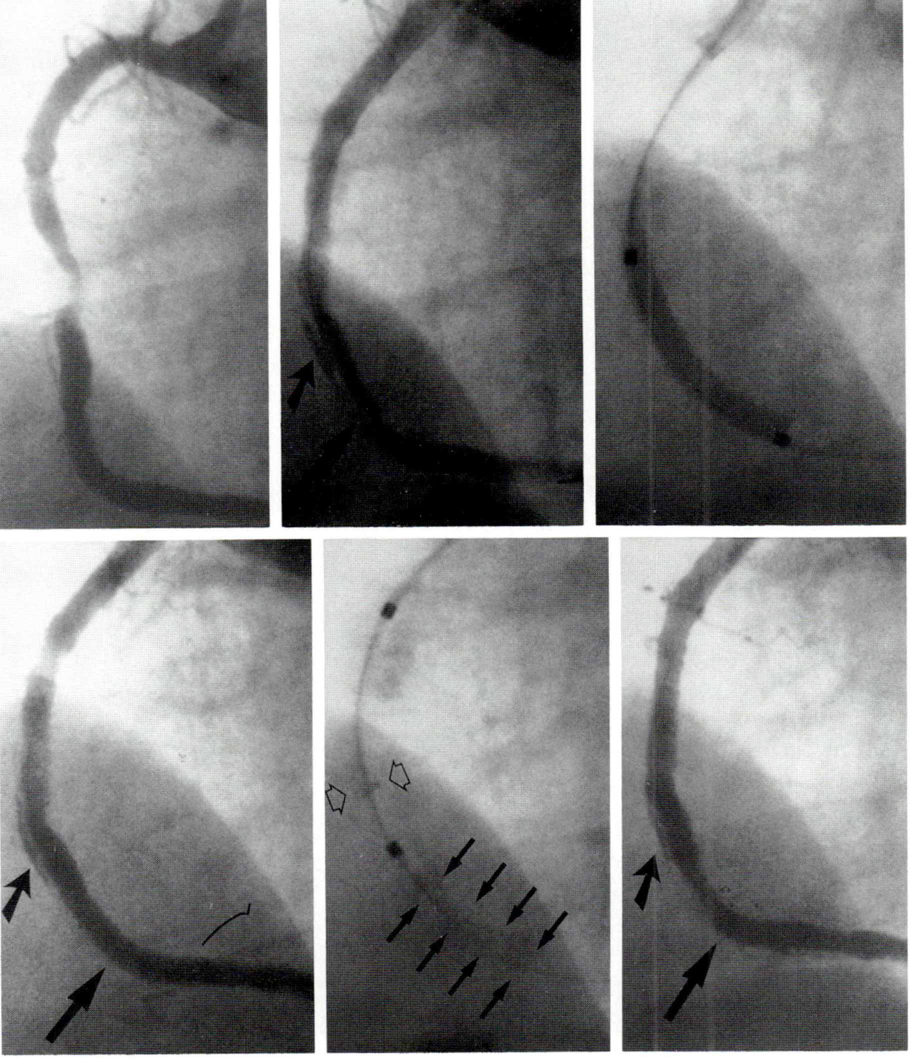

How can these problems be avoided?

Gary Roubin, MD, PhD, USA: This problem will be avoidable with availability of the GR-II stent. Not only is the GR-II vastly more trackable but it will be available in 40 mm lengths and diameters up to 5.0 mm. This stent has proximal and distal markers that allow great precision in placement. It also has a flatwire construction that prevents the stent coils from separating during deployment and it prevents the "accordion-effect" when a second stent is placed inside the first. With the original Gianturco-Roubin stent, this problem can be avoided as follows: The first stent should be deployed well distal to the lesion, at 4-5 ATM. The deployment balloon should be withdrawn 2-3 mm so the distal end of the delivery balloon is inside the stent, and inflated to 8 ATM for 30-60 seconds. This ensures that the coils are well-embedded into the wall prior to additional stent placement. Before placing the second stent, a 4.0 mm balloon should be advanced into the first stent and inflated at 16 ATM. The second stent can then be advanced into the first stent without concern.

Ulrich Sigwart, MD, England: The 4.0 mm Gianturco-Roubin stent is placed slightly more distally than I would have preferred As the dissection has happened at the site of the original lesion, it is most important to cover this lesion perfectly. The lesion distal to the dissection (in the upper middle panel) is most likely an intralumural hematoma, and it is not necessary to cover this lesion with a stent. It is most important to cover the dissection at the original lesion; a stent with good radial force (Palmaz-Schatz, Wallstent) would have done a better job if placed in the original dissection.

Dean Kereiakes, MD, USA: This case illustrates a problem sometimes encountered during placement of multiple coil stents. Migration of the distal stent and telescoping of the proximal stent can be successfully dealt with, but are best avoided. I recommend returning to the fourth angiographic frame of this sequence, at which time a 4.0 mm Gianturco-Roubin stent has been successfully deployed and encompasses most of the dissection, but there is an area of persistent dissection at the proximal end of the stent. At this point, I recommend postdilation with a 4.0 x 9 mm Titan balloon at ≥ 18 ATM. If a 20 minute observation is associated with continued normal flow, normal wash-out, no contrast staining, and no evidence of progressive lumen compromise, I would not place a second (proximal) stent in this vessel. I believe that mild residual dissection that does not cause lumen compromise or impede flow does not mandate placement of a second coil stent. Following optimal high-pressure dilation, adjunctive ReoPro is recommended. If the decision is made to place a second coil stent, it is mandatory to postdilate the first stent to prevent the coils from "catching" each other. Every attempt should be made to limit the force applied in delivering the second stent. If maximal dilation of the first stent does not eliminate "drag" during placement of the second stent, I would pull back the second stent, rotate the catheter, and attempt to realign the approach by having the patient take a deep breath or cough. Finally, a prominent angle can be fashioned on the guidewire, in an attempt to deflect the nose of the second delivery balloon to facilitate crossing.

What do you recommend now?

Gary Roubin, MD, PhD, USA: Vessels larger than 4 mm should not be treated with the Gianturco-Roubin stent, which can achieve a maximal diameter of 3.8 mm. In the current situation as shown, I would advance a trackable 4 mm balloon (Cordis Olympix II, Scimed Bandit) into the stented segment and inflate at 14-15 ATM. Over an extra-support wire, I would attempt to deploy another stent inside the suboptimal segment.

Dean Kereiakes, MD, USA: I recommend using a double-ply balloon such as the short Mongoose or Titan. These catheters have the strength to adequately expand the telescoped stent. Multiple high-pressure balloon inflations would be performed throughout the length of both stents.

If CABG is not recommended, please detail your medical therapy.

Gary Roubin, MD, PhD, USA: Regardless of the result, I would manage the patient on aspirin, ticlopidine, and low molecular weight heparin (30 mg BID). Unless the case is done very late in the day, I would remove the sheath 4 hours later. ReoPro appears to be useful in a wide range of suboptimal results after stenting.

Ulrich Sigwart, MD, England: I would not send the patient to surgery automatically, but place him on a regular anticoagulation regimen.

Dean Kereiakes, MD, USA: Adjunctive ReoPro is very useful. I also recommend repeat angiography in 3-4 months to reassess coronary patency.

Editors' Perspective: On occasion, stenting becomes extremely challenging for the operator; in these situations, it is important to stay calm, be flexible, and tackle problems as they arise. In this particular case, multiple technical errors and unforgiving hardware conspired to make a difficult case even more difficult. In contemporary stenting, this lesion could be treated with a variety of newer and improved stent designs, including the GR-II stent and the Wallstent. Other balloon-expandable stents could be used, but multiple stents would be necessary to cover such a lengthy dissection.

*****

STENT: FILLING DEFECTS

A lesion in the proximal vein graft to the OM (reference vessel = 5.5 mm, left panel) is treated by implantation of a 5.0 mm PS204 biliary stent (middle panel; small arrows indicate margins of stent). After adjunctive PTCA with a 5.0 x 20 mm balloon at 14 ATM (right panel), there is mild haziness inside the stent segment and a small filling defect at the distal end of the stent (open arrow). The patient is asymptomatic.

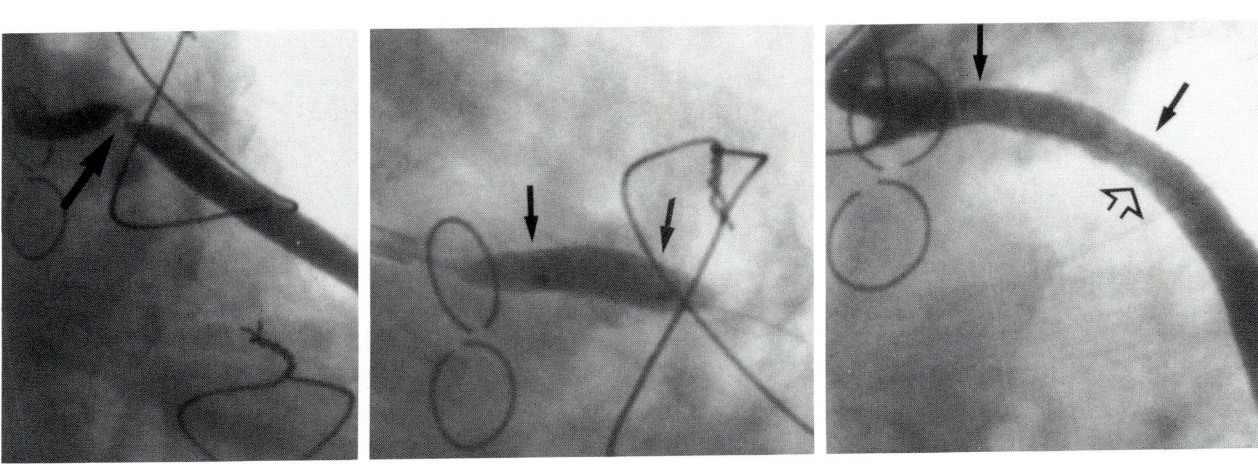

What do you recommend now?

Richard Heuser, MD, USA: I don't like the PS204 biliary stent because the articulation is too long. Specifically, haziness often occurs, sometimes requiring a second stent inside the PS204. The haziness in the stent can be studied with an angioscope to determine if this is thrombus. I would use prolonged balloon inflations inside the stent, a Dispatch catheter to infuse urokinase (250,000 to 500,000 units), or the Localmed catheter with heparin infusion. Other considerations are ReoPro infusion or an overnight infusion of urokinase. However, in most cases, I feel that prolonged balloon inflation or the Dispatch catheter would resolve the problem. I would keep the sheaths in place and repeat angiography the next day. I would then stop the heparin and send the patient home on aspirin and ticlopidine.

Richard Schatz, MD, USA: This no doubt represents grumous disrupted by the balloon following stent placement, with or without associated clot. I would perform additional PTCA for at least 3-5 minutes. If the defect persists or worsens, a second stent is indicated. More importantly, the stent appears undersized compared to the remaining vessel. The vessel looks much more like a 6.0 mm vessel. Once taken to 6.0 mm, this patient could be discharged within 6-24 hours on aspirin and ticlopidine. Intravascular ultrasound is of little use if the operator takes the stent to high pressure (at least 15 ATM with a Total Cross). There is no role for ReoPro in this case.

Masakiyo Nobuyoshi, MD, USA: The mild haziness inside the stent represents thrombus in the vein graft. There is no residual stenosis, and antegrade flow is good. I would not perform any intervention, other than administer urokinase (96,000 units over 12 hours) and heparin. I would repeat angiography the next day; if haziness has resolved, the usual therapy is recommended. If haziness persists, I would administer more urokinase (96,000 units IV over 24 hours).

> **Editors' Perspective: This type of haziness in and adjacent to the distal stent margin is characteristic of a suboptimal result, and may be due to unstented residual plaque, dissection, or thrombus; unfortunately, contrast angiography is not particularly reliable in distinguishing these problems. The operator has several options at this point, but terminating the procedure without further intervention is not a good idea. A simple first measure is to redilate the lesion with a prolonged balloon inflation. On-line quantitative coronary angiography or IVUS can be useful to estimate vessel diameter and assist in selecting the proper size balloon. Second, another overlapping stent can be implanted to clean-up the angiographic result, and tack-up residual plaque or dissection within the articulation or at the stent margin. Third, IVUS or angioscopy can be used to assess the nature of the lesion and determine the most appropriate intervention. However, IVUS is insensitive to thrombus and angioscopy does not provide quantitative information or confirm optimal stent deployment. Finally, if thrombus is highly suspected or confirmed, adjunctive lytic therapy or ReoPro may be useful.**

*****

STENT: SUBACUTE THROMBOSIS

A 60-year-old man had multiple biliary stents implanted in the SVG to the LAD 4 days ago. Despite treatment with aspirin and a continuous heparin infusion (PTT = 90 seconds), he develops abrupt chest pain and anterior ST segment elevation. Angiography demonstrates stent thrombosis (reference diameter = 4.5 mm). Other grafts and left ventricular function are normal.

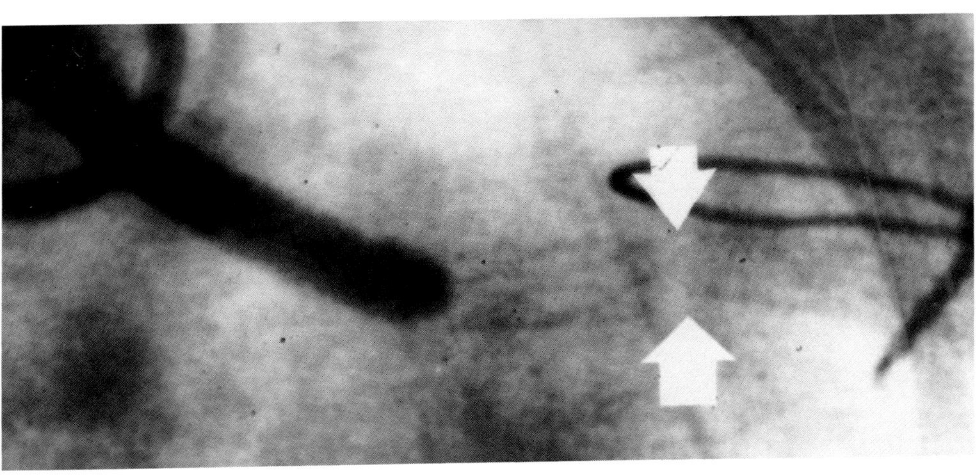

How would you manage this patient?

Gary Roubin, MD, PhD, USA: I would use a Lumax 8F AL1 or AL2 guide, a 4.0 mm Cobra (0.018-inch compatible), and a 0.016-inch Hyperflex wire, using the balloon to support the wire. I would advance a J-tip wire through the stent to the distal vessel. Having crossed the stent, I would advance the balloon into the distal vessel and inject contrast through the balloon, to confirm proper position in the distal vessel. Prolonged inflations will often eliminate the thrombus. Depending on left ventricular function, an intraaortic balloon pump is often very useful for augmenting flow. I would also administer liberal amounts of nitroglycerin and verapamil. I would exchange the 4.0 mm Cobra balloon for a 5.0 mm Total Cross and perform additional low-pressure inflations inside the stent.

Richard Schatz, MD, USA: This patient presents with subacute stent thrombosis despite anticoagulation; acute intervention carries a high success rate and a low complication rate, but the impact on restenosis is unknown. This patient will benefit from immediate reperfusion; a Cordis Stabilizer wire is my first choice. The wire tip should have a generous curve to prolapse across the clotted stent. This is the safest way to cross a stent and prevent the rare passage of a wire between the stent and the vessel wall. I would use a 4.5 mm Schwarten or 5.0 mm Total Cross and inflate to 10-15 ATM. If the patient is hemodynamically unstable, I would use a perfusion balloon. If the vein graft has a superior takeoff, I would use an Amplatz guide; for horizontal takeoff, a hockey stick guide; and an inferior takeoff, a multipurpose guide.

Antonio Colombo, MD, Italy: The thrombosed stent should be reopened with a 0.014-inch Hi-torque floppy guidewire and PTCA. Following an adequate final result by angiography, IVUS should be performed to fully evaluate optimal stent deployment. It is extremely important to identify the cause of stent thrombosis. Considerations include inadequate stent expansion, unstented residual dissection or stenosis, patient-failure to properly take antiplatelet therapy, etc. Once the problem is identified, it must be corrected.

There appears to be an unstented "gap" between two stents (arrowheads), which is not an articulation site. Is this relevant to the development of stent thrombosis?

Gary Roubin, MD, PhD, USA: If a significant residual lesion exists between the two stents, I would deploy a 10 mm biliary stent on a Total Cross balloon.

Richard Schatz, MD, USA: The most common cause of stent thrombosis is operator error at the time of initial placement, due to incomplete stent expansion or untreated residual dissection. When stent thrombosis occurs, I always proceed with the idea that further PTCA or stent implantation is necessary. Another common mistake is to leave residual thrombus in the stent; I would be extremely aggressive with intramural lytics with or without overnight infusion. In this particular case, I would consider deploying another biliary stent mounted on a Schwarten balloon. I do not recommend stent deployment with a Total Cross balloon, because of the risk of balloon rupture. The gap between the two stents is not relevant unless the culprit lesion is at the gap. In this case, I would place a P104 biliary stent at this site.

Antonio Colombo, MD, Italy: Single or multiple biliary stents should be implanted to correct the problems. In addition to the stent gap, it appears that the more distal stent is less expanded, and I recommend a larger balloon or higher inflation pressure to optimize the result. Incomplete lesion coverage and stent underexpansion may have contributed to stent thrombosis.

What is your medical regimen?

Gary Roubin, MD, PhD, USA: If there is evidence for residual thrombus, I would administer urokinase (80,000 units/hr for 12 hrs) through a multihole infusion catheter, maintain the PTT at 45-50 seconds, and perform repeat angiography the next day. After sheaths are removed, I would restart heparin 4 hours later. I would discharge the patient on aspirin, ticlopidine, subcutaneous low molecular weight heparin (for 10 days), and Coumadin.

Richard Schatz, MD, USA: Intravenous lytic therapy is not recommended (unless the cath lab is absolutely unavailable) because of access site bleeding. Lytics are valuable, but I save them for intracoronary use once the vessel is open, where a higher concentration of drug can be delivered through a Dispatch catheter (250,000 units of urokinase or 10 mg of tPA). Once the vessel is open, the operator must ask himself "Why did this stent clot?" If there is a lapse in anticoagulation, then that should be remedied. If there is unrecognized dissection, that should be repaired with another stent. If the result is excellent with the addition of one or two more stents and I have solved the problem, I would treat the patient with aspirin, ticlopidine, and Coumadin for 30 days. Although unproven, there may be a role for ReoPro (standard bolus and infusion) in stent thrombosis. I would keep the ACT between 250-300 seconds, and remove the vascular sheaths when the ACT is below 150 seconds. I would not use ReoPro if thrombolytic drugs had been given. This patient should be treated with maximum anticoagulation between Day 3 and Day 7, which is the time period during which rethrombosis may occur.

Antonio Colombo, MD, Italy: Following the achievement of a good final result confirmed by IVUS, I would continue overnight heparin. The patient will be discharged on aspirin and 2 weeks of ticlopidine (optional).

Editors' Perspective: In the past, stent thrombosis was viewed as a clotting disorder and was blamed on "inadequate" anticoagulation in the setting of a metal implant in the

coronary artery. Due to the pioneering work of Dr. Colombo and others, stent thrombosis is now viewed as a mechanical problem caused by suboptimal stent deployment. With better understanding of stent deployment technique, the incidence of stent thrombosis has decreased dramatically despite elimination of potent anticoagulant drugs. The risk of stent thrombosis can be minimized by ensuring complete stent expansion, full apposition to the wall, and complete coverage of dissection and residual plaque at the time of initial stent implantation. Intravascular ultrasound is a useful tool for assessing the adequacy of stent implantation, and should be strongly considered if there is any uncertainty about stent deployment.

If stent thrombosis does occur, the patient must be returned immediately to the cath lab to restore vessel patency; intravenous thrombolytic therapy is not appropriate treatment. A large "J" should be placed on the guidewire so it prolapses across the occlusion rather than inadvertently passes under the stent struts; steering the guidewire to avoid the struts is impossible. In addition, the operator must identify and reverse the cause of stent thrombosis. Residual unstented disease or dissection, and incomplete stent expansion or apposition should be specifically sought and corrected, even if additional stents are required.

Useful adjunctive therapies include intracoronary lytic therapy and intracoronary ReoPro for residual filling defects or thrombus after successful recanalization. Neither has been proven to be beneficial, but anecdotal experience is positive. Rheolytic thrombectomy devices such as the Possis AngioJet may be useful, but have not been widely tested for stent thrombosis, and cutting and aspiration devices (such as TEC) should probably be avoided due to the risk of stent disruption. If mechanical deficiencies are corrected and the subsequent result is excellent, appropriate medical therapy includes aspirin and ticlopidine. Subcutaneous heparin and/or oral Coumadin are reasonable, but of unproven benefit.

*****

STENT: RESIDUAL DISSECTION

PTCA of the proximal RCA with a 3.5 x 20 mm balloon results in extensive spiral dissection from the ostium to the PDA. Seven overlapping Cook stents (2 x 3.0 mm stents distal, 3 x 3.5 mm stents mid, and 2 x 4.0 mm stents proximal) are implanted and dilated at 14-16 ATM. Final angiography shows a patent lumen and TIMI-3 flow, with residual dissection outside the stent coils (black arrows) and contrast staining of the right Sinus of Valsalva. The patient is asymptomatic and the ECG is normal.

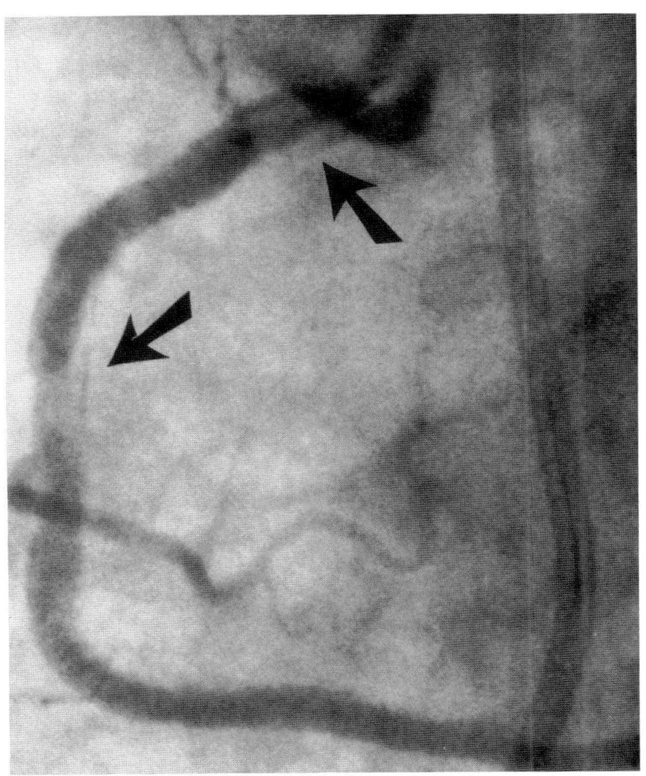

What do you recommend now?

Gary Roubin, MD, PhD, USA: Generally, this appearance in the mid-RCA results from undersizing the stent or not overlapping the stent sufficiently to assure good radial support. I would pass a flexible J-tip wire through the stents, followed by a 4.0 mm Cordis Olympix balloon. Having placed the balloon distally, I would exchange for a 0.018-inch Roadrunner wire, and dilate the residual dissection and proximal vessel at 15 ATM. I would attempt to place a 4.0 x 12 mm Cook stent into the dissected segment. Be prepared to use good push/pull technique and allow time for the stents to "wriggle" across one another to get the short stent into the offending segment. The new 10 mm GR-II stent will work nicely for this situation in the future. Deploy the stent in that place and perform additional high pressure inflations with the Olympix balloon. I would then implant a 10 mm biliary stent in the ostium of the RCA, and postdilate with a 4.0 mm Titan at 20 ATM. I recommend aspirin, ticlopidine, and low-molecular weight heparin (for 10 days).

Dean Kereiakes, MD, USA: My recommendation is to redilate areas of residual dissection with a quarter-size larger balloon or slightly higher pressure in the mid and proximal regions, to minimize the degree of residual dissection. The presence of residual dissection per se does not preclude successful short and long-term outcome. I strongly recommend adjunctive intravenous ReoPro (weight-adjusted bolus and 12-hour infusion), aspirin, and ticlopidine. I recommend repeat angiography in 3-4 months to detect restenosis.

John Douglas Jr., MD, USA: Although multiple stents were effective in restoring flow, there are two areas with suboptimal lumen and residual dissection, with some extravasation of dye outside the proximal RCA. Fortunately, the extravasation appears to be contained. I am concerned about the two areas marked by arrows and would treat further by placing a 4.0 mm Palmaz-Schatz stent over a Platinum-Plus guidewire at each site. I would expand each stent with a 4.0 mm balloon at 18-20 ATM. Echocardiography would be considered to evaluate possible pericardial effusion. If the patient remains stable, I recommend aspirin (80 mg QD), ticlopidine (250 mg BID), and low molecular weight heparin (for 10 days).

Editors' Perspective: Residual dissection and stenosis are characteristic of a suboptimal result after bailout stenting for abrupt closure. It is unclear whether anticoagulation alone (without further intervention) is sufficient to prevent stent thrombosis or recurrent ischemic complications when this type of result is obtained. It is also unclear whether these patients should be referred for urgent bypass surgery. In our opinion, the patient should leave the cath lab with either a reasonable result after multiple stent implantation or on their way to the operating room for definitive revascularization. In cases where bailout stents are implanted for long, complex dissections, it is not unusual to require overlapping stents to "seal" residual dissection; it is better to insert more stents and achieve a secure result than leave residual dissection. If additional stents

cannot be implanted, the operator must decide between relying on medical therapy to prevent stent thrombosis or referring the patient for bypass surgery. The correct answer to this dilemma is unknown, but we favor bypass surgery if the patient has normal wall motion in the distribution of the target vessel. If medical therapy is selected, aspirin and ticlopidine should be prescribed, and we favor subcutaneous heparin over Coumadin anticoagulation.

*****

NO-REFLOW

TEC atherectomy is performed on this degenerated saphenous vein graft (reference vessel = 4.2 mm) with a 7.5F cutter, but is complicated by chest pain, ST elevation, and no-reflow (TIMI flow =1).

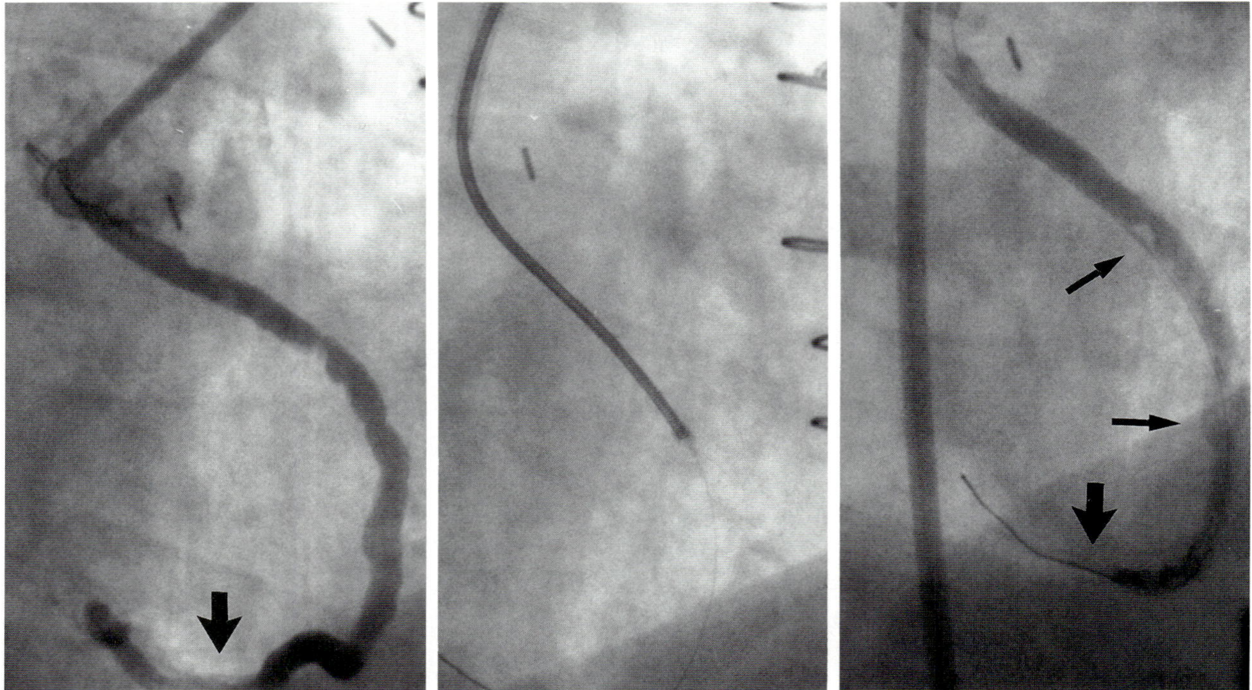

What do you recommend now?

Michael Mooney, MD, USA: I would administer diltiazem (2-4 mg IC), heparin (2,000-3,000 units IC), and nitroglycerin (200 mcg IC) directly into the vein graft. A temporary pacemaker should be readily available. I would measure a translesional pressure gradient to confirm no-reflow. I would not send the patient to surgery, since it is completely ineffective for no-reflow.

If no-reflow persists, I would administer intracoronary adenosine.

Spencer King III, MD, USA: This patient has no-reflow after TEC, likely due to distal microembolization. I would advance a deflated balloon catheter into the distal vessel, and administer a calcium antagonist.

Bernhard Meier, MD, Switzerland: In an old vein graft, TEC atherectomy results in distal embolization and poor distal flow; mechanical and pharmacologic approaches should be utilized to reestablish flow. The first consists of advancing the nonactivated TEC device or a deflated balloon as far distal as possible, to push embolized fragments into the periphery. The latter consists of generous administration of intracoronary nitrates and calcium blockers and vigorous flushing with heparinized saline. In some cases, flow will not be reestablished, and infarction will ensue. Emergency bypass surgery is of no value under these circumstances. Thrombolytic therapy or ReoPro is probably not helpful, because the embolized fragments consist of old grumous from the degenerated vein graft, rather than fresh thrombus.

Editors' Perspective: Operators who perform percutaneous interventions on saphenous vein grafts should always anticipate the possibility of no-reflow, keeping a consistent treatment strategy in mind. It is of paramount importance to clearly distinguish no-reflow from abrupt closure of the target vessel, since treatment strategies are totally different. There are no prospective randomized trials comparing treatments of no-reflow, although several observational studies permit reasonable recommendations. First and foremost is the observation that many cases of no-reflow can be reversed by intracoronary calcium antagonists. Most experience is with verapamil (100-250 mcg bolus every 2-4 minutes up to 2 mg as needed), but diltiazem is also effective (1-2 mg bolus every 2-4 minutes, not to exceed 10 mg). The key point is to ensure drug delivery to the distal capillary bed: If there is TIMI flow $\leq$ 1, drug administered through the guiding catheter (particularly those with sideholes) will never reach the distal capillary bed. In these circumstances, it is best to advance a deflated balloon catheter, infusion catheter, or any suitable transfer catheter into the distal vessel, and administer an intracoronary calcium antagonist through the central lumen. A very nice catheter for this purpose is the Ultrafuse-X, which is a double lumen catheter that allows distal drug delivery without relinquishing guidewire access. If there is "slow-flow" (TIMI flow = 2), a calcium antagonist can be delivered through the guiding catheter. The second point is that intracoronary nitroglycerin has not been shown to effectively reverse no-reflow, and should not be used as sole therapy. However, since it is not deleterious, may reverse associated epicardial spasm, and is not associated with any delays, intracoronary nitroglycerin is a reasonable adjunct. Third, while intracoronary lytics are potentially useful for distal embolization of thrombus to epicardial vessels, they are much less useful for the distal microembolization characteristic of no-reflow; in our experience, intracoronary urokinase restores flow in < 10% of no-reflow cases, and increases the risk of bleeding and femoral vascular injury. Fourth, the value of intraaortic balloon pump counterpulsation is a matter of debate; it is clearly useful when there is

hemodynamic compromise, possibly useful in milder degrees of "slow-flow," and probably not useful for true no-reflow. Fifth, limited anecdotal experience with ReoPro is positive, but further study is needed. Finally, conventional approaches to abrupt closure (prolonged balloon inflations, stents, emergency bypass surgery) have no role in the treatment of no-reflow.

*****

LATE ANEURYSM

Directional atherectomy was performed on this focal stenosis in the LCX (left panel reference vessel = 3.1 mm), leaving an excellent angiographic result (middle panel). Six months later the patient developed atypical chest pain. Repeat angiography shows a focal aneurysm just proximal to the original lesion (right panel). Other coronary arteries and left ventricular function are normal.

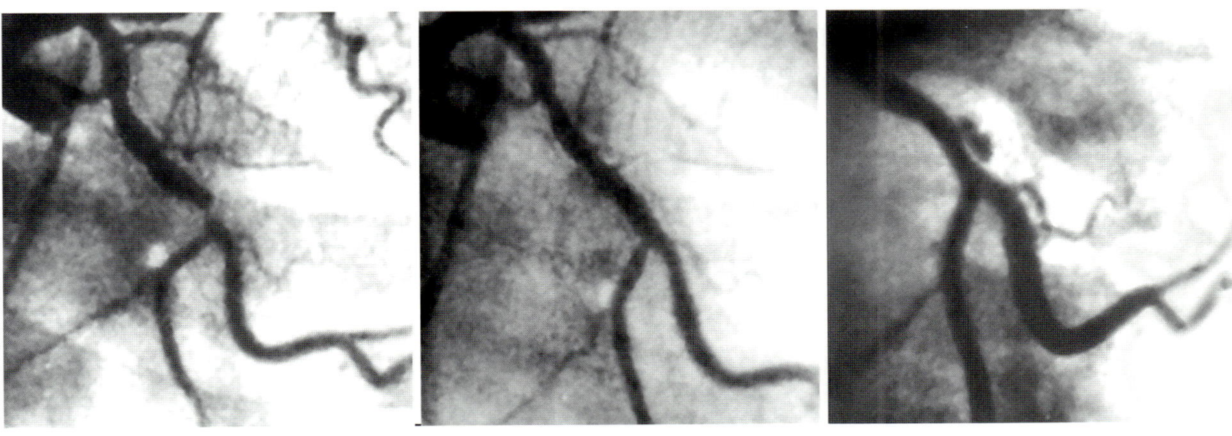

How would you manage this patient now?

David Faxon, MD, USA: Angiography demonstrates an aneurysm at the site of successful directional atherectomy. I would not perform intervention at this time. It seems very unlikely that this is a psuedoaneurysm, and is more likely to be an aneurysm localized to the atherosclerotic plaque on the superior surface of the artery. Thus, conservative management is best. I expect the aneurysm to fill-in and heal over several months.

David Holmes, MD, USA: There is a focal aneurysm just proximal to the initial stenosis. There are limited data on guidelines for management of these patients. If the patient has atypical chest pain, I would manage the patient conservatively. There is no evidence for restenosis.

Dean Kereiakes, MD, USA: This is a small focal aneurysm involving the site of prior directional atherectomy, but no evidence for restenosis. In the absence of significant restenosis, I recommend continued medical therapy.

Are any other imaging modalities indicated or useful?

David Faxon, MD, USA: Ultrasound is useful to assess the extent and nature of the aneurysm. If the aneurysm is localized to the arterial wall (not a psuedoaneurysm), I recommend antiplatelet therapy alone. If the aneurysm extends through the wall (false aneurysm), I would consider bypass surgery, since I would be concerned about rupture into the pericardial space.

David Holmes, MD, USA: Intravascular ultrasound is ideal. If this is a narrow-neck aneurysm, then conservative medical therapy is indicated. If this is a broad-based aneurysm, I would implant a coated stent. If conservative management is selected, I would repeat angiography in 1-3 months.

Dean Kereiakes, MD, USA: I do not recommend intravascular ultrasound or other diagnostic modalities.

> **Editors' Perspective: This is a rather unusual finding several months after successful atherectomy, and could represent a true or false aneurysm. There are little data to guide appropriate therapy in this case, and this lack of information is reflected by the lack of consensus among the experts. This particular patient did well with conservative therapy without further imaging or repeat angiography.**

*****

CORONARY ECTASIA

Directional atherectomy was performed on a focal stenosis in the mid-RCA (reference diameter = 3.5 mm). After multiple passes and cuts, large amounts of tissue were retrieved. The final angiogram shows a symmetric zone of coronary ectasia, but no contrast extravasation or staining.

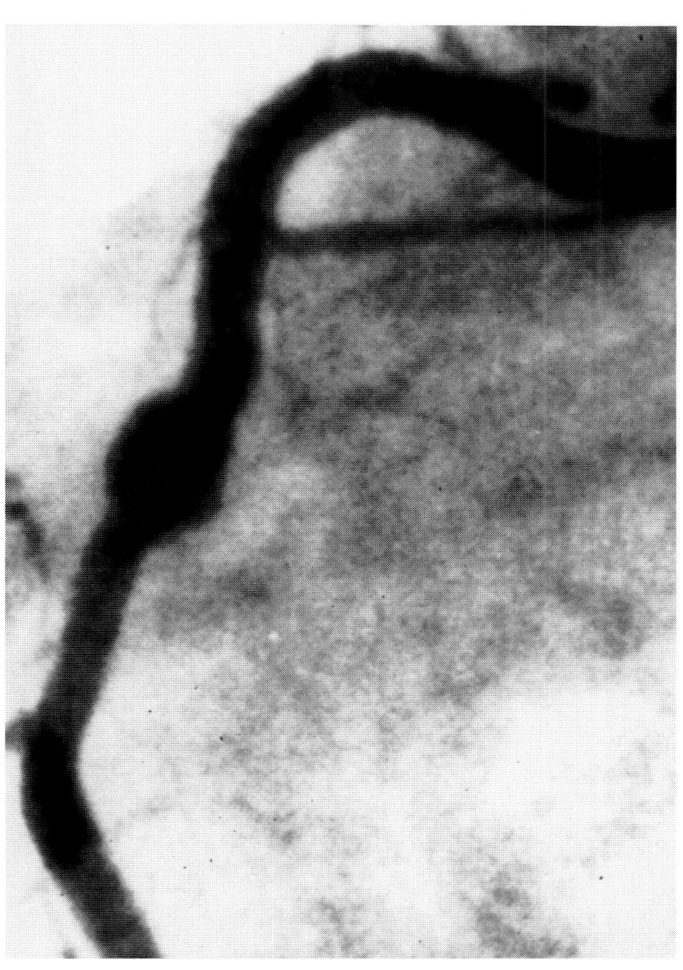

What do you recommend now?

John Douglas Jr., MD, USA: This is an example of "ultra-optimal" atherectomy with bulbous ectasia, due to stretching of the vessel wall which has been thinned by atherectomy. There is potential for development of a false aneurysm and free perforation, but I believe the risk is small. I would stop heparin, and recommend repeat angiography in a few months, to reassess the stability of this angiographic finding.

Dean Kereiakes, MD, USA: This patient has ectasia following directional atherectomy. I recommend discontinuation of heparin, but continuation of aspirin. I recommend avoidance of competitive sports for 1 month, and repeat angiography at that time.

Bernhard Meier, MD, Switzerland: Overzealous directional atherectomy results in circumferential ectasia. The risk of subsequent rupture is not known; I assume the risk is small and that no further treatment is necessary. It is wise to withhold further anticoagulation. A decrease in ectasia during followup is just as likely as a further expansion; I do not favor routine angiographic followup in the absence of symptoms.

Are adjunctive imaging modalities useful?

John Douglas Jr., MD, USA: I would not perform intravascular ultrasound. Transesophageal echocardiography can be used to assess late expansion.

Dean Kereiakes, MD, USA: Ultrasound is not needed; I recommend repeat angiography in 1 month.

> <u>Editors' Perspective</u>: **The mechanism of coronary ectasia immediately after directional atherectomy is probably deep tissue resection, altered vessel compliance, and aneurysmal dilatation initiated by the balloon on the AtheroCath. Although long-term natural history studies of these types of lesions are not available, published data suggest that the risk of perforation is low. The impact of deep tissue resection on restenosis is more controversial, although most contemporary studies suggest no impact.**

*****

FREE PERFORATION

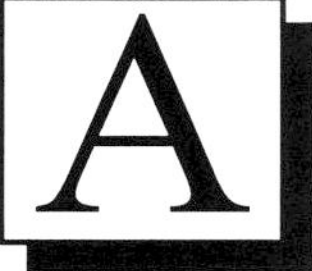

A 60-year-old woman undergoes atherectomy of the RCA (reference diameter = 2.4 mm), resulting in a jet of free contrast into the pericardium and staining of the right ventricular outflow tract. Other vessels and left ventricular function are normal.

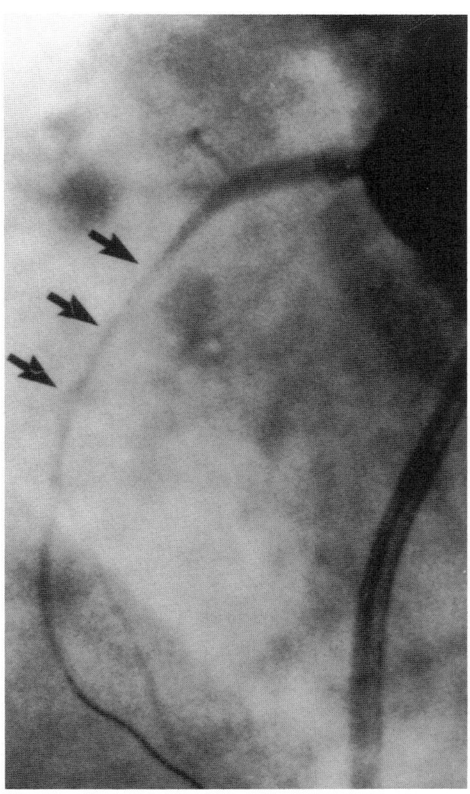

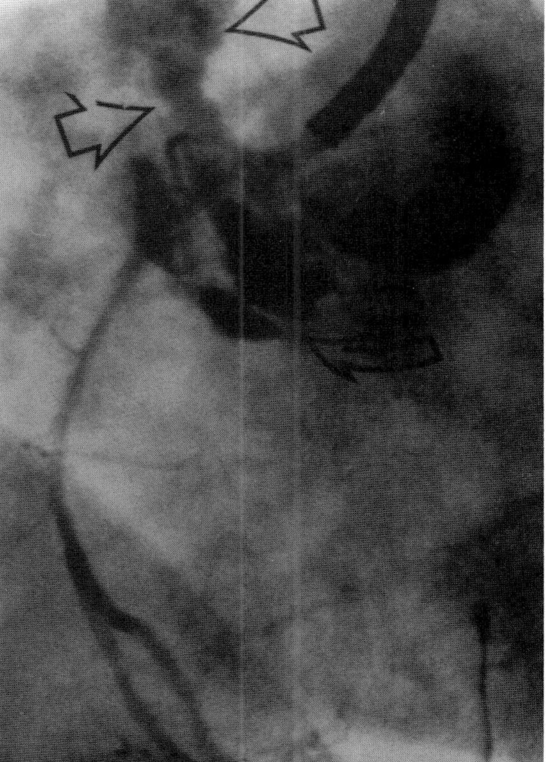

What is your immediate management of this patient?

Richard Heuser, MD, USA: This is a nightmare. First, I would type and crossmatch for blood transfusion. Second, I would notify the operating room. If the patient has tamponade, I would reverse the heparin immediately. If necessary, I would place a pacer and intraaortic balloon pump to support the blood pressure. I would inflate a 3.0 x 20 mm perfusion balloon for 10-15 minutes. This appears to be a nondominant or small RCA that could be occluded without mortality or significant infarction. If shock persists, percutaneous cardiopulmonary support may be necessary. If I could not effectively seal this perforation, I would refer the patient for emergency surgery. Other options are an endoluminal graft or a vein-covered biliary stent to seal the tear, but this vessel is much too small for either consideration. A Gianturco-Roubin stent, Wallstent, or Palmaz-Schatz stent are not warranted, since they would not seal the perforation.

David Holmes, MD, USA: With a large perforation like this, immediate management is balloon inflation. If the patient is unstable, an intraaortic balloon pump is indicated. If the patient is stable and there is no evidence for further extravasation, conservative management is indicated (but I think that would be unlikely) and anticoagulation should be discontinued. Given the large size of the perforation, it may be related to removal of a portion of the arterial wall. Implantation of a vein-covered stent has some appeal, although it is a very long lesion and I do not think it would very effective.

Gary Roubin, MD, PhD, USA: My immediate management of this problem is to place a 3.0 x 30 mm perfusion catheter in the proximal RCA, inflated to 2-3 ATM for 30 minutes. I would give small doses of Protamine to bring the ACT down to 150 seconds. After 30 minutes, I would remove the balloon catheter and check for additional contrast extravasation. Invariably, the problem is solved after a 30 minute inflation.

The patient remains stable and there is no further contrast extravasation. Describe your approach for the next 72 hours.

Richard Heuser, MD, USA: I would not heparinize this patient. I would observe the patient in the ICU with a right heart catheter in place.

Gary Roubin, MD, PhD, USA: I would not anticoagulate after the procedure and would obtain an echocardiogram immediately and 2-3 hours later in the coronary care unit. I would manage the patient with aspirin alone.

Editors' Perspective: This rare but catastrophic complication is more common after lasers and atherectomy than after PTCA. Regardless of the cause of perforation, immediate attention must be devoted to hemodynamic stabilization — ischemia is a secondary issue. An inflated balloon should be immediately positioned at the site of perforation. If the exact location of the perforation cannot be ascertained, a long (30-40 mm) balloon should be inserted to ensure coverage. A properly positioned balloon will prevent any further extravasation into the pericardium, and afford the operator more time to resuscitate the patient. Subsequent preparation and insertion of a perfusion balloon can follow, if appropriate. If there is hemodynamic collapse, the operator should do 4 more things at the same time: Protect the airway, initiate CPR, notify the surgeons, and perform immediate pericardiocentesis, leaving the pericardial drainage catheter in place. If there is any more than a moments delay in retrieving the pericardiocentesis tray, intravenous pressors and fluids should be administered to support the blood pressure. Heparin-induced anticoagulation should be reversed slowly (e.g., protamine 5-10 mg IV every 5 minutes, aiming for an ACT of 150-180 seconds). Although percutaneous CPS can be lifesaving, it can rarely be primed and instituted within minutes, and efforts are better directed at evacuating the pericardium, even by emergency pericardial window. If the patient is not in hemodynamic collapse initially, or once the patient is successfully resuscitated, further attention can be devoted to the coronary artery. Approximately two-thirds of perforations can be managed without emergency surgery, but the need for surgery is higher after free perforations caused by laser and atherectomy devices compared to those caused by PTCA. Indications for surgery include persistent (or recurrent) extravasation of contrast despite prolonged balloon inflations, and severe ischemia from vessel injury or as a consequence of balloon inflations. If the patient can be stabilized without surgical intervention, continuous monitoring of right heart filling pressures, observation in the coronary care unit, continuous pericardial drainage, and serial echocardiograms are recommended. There are a few investigational approaches to perforation, including implantation of stents covered with autologous veins or synthetic materials such as PTFE (Teflon), and coil embolization of perforated vessels that supply small areas of viable myocardium.

*****

CONTAINED PERFORATION

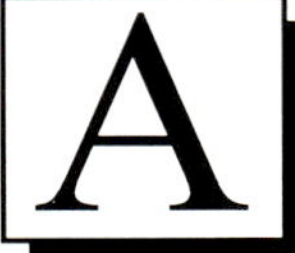

A 60-year-old woman undergoes atherectomy. After atherectomy of the proximal LCX (reference diameter = 2.8 mm), there is a small cloud of contrast in the periadventitial space. Other vessels and left ventricular function are normal.

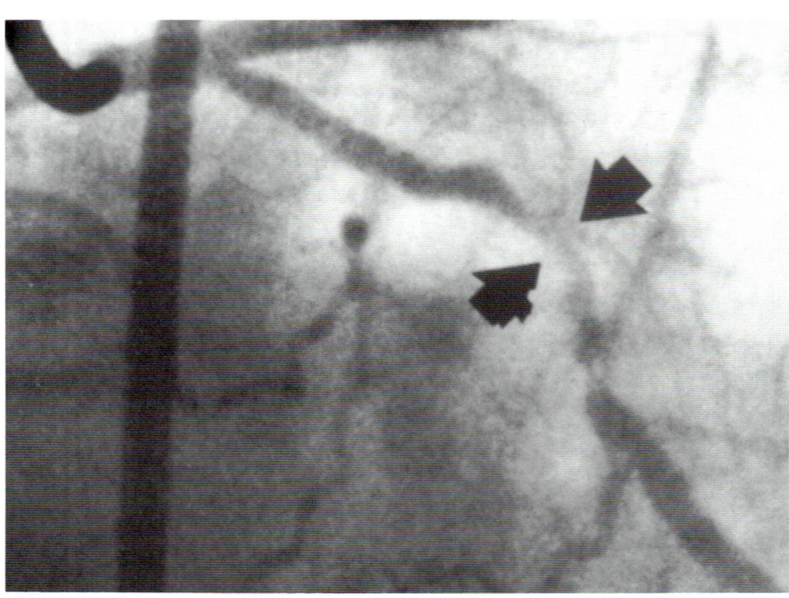

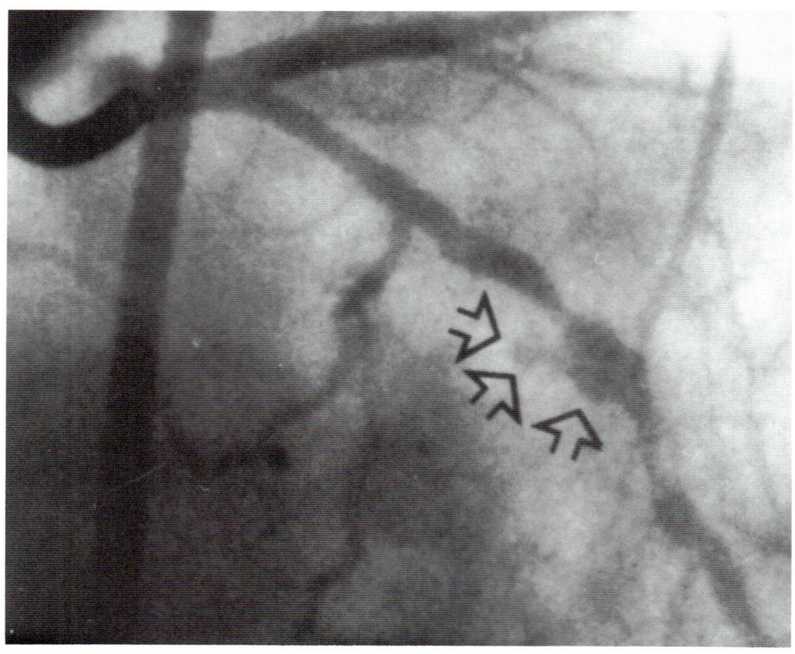

What is your immediate management of this patient?

Richard Heuser, MD, USA: This patient has contrast in the periadventitial space, but will probably do well and will not develop tamponade. However, I would place a Swan-Ganz catheter and monitor hemodynamics in the catheterization laboratory. If the dye slowly resorbs over several minutes, chances are that this problem could be solved by deploying a Palmaz-Schatz stent. A perfusion balloon might be advantageous for 15-20 minutes not only to postdilate the stent but also to clear the contrast in the periadventital space. In the majority of these cases, a stent is all that is necessary.

David Holmes, MD, USA: After atherectomy, there is a small cloud of contrast in the periadventitial space. I would place a 3.0 mm perfusion balloon at low-pressure for 15-20 minutes. I think the patient will do well without surgery. If the artery looks well-sealed, I would discontinue anticoagulation. If there is a residual area of ectasia, I would bring the patient back the next day for repeat angiography. If the patient is unstable or the perforation is enlarging, then immediate surgery is recommended. Intravascular ultrasound can be helpful in this case to see what the local anatomy is like: If there is a small tear in the artery, a vein-covered stent can be used. This takes a while to prepare and is not indicated if the patient is unstable.

Gary Roubin, MD, PhD, USA: The first point with such a complication is not to panic. In this case, I would inflate a 3.0 x 30 mm perfusion balloon at 3-4 ATM so the area of extravasation is well-covered. I would slowly reverse anticoagulation with protamine, and after 30 minutes, withdraw the balloon and repeat angiography. If there is TIMI-3 flow and no further dye extravasation (this is invariably the case), I would complete the case at this point and manage the patient with aspirin alone.

The patient remains stable. How would you manage this patient over the next 72 hours?

Richard Heuser, MD, USA: After the periadventitial space has cleared, I would keep the patient in the hospital for an extra day, discharging her within 48 hours on aspirin and ticlopidine. These are the types of cases for which we may eventually use endoluminal grafts to seal perforations.

Gary Roubin, MD, PhD, USA: I would obtain an echocardiogram immediately after leaving the catheterization laboratory and 2-3 hours later. I recommend followup angiography in 2-months.

Editors' Perspective: Although contained perforations may heal spontaneously, their natural history is uncertain. In our experience with new devices, we have learned that some patients with this angiographic appearance may develop delayed (8-24 hours later) free perforation and tamponade, despite the fact that free perforation was not present at the time of angiography. For this reason, we believe that further therapy is warranted, which at a minimum includes repeat PTCA with a prolonged (10-30 minute) balloon inflation (perfusion balloons are ideal for this task). Further anticoagulation should be withheld. If the angiographic appearance improves and remains stable, the patient should be observed in-hospital for at least 36 hours, and serial echocardiograms should be obtained, looking for an enlarging pericardial effusion.

*****

— Section 6 —

Miscellaneous

STENT EMBOLIZATION

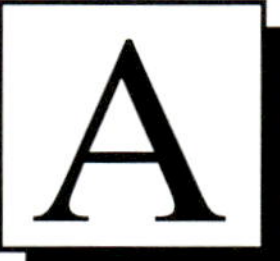

Attempted biliary stent implantation in the ostium of the SVG to the OM (left panel) is complicated by distal embolization of the stent to the iliac artery bifurcation (fluoroscopic image in middle panel; contrast in ureter).

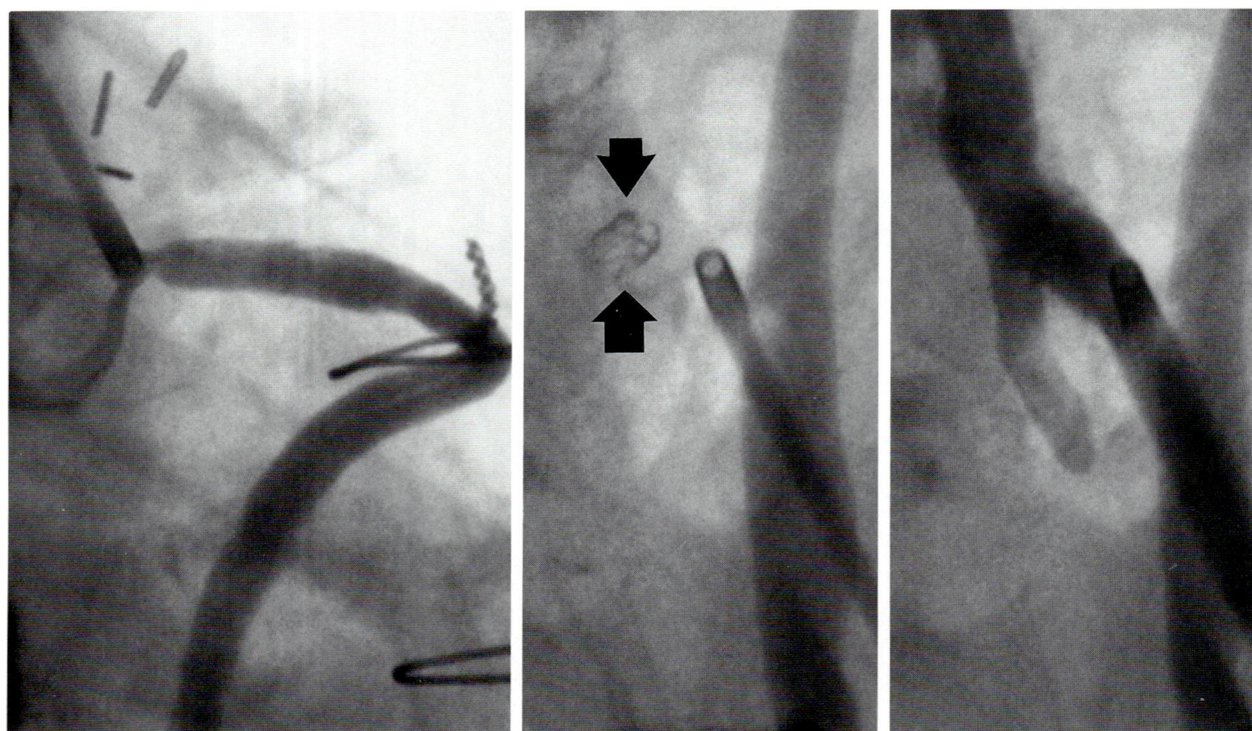

How would you manage this problem now?

Richard Schatz, MD, USA: This unfortunate complication is frequently "overstated" and "overmanaged." The stent appears to be partially expanded. If this situation occurs, one should use every precaution to ensure that the stent stays on the wire, enabling the operator to fully deploy the stent wherever it lands in the peripheral circulation. Attempts to retrieve the stent are usually fruitless, fraught with hazard, and time consuming. The safest place for an embolized stent is in the iliac or femoral artery once it is fully deployed. Since the stent is awkwardly teetering at the bifurcation, is no longer threaded by the wire, and appears expanded, there is no way to safely retrieve it. Fortunately, since it is porous and 90% air, it is unlikely to cause significant ischemia; therefore, it should be left alone. The trick is to never get into this situation by losing wire position!

Antonio Colombo, MD, Italy: In this case it seems that the sheath tip is still distal to the stent. I would exchange for a 10F sheath to allow easier entry of the stent into the sheath and try to retrieve the stent with a gooseneck device. If the stent migrates distal to the introducer, a contralateral approach can be used. Antegrade puncture of the common femoral artery would be another option if the stent migrates distally. In case the stent cannot be retrieved, crushing the stent with a balloon against the wall of a large vessel is an option. If a dedicated retrieval system is not available, 2 coronary guidewires can be used to wrap the stent and to pull it out.

Ulrich Sigwart, MD, England: One should try to get the stent out or deploy it. I think that threading a Wholey wire or a Magnum wire through this biliary stent would not be so difficult. The Wholey wire has the advantage of making stent deployment easy since it accepts large peripheral balloons. Since this stent is partially expanded, I would try to deploy it, rather than remove it.

Editors' Perspective: Stent embolization to the peripheral circulation can be managed in several ways. First, an attempt can be made to remove the stent. This is far easier if the stent is still on the guidewire and not expanded: A low-profile balloon can be threaded through the stent, inflated, and pulled back to "capture" and withdraw the stent into the arterial sheath. A second approach is to use a balloon of sufficient diameter to fully deploy the stent at the site of embolization; this can be accomplished with the stent partially expanded or unexpanded. Third, if the stent cannot be retrieved or expanded, it can be left alone or "crushed" against the vessel wall by another balloon outside the stent. In this patient, the stent was deployed in the iliac artery using a peripheral angioplasty balloon and a 0.035-inch J-wire.

*****

CATHETER EMBOLIZATION

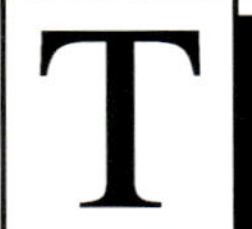

The distal end of a central venous catheter was sheared off and embolized to the left pulmonary artery (LAO projection).

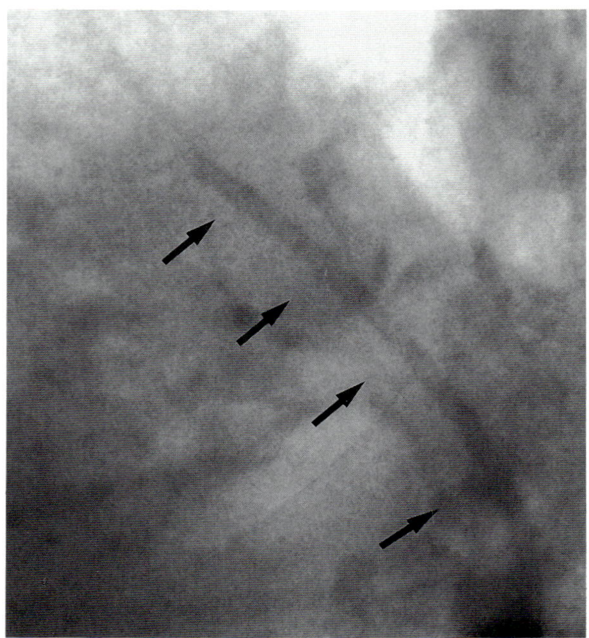

How would you manage this problem now?

David Williams, MD, USA: This patient has experienced embolization of a central venous catheter to the left pulmonary artery. These catheters can be retrieved by intravascular snares. Access from the internal jugular provides the greatest chance of reaching the fragment, which can be retrieved with a 6F catheter and a 15 mm Nitinol snare.

Patrick Whitlow, MD, USA: This interesting problem could probably be solved by utilizing a Microvena gooseneck snare through a multipurpose diagnostic catheter. I would place an 8F venous sheath in the right femoral vein, and manipulate a multipurpose catheter into the right heart and pulmonary outflow tract (a Goodale-Luben catheter can be utilized if the multipurpose catheter fails). Once in the pulmonary outflow tract, I would advance a 0.035-inch J-wire or Wholey wire and multipurpose catheter proximal to the venous line. The guidewire would then be removed and replaced by a 15 mm gooseneck snare. The snare can be manipulated around the proximal end of the venous line and the catheter advanced to the tip of the gooseneck. Once this position is achieved, the entire system can be pulled back through the right heart and into the femoral vein. If the orientation of the snare and venous line is optimal, it could be retracted into the 8F sheath and removed as a unit.

Masakiyo Nobuyoshi, MD, Japan: I would use an 8F sheath in the femoral vein, and advance an 8F JR4 catheter to the left pulmonary artery over a guidewire. The guidewire should be withdrawn and replaced with the basket retriever. With the basket inside the guiding catheter, both should be advanced beyond the embolized catheter; the basket should then be opened and manipulated so that the lost catheter fragment is engaged between the basket wires. Sometimes the catheter fragment attaches to the pulmonary wall and cannot be engaged with the basket. If this is the case, the basket should be withdrawn and bent slightly at the base to form a 15-20° angle to facilitate capture. Once the foreign body is engaged, the guide catheter should be slowly advanced until the basket is closed with the foreign body trapped inside, and the entire assembly should be withdrawn while tension is applied to the basket wire. Loop snares are less successful in retrieving pulmonary artery catheter fragments.

Editors' Perspective: Gooseneck snares and basket retrieval devices are occasionally needed to remove catheter fragments in the central circulation. If the fragment cannot be removed through the femoral venous sheath, cutdown on the femoral vein can facilitate removal of the fragment under direct vision. In this case, the catheter fragment was withdrawn into the femoral vein using a 7F Multipurpose catheter and a Microvena gooseneck snare. Femoral vein cutdown was required, since the fragment could not be withdrawn through the sheath.

*****

SHEATH EMBOLIZATION

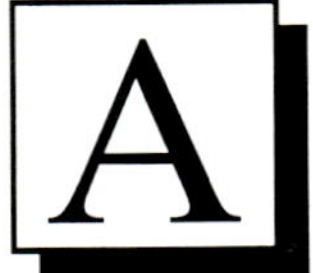

A 6F vascular sheath was sheared off and embolized distally in the femoral artery.

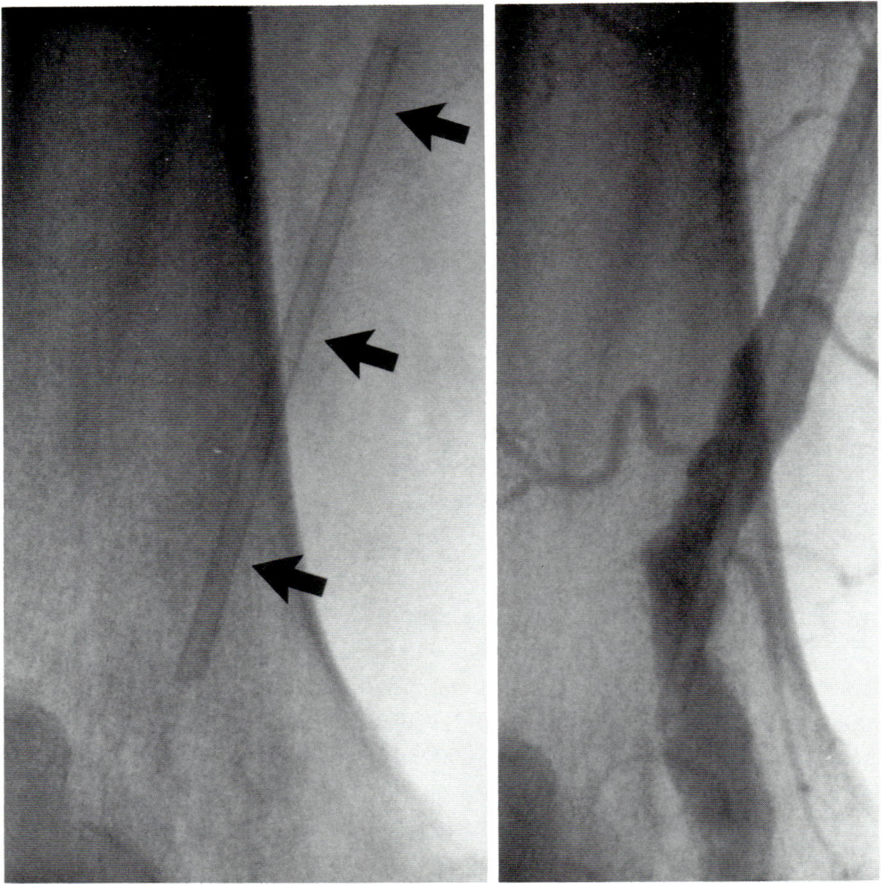

How would you manage this problem?

Nicolaus Reifart, MD, Germany: I would access the left groin, introduce an 8F sheath, and enter the right iliac artery with an 8F JR3 or multipurpose guiding catheter. The vascular sheath could be engaged with a Microvena snare and pulled into the guiding catheter.

Gary Roubin, MD, PhD, USA: I would access the contralateral femoral artery with a 9F sheath and place a 90 cm 8F IMA catheter around the horn of the iliac bifurcation over a Wholey wire, down the common iliac artery. I would then advance a Microvena snare through the guiding catheter to catch the femoral sheath fragment. If the sheath cannot be snared using this technique, an alternative technique is to place a 9 French multipurpose catheter over the Wholey wire, and use Cook retrieval forceps to grab the end of the sheath. The sheath can then be pulled back around the horn and through the 9 French sheath.

Paul Teirstein, MD, USA: This vascular sheath has embolized distally in the femoral artery. I have no personal experience in peripheral angioplasty below the iliac arteries. Therefore, I would refer this patient to an interventional radiologist for help. I would also fire the fellow who allowed this problem to occur!

Editors' Perspective: Retrieval of catheter fragments and other foreign bodies is occasionally required and has been simplified by the availability of a variety of gooseneck snares. If the embolized sheath cannot be retrieved through the contralateral femoral sheath, it may be possible to withdraw the catheter up to the common femoral artery, where direct cutdown on the femoral artery can facilitate removal of the fragment under direct vision (which was necessary in this patient).

*****

PSEUDOLESION

A target lesion in the mid-RCA (left panel) is crossed with a guidewire, and multiple severe stenoses appear throughout the vessel (middle panel). After PTCA and removal of the guidewire, there is a mild residual stenosis in the target lesion (right panel), but the other stenoses are no longer apparent.

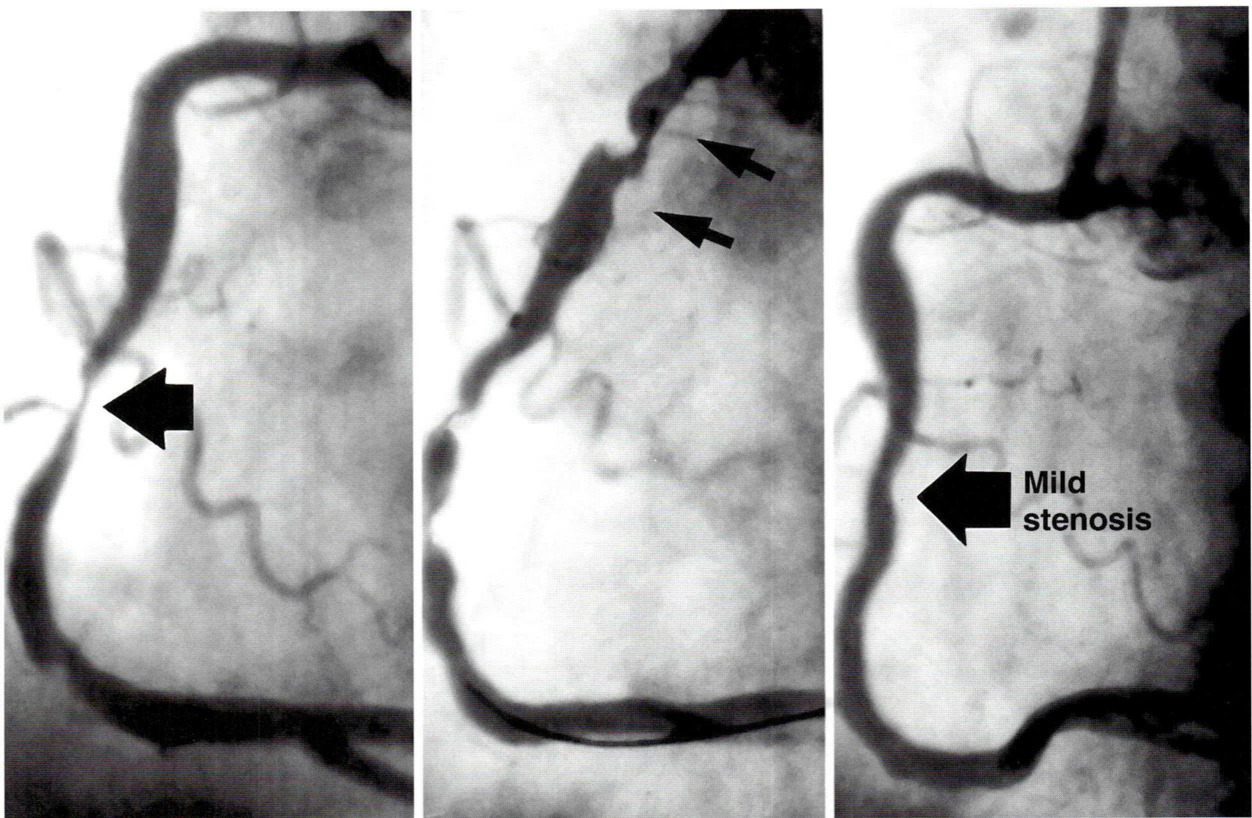

How do you distinguish pseudolesions from true lesions induced by PTCA hardware?

David Faxon, MD, USA: This patient illustrates one of the problems with stiff guidewires, namely, artificial straightening of the artery and the creation of pseudolesions. This poses a significant problem in assessing the progress of the procedure. In general, I try to ignore pseudolesions and concentrate on the primary lesion. Once that has been satisfactorily treated, the stiff guidewire should be pulled back to allow the more flexible portion to traverse these lesions to determine if they are real or not. Alternatively, a stiff guidewire can be exchanged for a floppy guidewire, which will not straighten the artery.

John Douglas Jr., MD, USA: Pseudolesions are commonly seen when tortuous native coronary arteries, internal mammary artery grafts, or other arteries are straightened by wires or catheters. These invaginations or "buckling" of the vessel wall occur at points of maximal tortuosity and may be associated with vessel spasm that responds to nitroglycerin. The stiffer the wire (or catheter) and the more tortuous the vessel, the more likely one will encounter pseudolesions. The best way to confirm the presence of a pseudolesion is to reduce or remove the straightening effect. This may be accomplished by replacing the stiff guidewire with a flexible one, or the operator can withdraw the guidewire so the distal flexible portion is across the segment in question. The wire (or catheter) may be removed completely, allowing the vessel to resume its usual shape.

Michael Mooney, MD, USA: The proximal RCA has multiple pseudolesions, due to excessive straightening by PTCA hardware. I would not like to lose access to the distal artery by removing equipment, without being certain as to the exact origin of the changes in the appearance of the artery. Staining within the presumed pseudolesion is uncommon, and if present, suggests dissection. If an extra-support wire has been used, I would exchange it for a floppy wire, which allows the artery to assume its more natural contour. The defects should improve dramatically if due to pseudolesions.

Editors' Perspective: Pseudolesions are frequently observed when stiff guidewires are used in tortuous vessels, including TEC and Rotablator wires, extra-support wires, and heavy-duty guidewires such as the Platinum-Plus. These "pseudolesions" are due to invagination of the vessel wall around a stiff guidewire, with a possible component of vasospasm. Initially, it is best to "ignore" these lesions and concentrate on the target lesion. After revascularization of the target lesion, it is reasonable to exchange for a flexible guidewire, to be sure the pseudolesions improve or resolve before removing the guidewire completely.

*****

— Section 7 —

References

Brachial & Radial PTCA

1. Sones FM, Shirey EK: Cine coronary arteriography. Mod Conc. Cardiovasc Dis. 31:735, 1962.
2. Judkins MP: Selective coronary arteriography: A percutaneous transfemoral technique. Radiology 89:815-824, 1967.
3. Stertzer SH: Brachial approach to transluminal coronary angioplasty. In Angioplasty. New York, McGraw-Hill, 1986, pp 260-294.
4. Yakubov SJ, George, BS: Coronary Intervention: Brachial Technique. In interventional Cardiovascular Medicine: Principles and Practice. New York, Churchill-Livingston Co., 1994, pp 451-64.
5. Huepler F: Coronary arteriography and left ventriculography: Sones technique. In Coronary Arteriography and Angioplasty. Hew York, McGraw-Hill, 1985, pp 137-181.
6. Kamada RO, Fergusson DJ, Itagaki RK: Percutaneous entry of the brachial artery for transluminal coronary angioplasty. Cathet Cardiovasc Diagn 15:132-133, 1988.
7. George BS: Brachial Technique to Intervention. In Textbook of Interventional Cardiology. Vol. 2. Philadelphia, W.B. Saunders Company, 1994, pp 549-564.
8. Kiemeneij F, Laarman, GJ. Percutaneous transradial artery approach for coronary stent implantation. Cath Cardiovasc Diagn. 30:173-178, 1993.
9. Keimeneij F, Laarman GJ, Slagboom T, Stella P. Transradial Palmaz-Schatz coronary stenting on an outpatient basis: Results of a prospective pilot study. J Invas Cardiol 7:5A-11A, 1995.
10. Barbeau GR, Carrier G, Ferland S, Larriviere MM. Transradial approach for coronary angiography, angioplasty and stent delivery: Procedural results. Circulation 1995;92:I-196.
11. Kiemeneij F, Laarman GJ, Slagboom T, van der Wieken R. Transradial coronary stenting in outpatients. Circulation 1995;92:I-535.
12. Vallabhan RC, Anwar A, Bret JR, et al. Radial artery access for cardiac catheterization and coronary angioplasty. Circulation 1995;92:I-602.
13. Johnson LW, Esenta P, Giambartolomei A, et al. Peripheral vascular complications of coronary angioplasty by the femoral and brachial techniques. Cath Cardiovasc Diagn. 1994;31:165-172.
14. George BS, Candela RJ, Topol EJ, et al. The brachial approach to emergency cardiac catheterization during thrombolytic therapy for acute myocardial infarction. Cathet Cardiovasc Diagn 1990;20:221-226.
15. Topol EJ, Califf RM, George BS, et al. A randomized trial of immediate vs. delayed elective angioplasty after intravenous tissue plasminogen activator in acute myocardial infarction. N. Engl J Med 317:581-588, 1987.
16. Topol EJ Califf RM, George BS, et al. Coronary arterial thrombolysis with combined infusion of recombinant tissue-type plasminogen activator and urokinase in patients with acute myocardial infarction. Circulation 77:1100-1107, 1988.
17. Topol EJ, George BS, Kereiakes DJ, et al. A randomized controlled trial of intravenous tissue plasminogen activator and early intravenous heparin in acute myocardial infarction. Circulation 79:281-286, 1989.
18. Kiemeneij, F, Laarman GJ, de Melker E. Tranradial artery coronary angioplasty. AM Heart J 1995;129:1-7.
19. Lotan C, Hasin Y, Mosseri M, Rozenman Y, et al. Transradial approach to coronary angiography and angioplasty. Am J Cardiol 76:164-167, 1995.
20. Stella P, Kiemeneij F, Laarman G, et al. Incidence and outcome of radial artery occlusion following transradial artery coronary angioplasty. Circulation 1995;92:I-225.
21. Kiemeneij F, Laarman GJ, Odekerken D, et al. Interim analysis of the ACCESS-study: A randomized comparison of transradial,-brachial and -femoral coronary angioplasty with 6-French guiding catheters. Circulation 1995;92:I-476.
22. Cubeddu MG, Arrowood ME, Mann JT. Right radial access for PTCA: A prospective study demonstrates reduced complications and hospital charges. Circulation 1995;92:I-662.
23. Fajadet J, Brunel P, Cassagneau B, et al. Transradial approach for interventional coronary procedures: analysis of complications. J Am Coll Cardiol 1996;27:392A.

Single & Multivessel PTCA

24. Hueb WA, Bellotti G, de Oliveira SA, et al. The Medicine, Angioplasty, or Surgery Study (MASS): A prospective, randomized trial of medical therapy, balloon angioplasty, or bypass surgery for single proximal LAD stenoses. J Am Coll Cardiol 1995;26:1600-1605.
25. Henderon RA, Pocock SJ, Hampton JR. Revascularization for patients with single vessel disease: Results from the randomized interventional treatment of angina (RITA) trial at 4.7 years. Circulation 1995;92:I-476.
26. Goy JJ, Eckhout E, Burnand B, et al. Coronary angioplasty versus left internal mammary artery grafting for isolated proximal left anterior descending artery stenosis. Lancet 1994;343:1149-1453.
27. Mark DB, Nelson CL, Califf RM, et al. Continuing evolution of therapy for coronary artery disease. Initial results from the era of coronary angioplasty. Circulation 1994;89:2015-2025.
28. Cameron J, Mahanonda N, Aroney C, et al. Outcome five years after percutaneous transluminal coronary angioplasty or coronary artery bypass grafting for significant narrowing limited to the left anterior descending coronary artery. Am J Cardiol 1994;74:544-549.
29. Parisi A, Folland E, Hartigan P. A comparison of angioplasty with medical therapy in the treatment of single-vessel coronary artery disease. N Engl J Med 1992;326:10-16.
30. Morris KG, Folland ED, Hartigan PM, et al. Unstable angina in late follow-up of the ACME trial. Circulation 1995;92:I-725.
31. Frierson JH, Dimas AP, Whitlow PL, Hollman JL. Angioplasty of the proximal left anterior descending coronary artery: Initial success and long-term follow-up. J Am Coll Cardiol 1992;19:745-751.
32. Henderson RA, Karani S, Dritsas A, et al. Long-term results of coronary angioplasty for single vessel, proximal left anterior

descending disease. Eur Heart J 1991;12:642-47.
33. Kramer JR, Proudfit W, Loop FD, et al. Late follow-up of 781 patients undergoing PTCA or bypass surgery for an isolated obstruction in the left anterior descending coronary artery. Am Heart J 1989;118:1144-53.
34. Coronary angioplasty versus coronary artery bypass surgery: The randomized intervention treatment of angina (RITA) trial. RITA Trial Participants. Lancet 1993;341:573-80.
35. Rodriguez A, Boullon F, Perez-Balino N. Argentine randomized trial of percutaneous transluminal coronary angioplasty versus coronary artery bypass surgery in multivessel disease (ERACI): In-hospital results and 1-year follow-up. J Am Coll Cardiol 1993;22:1060-1067.
36. Hamm C, Reimers J, Ischinger T, Rupprecht H. A randomized study of coronary angioplasty compared with bypass surgery in patients with symptomatic multivessel coronary disease. N Engl J Med 1994;331:1037-1043.
37. First-year results of CABRI Coronary Angioplasty versus Bypass Revascularization Investigation). CABRI Trial Participants. Lancet 1995;346:1179-84.
38. King S, Lembo N, Weintraub W, Kosinski A. A randomized trial comparing coronary angioplasty with coronary bypass surgery. N Engl J Med 1994;331:1044-1150.
39. The Bypass Angioplasty Revascularization Investigation (BARI): Five-year mortality and morbidity in a randomized study comparing CABG and PTCA in patients with multivessel coronary disease. The BARI Investigators. N Engl J Med (submitted).
40. Ellis S, Cowley M, Whitlow P, et al. Prospective case-control comparison of percutaneous transluminal coronary revascularization in patients with multivessel disease treated in 1986-1987 versus 1991: Improved in-hospital and 12-month results. J Am Coll Cardiol 1995;25:1137-42.
41. Danchin N, Cador R, Dibon O, et al. Changes in immediate outcome of PTCA in multivessel coronary artery disease: Implications for the interpretation of randomized trials of PTCA versus CABG. Circulation 1995;92:I-475.
42. O'Keefe JH, Allan JJ, McCallister BD, McConahay DR. Angioplasty versus bypass surgery for multivessel Coronary artery disease with left ventricular ejection fraction <40%. Am J Cardiol 1993;71:897-901.
43. Ellis SG, Vandormael MG, Cowley MJ, et al. Coronary morphologic and clinical determinants of procedural outcome with angioplasty for multivessel coronary disease: Implications for patient selection. Circulation 1990;82:1193-1202.
44. Ellis SG, Cowley MK, DiSciascio G, et al. Determinants of 2-year outcome after coronary angioplasty in patients with multivessel disease on the basis of comprehensive preprocedural evaluation: Implications for patient selection. Circulation 1991;82:1905-1914.
45. LaVee J, Rath S, Hoa, et al. Does complete revascularization by the conventional method truly provide the best possible results? Analysis of results and comparison with revascularization of infarct-prone segments (systematic segmental myocardial revascularization): The Sheba Study. J Thorac Cardiovasc Surg 1986;92:279-290.
46. Schaff HV, Gersh BJ, Pluth JR, et al. Survival and functional status after coronary artery bypass grafting: Results 10 to 12 years after surgery in 500 patients. Circulation 1983;68:II-200-204.
47. Lawrie GM, Morris GC, Silvers A, et al. The influence of residual disease after coronary bypass on the 5-year survival rate of 1274 men with coronary artery disease. Circulation 1982;66:717-723.
48. Jones EL, Craver JM, Guyton RA, et al. Importance of complete revascularization in performance of the coronary bypass operation. Am J Cardiol 1983;51:7-12.
49. Cukingham RA, Carey JS, Wittig JH, et al. Influence of complete coronary revascularization on relief of angina. J Thorac Cardiovasc Surg 1980;79:188-193.Mabin TQA, Holmes DR, Smith HC, et al. Follow-up clinical results in patients undergoing percutaneous transluminal coronary angioplasty. Circulation 1985;71:754-760.
50. Vandormael MG, Chaitman BR, Ischinger T, Aker UT. Immediate and short-term benefit of multilesion coronary angioplasty: Influence of degree of Revascularization. J Am Coll Cardiol 1985;6:983-991.
51. Bourassa MG, Yeh W, Detre K, for the NHLBI PTCA Investigators. Five-year event rates after multivessel PTCA when complete revascularization is not possible or not intended. J Am Coll Cardiol 1994;February:223A.
52. Bell M, Bailey K, Reeder G, Lapeyre A, Holmes D. Percutaneous transluminal angioplasty in patients with multivessel coronary disease: How important is complete revascularization for cardiac event-free survival? J Am Coll Cardiol 1990;16:553-562.
53. Reeder GS, Holmes DR, Detre K, et al. Degree of revascularization in patients with multivessel coronary disease: A report from the National Heart, Lung and Blood Institute Percutaneous Transluminal Coronary Angioplasty Registry. Circulation 1988;3:638-644.
54. Cowley M, Vandermael M, Topol E, et al. Is traditionally defined complete revascularization needed for patients with multivessel disease treated by elective coronary angioplasty? J Am Coll Cardiol 1993;22:1289-1297.
55. Weintraub W, King S, Douglas J, Kosinski A. Percutaneous transluminal coronary angioplasty as a first revascularization procedure in single-, double, and triple-vessel coronary artery disease. J Am Coll Cardiol 1995;26:142-151.
56. Le Feuvre C, Bonan R, Cote Gilles, et al. Five-to-10 year outcome after multivessel percutaneous transluminal coronary angioplasty. Am J Cardiol 1993;71:1153-1158.
57. Lafont A, Dimas AP, Grigera F, Pearce G. Percutaneous transluminal coronary angioplasty of one major coronary artery when the contralateral vessel is occluded. J Am Coll Cardiol 1993;22:1298-1303.
58. De Bruyne B, Renkin J, Col J, Wijns W. Percutaneous transluminal coronary angioplasty of the left coronary artery in patients with chronic occlusion of the right coronary artery: Clinical and functional results. Am Heart J 1991;122:415.
59. Teirstein P. Giorgi L, Johnson W, et al. PTCA of the left coronary artery when the right coronary artery is chronically occluded. Am Heart J 1990;119:479.
60. Le Feuvre C, Bonan R, Lesperance J, et al. Predictive factors of restenosis after multivessel percutaneous transluminal coronary angioplasty. Am J Cardiol 1994;73:840-844.
61. Mock M, Ringqvist I, Fisher L, et al. Survival of medically treated patients in the Coronary Artery Surgery Study (CASS) Registry. Circulation 1982;66:562-8.
62. Hueb WA, Bellotti G, de Oliveira A, et al. The Medicine, Angioplasty or Surgery Study (MASS): A prospective, randomized trial

of medical therapy, balloon angioplasty or bypass surgery for single proximal left anterior descending artery stenoses. J Am Coll Cardiol 1995;26:1600-5.
63. Breeman A, Boersma E, Deckers JW, et al. The impact of the completeness of revascularization on adverse cardiac events at 1 year follow-up in 1021 CABRI patients. J Am Coll Cardiol 1996;27:55A.
64. Ellis SG, Whitlow PL, Guetta V, et al. A highly significant 40% reduction in ischemic complications of percutaneous coronary intervention in 1995: Beginning of a new era? J Am Coll Cardiol 1996;27:253A.
65. Rodriquez A, Mele E, Peyregne E, et al. Three-year follow-up of the Argentine Randomized Trial of PTCA vs. CABG in multivessel disease (ERACI). J Am Coll Cardiol 1996;27:1178-84.
66. Sim I, Gupta M, McDonald K, Bourassa MG, Hlatky MA. A meta-analysis of randomized trials comparing CABG with PTCA in multivessel coronary artery disease. Am J Cardiol 1995;76:1025-9.

High-Risk Intervention

67. Kahn JK, Rutherford BD, McConahay DR, et al. In-hospital death following PTCA: complex patients or complex morphology. Circulation 1990;82:III-509.
68. Kimmel SE, Berlin JA, Strom BL, Laskey WK. Development and validation of a simplified predictive index for major complications in contemporary percutaneous transluminal coronary angioplasty practice. J Am Coll Cardiol 1995;26:931-938.
69. Ellis SG, Roubin GS, King SP III et al. In-hospital cardiac mortality after acute closure after coronary angioplasty: Analysis of risk factors from 8,207 procedures. J Am Coll Cardiol 1988;11:211.
70. Anto HR, Chou SY, Porush JG, et al. Infusion intravenous pyelography and renal function: Effects of hypertensic mannitol in patients with chronic renal insufficiency. Arch Intern Med 1981;141:1652.
71. Stack RS, Quigley PJ, Collins G, et al. Perfusion balloon catheter. Am J Cardiol 1988;61:77G.
72. Turi ZG, Campbell CA, Gottimukkala MV, et al. Preservation of distal coronary perfusion during prolonged balloon inflations with an autoperfusion angioplasty catheter. Circulation 1987;75:1275.
73. Zalewski A, Goldberg A, Dervan JP, et al. Myocardial protection during transient coronary artery occlusion in man: beneficial effects of regional β-adrenergic blockade. Circulation 1986;73:734.
74. Kern MJ, Pearson A, Woodruff R, et al. Hemodynamic and echocardiographic assessment of the effects of diltiazem during transient occlusion of the left anterior descending coronary artery during percutaneous transluminal coronary angioplasty. Am J Cardiol 1989;64:849.
75. Hombach V, Hopp HW, Fuchs M, et al. Beneficial effects of intracoronary nifedipine during percutaneous transluminal coronary angioplasty. Herz. 1986;11:232.
76. Hanet C, Rousseau M-F, Vincent MF, et al. Myocardial protection by intracoronary nicardipine administration during percutaneous transluminal coronary angioplasty. Am J Cardiol 1987;59;1035.
77. Banka VS, Trivedi A, Patal R, et al. Prevention of myocardial ischemia during coronary angioplasty: A simple new method for distal antegrade arterial blood perfusion. Am Heart J 1989;118:830-836.
78. Gabliani G, Deligonul U, Kern MJ, et al. Acute coronary occlusion occurring after successful percutaneous transluminal coronary angioplasty: Temporal relationship to discontinuation of anticoagulation. Am Heart J 1988;16:696.
79. Caracciolo EA, Davis KB, Sopko G, et al. Comparison of surgical and medical group survival in patients with left main coronary artery disease. Long-term CASS experience. Circulation 1995;91:2325-2334.
80. Conley MJ, Ely RI, Kisslo J, et al. The prognostic spectrum of left main stenosis. Circulation 178;57:947-952.
81. O'Keefe JH Jr., Hartzler GO, Rutherford BD, et al. Left main coronary angioplasty: early and late results of 127 acute and elective procedures. Am J Cardiol 1989;64:144-7.
82. Fajadet J, Brunel P, Jordan C, et al. Is stenting of left main coronary artery a reasonable procedure? Circulation 1995;92:I-355.
83. Itoh A, Colombo A, Hall P, et al. Stenting in protected and unprotected left main coronary artery: Immediate and follow-up results. J Am Coll Cardiol 1996;27:277A.

Unstable Ischemic Syndromes

84. Zijlstra F, Jan de Boaer M, Hoorntje JCA, Reiffer S, Reiber JHC, Suryapranata H. A comparison of immediate coronary angioplasty with intravenous streptokinase in acute myocardial infarction. N Engl J Med 1993;328:680-684.
85. Griffin J, Grines CL, Marsales D, et al. A prospective, randomized trial evaluating the prophylactic use of balloon pumping in high risk myocardial infarction patients: PAMI-2. J Am Coll Cardiol 1995;25:86A.
86. Brodie BR, Grines CL, Ivanhoe R, Knopf W, Taylor G, O'Keefe J, Weintraub RA, Berdan LG, Tcheng JE, Woodlief LH, Califf RM, O'Neill WW. Six-month clinical and angiographic follow-up after direct angioplasty for acute myocardial infarction. Circulation 1994;90:156-162.
87. O'Neill WW, Weintraub R, Grines CL, Meany TB, Brodie BR, Friedman HZ, Ramos RG, Gangadharan V, Levin RN, Choksi N, Westveer DC, Strzelecki RN, Timmis GC. A prospective placebo-controlled randomized trial of intravenous streptokinase and angioplasty therapy of acute myocardial infarction. Circulation 1992;86:1710-1717.
88. Weaver WD, Parsons L, Every N. Primary coronary angioplasty in hospitals with and without surgery backup. J Invas Cardiol 1995;7:34F-39F.
89. Ayres M. Coronary angioplasty for acute myocardial infarction in hospitals without cardiac surgery. J Invas Cardiol 1995;7:40F-46F.
90. Weaver W, Parsons L, Martin JS, Every N. Direct PTCA for treatment of acute myocardial infarction: A community experience in hospitals with and without surgical back-up. Circulation 1995;92:I-138.

91. Wharton TP, Schmitz JM, Fedele FA, McNamara NS, Gladstone AR, Jacobs MI. Primary angioplasty in acute myocardial infarction at community hospitals without cardiac surgery: Experience in 195 cases. Circulation 1995;92:I-138.
92. Ohnishi Y, Saffitz J, Sobel B, Coor P, Goldstein J. Primary angioplasty minimizes reperfusion injury and enhances recovery of myocardial function compared with thrombolysis. J Am Coll Cardiol 1995:219A.
93. Kinn J, Benzuly K, Sachs D, O'Neill W. Primary angioplasty results in less myocardial rupture than thrombolytics in patients recently treated for acute myocardial infarction. Circ 1995;92:I-139.
94. Krikorian R, Vacek J, Rosamont T, Beauchamp G. Timing, mode and predictors of death after direct angioplasty for acute myocardial infarction. J Am Coll Cardiol 1995:296A.
95. O'Keefe JO, Bailey WL, Rutherford BD, Hartzler GO. Primary angioplasty for acute myocardial infarction in 1000 consecutive patients. Am J. Cardiol 1993;72:107-G-115G.
96. Brodie BR, Weintraub RA, Stuckey TD, et al. Outcomes of direct coronary angioplasty for acute myocardial infarction in candidates and non-candidates for thrombolytic therapy. Am J Cardiol 1991;67:7-12.
97. Beauchamp GD, Vacek JL, Robuck W. Management comparison for acute myocardial infarction: direct angioplasty versus sequential thrombolysis-angioplasty. Am Heart J 1990;120:237-242.
98. Nakagawa Y, Iwasaki Y, Takeshi, Nobuyoshi M. Serial angiographic follow-up after successful direct angioplasty for acute myocardial infarction; single center experience. Circulation 1993;88(Suppl I):I-106 (abstr).
99. Rothbaum DA, Linnemeier TJ, Landin RJ, et al. Emergency percutaneous transluminal coronary angioplasty in acute myocardial infarction: a 3 year experience. J Am Coll Cardiol 1987;10:264-272.
100. Miller PF, Brodie BR, Weintraub RA, et al. Emergency coronary angioplasty for acute myocardial infarction. Arch Intern Med 1987;147:1565-1570.
101. Dageford DA, Genovely HC, Goodin RR, Allen RD. Emergency percutaneous transluminal coronary angioplasty in acute myocardial infarction. J Kentucky Med Assn 1987;85:368-372.
102. Kimura T, Nosaka H, Ueno K, Nobuyoshi M. Role of coronary angioplasty in acute myocardial infarction. Circulation 1986;74(Suppl II):II-22(abstr).
103. Marco J, Caster L, Szatmary LJ, Fajadet J. Emergency percutaneous transluminal coronary angioplasty without thrombolysis as initial therapy in acute myocardial infarction. Int J Cardiol 1987;15:55-63.
104. O'Neill W, Timmis GC, Bourdillon PD, et al. A prospective randomized clinical trial of intracoronary streptokinase versus coronary angioplasty for acute myocardial infarction. N Engl J Med 1986;314:812-818.
105. Stone GW, Rutherford BD, McConahay DR, et al. Direct coronary angioplasty in acute myocardial infarction: outcome in patients with single vessel disease. J Am Coll Cardiol 1990;15:534-43.
106. Stone GW, Grines CL, Topol EJ. Update on percutaneous transluminal coronary angioplasty for acute myocardial infarction. Book chapter. Current Review of Interventional Cardiology. Ed. E. Topol, M.D., P. Serruys, M.D., Current Medicine, Philadelphia, PA, 1995. 1-56.
107. Stone CW, Grines CL, Browne KF, Marco J, Rothbaum D, O'Keefe J, Hartzler GO, Overlie P, Donohue B, Chelliah N, Timmis GC, Vlietstra R, Strzelecki M, Puchrowicz-Ochocki S, O'Neill WW. Predictors of in-hospital and 6 month outcome after acute myocardial infarction in the reperfusion era: The Primary Angioplasty in Myocardial Infarction (PAMI) trial. J Am Coll Cardiol 1995;25:370-377.
108. Waldecker B, Waas W, Haberbosch W, Voss R, Kistler P, Tillmanns H. Long-term follow-up (2.5 years) of 300 consecutive patients with primary angioplasty for acute myocardial infarction. Circulation 1995;92:I-461.
109. Maynard C, Weaver D, Litwin PE, et al. Hospital mortality in acute myocardial infarction in the era of reperfusion therapy (the Myocardial Infarction Triage and Intervention Project). Am J Cardiol 1993;72:877-82.
110. Rogers WJ, Chandra NC, Gore JM for the NMRI Investigators. National registry of myocardial infarction (NMRI): What have we leaned from the first 100,000 patients? J Am Coll Cardiol 1993;21:349A.
111. Cragg DR, Friedman HZ, Bonema JD, et al. Outcome of patients with acute myocardial infarction who are ineligible for thrombolytic therapy. Ann Int Med 1991;115:173-177.
112. Grines CL, Browne KF, Marco J, Rothbaum D, Stone GW, O'Keefe J, Overlie P, Donohue B, Chelliah N, Timmis GC, Vlietstra RE, Strzelecki M, Puchrowicz-Ochocki S, O'Neill W. A comparison of immediate angioplasty with thrombolytic therapy for acute myocardial infarction. N Engl J Med 1993;328:673-679.
113. Grines CL, Griffin JJ, Brodie BR, Stone GW, Donohue BC, Balestrini CE, Wharton TP, Spain MG, Shimshak T, Jones D, Mason D, Sachs D, O'Neill WW. The second Primary Angioplasty for Myocardial Infarction study (PAMI-II): Preliminary Report. Circulation 1994;90:I-433.
114. Grines C, Marsalese D, Brodie B, Griffin J, Donohue B, Sampaolesi A, Costantini C, Stone G, Spain M, Jones D, Sachs D, Mason D, O'Neill W. Acute cath provides the best method of risk stratifying MI patients. Circulation, 1995;92:I-531.
115. Stone GW, Grines CL, Browne KF, Marco J, Rothbaum D, O'Keefe J, Overlie P, Donohue B, Puchrowicz S, O'Neill WW. Outcome of different reperfusion strategies in thrombolytic "eligible" versus "ineligible" patients with acute myocardial infarction. J Am Coll Cardiol February 1995;401A.
116. Grines CL, Booth D, Nissen S, Gurley J, Bennett K, O'Connor WN, DeMaria A. Mechanism of acute myocardial infarction in patients with prior coronary artery bypass grafting and therapeutic implications. Am J Cardiol 1990;65:1292-96.
117. McKendall GR, Drew TM, Kelsey SF, et al. What is the optimal treatment for thrombolytic ineligible AMI Preliminary results of the Study of Medicine vs. Angioplasty Reperfusion Trial (SMART). J Am Coll Cardiol 1994;1A-484A:225A.
118. Kaplan AJ, Bengtson JR, Aronson LG, et al. Reperfusion improves survival in patients with cardiogenic shock after acute myocardial infarction. J Am Coll Cardiol 1990;15:155 (abstr).
119. Lee L, Erbel R, Brown TM, et al. Multicenter registry of angioplasty therapy of cardiogenic shock: initial and long-term survival. J Am Coll Cardiol 1991;17:599-603.
120. Gacioch GM, Ellis SG, Lee L, et al. Cardiogenic shock complicating acute myocardial infarction: the use of coronary angioplasty

and the integration of the new support devices into patient management. J Am Coll Cardiol 1992;19:647-653.Bengtson JR, Kaplan AJ, Pieper KS, et al. Prognosis in cardiogenic shock after acute myocardial infarction in the interventional era. J Am Coll Cardiol 1992;20:1482-1489.

121. Hibbard MD, Holmes DR, Gersh BJ, Reeder GS. Coronary angioplasty for acute myocardial infarction complicated by cardiogenic shock. Circulation 1990;82:III-511.
122. Moosvi AR, Villaneuva L, Gheorghiade M, et al. Early revascularization improves survival in cardiogenic shock. Circulation
123. Eltchaninoff H, Simpendorfer C, Whitlow PL. Coronary angioplasty improves both early and 1 year survival in acute myocardial infarction complicated by cardiogenic shock. J Am Coll Cardiol 1991;17:167.
124. Brown TM, Lannone LA, Gordon DF, et al. Percutaneous myocardial reperfusion reduces mortality in acute myocardial infarction complicated by cardiogenic shock. Circulation 1995;72:III-309.
125. O'Neill WW, Erbel R, Laufer N, et al. Coronary angioplasty therapy of cardiogenic shock complicating acute myocardial infarction. Circulation 1995;72:III-309.
126. Meyer P, Blanc P, Badouy M, Morand P. Treatment de choc cardiogenique primaire par angioplastie transluminale coronarienne a la phase aigue de l'Infarctus. Arch Mal Coeur 1990;83:329-334.
127. Lee L, Bates ER, Pitt B, Walton JA, et al. Percutaneous transluminal coronary angioplasty improves survival in acute myocardial infarction complicated by cardiogenic shock. Circulation 1988;78:145-151.
128. Seydoux C, Goy J-J, Beuret P, et al. Effectiveness of percutaneous transluminal coronary angioplasty in cardiogenic shock during acute myocardial infarction. Am J Cardiol 1992;68:968-969.
129. Heuser RR, Maddoux GL, Goss JE, et al. Coronary angioplasty in the treatment of cardiogenic shock: the therapy of choice. J Am Coll Cardiol 1986;7:219.
130. Shani J, Rivera M, Geengart A, et al. Percutaneous transluminal coronary angioplasty in cardiogenic shock. J Am Coll Cardiol 1986;7:149.
131. Disler L, Haitas B, Benjamin J, et al. Cardiogenic shock in evolving myocardial infarction: treatment by angioplasty and streptokinase. Heart Lung 1987;16:649.
132. Verna E, Repetto S, Boscarina M, et al. Emergency coronary angioplasty in patients with severe left ventricular dysfunction of cardiogenic shock after acute myocardial infarction. Eur Heart J 1989;10:958-966.
133. Hochman JS, Boland J, Sleeper LA, Porway M, Brinker J, Col J, Jacobs A, Slater J, Miller D, Wasserman H, Menegus MA, Talley D, McKinlay S, Sanborn T, LeJemtel T, and the SHOCK Registry Investigators. Current spectrum of cardiogenic shock and effect of early revascularization on mortality. Circulation 1995;91:372-881.
134. Holmes DR, Bates ER, Kleiman NS, Sadowski Z, Horgan JHS, Morris DC, Califf RM, Berger PB, Topol EJ. Contemporary reperfusion therapy for cardiogenic shock: The GUSTO-I trial experience. J Am Coll Cardiol 1995;26:668-674.
135. Anderson RD, Stebbins AL, Bates E, Stomel R, Granger CB, Ohman EM. Underutilization of aortic counterpulsation in patients with cardiogenic shock: Observations from the GUSTO-1 study. Circulation 1995;92:I-139.
136. O'Neill WW, Brodie BR, Ivanhoe R, Knopf W, Taylor G, O'Keefe J, Grines CL, Weintraub R, Sickinger B, Berdan LG, Tcheng JE, Woodlief LG, Strzelecki M, Hartzler G, Califf RM. Primary Coronary Angioplasty for Acute Myocardial Infarction (The Primary Angioplasty Registry). Am J Cardiol 1994;73:627-634.
137. Gruppo Italiano per lo Studio della Streptochinasi nell'Infarto Miocardico (GISSI): Effectiveness of intravenous thrombolytic treatment in acute myocardial infarction. Lancet 1986;1:397-402.
138. ISIS-2 (Second International Study Group of Infarct Survival) collaborative group: Randomized trial of intravenous streptokinase, oral aspirin, both, or neither among 17,187 cases of suspected acute myocardial infarction. Lancet 1988;2:349-360.
139. Wilcox RG, Olsson CG, Skene AM, Von Der Lippe G, Jensen G, Hampton JR. Trial of tissue plasminogen activator for mortality reduction in acute myocardial infarction. Anglo Scandinavian Study of Early Thrombolysis (ASSET). Lancet 1988;2:525-530.
140. AIMS Trial Study Group: Effect of intravenous APSAC on mortality after acute myocardial infarction: Preliminary report of a placebo-controlled clinical trial. Lancet 1988;1:515-549.
141. Chesebro JH, Knatterud G, Roberts R, et al. Thrombolysis in Myocardial Infarction (TIMI) Trial, phase I: a comparison between intravenous tissue plasminogen activator and intravenous streptokinase. Circulation 1987;76:142-154.
142. Topol EJ, Califf RM, George BS, Kereiakes DJ, Lee KL. Insights derived from the Thrombolysis and Angioplasty in Myocardial Infarction (TAMI) trials. J Am Coll Cardiol 1988;12:24A-31A.
143. Grines CL, Nissen SE, Booth DC, et al. A prospective, randomized trial comparing half-dose tissue-type plasminogen activator with streptokinase to full-dose tissue-type plasminogen activator. Circulation 1991;84:540-549.
144. Califf RM, Topol EJ, Stack RS, et al. Evaluation of combination thrombolytic therapy and timing of cardiac catheterization in acute myocardial infarction: results of Thrombolysis and Angioplasty in Myocardial Infarction-Phase 5 randomized trial. Circulation 1991;83:1543-1556.
145. Carney RJ, Murphy GA, Brandt TR, et al. Randomized angiographic trial of recombinant tissue-type plasminogen activator (alteplase) in myocardial infarction. J Am Coll Cardiol 1992;20:17-23.
146. Granger CB, Ohman EM, Bates E. Pooled analysis of angiographic patency rates from thrombolytic therapy trials. Circulation 1992;86(suppl I):I-269(abstr).
147. Kennedy JW, Martin GV, Davis KB, et al. The Western Washington Intravenous Streptokinase in Acute Myocardial Infarction randomized trial. Circulation 1988;77:345-352.
148. Schroder R, Neuhaus K-L, Leizorovicz A, Linderer T, Tebbe U. A prospective placebo-controlled double-blind multicenter trial of intravenous streptokinase in acute myocardial infarction (ISAM): long-term mortality and morbidity. J Am Coll Cardiol 1987;9:197-203.
149. Meinertz T, Kasper W, Schumacher M, Just H. The German multicenter trial of anisoylated plasminogen streptokinase activator complex versus heparin for acute myocardial infarction. Am J Cardiol 1988;62:347-351.
150. Gibbons RJ, Holmes DR, Reeder GS, Bailey KR, Hopenspirger MR, Gersh BJ. Immediate angioplasty compared with the

administration of a thrombolytic agent followed by conservative treatment for myocardial infarction. N Engl J Med 1993;328:685-691.

151. O'Neill W, Timmis GC, Bourdillon PD, Lai P, Ganghadarhan V, Walton J, Ramos R, Laufer N, Gordon S, Schork MA, Pitt B. A prospective randomized clinical trial of intracoronary streptokinase versus coronary angioplasty for acute myocardial infarction. N Engl J Med 1986;314:812-818.
152. DeWood MA, Fisher MJ, for the Spokane Heart Research Group. Direct PTCA versus intravenous rtPA in acute myocardial infarction: Preliminary results from a prospective randomized trial. Circulation 1989;80:II-418.
153. Ribeiro EE, Silva LA, Carneiro R, D'Oliveria LG, Gasquez A, Jose GA, Tavares JR, Petrizzo A, Torossian S, Duprat R, Buffolo E, Ellis SG. Randomized trial of direct coronary angioplasty versus intravenous streptokinase in acute myocardial infarction. J Am Coll Cardiol 1993;22:376-380.
154. Elizaga J, Garcia EJ, Delcan JL, Garcia-Robles JA, Bueno H, Soriano J, Abeytua M, Lopez-Bescos L. Primary coronary angioplasty versus systemic thrombolysis in acute anterior myocardial infarction: in-hospital results from a prospective randomized trial. Circulation 1993;88:I-411.
155. Michels KB, Yusif S. Does PTCA in acute myocardial infarction affect mortality and reinfarction rates? A quantitative overview (meta-analysis) of the randomized clinical trials. Circulation 1995;91:476-485.
156. O'Neill WW, de Boaer MJ, Gibbons RJ, Holmes DR, Timmis GC, Sachs D, Griens CL, Zijlstra F. Data from three prospective randomized clinical trials of thrombolytic versus angioplasty therapy of acute myocardial infarction. Preliminary results from a pooled analysis. Book chapter in Primary Coronary Angioplasty in Acute Myocardial Infarction. Ed. Menko Jan de Boer, Proefschrift Rotterdam: Erasmus University, 1994, pp. 165-171.
157. The GUSTO Angiographic Investigators. The effects of tissue plasminogen activator, streptokinase, or both on coronary-artery patency, ventricular function, and survival after acute myocardial infarction. N Engl J Med 1993;329:1615-1622.
158. Topol EJ, Califf RM, Vandormael M, et al, the the Thrombolysis and Angioplasty in Myocardial Infarction (TAMI-6) Study Group. A randomized trial of late reperfusion therapy for acute myocardial infarction. Circulation 1992;85:2090-2099.
159. Meijer A, Verheugt FWA, Werter CJPJ, Lie KI, vander Pol JMJ, van Eenige MJ. Aspirin versus coumadin in the prevention of reocclusion and recurrent ischemia after successful thrombolysis: A prospective placebo-controlled angiographic study. Results of the APRICOT study. Circulation 1993;87:1524-1530.
160. Meijer A, Verheugt F, Eenigem M, Werter C. Left ventricular function at 3 months after successful thrombolysis. Impact of reocclusion without reinfarction on ejection fraction, regional function and remodeling. Circulation 1994;90:1706-1714.
161. Veen G, Meyer A, Verheugt F, et al. Culprit lesion morphology and stenosis severity in the prediction of reocclusion after coronary thrombolysis: Angiographic results of the APRICOT study. J Am Coll Cardiol 1993;22:1755-62.
162. White H, French J, Hamer A, et al. Frequent reocclusion of patent infarct-related arteries between 4 weeks and 1 year: Effects of antiplatelet therapy. J Am Coll Cardiol 1995;25:218-23.
163. Mark DB, O'Neill WW, Brodie B, Ivanhoe R, Knopf W, Taylor G, O'Keefe JH, Grines CL, Davidson-Ray L, Knight JD, Califf RM. Baseline and six-month costs of primary angioplasty therapy for acute myocardial infarction: Results from the primary angioplasty registry. J Am Coll Cardiol 1995;26:688-695.
164. Eckleberg T, Vlietstra R, Brenner A, Grines C, O'Neill W, Browne K. Cost comparison of primary angioplasty versus thrombolytic therapy for acute myocardial infarction. J Am Coll Cardiol 1993;21:347A.
165. Brodie B, Grines CL, Spain M, et al. A prospective, randomized trial evaluating early discharge (day 3) without non-invasive risk stratification in low risk patients with acute myocardial infarction: PAMI-2. J Am Coll Cardiol 1995;25:5A.
166. Donohue BC, O'Neill WW, Jackson EJ, Brodie B, Griffin J, Balestrini C, Stone G, Wharton T, Jones DE, Grines CL. Cost analysis of different management strategies for myocardial infarction. J Am Coll Cardiol 1996;27:221A.
167. Ellis SG, Vande Weft F, DaSilva ER, et al. Present status of rescue coronary angioplasty: Current polarization of opinion and randomized trials. J Am Coll Cardiol 1992;19:681-686.
168. Califf RM, Topol EJ, George BS, et al. Characteristics and outcomes of patients in whom reperfusion with tissue-type plasminogen activator fails: results of the Thrombolysis and Angioplasty in Myocardial Infarction TAMI) trial. Circulation 1988;77:1090-1099.
169. Fung AY, Lai P, Topol EJ, et al. Value of percutaneous transluminal coronary angioplasty after unsuccessful intravenous streptokinase therapy in acute myocardial infarction. Am J Cardiol 1986;58:686-691.
170. Topol EJ, Califf RM, George BS, et al and the TAMI Study Group. Coronary arterial thrombolysis with combined infusion of recombinant tissue-type plasminogen activator and urokinase in patients with acute myocardial infarction. Circulation 1988;77:1100-1107.
171. Grines CL, Nissen SE, Booth DC, et al and the KAMIT study group. A new thrombolytic regimen for acute myocardial infarction using combination half dose tissue-type plasminogen activator with full dose streptokinase: a pilot study. J Am Coll Cardiol 1989;14:573-580.
172. Holmes DR, Gersh BJ, Baily KR, et al. "Rescue" percutaneous transluminal coronary angioplasty after failed thrombolytic therapy: 4-year follow-up. J Am Coll Cardiol 1989;13:193 (abstr).
173. Grines CL, Nissen SE, Booth DC, et al and the Kentucky Acute Myocardial Infarction Trial (KAMIT) Group. A prospective, randomized trial comparing combination half-dose tissue-type plasminogen activator and streptokinase with full-dose tissue-type plasminogen activator. Circulation 1991;84:540-549.
174. O'Connor CM, Mark DB, Hinohara T, et al. Rescue coronary angioplasty after failure of intravenous streptokinase in acute myocardial infarction: in-hospital and long-term outcomes. J Invasive Cardiol 1989;1:85-95.
175. Baim DS, Diver DJ, Knatterud GL and the TIMI II-A Investigators. PTCA "salvage" for thrombolytic failures: implications from TIMI II-A. Circulation 1988;78(Suppl II):II-112(abstr).
176. Whitlow PL. Catheterization/rescue angioplasty following thrombolysis (CRAFT) study: results of rescue angioplasty. Circulation 1990;82(Suppl III):III-308(abstr).
177. Abbottsmith CW, Topol EJ, George BS, et al. Fate of patients with acute myocardial infarction with patency of the infarct-related

vessel achieved with successful thrombolysis versus rescue angioplasty. J Am Coll Cardiol 1990;16:770-778.
178. Gibson CM, Cannon CP, Piana RN, et al. Rescue PTCA in the TIMI 4 trial. J Am Coll Cardiol 1994;1A-484A:225A.
179. Wnqk A, Krupa H, Gasior M, Kalarus Z, Borkowski B, Wqs T, Lekston A, Wester A, Chodor P, Pasyk S. Results of rescue-angioplasty after unsuccessful intracoronary streptokinase therapy in patients with acute myocardial infarction. European Congress of Cardiology, abstract, 1995.
180. Ross AM, Reiner JS, Thompson MA, et al. Immediate and follow-up procedural outcome of 214 patients undergoing rescue PTCA in the GUSTO trial: no effect of the lytic agent. Circulation 1993;88(Suppl I):I-410(abstr).
181. Ellis SG, Ribeiro da Silva E, Heyndrickx G, Talley D, Cernigliaro C, Steg G, Spaulding C, Nobuyoshi M, Erbel R, Vassanelli C, Topol EJ. Randomized comparison of rescue angioplasty with conservative management of patients with early failure of thrombolysis for acute anterior myocardial infarction. Circulation 1994;90:2280-2284.
182. Belenkie I, Traboulsi M, Hall CA, Hansen JL, Roth DL, Manyari D, Filipchuck NG, Schnurr LR, Rosenal TW, Smith ER, Knudtson M. Rescue angioplasty during myocardial infarction has a beneficial effect on mortality: A tenable hypothesis. Can J Cardiol 1992;8:357-362.
183. The CORAMI Study Group. Outcome of attempted rescue coronary angioplasty after failed thrombolysis for acute myocardial infarction. Am J of Cardiol 1994;74:172174.
184. Rogers WJ, Baim DS, Gore JM, et al for the TIMI-IIA Investigators. Comparison of immediate invasive, delayed invasive, and conservative strategies after tissue-type plasminogen activator. Circulation 1990;81:1457-1476.
185. Topol EJ, Califf RM, George BS, et al and the Thrombolysis and Angioplasty in Myocardial Infarction Study Group. A randomized trial of immediate versus delayed elective angioplasty after intravenous tissue plasminogen activator in acute myocardial infarction. N Engl J Med 1987;317:581-588.
186. Simoons ML, Arnold AET, Bertriu A, et al. Thrombolysis with tissue plasminogen activator in acute myocardial infarction: No additional benefit from immediate percutaneous coronary angioplasty. Lancet 1988;1:197-202.
187. Gibson C, Cannon C, Piana R. Angiographic predictors of reocclusion after thrombolysis: Results from the thrombolysis in myocardial infarction (TIMI-4) trial. J Am Coll Cardiol 1995;25:589-9.
188. The TIMI Study Group. Comparison of invasive and conservative strategies after treatment with intravenous tissue plasminogen activator in acute myocardial infarction. Results of the Thrombolysis in Myocardial Infarction (TIMI) Phase II Trial. N Engl J Med 1989;320.
189. SWIFT (Should We Intervene Following Thrombolysis?) Trial Study Group. SWIFT trial of delayed elective intervention vs. conservative treatment after thrombolysis with anistreplase in acute myocardial infarction. Br Med J 1991;302:5550560.
190. Barbash GI, Roth A, Hod H, et al. Randomized controlled trial of late in-hospital angiography and angioplasty versus conservative management after treatment with recombinant tissue-type plasminogen activator in acute myocardial infarction. Am J Cardiol 1990;66:538-545.
191. Van den Brand MJ, Betrui A, Bescos LL, et al. Randomized trial of deferred angioplasty after thrombolysis for acute myocardial infarction. Coronary Artery Disease 1992;3:393-401.
192. Ozbek C, Dyckmans J, Sen S, et al. Comparison of invasive and conservative strategies after treatment with streptokinase in acute myocardial infarction: results of a randomized trial (SIAM). J Am Coll Cardiol 1990;15:63A (abstr).
193. Mueller HS, Cohen LS, Braunwald E, et al, for the TIMI Investigators. Predictors of early morbidity and mortality after thrombolytic therapy of acute myocardial infarction. Analyses of patient subgroups in the Thrombolysis in Myocardial Infarction (TIMI) Trial, Phase II. Circulation 1992;85:1254-1264.
194. Guerci AD, Gerstenblith G, Brinker JA, et al. A randomized trial of intravenous tissue plasminogen activator for acute myocardial infarction with subsequent randomization to elective coronary angioplasty. N Engl J Med 1987;317:1613-1618.
195. Danchin N, Angioi M, Cardar R, et al. Late percutaneous recanalization of chronic total coronary occlusion after myocardial infarction improves global and regional left ventricular function and avoids remodeling in the absence of subsequent reocclusion. Circulation 1995;92:I-74.
196. Meneveau N, Bassard J, Lablanche J, et al. Late reopening with angioplasty of totally occluded infarct related arteries prevents LV remodelling after myocardial infarction. Presented at the European Congress of Cardiology, 1995.
197. Van de Werf F. Discrepancies between the effects of coronary reperfusion on survival and left ventricular function. Lancet 1989;I:1367-1369.
198. Galvani M, Ottani F, Ferrini D, Sorbello F, Rusticali F. Patency of the infarct-related artery and left ventricular function as the major determinants of survival after Q-wave acute myocardial infarction. Am J Cardiol 1993;71:I-7.
199. Anderson JL. Overview of patency as an endpoint of thrombolytic therapy. Am J Cardiol 1991;67:11-16E.
200. Topol EJ, Califf RM, Vandormael M, Grines CL, George BS, Sanz ML, Wall T, O'Brien M, Schwaiger M, Aguirre FV, Young S. Popma JJ, Lee KL, Ellis SG and the Thrombolysis and Angioplasty in Myocardial Infarction-6 Study Group. A randomized trial of late reperfusion therapy for acute myocardial infarction. Circulation 1992,85:2090-2099.
201. DANAMI Study. Results presented at the American Heart Association, 1995 Plenary Session.
202. Braunwald E, Mark DB, Jones RH, Cheitlin MD, Fuster V, McCauley K, Edwards C, Green LA, Mushlin AL, Swain JA, Smith EE, Cowan M, Rose GC, Concannon CA, Grines CL, Brown L, Lytle BW, Goldman LA, Topol EJ, Willerson JT, Brown J, Archibald N. Unstable Angina: Diagnosis and Management - Clinical Practice Guidelines. U.S. Department of Health and Human Services. AHCPR Publication No. 94-0682, March 15, 1994.
203. Roberts W, Kragel A, Gertz S, Roberts S. Coronary arteries in unstable angina, acute myocardial infarction and sudden coronary death. Am J Cardiol 1994;127:1588-1593.
204. DeFeyter P, Serruys P. Percutaneous transluminal coronary angioplasty for unstable angina. In: Textbook of Interventional Cardiology. Ed. EJ Topol, M.D. W.B. Saunders Co., 1994, p. 274.
205. Steffenino G, Meier B, Finci L, et al. Follow-up results of treatment of unstable angina by coronary angioplasty. Br Heart J, 1987; 57:416.

206. Myler RK, Shaw RE, Stertzer SH, et al. Unstable angina and coronary angioplasty. Circulation 1990;82:II-88-95.
207. Stammen F, De Scheerder I, Glazier JJ, et al. Immediate and follow-up results of the conservative coronary angioplasty strategy of unstable angina pectoris. Am J Cardiol 1992;69:1533.
208. de Feyter PJ, Suryapranata H, Serruys PW, et al. Coronary angioplasty for unstable angina: Immediate and late results in 200 consecutive patients with identification of risk factors for unfavorable early and late outcome. J Am Coll Cardiol 1988;12:324.
209. Plokker HWT, Ernst SMPG, Bal ET, et al. Percutaneous transluminal coronary angioplasty in patients with unstable angina pectoris refractory to medical therapy. Cathet Cardiovasc Diagn 1988;14:15.
210. Perry RA, Seth A, Hunt A, et al. Coronary angioplasty in unstable angina and stable angina: A comparison of success and complications. Br Heart J 1988;60:367.
211. Bentivoglio LG, Holubkov R, Kelsey SF et al. Short and long term outcome of percutaneous transluminal coronary angioplasty in unstable versus stable angina pectoris: A report of the 1985-1986 NHLBI PTCA Registry. Cathet Cardiovasc Diagn 1991;23:227.
212. Rupprecht HJ, Brennecke R, Kottmeyer M, Bernhard G, Erbel R, Pop T, Meyer R. Short and long-term outcome after PTCA in patients with stable and unstable angina. Eur Heart J 1990;11:964.
213. Morrison DA. Coronary angioplasty for medically refractory unstable angina within 30 days of acute myocardial infarction. Am Heart J 1990;120:256.
214. Ambrose J, Almeida O, Sharma S, et al. Adjunctive thrombolytic therapy during angioplasty for ischemic rest angina. Results of the TAUSA trial. Circulation 1994;90:69-77.
215. Lincoff A, Califf R, Anderson K, et al. Striking clinical benefit with platelet GPIIb/IIIa inhibition by C7E3 among patients with unstable angina: Outcome of the EPIC trial. Circulation 1994;90:I-21.
216. Williams D, Sharaf B, Braunwald E, et al. Percutaneous transluminal coronary angioplasty (PTCA) for acute myocardial ischemia: The TIMI-3 experience. Circulation 1994;90:I-433.
217. Bittl J, Strong J, Brinker J, et al. Treatment with Bivalirudin (Hirulog) as compared with heparin during coronary angioplasty for unstable or post infarction angina. N Engl J Med 1995;333:764-9.
218. Serruys P, Herrman J, Simon R, et al. A comparison of Hirudin with heparin in the prevention of restenosis after coronary angioplasty. N Engl J Med 1995;333:757-63.
219. Bengtson J, Wilson J. Interventions in unstable angina. In: Interventional Cardiovascular Medicine - Prinicipals and Practice. Eds. Roubin, Califf, O'Neill, Phillips, Stack. Churchill Livingstone, Inc. New York, New York, 1996.
220. Chuang Y, Popma J, Satler et al. Increasing angina predicts an unfavorable outcome after new device angioplasty. J Am Coll Cardiol 1994:289A.
221. Hong M, Popma J, Wong S, et al. Incidence of and factors associated with abrupt closure in patients undergoing elective, new device angioplasty in native coronary arteries. J Am Coll Cardiol 1995;122A.
222. Harrington R, Holmes D, Berdan L, et al. Clinical characteristics and outcomes of patients with unstable angina undergoing percutaneous intervention in CAVEAT. J Am Coll Cardiol 1994;288A.
223. Ambrose J, Almeida D, Ratner D, et al. Heparin administered prior to angioplasty does not decrease angioplasty complications. Circulation 1994;90:I-374.
224. TIMI-3B Investigators. Effects of tissue plasminogen activator and a comparison of early invasive and conservative strategies in unstable angina and non Q-wave myocardial infarction. Circulation 1994;89:1545-1556.
225. Anderson H, Cannon C, Stone P, et al. One year results of the thrombolysis in myocardial infarction (TIMI)3B clinical trial. J Am Coll Cardiol 1995;26:1643-1650.
226. CABRI Trial Partipants. First-year results of CABRI (Coronary Angioplasty vs Bypass Revascularisation Investigation). Lancet 1995;346:1179-84.
227. RITA Trial Participants. Coronary angioplasty versus coronary artery bypass surgery: The Randomised Intervention Treatment of Angina (RITA) trial. Lancet 1993;343:573-80.
228. King SB, Lembo NJ, Kosinski AS, et al. A randomised trial comparing coronary angioplasty with coronary bypass surgery. N Engl J Med 1994;331:1044-50.
229. Hamm CW, Riemers J, Ischinger T, et al. A randomised study of coronary angioplasty compared with bypass surgery in patients with symptomatic multi-vessel coronary disease. N Engl J Med 1994;331:1037-1043.
230. Rodriguez A, Boullon F, Prez-Balino N, et al. Argentine randomised trial of percutaneous transluminal coronary angioplasty versus coronary artery bypass surgery in multi-vessel disease (ERACI): in-hospital results and 1-year follow-up. J Am Coll Cardiol 1993;22:1060-67.
231. Bypass Angioplasty Revascularization Investigation (BARI). N Engl J Med 1996, in press.
232. Kaplan B, Safian R, Grines C, et al. Differences in outcome after angioplasty for AMI: The left anterior descending artery vs the right coronary. J Am Coll Cardio 1996;27:166A.
233. Bates ER. Reperfusion therapy in inferior myocardial infarction. J Am Coll Cardiol 1988;12:44A-51A.
234. Gacioch GM, Topol EJ. Sudden paradoxic clinical deterioration during angioplasty of the occluded right coronary artery in acute myocardial infarction. J Am Coll Cardiol 1989;14:1202-9.
235. Kahn JK, Rutherford BD, McConahay DR, et al. Catheterization laboratory events and hospital outcome with direct angioplsty for acute myocardial infarction. Circulation 1990;82:1910-1915.
236. Ohman EM, Califf RM, Topol EJ, et al. Consequences of reocclusion after successful reperfusion therapy in acute myocardial infarction. Circulation 1990;82:781-91.
237. Stone GW, Griens CL, Browne KF, Marco J, Rothbaum D, O'Keefe J, Hartzler GO, Overlie P, Donohue B, Chelliah N, Vlietstra R, Puchrowicz-Ochocki S, O'Neill WW. Implications of recurrent ischemia after reperfusion therapy in acute myocardial infarction: A comparison of thromboytic therapy and primary angioplsty. J Am Coll Cardiol 1995;26:66-72.
238. Grines C, Brodie B, Griffin J, Donohue B, Sampaoiesi A, Costantini C, Sachs D, Wharton T, Esente P, Spain M, Stone G. Which primary PTCA patients may benefit from new technologies? Circulation, 1995;92:I-146.

239. Nunn C, O'Neill W, Rothbaum D, O'Keefe J, Overlie P, Donohue B, Mason D, Catlin T, Grines C. Primary angioplasty for myocardial infarction improves long-term survival : PAMI-1 follow-up. J Am Coll Cardiol 1996;27:153A.
240. Ohman GM, George B, White C, et al. Use of aortic counterpulsation to improve sustained coronary patency during acute MI. Results of a randomized trial. Circulation 1994;90:792-799.
241. Ishihara M, Sato H, Tateishi H, et al. Intraaortic balloon pumping as the postangioplasty strategy in acute myocardial infarction. Am Heart J 1991;122:385-389.
242. Grines CL, Brodie BR, Griffin JJ, Donohue BC, Costantini C, Balestrini C, Stone G, Jones DE, Sachs D, O'Neill WW. Prophylactic intraaortic balloon pumping for acute myocardial infarction does not improve left ventricular function. J Am Coll Cardiol 1996;27:167A.
243. Stone GW, Marsalese D, Brodie B, Griffin J, Donohue B, Costantini C, Balestrini C, Wharton, Jones D, Sachs D, Grines CL. The routine use of intra-aortic balloon pumping after primary PTCA improves clinical outcomes in very high risk patients with acute myocardial infarction - Results of the PAMI-2 trial. Circulation 1995;92:I-139.
244. Ghazzal ZMB, Hinohara T, Scott NA, et al. Directional coronary atherectomy in patients with recent myocardial infarction: a NACI Registry report. J Am Coll Cardiol 1993;21:32A.
245. Robertson G, hinohara T, Vetters J, et al. Directional coronary atherectomy for patients with recent myocardial infarction. J Am Coll Cardiol 1994:219A.
246. Abdelmeguid A. Sapp S, Lynch D, et al. Immediate and follow-up results of directional coronary atherectomy for the treatment of unstable angina. Circulation 1993;88:I-496.
247. Topol EJ, Leya F, Pinkerton CA, et al. A comparison of directional atherectomy with coronary angioplasty in patients with coronary artery disease. N Engl J Med 1993;329:221-7.
248. Smucker ML, Sarnat WS, Kil D, Scherb DE, Howard PF. Salvage from cardiogenic shock by atherectomy after failed emergency coronary artery angioplasty. Cath Cardiovasc Diagn 1990;21:23-5.
249. Lasorda DM, Incorvati DL, Randall RR. Extraction atherectomy during myocardial infarction in a patient with prior coronary artery bypass surgery. Cath Cardiovasc Diag 1992;26:117-121.
250. Larkin TJ, Niemyski PR, Parker MA, Kramer BL. Primary and rescue extraction atherectomy in patients with acute myocardial infarction. Circulation 1991;84:II-537.
251. Larkin TJ, O'Neill WW, Safian RD, Schreiber TL, May MA, Kazziha S, Niemyski PR, Parker MA, Kramer BL, Grines CL. A prospective study of transluminal extraction atherectomy in high risk patients with acute myocardial infarction. J Am Coll Cardiol 1994;226A.
252. Kaplan BM, O'Neill WW, Safian RD, Schreiber TL, Larkin TJ, Dooris M, May M, Grines CL. Clinical and angiographic follow-up to a prospective study of transluminal extraction atherectomy in high risk patients with acute myocardial infarction. J Am Coll Cardiol, 1995:331A.
253. Malosky S, Hirschfeld J, Herman H. Comparison of results of intracoronary stenting in patients with unstable vs stable angina. Cath and CV Diagn 1994;31:95-101.
254. Levy G, deBoisgelin, Volpiliere R, Bouvagnet P. Intracoronary stenting in direct infarct angioplasty: Is it dangerous? Circulation 1995;92:I-139.
255. Neumann F, Walter H, Schmitt C, Alt E, Schomig. Coronary stenting as an adjunct to direct balloon angioplasty in acute myocardial infarction. Circulation 1995;92:I-609.
256. Monassier JP, Elias J, Meyer P, et al. STENTIMI I: The French Registry of stenting at acute myocardial infarction. J Am Coll Cardiol 1996;27:68A.
257. Verna E, Castiglioni B, Onofri M, et al. Intracoronary stenting of the infarct-related artery without anticoagulation in acute myocardial infarction. Euro Heart J 1995;16:12.
258. Benzuly KH, Goldstein JA, Almany SL, et al. Feasibility of stenting in acute myocardial infarction. Circulation 1995;92:I-616.
259. Romero M, Medina A, Suarez J, et al. Elective Palmaz-Schatz stent implantation in acute coronary syndromes induced by thrombus-containing lesions. Euro Heart J 1995;16:179.
260. Van der Giessen WJ, Hardhammar P, Van Beusekom MM, et al. Reduction of thrombotic events using heparin-coated Palmaz-Schatz stents. Circulation 1993;88:I-661.
261. Serruys PW, Emanuelsson H, van der Giessen W, Lunn AC, Kiemeney F, Macaya C, Rutsch W, Heyndrickx G, Suryapranata H, Legrand V, Goy JJ, Materne P, Bonnier H, Morice M-C, Fajadet J, Belardi J, Colombo An, Garcia E, Ruygrok P, de Jaegere P, Morel M-A. Heparin-coated Palmaz-Schatz stents in human coronary arteries. Circulation 1996;93:412-422.
262. Topaz O. Holmium laser coronary thromboysis - a new treatment modality for revascularization in acute myocardial infarction: Review. J Clin Laser Med & Surg 1992;10:427-31.
263. De Marchena E, Mallon S, Posada JD, et al. Direct holmium laser-assisted balloon angioplasty in acute myocardial infarction. Am J Cardiol 1993;71:1223-5.
264. Topaz O, Rozenbaum EA, Battista S, Peterson C, Wysham DG. Laser facilitated angioplasty and thrombolysis in acute myocardial infarction complicated by prolonged or recurrent chest pain. Cath Cardiovasc Diag 1993;28:7-16.
265. Topaz O, Minisi A, Luxenberg M, et al. Laser angioplasty for lesions unsuitable for PTCA in acute myocardial infarction: Quantitative coronary angiography and clinical results. Circulation 1994;90:I-434.
266. Spears JR, Kundu SK, McMath LP. Laser balloon angioplasty: Potential for the reduction of the thrombogenicity of the injured arterial wall and for local application of bioprotective materials. J Am Coll Cardiol 1991;17:179B-188B.
267. Spears JR, Dsgisn TF, Douglas JS, et al. Multicenter acute and chronic results of laser balloon angioplasty for refractory abrupt closure after PTCA. Circulation 1991;84:II-517.
268. Reis GJ, Pomerantz RM, Jenkins RD, et al. Laser balloon angioplasty: clinical, angiographic and histologic results. J Am Coll Cardiol 1991;18:193-202.
269. Schwartz L, Andrus S, Sinclair IN, et al. Restenosis following laser balloon angioplasty - a randomized pilot multicenter trial.

Circulation 1991;84:II-361.
270. Makowski S, O'Neill B, Sarkis A, et al. Physiological low stress angioplasty at 60° C. Initial results and 6 month follow-up. J Am Coll Cardiol 1993;21:440A.
271. Saito S, Arai H, Kim K, et al. Initial experience of unipolar radio-frequency hot balloon angioplasty for bail-out from abrupt coronary closure after conventional balloon angioplasty. J Am Coll Cardiol 1993;21:338A.
272. Moura A, Lam JYT, Hebert D, Letchacovski G, Robitaille D, Grant G, Kaplan A. Local heparin delivery decreases the thrombogenicity of the balloon-injured artery. Circulation 1994;90:I-449.
273. Thomas CN, Barry JJ, King SB, Scott NA. Local delivery with heparin with a PTCA infusion balloon inhibits platelet-dependent thrombosis. J Am Coll Cardiol 1994;23:4A.
274. Azrin MA, Mitchel JF, Fram DB, Pedersen CA, Cartun RW, Barry JJ, Bow LM, Waters D, McKay RG. Decreased platelet deposition and smooth muscle cell proliferation following intramural heparin delivery with hydrogel-coated balloons. Circulation 1994;90:433-441.
275. Fram DB, Mitchel JF, Azrin MA, Schwedick MW, Waters DD, McKay RG. Local heparin delivery in porcine coronary arteries with the Dispatch catheter delivery, washout and effect on platelet deposition following balloon angioplasty. Circulation 1994;90:I-493.
276. Mitchel JF, Azrin MA, Schwedick MW, Bow LM, Waters DD, McKay RG. Local delivery of heparin with a novel iontophoretic catheter - quantitative heparin delivery and effect on platelet depositon following balloon angioplasty. Circulation 1994;90:I-492.
277. Lopez-Sendon J, Sobrino N, Gamallo C, Lorenzo A, Jimenez J, Calvo L, Sobrino JA, Rico J, de Miguel E. Locally delivered heparin reduces intimal hyperplasian and lumen stenosis following arterial balloon injury in swine. European Heart J 1993;14:191.
278. Camenzind E, van der giesen W, Ligthart J, Ruygrok P, de Jaegere P, de Feyter P, Serruys PW. Local, low pressure heparin delivery following angioplasty in man: the solution to restenosis? J Am Col Cardiol 1995:376A.
279. Steg P, Spaulding C, Makowski S, et al. A double blind randomized trial of hydrogel balloon delivery of urokinase during primary angioplasty for acute myocardial infarction. Circulation 1995;92:I-543.
280. Hartnell GG, Saxton JM, Friedl SE, et al. Ultasonic thrombus ablation: in vitro assessment of a novel device for intracoronary use. J Interven Cardiol 1993;6:69-76.
281. Steffen W, Luo H, Nita H, et al. Catheter delivered therapeutic ultrasound recanalizes thrombotically occluded canine coronary arteries. J Am Coll Cardiol 1993;21:338A.
282. Hamm C, Steffen W, Reimers J, et al. Ultrasound induced thrombolysis in patients with acute myocardial infarctions. Circulation 1995;92:I-416.
283. Coller BS. Platelets and thrombolytic therapy. N Engl J Med 1990;322:33-42.
284. Lacoste L, Lam JYT, Letchacovski G. Comparative antithrombotic efficacy of aspirin: 80mg vs 325mg daily. Circulation 1994;90:I-552.
285. Dabaghi SF, Damat S, Hendricks O, Payne J, Kleiman NS. Low dose aspirin inhibits in vitro platelet aggregation within minutes after ingestion. Circulation 1992;86:I-261.
286. Lacoste L, Lam JYT. Enhanced platelet thrombus formation in unstable angina. Circulation 1994;90:1374.
287. Hardisty RM, Powling MJ, Nokes TJC. The action of ticlopidine on human platelets; studies on aggregation, secretion, calcium mobilization, and membrane glycoproteins. Thromb Haemost. 1990;64:105-115.
288. Khurana S, Westley S, Mattson J, Safian R. Is it possible to expedite the antiplatelet effect of ticlopidine? Presented at the TCT, February, 1996.
289. Sadowski Z, Kuczak D, Dyduszynski. Comparison of ticlopidine and aspirin in unstable angina, presented at European Congress of Cardiology, 1995.
290. Jeong M, Owen W, Staabon, et al. Does ticlopidine effect platelet deposition and acute stent thrombosis? Circulation 1995;92:I-489.
291. Gregorini L, Marco J, Fajadet J, et al. Ticlopidine alternates post-angioplasty thrombin generation . Circulation 1995;92:I-608.
292. EPIC Investigators. Use of a monoclonal antibody directed against the platelet glycoprotein IIb/IIIa receptor in high-risk coronary angioplasty. N Engl J Med 1994;330:956-961.
293. Topol EJ, Califf RM, Weisman HF, Ellis SG, Tcheng JE, Worley S, Ivanhoe R, George BS, Fintel D, Weston M, Sigmon K, Anderson KM, Lee KL, Willerson JT; on behalf of the EPIC investigators. Randomised trial of coronary intervention with antibody against platelet IIb/IIIa integrin for reduction of clinical restenosis: Results at six months. Lancet 1994;343:881-886.
294. Lefkovits J, Ivanhoe R, Anderson K, et al. Platelet IIb/IIIa receptor inhibition during PTCA for acute myocardial infarction: Insights from the EPIC trial. Circulation 1994;90:I-564.
295. Linoff AM, Califf R, Anderson , et al. Striking clinical benefit with platelet IIb/IIIa inhibition by C7E3 among patients with unstable angina: Outcome in the EPIC trial. Circulation 1994;90:I-21.
296. Moliterno D, Califf R, Anderson K, et al. Activated clotting time is increased during coronary interventions with platelet IIb/IIIa antagonism: Results from the EPIC trial. J Am Coll Cardiol 1994:106A.
297. EPILOG study results. Press release, December, 1995.
298. Muhlestein J, Gomez M, Karagounish L. Rescue ReoPro: Acute utilization of Abciximab for the dissolution of coronary thrombus developing as a complication of coronary angioplasty. Circualtion 1995;92:I-607.
299. Tcheng J, Lincoff AM, Sigmon K. Platelet glyprotein IIb/IIIa inhibition with integrelin during PTCA: The Impact II trial. Circulation 1995;92:I-543.
300. Kereiakes D, Kleiman N, Ambrose J. A dosing study in high risk PTCA of MK-383, a platelet IIb/IIIa antagonist. Circulation 1994;90:I-21.
301. Hettleman BD, Aplin RA, Sullivan PR, et al: Three days of heparin pretreatment reduces major complications of coronary angioplasty in patients with unstable angina. J Am Coll Cardiol 1990;15:154.
302. Lasky MAL, Deutsch E, Barnathan E, et al. Influence of heparin therapy on percutaneous transluminal coronary angioplasty

outcome in unstable angina pectoris. Am J Cardiol 1990;65:1425.

303. Pow TK, Varricchione TR, Jacobs AK, et al. Does pretreatment with heparin prevent abrupt closure following PTCA? J Am Coll Cardiol 1988;11:238A.

304. Lukas MA, Deutsch E, Hirschfeld JW, et al. Influence of heparin on percutaneous transluminal coronary angioplasty outcome in patients with coronary arterial thrombus. Am J Cardiol 1990;65:179.

305. Myler RK, Shaw RE, Stertzer SH, et al. Unstable angina and coronary angioplasty. Circulation 1990;82:II-95.

306. Ambrose J, Almeida D, Ratner D, et al. Heparin administered prior to angioplasty does not decrease angioplasty complications. TAUSA trial results. Circulation 1994;90:I-374.

307. Wharton TP, Marsalese D, Brodie BR, Griffin JJ, Donohue BC, Costantini CRF, Balestrini CE, Stone GW, Esente P, Moses J, McNamara NS, Jones D, Sachs D, Grines CL. How often do infarct-related arteries show early perfusion without prior thrombolytic therapy, and should these vessels be dilated acutely? Results from PAMI-2. Circulation 1995:92:I-530.

308. Verheugt F, Marsh R, Veen G. Megadose bolus heparin as reperfusion therapy for acute myocardial infarction: Results of the HEAP pilot study. Circulation 1995;92:I-41.

309. Ferguson J, Dougherty K, Gaos C, et al. Relation between procedural activated coagulation time and outcome after percutaneous transluminal coronary angioplasty. J Am Coll Caridol 1994;23:1061-1065.

310. Snitzer R, Hiremath Y, Lee J, et al. Suppression of intracoronary thrombin activity by weight-adjusted heparin administration during coronary interventions. Circulation 1995;92:I-609.

311. Winters K, Oltrona L, Hiremath Y, et al. Heparin-resistant thrombin activity is associated with acute ischemic events during high risk coronary interventions. Circulation 1995;92:I-608.

312. Harrington Ra, Leimberer JD, Berdan L, Topol EJ, Califf RM for the CAVEAT Investigators. The ACT index: A method for stratifying likelihood of success and risk of acute complications in coronary intervention. Circulation 1993;88:I-208.

313. Naqvi T, Ivy P, Linn P, et al. Low dose heparin enhances and high dose heparin suppresses platelet P-selection expression and platelet aggregation. Circulation 1995;92:I-673.

314. Ahmed W, Meckel C, Grines C, et al. Relation between ischemic complications and activated clotting times during coronary angioplasty: Different profiles for heparin and Hirulog. Circulation 1995;92:I-608.

315. Nairns CR, Hillegass WG, Nelson CL, et al. Activated clotting time predicts abrupt closure risk during angioplasty. J Am Coll Cardiol 1994;23:470A.

316. Hillegass W, Narins C, Brott B, et al. Activated clotting time predicts bleeding complications from angioplasty. J Am Coll Cardiol 1994;184A.

317. Blumenthal R, Wolff M, Resar J, et al. Preprocedural anticoagulation does not reduce angioplasty heparin requirments. Am Heart J 1993;125:1221.

318. Kander NH, Holland KJ, Pitt B, Topol EJ. A randomized pilot trial of brief versus prolonged heparin after succerssful reperfusion in acute myocardial infarction. Am J Cardiol 1990;65:139-142.

319. Granger C, Armstrong P. For the GUSTO IIa investigators. Reinfarction following discontinuation of intravenous heparin or hirudin for unstable angina and acute myocardial infarction. Circulation 1995;92:I-460.

320. Granger C, Miller J, Bovill E, et al. Rebound increase in thrombin generation and activity after cessation of intravenous heparin in patients with acute coronary syndromes. Circulation 1995;91:1929-35.

321. Flather M, Weitz J, Campeau J, et al. Evidence for rebound activation of the coagulation system after cessation of intravenous anticoagulant therapy for acute MI. Circulation 1995;92:I-485.

322. Strony J, Ahmed W, Meckel C, et al. Clinical evidence for thrombin rebound after stopping heparin but not hirulog. Circulation 1995;92:I-609.

323. Khan M, Sepulveda J, Jeroudi M, et al. Rebound increase in thrombin activity with associated decrease in antithrombin III levels after PTCA. Circulation 1995;92:I-785.

324. Spielberg C, Schnitzer L, Linderer T, et al. Influence of catheter technology and adjuvant medication on acute complications in percutaneous coronary angioplasty. Cathet Cardiovasc Diagn, 1990;21:72.

325. Ambrose JA, Torre SR, Sharma SK, et al. Adjuvant urokinase for PTCA in unstable angina: final angiographic results of TAUSA pilot study. Circulation, 1991;84:II-590.

326. Buller CE, Fung AY, Thompson CR, Ricci DR, Thompson B, Schrachtman M, Williams DO. Does pre-treatment with tPA improve safety of coronary angioplasty in acute coronary syndrome? Results from TIMI II-B. Circulation 1994;90:I-22.

327. Ambrose JA, Almeida OD, Sharma SK, Torre SR, Marmur JD, Israel DH, Ratner DE, Weiss MB, Hjemdahl-Monsen CE, Myler TK, Moses J, Unterecker WJ, Grunwald AM, Garrett JS, Cowley MJ, Anwar A, Sobolski J for the TAUSA Investigators. Adjunctive thrombolytic therapy during angioplasty for ischemic rest angina. Results of the TAUSA Trial. Circulation 1994;90:69-77.

328. Mehran R, Ambrose JA, Bongu RM, Almeida OD, Israel DH, Torre S, Sharma SK, Ratner ED for the TAUSA study group. Angioplasty of complex lesions in ischemic rest angina: Results of the Thrombolysis and Angioplasty in UnStable Angina (TAUSA) trial. J Am Coll Cardiol 1995;26:961-966.

329. Kerins DM, Roy L, FitzGerald GA, Pitzgerald DJ. Platelet and vascular function during coronary thrombolysis with tissue-type plasminogen activator. Circulation, 1989;80:1718.

330. Bennett WR, Yawn DH, Migliore PJ, et al. Activation of the complement system by recombinant tissue plasminogen activator. J Am Coll cardiol, 1987;10:627.

331. Fitzgerald DJ, Roy L, Wright F, Fitzgerald GA. Functional significance of platelet activation following coronary thrombolysis. Circulation, 1987;76:IV-153.

332. Castaneda-Zuniga WR, Sibley R, Amplatz K. The pathologic basis of angioplasty. Angiology, 1984;35:195.

333. Kohchi K, Taebayashi S, Block PC. Arterial changes after percutaneous transluminal coronary angioplasty: results at autopsy. J Am Coll Cardiol, 1987;10:592.

334. Waller BF, Rothbaum DA, Pinkerton CA, et al. Status of the myocardium and infarct-related coronary artery in 19 necropsy patients

with acute recanalization using pharmacologic (streptokinase, r-tissue plasminogen activator), mechanical (percutaneous transluminal coronary angioplasty) or combined types of reperfusion therapy. J Am Coll Cardiol, 1987;9:785.

335. Colavita PG, Ideker RE, Reimer KA, et al. The spectrum of pathology associated with percutaneous transluminal coronary angioplasty during acute myocardial infarction. J Am Coll Cardiol, 1986;8:855.
336. Grines C, Schreiber T, Savas V, et al. A randomized trial of low osmolar ionic versus nonionic contrast media in patients with acute myocardial infarction or unstable angina undergoing PTCA. J Am Coll Cardiol 1996;27:1381-6.
337. Piessens JH, Stammen F, Brolix MC, et al. Effects of an ionic versus a nonionic low osmolar contrast agent on the thrombotic complications of coronary angioplasty. Catheterization and Cardiovascular Diagnosis 1993;28:99-105.
338. Aguirre F, Topol EJ, Donohue T. Impact of ionic and non inoic contrast media on post PTCA ischemic complications: Results from the EPIC trial. J Am Coll Cardiol 1995;25:8A.
339. Ellis S, Gusto IIB Angioplasty Substudy. Presented at the ACC Scientific Sessions, March, 1996.
340. Faxon DP, Detre KM, McCabe CH, et al. Role of percutaneous transluminal coronary angioplasty in the treatment of unstable angina. Report from the National Heart, Lung, and Blood Institute Percutaneous Transluminal Coronary Angioplasty and Coronary Artery Surgery Study Registries. Am J Cardiol 1994;53:131C.
341. Kamp O, Beatt KJ, de Feyter PJ, et al. Short-, medium-, and long-term follow-up after percutaneous transluminal coronary angioplasty for stable and unstable angina pectoris. Am Heart J 1989;117:991.
342. Erbel R, Pop T, Diefenbach C, Meyer J. Long-term results of thrombolytic therapy with and without percutaneous transluminal coronary angioplasty. J Am Coll Cardiol 1989;14:276-285.
343. Verna E, Castiglioni B, Onofri M, et al. Intracoronary stenting of the infarct-related artery without anticoagulation in acute myocardial infarction. Euro Heart J 1995;16:12.
344. Levy G, deBoisgelin, Volpiliere R, Bouvagnet P. Intracoronary stenting in direction infarct angioplast: Is it dangerous? Circulation 1995;92:I-139.
345. Romero M, Medina A, Suarex J, et al. Elective Palmaz-Schatz stent implantation in acute coronary syndromes induced by thrombus-containing lesions. Euro Heart J 1995;16:179.
346. Repetto S, Onofri M, Castiglioni B, et al. Stenting of the infarct related artery during complicated angioplasty in acute myocardial infarction. J Invas Cardiol 1996;8:177-183.
347. Rodriguez A, Fernandex M, Santaera O, et al. Coronary stenting in patients undergoing PTCA during acute myocardial infarction. Am J Cardiol 1996;77:685-689.
348. Steinhubl S, Moliterno O, Teirstein P, et al. Stenting for acute myocardial infarction: The early United States multicenter experience. J Am Coll Cardiol 1996;22:279A.
349. Benzuly K, Allen D, Mason D, et al. A prospective pilot study of primary stenting for acute myocardial infarction (STAMI). J Invas Cardiol 1996;8:38.
350. Stone G, Marice M, Brodie B, et al. Primary stenting in acute MI: Interim report from the PAMI-3 stent pilot study. European Congress of Cardiology. August, 1996.
351. Lefkovits J, Anderson K, Weisman H, Topol E. Increased risk of non-Q-MI following DCA: Evidence for a platelet dependant mechanism from the EPIC Trial. Circulation 1994;90:I-214.
352. Dooris M, Hoffman M, Glazier S, et al. Comparative results of transluminal extraction coronary atherectomy in saphenous vein graft lesions with and without thrombus. J Am Coll Cardiol 1995;25:1700-1705.

LV Dysfunction

353. Gruentzig AR, Senning A, Siegenthaler WE. Nonoperative dilation of coronary artery stenosis: percutaneous transluminal coronary angioplasty. N Engl J Med 1979;301:61-68.
354. Stevens T, Kahn JK, McCallister BD, et al. Safety and efficacy of percutaneous transluminal coronary angioplasty in patients with left ventricular dysfunction. Am J Cardio 1991;68:313-319.
355. Serota H, Deligonul U, Lee WH, et al. Predictors of cardiac survival after percutaneous transluminal coronary angioplasty in patients with severe left ventricular dysfunction. Am J Cardiol 1991;67:367-372.
356. Kohli RS, DiSciascio G, Cowley MJ, et al. Coronary angioplasty in patients with severe left ventricular dysfunction. J Am Coll Cardiol 1990;16:807-811.
357. Eltchaninoff H, Franco I, Whitlow PK, et al. Late results of coronary angioplasty in patients with left ventricular ejection fractions < or =40%. Am J Cardiol 1994;73:1047-52.
358. O'Keefe JH, Allan JJ, McCallister, et al. Angioplasty versus bypass surgery for multivessel coronary artery disease with left ventricular ejection fraction < 40%. Am J Cardiol 1993;71:897-901.
359. Holmes DR, Detre KM, Williams DO, et al. Long term outcome of patients with depressed left ventricular function undergoing percutaneous transluminal coronary angioplasty. The NHLBI PTCA Registry. Circulation 1993;87:21-9.
360. Terrien EF, Siegel N, O'Neill WW, et al. Angioplasty in patients with severe left ventricular dysfunction an analysis of immediate and long term survival. J Am Coll Cardiol 1993;21:272A.
361. Pigott JD, Kouchoukos NT, Oberman A, et al. Late results of surgical and medical therapy for patients with coronary artery disease and depressed left ventricular function. J Am Coll Cardiol 1985;5:1036-1045.
362. Alderman EL, Fisher LD, Litwin P, et al. Results of coronary artery surgery in patients with poor left ventricular function (CASS). Circulation 1983;68:785-795.
363. Miller TD, Christian TF, Taliercio CP, et al. Impaired left ventricular function, one- or two-vessel coronary artery disease, and severe ischemia: outcome with medical therapy versus revascularization. Mayo Clin Proc 1994;69:626-31.
364. Hochberg MS, Parsonnet V, et al. Coronary artery bypass grafting in patients with ejection fractions below forty percent. J Thorac Cardiovasc Surg 1983;86:519-527.

365. Rahimtoola SH, Nunley D, Grunkemeier G, et al. Ten year survival after coronary artery bypass surgery for unstable angina. N Engl J Med 1983;308:676-681.
366. The Veterans Administration Coronary Artery Bypass Surgery Cooperative Group. Eleven year survival in the Veterans Administration trial of coronary bypass surgery for stable angina. N Engl J Med 1995;311:1333-1339.
367. Elefteriades JA, Tolis G, Levi E, et al. Coronary artery bypass grafting in severe left ventricular dysfunction: excellent survival with improved ejection fraction and functional state. J Am Coll Cardiol 1993;22:1411-7.
368. BARI Investigators. The bypass angioplasty revascularization investigation (BARI): five year mortality and morbidity in a randomized study comparing CABG and PTCA in patients with multivessel coronary artery disease. N Engl J Med (in-press).
369. Califf R, Phillips H, Hindman M, et al. Prognostic value of a coronary artery jeopardy score. J Am Coll Cardiol 1985;5:1055-63.
370. Ellis SG, Roubin GS, King SB III, et al. In-hospital cardiac mortality after acute closure after coronary angioplasty: analysis of risk factors from 8207 procedures. J Am Coll Cardiol 1988;11:211-216.
371. Kaltenbach M, Gruentzig A, Rentrop P, et al. In: Transluminal Coronary Angioplasty and Intracoronary Thrombolysis, 1982;145-150.
372. Alderman JD, Gabliani GI, McCabe CH, et al. Incidence and management of limb ischemia with percutaneous wire-guided intraaortic balloon catheters. J Am Coll Cardiol 1987;9:524-530.
373. Fuchs RM, Brin KP, Brinker JA, et al. Augmentation of regional coronary blood flow by intra-aortic balloon counterpulsation in patients with unstable angina. Circulation 1983;68:117-123.
374. Kahn JK, Rutherford BD, McConahay DR, et al. Supported "high risk" coronary angioplasty using intraaortic balloon pump counterpulsation. J Am Coll Cardiol 1990;15:1151-1155.
375. Meany TB, Pavlides G, Cragg D, et al. Prophylactic percutaneous cardio- pulmonary bypass versus intraaortic balloon pump support for high risk angioplasty. J Am Coll Cardiol 1992;19:349A.
376. Murphy DA, Craver JM, Jones EL, et al. Surgical management of acute myocardial ischemia following percutaneous transluminal coronary angioplasty. J Thorac Cardiovasc Surg 1984;87:332-339.
377. Ishihara M, Sato H, Tateishi H, et al. Intraaortic balloon pumping as the postangioplasty strategy in acute myocardial infarction. Am Heart J 1991;122:385-388.
378. Ohman EM, George BS, White CJ, et al. Use of aortic counterpulsation to improve sustained coronary artery patency during acute myocardial infarction. Results of a randomized trial. Circulation 1994;90:792-9.
379. Ohman EM, Califf RM, George BS, et al. The use of intraaortic balloon pumping as an adjunct to reperfusion therapy in acute myocardial infarction. Am Heart J 1991; :895-901.
380. Leinbach RC, et al. Early intraaortic balloon pumping for anterior myocardial infarction without shock. Circulation 1978;58:204.
381. Hanson EC, et al. Control of post infarction ventricular irritability with intraaortic balloon pump. Circulation 1978;62:30.
382. Aroesty J, Weintraub R, Paulin S, et al. Medically refractory unstable angina pectoris. Ii. Hemodynamic and angiographic effects of intraaortic balloon counterpulsation. Am J Cardiol 1979;43:887.
383. DeWood MA, Notske RN, Hensley GR, et al. Intraaortic balloon counterpulsation with and without reperfusion for myocardial infarction shock. Circulation 1980;61:1105-1112.
384. Tomasso CL. Use of percutaneously inserted cardiopulmonary bypass in the cardiac catheterization laboratory. Cathet Cardiovasc Diagn 1990;20:32-38.
385. Sturm JT, McGee MG, Fuhrman TM, et al. Treatment of postoperative low output syndrome with intraaortic balloon pumping: experience with 419 patients. Am J Cardiol 1980;45:1033-1036.
386. Vogel RA, Shawl F, Tommaso C, et al. Initial report of the national registry of elective cardiopulmonary bypass supported coronary angioplasty. J Am Coll Cardiol 1990;15:23-29.
387. Stack RK, Pavlides GS, Miller R, et al. Hemodynamic and metabolic effects of venoarterial cardiopulmonary support in coronary artery disease. Am J Cardiol 1991;67:1344-1348.
388. Vogel RA et al. Chapter 26 in Textbook of Interventional Cardiology 1994. Editor Topol (W.B. Saunders).
389. Shawl FA, et al. Cardiopulmonary bypass supported PTCA: long term follow-up of 85 consecutive patients. Circulation 1990;82:III-653A.
390. Overlie PA, Walter PD, Hurd HP, et al. Emergency cardiopulmonary support with circulatory support devices. Cardiology 1994;84(3):231-7.
391. Overlie PA. Emergency use of portable cardiopulmonary bypass. Cathet Cardiovasc Diagn 1990;20:27-31.
392. Loisance D, Dubois-Rande JL, et al. Prophylactic use of Hemopump in high risk coronary angiography. J Am Coll Cardiol 1990;15:249A.
393. Wampler RK, Moise JC, Frazier OH, et al. In vivo evaluation of a peripheral vascular access axial flow blood pump. Trns Am Soc Artif Intern Organs Trans 1988;34:450-454.
394. Smalling RW, Cassidy DB, Merhige M, et al. Improved hemodynamic and left ventricular unloading during acute ischemia using the Hemopump left ventricular assist device compared to intra aortic balloon counterpulsation. J Am Coll Cardiol 1989;13:160A.
395. Babic UU, Grujicic S, Djurisic Z, et al. Percutaneous left atrial aortic bypass with a roller pump. Circulation 1989;80:II-272.
396. Stack RS, Quigley PJ, Collins G, et al. Perfusion balloon catheter. Am J Cardiol 1988;61:77G-80G.
397. Turi ZG, Campbell CA, Gottimukkala MV, et al. Preservation of distal coronary perfusion during prolonged balloon inflation with an autoperfusion angioplasty catheter. Circulation 1987;75:1273-1280.
398. Banka VS, Trivedi A, Patel R, et al. Prevention of myocardial ischemia during coronary angioplasty: a simple new method for distal antegrade arterial blood perfusion. Am Heart J 1989;118:830-836.
399. Bell MR, Nishimura RA, Holmes DR, et al. Does intracoronary infusion of Fluosol-Da.. 20% prevent left ventricular diastolic dysfunction during coronary balloon angioplasty? J Am Coll Cardiol 1990;16;4:959-966.
400. Robalino BD, Marwick T, Lafont A, et al. Protection against ischemia during prolonged balloon inflation by distal coronary perfusion with use of an autoperfusion catheter or Fluosol. J Am Coll Cardiol 1992;20:1378-84.

401. Christensen CW, Reeves WC, Lassar TA, et al. Inadequate subendocardial oxygen delivery during perfluorocarbon perfusion in a canine model of ischemia. Am Heart J 1988;115:30-37.
402. Hajduczki I, Kar S, Areeda J, et al. Reversal of chronic regional myocardial dysfunction (hibernating myocardium) by synchronized diastolic coronary venous retroperfusion during coronary angioplasty. J Am Coll Cardiol 1990;15:238-242.
403. Drury JK, Yamazaki S, Fishbein MC, et al. Synchronized diastolic coronary venous retroperfusion: results of a preclinical safety and efficacy study. J Am Coll Cardiol 1985;6:328-335.
404. Incorvati RL, Tauberg SG, Pecora MJ, et al. Clinical applications of coronary sinus retroperfusion during high risk percutaneous transluminal coronary angioplasty. J Am Coll Cardiol 1993;22:127-34.
405. Nanto S, Nishida K, Hirayama A, et al. Supported angioplasty with synchronized retroperfusion in high risk patients with left main trunk or near left main trunk obstruction. Am Heart J 1993;125:301-9.
406. Carday E, Kar S, Drury JK, et al. Coronary venous retroperfusion for support of ischemic myocardium. Cardiovascular Rev Rep 1988:9:50-53.
407. Kar S, et al. Reduction of PTCA induced ischemia by Synchronized Coronary Venous Retroperfusion: Results of a Multicenter Clinical Trial. J Am Coll Cardiol 1990;15:250A.
408. Zalewski A, Goldberg S, Dervan JP, et al. Myocardial protection during coronary occlusion in man: beneficial effects of regional b blockade. J Am Coll Cardiol 1985;5:445.
409. Zalewski A, Savage M, Goldberg S. Protection of the ischemic myocardium during percutaneous transluminal coronary angioplasty. Am J Cardiol 1988;61:54-60G.

Special Patient Populations

410. Kahn JW, Hartzler GO. Saphenous vein graft angioplasty in a teenager. Am J Cardiol 1990;65:25-260.
411. Mehan V, Urban P, et al. Coronary angioplasty in the young: Procedural results and late outcome. J Invas Cardiol 1994;6:202-208.
412. Buffet P, Colasante B, et al. Long-term follow-up after coronary angioplasty in patients younger than 40 years of age. Am Heart J 1994;127:509-513.
413. Kofflard M, van Dombur R, van den Brand M, de Jaegere P. 5-year follow-up of coronary angioplasty in patients aged 35 years or younger. Circulation 1994;88(Part II):I-218.
414. Stone GW, Ligon RW, Rutherford BD, et al. Short-term outcome and long-term follow-up following coronary angioplasty in the young patient: An 8-year experience. Am Heart J 1989;118:873-877.
415. Hannan E, and Burke J. Effect of age on mortality in coronary artery bypass surgery in New York, 1991-1992. Am Heart J 1994;128:1184-91.
416. O'Keefe J, Sutton M, et al. Coronary angioplasty versus bypass surgery in patients >70 years old matched for ventricular function. J Am Coll Cardiol 1994;24:425-430.
417. Peterson ED, Gollis JG, Bebchuk JD, DeLong ER, et al. Chances in mortality after myocardial revascularization in the elderly. The National Medicare experience. Ann Intern Med. 1994;121:919-927.
418. Mick MJ, Simpfendorfer C, et al. Early and late results of coronary angioplasty and bypass in octogenarians. Am J Cardiol 1991;68:1316-1320.
419. Lindsay J, Reddy V, et al. Morbidity and mortality rates in elderly patients undergoing percutaneous coronary transluminal angioplasty. Am Heart J 1994;128:697-702.
420. Burnstein S, Sun GW, Hammer JS, Mann JD, et al. Adjusted influence of age and gender on PTCA outcomes and hospital resource consumption. J Am Coll Cardiol 1994;March Special Issue:223A.
421. Jollis JG, Peterson ED, Bebchuk JD, DeLong ER, et al. Coronary angioplasty in 20,006 patients over age 80 in the United States. J Am Coll Cardiol 1995; February Special Issue:47A.
422. Thompson RC, Holmes DR, Grill DR, Bailey KR. Changing outcome of angioplasty in elderly. J Am Coll Cardiol 1996;27:8-14.
423. Little T, Milner M, Lee K, Contantine J, Pichard AD, Lindsay JJ. Late outcome and quality of life following percutaneous transluminal coronary angioplasty in octogenarians. Cathet Cardiovasc Diagn 1993;29:261-266.
424. Forman DE, Berman AD, McCabe CH, et al. PTCA in the elderly: The "young-old" versus the "old-old". J Am Geriatr Soc 1992;40:19-22.
425. ten Berg J, Bal E, et al. Initial and long-term results of percutaneous transluminal coronary angioplasty in patients 75 years of age and older. Cathet Cardiovasc Diagn 1992;26:165-170.
426. Thompson RC, Holmes DR, Gersh B, Mock MB. Percutaneous transluminal coronary angioplasty in the elderly: Early and long-term results. J Am Coll Cardiol 1991;17:1245-1250.
427. Yokoi H, Kimur T, Sawada Y, Nosaka H, et al. Efficacy and safety of Palmaz-Schatz stent in elderly (≥ 75 years old) patients: Early and follow-up results. J Am Coll Cardiol 1995; February Special Issue:47A.
428. Fishman RF, Kuntz RE, Carrozza JP, et al. Acute and long-term results of coronary atherectomy in women and the elderly. Circulation (in-press).
429. Movsowitz H, Manginas A, et al. Directional coronary atherectomy can be successfully performed in the elderly. Am J Cardiol 1994;31:261-263.
430. Elliot JM, MacIsaac AI, Lefkovits J, Horrigan MCG, Franco I, Whitlow PL. New coronary devices in the elderly: Comparison with angioplasty. Circulation 1994;90:4:I-333.
431. Henson, K. D., J. J. Popma, et al. Comparison of results of rotational coronary atherectomy in three age groups (<70,70 to 79 and >80 years). Am J Cardiol 1993;71:862-864.
432. Weyrens F, Goldberg I, et al. Percutaneous transluminal coronary angioplasty in patients aged >90 years. Am J Cardiol 1994;74:397-398.
433. Santana J, Haft J, LaMarche N, Goldstein J. Coronary angioplasty in patients eighty years of age or older. Am Heart J 1992;124:13-

18.
434. Bedotto JB, Rutherford BD, McConahay DR, et al. Results of multivessel percutaneous transluminal coronary angioplasty in persons aged 65 years and older. Am J Cardiol 1991;67:1051-1055.
435. Jackman JD, Navetta FI, Smith JE, et al. Percutaneous transluminal coronary angioplasty in octogenarians as an effective therapy for angina pectoris. Am J Cardiol 1991;116-119.
436. Myler RK, Webb JG, Nguyen KPV, et al. Coronary angioplasty in octogenarians: Comparison to coronary bypass surgery. Cathet Cardiovasc Diagn 1991;23:3-9.
437. Jeroudi OM, Kleiman NS, Minor ST,et al. Percutaneous transluminal coronary angioplasty in octogenarians. Ann Intern Med 1990;113:423-428.
438. Rizo-Patron C, Hamad N, Paulus R, et al. Percutaneous transluminal coronary angioplasty in octogenarians with unstable coronary syndromes. Am J Cardiol 1990;66:857-858.
439. Rich JJ, Crispino CM, Saporito JJ, et al. Percutaneous transluminal coronary angioplasty in octogenarians. Am J Cardiol 1988;61:457-458.
440. Kern MJ, Deligonoul U, Galan K, et al. Percutaneous transluminal coronary angioplasty in octogenarians. Am J Cardiol 1988;61:457-458.
441. Weyrens EJ, Goldenberg I, Fishman MJ, et al. Percutaneous transluminal coronary angioplasty in patients aged > 90 years. Am J Cardiol 1994;74:397-398.
442. Lerner DJ, Kannel WB. Patterns of coronary heart disease morbidity and mortality in the sexes: A 26-year follow-up of the Framingham population. Am Heart J 1986;111:383-390.
443. Harper R, Kennedy G, DeSanctis R, et al. The incidence and pattern of angina prior to acute myocardial infarction: A study of 577 cases. Am Heart J 1979;97:178-183.
444. Weiner DA, Ryan TJ, McCabe CH, et al. Exercise stress testing: Correlations among history of angina, ST-segment response and prevalence of coronary-artery disease in the Coronary Artery Surgery Study (CASS). N Engl J Med 1979;301:230-235.
445. Stone G, Grines C, Browne K, et al. Comparison of in-hospital outcome in men versus women treated by either thrombolytic therapy or primary coronary angioplasty for acute myocardial infarction. Am J Cardiol 1995;75:987-992.
446. Malenka DJ, O'Connor GAT, Robb J, Kellett M Jr., et al. Is female gender a risk factor for adverse outcomes following PTCA? Circulation 1995;92:I-437.
447. Weintraub WS, Wenger NK, Kosinski AS, et al. Percutaneous transluminal coronary angioplasty in women compared with men. J Am Coll Cardiol 1994;24:81-90.
448. Arnold A, Mick M, et al. Gender differences for coronary angioplasty. Am J Cardiol 1994;74:18-21.
449. Cavero PG, O'Keefe JH, McCallister B, Cochran V, et al. Effect of gender on early and longterm outcome after multiple vessel revascularization with coronary bypass surgery or balloon angioplasty. J Am Coll Cardiol 1994;February Special Issue:351A.
450. Kelsey S, James M, Holubkov AL, Holubkov R. Results of percutaneous transluminal coronary angioplasty in women. 1985-1986 National Heart, Lung, and Blood Institute's Coronary Angioplasty Registry. Circulation 1993;87:720-727.
451. Bell MR, Holmes DR, Berger PB, et al. The changing in-hospital mortality in women undergoing percutaneous transluminal coronary angioplasty. JAMA 1993;269:2091-2095.
452. Kahn JK, Rutherford BD, McConahay DR, et al. Comparison of procedural results and risks of coronary in men and women for conditions other than acute myocardial infarction. Am J Cardiol 1992;69:1241-1242.
453. Bell M, Grill D, Garratt K, Berger P, Gersh B, Holmes D. Long-term outcome of women compared with men after successful coronary angioplasty. Circulation 1995;91:2876-2881.
454. Erne P, Evequoz D, Zuber M, Yoon S, Burckhardt D. Swiss interventional study on silent ischemia II (SWISSI II): Study design and preliminary results. Circulation 1995;92:I-80.
455. Baumbach A, Bittl J, Fleck E, et al. Acute complications of excimer laser coronary angioplasty: A detailed analysis of multicenter results. J Am Coll Cardiol 1994;23:1305-1313.
456. Combs WG, Rothenberg MD, Burke JA, et al. Gender does not influence the morbidty and mortality associated with diagnostic and interventional cardiac catheterization procedures. J Am Coll Cardiol 1994;February Special Issue:401A.
457. Dean LS, Voorhees WD, Sutor C, Roubin GS. Female gender: A risk factor for complications following intracoronary stenting? A Cook multicenter Registry Report. Circulation 1994;90:4:I-620.
458. Ellis, S., J. Popma, et al. Relation of clinical presentation, stenosis morphology, and operator technique to the procedural results of rotational atherectomy-facilitated angioplasty. Circulation 1994;89:882-892.
459. Bowling BA, May M, Lichtenberg A, et al. Clinical and angiographic outcome of new interventional devices in men and women. Circulation 1994;88:I-448.
460. Casale PN, Marco J, Warth D, Buchbinder M. Women have a lower success rate and higher complication rate with percutaneous rotational atherectomy. Circulation 1994;88:I-448.
461. Henson KD, Popma JJ, Satler LF, Kent KM, et al. Late clinical outcome after new device angioplasty in women. J Am Coll Cardiol 1993;21:2:233A.
462. Mehta S, Margolis JR, Bejarano J, et al. Acute and long-term results with new devices do not demonstrate significant gender differences: Results from the NACI Registry. Circulation 1994;88:I-448.
463. Movsowitz H, Emmi R, Manginas A, et al. Does female gender affect the success rate and outcome of directional coronary atherectomy? Circulation 1994;88:I-448.
464. Sempos C, Cooper R, Kovear MD, McMullen M. Divergence of the recent trends in coronary mortality for the four major race-sex groups in the United States. Am J Public Health 1988;78:1422-1427.
465. Maynard C, Fisher LD, Passamani ER. Survival of black persons compared with white persons in the Coronary Artery Surgery Study (CASS). Am J Cardiol 1987;60:513-518.
466. Scott, N, Kelsey S, et al. Percutaneous transluminal coronary angioplasty in African-American patients (The National Heart, Lung,

and Blood Institute 1985-1986 percutaneous transluminal coronary angioplasty registry). Am J Cardiol 1994;73:1141-1146.
467. Chuang YC, Merritt AJ, Popma JJ, Bucher TA, et al. Do racial differences affect outcome after new device angioplasty? J Am Coll Cardiol 1994;February Special Issue:301A.
468. Scott NA, Capers Q, Weintraub WS, Liberman HA, et al. In hospital and long term outcome of PTCA in African-American women and men. Circulation 1994;88:I-448.
469. The BARI Investigators. The Bypass Angioplasty Revascularization Investigation (BARI): five year mortality and morbidity in a randomized study comparing CABG and PTCA in patients with multivessel coronary disease. N Engl J Med 1996 (Submitted).
470. Uthoff K, Schuerholz T, Mϋgge A, Schaefers JH, et al. Coronary revascularization in renal risk patients —coronary angioplasty (PTCA) or coronary artery bypass grafting (CABG)? Circulation 1995;92:I-643.
471. Stein B, Weintraub W, et al. Influence of diabetes mellitus on early and late outcome after percutaneous transluminal coronary angioplasty. Circulation 1995;91:979-989.
472. Faxon DP, Kip KE, Currier JW, Yeh W, et al. Diabetics have a significantly poorer eight year outcome after angioplasty. Circulation 1995;92:I-76.
473. Tan K, Sulke N, et al. Clinical and lesion morphologic determinants of coronary angioplasty success and complications: Current experience. J Am Coll Cardiol 1995;25:855-65.
474. Bailey WL, Westerhausen DR, Rutherford BD, McConahay DR, et al. Characteristics and long term outcomes of diabetic patients presenting for coronary angioplasty. J Am Coll Cardiol 1993;21:2:273A.
475. Carrozza J, Kuntz R, et al. Angiographic and clinical outcome of intracoronary stenting: Immediate and long-term results from a large single-center experience. J Am Coll Cardiol 1992;20:328-337.
476. Rensing BJ, Hermans WR, Strauss BH, Serruys PW. Regional differences in elastic recoil after percutaneous transluminal coronary angioplasty: A quantitative angiographic study. J Am Coll Cardiol 1991;17:34B-8B.
477. Weintraub WS, Kosinski AS, Brown CL, King SB III. Can restenosis after coronary angioplasty be predicted from clinical variables? J Am Coll Cardiol 1993;21:6-14.
478. Levin GN, Leya F, Keeler G, Berdan LG, Jacobs AK. The impact of diabetes mellitus on restenosis following directional coronary atherectomy and PTCA: A report from CAVEAT-1. Circulation 1994;90:4:I-652.
479. Faxon DP. Effect of high dose angiotensin-converting enzyme inhibition on restenosis: Final results of the MARCATOR study, a multicenter, double-blind, placebo-controlled trial of cilazapril. J Am Coll Cardiol 1995;2:362-9.
480. Bourassa MG, Lesperance J, Eastwood C, et al. Clinical, physiologic, anatomic and procedural factors predictive of restenosis after percutaneous transluminal coronary angioplasty. J Am Coll Cardiol 1991;18:368-76.
481. Kahn JK, Rutherford BD, McConahay DR, et al. Short and longterm outcome of percutaneous transluminal coronary angioplasty in chronic dialysis patients. Am Heart J 1990;119:484-489.
482. Reusser LM, Osborn LA, White HJ, et al. Increased morbidity after coronary angioplasty in patients on chronic hemodialysis. Am J Cardiol 1994;73:965-6.
483. Ahmed WH, Pashos CL, Ayanian JZ, Bittle JA. 30-day and one-year mortality in hemodialysis patients undergoing coronary revascularization: Results from a national cohort. Circulation 1995;92:I-75.
484. Schroeder J, Gao SZ, et al. A preliminary study of diltiazem in the prevention of coronary artery disease in heart-transplant recipients. N Engl J Med 1993;328:164-170.
485. Halle A, DiSciascio G, et al. Coronary angioplasty, atherectomy and bypass surgery in cardiac transplant recipients. J Am Coll Cardiol 1995;26:120-8.
486. Swan JW, Norell M, Yacoub M, et al. Coronary angioplasty in cardiac transplant recipients. Eur Heart J 1993;14:65-70.
487. Sandhu JS, Uretsky BF, Reddy S, et al. Potential limitations of percutaneous transluminal coronary angioplasty in heart transplant recipients. Am J Cardiol 1992;69:1234-1237.
488. Mullins PA, Shapiro LM, Aravot DA, et al. Experience of percutaneous transluminal coronary angioplasty in orthotopic transplant recipients. Eur Heart J 1991;12:1205-1207.
489. Chaitman B, Stone P, Knatterud G, et al. Asymptomatic cardiac ischemia pilot (ACIP) study: Impact of anti-ischemia therapy on 12-week rest electrocardiogram and exercise test outcomes. J Am Coll Cardiol 1995;26:585-593.
490. Rogers W, Bourassa M, Andrews T, et al. Asymptomatic cardiac ischemia pilot (ACIP) study: Outcome at 1-year for patients with asymptomatic cardiac ischemia randomized to medical therapy or revascularization. J Am Coll Cardiol 1995;26:594-605.
491. Bourassa M, Pepine C, Forman S, et al. Asymptomatic cardiac ischemia pilot (ACIP) study: Effects of coronary angioplasty and coronary artery bypass graft surgery on recurrent angina and ischemia. J Am Coll Cardiol 1995;26:606-614.
492. Knatterud GL, Bourassa MG, Pepine CJ, et al. Effects of treatment strategies to suppress ischemia in patients with coronary artery disease: 12-week results of the Asymptomatic Cardiac Ischemia Pilot (ACIP) study. J Am Coll Cardiol 1994;24:11-20.
493. Stone GW, Spaude D, Ligon RW, et al. Usefulness of percutaneous transluminal coronary angioplasty in alleviating silent myocardial ischemia in patients with absent or minimal painful myocardial ischemia. Am J Cardiol 1989;64:560-564.
494. Lefevre T, Morice MC, Labrunie B, et al. Coronary stenting in elderly patients. Results from the stent without coumadin French Registry. J Am Coll Cardiol 1996;27:252A.
495. Hermiller J, Fry E, Berkompas D, et al. Effect of gender on acute outcome following intracoronary bailout stenting. J Invas Cardiol 1996;8.
496. Thompson RC, Holmes DR, Grill DE, Mock MB, Bailey KR. Changing outcome of angioplasty in the elderly. J Am Coll Cardiol 1996;27:8-14.
497. Laster SB, Rutherford BD, Giorgi LV, et al. Results of direct PTCA in octogenarians. Am J Cardiol 1996;77:10-13.

Overview of New Devices

498. Adelman A, Eric C, Kimball B, et al. A comparison of directional atherectomy with balloon angioplasty for lesions of the left anterior descending coronary artery. N Engl J Med 1993;329:228-233.
499. Topol E, Leya F, Pinkerton C, et al. A comparison of directional atherectomy with coronary angioplasty in patients with coronary artery disease. N Engl J Med 1993;329:221-227.
500. Vandormael M, Reifart N, Preusler W, et al. Six months following excimer laser angioplasty, rotational atherectomy and balloon angioplasty for complex lesions: ERBAC study. Circulation 1994;90:I-213.
501. Serruys P, deJegere P, Kiemeneij F, et al. A comparison of balloon expandable stent implantation with balloon angioplasty in patients with coronary artery disease. N Engl J Med 1994;331:489-495.
502. Fischman D, Leon M, Baim D, et al. A randomized comparison of coronary stent placement and balloon angioplasty in the treatment of coronary artery disease. N Engl J Med 1994:496-501.
503. Safian R, Freed M, Lichtenberg A, et al. Usefulness of percutaneous transluminal coronary angioplasty after new device coronary interventions. Am J Cardiol 1994;73:642-646.
504. Safian R, May M, Lichtenberg A, Schreiber T, Pavlides G. Detailed clinical and angiographic analysis of transluminal extraction coronary atherectomy for complex lesions in native coronary arteries. J Am Coll Cardiol 1995;25:848-854.
505. McCullough PA, O'Neill WW, May M, et al. Predictors of acute complications after percutaneous coronary revascularization with new devices. J Am Coll Cardiol 1995;25:122A.
506. Safian R, Freed M, Lichtenberg A, et al. Are residual stenoses after excimer laser angioplasty and coronary atherectomy due to inefficient or small devices? Comparison with balloon angioplasty. J Am Coll Cardiol 1993;22:1628-1634.
507. Kuntz RE, Safian RD, Carrozza JP, Fishman RF, Mansour M, Baim D. The importance of acute luminal diameter in determining restenosis after coronary atherectomy or stenting. Circulation 1992;86:1827-1835.
508. Kuntz R, Gibson C, Nobuyoshi M, Baim D. Generalized model of restenosis after conventional balloon angioplasty and new devices. J Am Coll Cardiol 1993;21:15-25.
509. Umans V, Melkert R, de Jaegere P, de Feyter P, Serruys P. A matched comparison of the long-term outcome of directional coronary atherectomy versus coronary stenting. J Am Coll Cardiol 1995;25:393A.
510. Foley DP, Appleman YE, Piek JJ. Comparison of angiographic restenosis propensity of excimer laser coronary angioplasty (ELCA) and balloon angioplasty (BA) in the Amsterdam Rotterdam (AMRO) trial. Circulation 1995;92:I-477.
511. Duerr RL, Topol EJ. Dissociation between minimal luminal diameter and clinical outcome at 6 month follow-up in randomized trials of percutaneous revascularization. J Am Coll Cardiol 1995;25:36A.
512. Miyazaki S, Nakao K, Itoh A, Daikoku S, et al. Correlation of residual stenosis immediately after coronary angioplasty with long-term prognosis. J Am Coll Cardiol 1995;25:269A.
513. Cohen EA, Foley B, Kimball BP, et al. Evidence for a device specific effect on late changes in lumen dimensions after directional atherectomy or intracoronary stenting. Circulation 1994;90:I-58.
514. Nio C, Freed M, Blankenship L. Procedural cost of new interventional devices. Am J Cardiol 1994;74:1165-1166.
515. Dick RJ, Popma JJ, Muller DWM, Burek KA. In-hospital costs associated with new percutaneous coronary devices. Am J Cardiol 1991;68:879-885.
516. Guzman L, Simpfendorfer C, Fix J, Franco I, Whitlow P. Comparison of costs of new atherectomy devices and balloon angioplasty for coronary artery disease. Am J Cardiol 1994;74:22-25.
517. Vandormael M, Reifart N, Preusler W, et al. In-hospital costs comparison of excimer laser angioplasty, Rotational atherectomy (Rotablator) and balloon angioplasty for complex coronary lesions: A randomized trial (ERBAC). J Am Coll Cardiol 1994;23:223A.
518. Weintraub WS, Waksman R, Bernard J, Hicks F, et al. The influence of new devices on the costs of interventional procedures. Circulation 1994;90:I-44.
519. Appleman YE, Birnie E, Piek JJ, de Feyter PJ, Koolen JJ, et al. Excimer laser angioplasty versus balloon angioplasty in longer coronary lesions: A cost-effectiveness analysis. Circulation 1995;92:I-512.
520. Adbelmeguid AE, Sapp SK, Topol EJ. Long-term outcome of transient uncomplicated in-lab coronary closure. Circulation 1994;90:I-43.
521. Waksman R, Ziyad MBG, Steenkiste AR, Detre K. Predictors and significance of myocardial infarction as a complication of new interventional devices: Report from the NACI Registry. Circulation 1994;90:I-43.
522. Tauke JT, Kong TQ, Meyers SN, Srinivasan G, et al. Prognostic value of creatinine kinase elevation following elective coronary artery interventions. J Am Coll Cardiol 1995;25:269A.
523. Kong TQ, Tauke JT, Meyers SN, Parker MA, Davidson, CJ. Late outcomes after elective coronary angioplasty: Impact of patient characteristics, lesion morphology and creatine kinase elevation. Circulation 1995;92:I-88.
524. Tardiff BE, Granger CB, Woodlief L, Mahaffey KW, et al. Prognostic significance of post-intervention isozyme elevations. Circulation 1995;92:I-544.
525. Redwood SR, Popma JJ, Kent KM, Pichard AD, et al. "Minor" CPK-MB elevations are associated with increased late mortality following ablative new-device angioplasty in native coronary arteries. Circulation 1995;92:I-544.
526. Hong MK, Popma JJ, Wong SC, Kent KM, et al. Incidence of and factors associated with abrupt closure in patients undergoing elective, new device angioplasty in native coronary arteries. J Am Coll Cardiol 1995;25:122A.
527. McCullough PA, O'Neill WW, Hoffman M, Glazier S, et al. The "protective effect" of restenosis lesions on angiographic complications with new devices. Circulation 1995;92:I-346.
528. Safian RD, Freed M, Reddy V, Kuntz RE, Baim DS, Grines CL, O'Neill WW. Do excimer laser and rotational atherectomy facilitate balloon angioplasty? Implications for lesion-specific coronary intervention. J Am Coll Cardiol (in-press).
529. Henson KD, Flood R, Javier SP, Popma JJ, et al. Transcatheter device synergy: Use of adjunct directional atherectomy after rotational atherectomy vs. excimer laser angioplasty. J Am Coll Cardiol 1994;23:220A.

530. De Franco AC, Tuzcu EM, Moliterno DJ, Guyer S, et al. Do new interventional devices "facilitate" balloon angioplasty? Ultrasound evidence of no reduction in vessel recoil. Circulation 1994;90:I58.
531. Israel D, Marmur J, Sanborn T. Excimer laser-facilitated balloon angioplasty of a nondilatable lesion. J Am Coll Cardiol 1991;18:1118-1119.
532. Berger PB, Bresnaha J. Use of excimer laser in the treatment of chronic total occlusion of a coronary artery that cannot be crossed with a balloon catheter. Cathet Cardiovasc Diagn. 1993;28:44-46.
533. Wolfe C, Landin R, Linnemeier T, et al. Successful excimer laser angioplasty following unsuccessful primary balloon angioplasty. Cathet Cardiovasc Diagn 1993;28:273-278.
534. Rosenblum J, O'Donnell MJ, Stertzer SH, Schechtmann NS. Rotational ablation of a severely angulated stenosis previously not amenable to balloon angioplasty. Am Heart J 1991;122:1766-1768.
535. Brown RIG, Penn IM. Coronary rotational ablation for unsuccessful angioplasty due to failure to cross the stenosis with a dilatation catheter. Cathet Cardiovasc Diagn. 1992;26:110-112.
536. Rosenblum J, Stertzer S, Shaw R, et al. Rotational ablation of balloon angioplasty failures. J Inv Cardiol 1992;4:312-318.
537. Brogan W, Popma J, Pichard A, et al. Rotational coronary atherectomy after unsuccessful coronary balloon angioplasty. Am J Cardiol 1993;71:794-798.
538. McCluskey E, Cowley M, Whitlow P. Multicenter clinical experience with rescue atherectomy for failed angioplasty. Am J Cardiol 1993;72:42E-46E.
539. Hofling B, Gonschior P, Simpson L, Bauriedel G. Efficacy of directional coronary atherectomy in cases unsuitable for percutaneous transluminal coronary angioplasty (PTCA) and after unsuccessful PTCA. Am Heart J 1992;124:341-348.
540. Bergelson B, Fishman R, Tomaso C, et al. Acute and long-term outcome of failed percutaneous transluminal coronary angioplasty treated by directional coronary atherectomy. Am J Cardiol 1994;73:1224-1226.
541. Harris W, Berger P, Holmes D, Garratt K. "Rescue" directional coronary atherectomy after unsuccessful percutaneous transluminal coronary angioplasty. Mayo Clin Proc 1994;69:717-722.
542. Macaya C, Alfonso F, Iniguez A, Goicolea J. Stenting for elastic recoil during coronary angioplasty of the left main coronary artery. Am J Cardiol 1992;70:105-107.
543. Kahn JK, Hartzler GO. Frequency and causes of failure with contemporary balloon coronary angioplasty and implications for new technologies. Am J Cardiol 1990;66:858-860.
544. Appleman YE, Piek JJ, Redekop WK, deFeyter PJ, et al. Excimer laser angioplasty versus balloon angioplasty in longer coronary lesions: A multivariate analysis. Circulation 1995;92:I-74.
545. Strikwerda S, van Swijndregt EM, Foley DP, Boersma E, et al. Immediate and late outcome of excimer laser and balloon coronary angioplasty: A quantitative angiographic comparison based on matched lesions. J Am Coll Cardiol 1995;26:939-946.
546. EPIC Investigators, Topol EJ. Use of a monoclonal antibody directed against the platelet glycoprotein IIb/IIIa receptor in high-risk coronary angioplasty. N Engl J Med 1994;330:956-61.
547. Bittl J, Strony J, Brinker J, et al. Treatment with Bivalirudin (hirulog) as compared with heparin during coronary angioplasty for unstable or postinfarction angina. N Engl J Med 1995;333:764-9.
548. Serruys P, Herrman J-P, Simon R, et al. A comparison of Hirudin with heparin in the prevention of restenosis after coronary angioplasty. N Engl J Med 1995;333:757-63.
549. Tcheng J, Harrington R, Kottke-Marchant J, Kleiman N. Multicenter, randomized, double-blind, placebo-controlled trial of the platelet integrin glycoprotein IIb/IIIa blocker integrelin in elective coronary intervention. Circulation 1995;91:2151-2157.
550. Lincoff AM, Topol EJ, Califf RM, Weisman HF, et al. Influence of platelet GP IIb/IIIa receptor inhibition with c7E3 on the sequelae of dissection during percutaneous coronary revascularization. J Am Coll Cardiol 1995;25:390A.
551. Challapalli RM, Eisenberg MJ, Sigmon K, Lemberger J. Platelet glycoprotein IIb/IIIa monoclonal antibody (c7E3) reduces distal embolization during percutaneous intervention of saphenous vein grafts. Circulation 1995;92:I-607.
552. Van Ommen V, Veen E, Daemen M, Habets J, et al. In vivo evaluation of the safety to the vessel wall of the hydrolyser (a hydrodynamic thrombectomy catheter). J Am Coll Cardiol 1994;23:406A.
553. Fajadet J, Bar O, Jordan C, Robert G, et al. Human percutaneous thrombectomy using the new hydrolyser catheter: Preliminary results in saphenous vein grafts. J Am Coll Cardiol 1994;23:220A.
554. Meltzer RS, Schwarz KQ, Mottley JG, Everbach EC. Therapeutic cardiac ultrasound. Am J Cardiol 1991;67:422-424.
555. Eccelston DS, Cumpston GN, Hodge AJ, Pearne-Rowe D, Don Michael TA. Ultrasonic coronary angioplasty during bypass grafting: A new method of atherectomy: Initial results. Circulation 1993;88:I-640.
556. Steffen W, Siegel RJ. Ultrasound angioplasty-a review. J Interven Cardiol 1993;6:77-88.
557. Ernst A, Schenk EA, Woodlock TJ. Feasibility of recanalization of human coronary arteries using high-intensity ultrasound. Am J Cardiol 1994;73:126-132.
558. Hartnell GG, Saxton JM, Friedl SE, Abela GS. Ultrasonic thrombus ablation: In vitro assessment of a novel device for intracoronary use. J Interven Cardiol 1993;6:69-76.
559. Hamm CW, Steffen W, Reimers J, Terres W. Ultrasound induced thrombolysis in patients with acute myocardial infarction. Circulation 1995;92:I-416.
560. Hamm CW, Bertrand ME, de Scheerder I, Gunn J, et al. Initial multicenter experience with therapeutic ultrasonic coronary angioplasty in patients. J Am Coll Cardiol 1995;25:268A.
561. Steffan W, Bertrand ME, Hamm CW, de Scheerder I, et al. Multicenter experience with therapeutic ultrasound coronary angioplasty in symptomatic patients. Circulation 1995;92:I-330.
562. Spears JR, Reyes VP, Wynne J et al. Percutaneous coronary laser balloon angioplasty: Initial results of a multicenter experience. J Am Coll Cardiol 1990;16:293.
563. Reis GJ, Pomerantz RM, Jenkins RD, et al. Laser balloon angioplasty: Clinical, angiographic and histologic results. J Am Coll Cardiol 1991;18:193.

564. Yamashita K, Satake S, Omira H, Ohtomo K. Radiofrequency thermal balloon coronary angioplasty: A new device for successful percutaneous transluminal coronary angioplasty. J Am Coll Cardiol 1994;23:336-340.
565. Saito S, Arai H, Kim K, Aoki N. Initial clinical experiences with rescue unipolar radiofreqency thermal balloon angioplasty after abrupt or threatened vessel closure complicating elective conventional balloon coronary angioplasty. J Am Coll Cardiol 1994;24:1220-8.
566. Becker GJ, Lee BI, Waller BF, Barry KJ. Radiofrequency balloon angioplasty-rationale and proof of principle. Invest. Radiology 1988;23:810-17.
567. Lee BI, Becker GJ, Waller BF, Barry KJ. Thermal compression and molding of atherosclerotic vascular tissue with use of radiofrequency energy: Implications for radiofrequency balloon angioplasty. J Am Coll Cardiol 1989;13:1167-75.
568. Walinsky P, Rose A, Martinez-Hernandez A, Smith DL. Microwave balloon angioplasty. J Inv Cardiol 1991;3:152-156.
569. Resar JR, Wolff ME, Hruban R, Brinker JA. Endoluminal sealing of vascular wall disruptions with radiofrequency-heated balloon angioplasty. Cathet Cardiovasc Diagn. 1993;29:161-167.
570. Fram DB, McKay RG. "Hot" balloon angioplasty: Radiofrequency, neodymium: YAG, and microwave. In Topol EJ (ed): Textbook of Interventional Cardiology, 2nd Edition. Philadelphia, WB Sauders Company, 1994, pp 819-839.
571. Makowski S, O'Neill B, Sarkis A, et al. Physiological low stress angioplasty at 60°C. Initial results and 6 month follow-up. J Am Coll Cardiol 1993;21:440A.
572. McMath LP, Kundu SK, Spears JR: Experimental application of bioprotective materials to injured arterial surfaces with laser balloon angioplasty, abstracted. Circulation 1990;82:III-72.
573. Rees ME, Michalis LK. Vibrational coronary angioplasty for chronic total occlusions. A novel approach. J Am Coll Cardiol 1994;23:58A.
574. Rees ME, Michalis LK. Vibrational coronary angioplasty; Challenging chronic total occlusions. Preliminary clinical data. J Am Coll Cardiol 1995;25:268A.
575. Rees ME, Michalis LK. Activated-guidewire technique for treating chronic coronary artery occlusion. Lancet 1995;346:943-944.
576. Barath P, Fishbein MC, Vari S, Forrester JS. Cutting balloon: A novel approach to percutaneous angioplasty. Am J Cardiol 1991;68:1249-1252.
577. Unterberg C, Buchwald AB, Barath P, Schmidt T, et al. Cutting balloon coronary angioplasty--initial clinical experience. Clin Cardiol 1993;16:660-664.
578. Popma JJ, Knopf WD, Davidson C, Feldman RC, Eisenhauer AC, et al. Angiographic outcome after "cutting" balloon angioplasty. J Am Coll Cardiol 1995;25:268A.
579. Solar RJ, Meaney DF, Miller RT, Rahdert DA, et al. Enhanced lumen enlargement with new focused force angioplasty device. Circulation 1995;92:I-147.
580. Drexler H, Fischell TA. Initial clinical experience using a novel pullback atherectomy catheter (PAC) in the treatment of obstructive coronary artery disease. Circulation 1995;92:I-147.
581. Agmon M, Scheinowitz M, Beitner S, et al. The Bard Rotary Atherectomy System (BRAS): Initial experience in patients with peripheral vascular disease. J Interven Cardiol 1993;6:51-59.
582. Wilson BH, Tuntelder J, Thompson M, Dezern K, et al. A coring device: Intracoronary rotational excision. J Am Coll Cardiol 1994;23:406A.
583. Kaltenbach M, Vallbracht C. Reopening of chronic coronary artery occlusions by low speed rotational atherectomy. J Interven Cardiol 1989;2:137-145.
584. Kaltenbach M, Vallbracht C, Hartmann A. Recanalization of chronic coronary occlusions by low speed rotational angioplasty (ROTACS). J Interven Cardiol 1991;4:155-165.
585. Vallbracht C, Liermann D, Prignitz I, et al. Results of low speed rotational angioplasty for chronic peripheral occlusions. Am J Cardiol 1988;62:935-940.
586. Serruys PW, Hamburger J, Fleck E, Koolen JJ, Teunissen Y. Laser guidewire: A powerful tool in recanalization of chronic total coronary occlusion. Circulation 1995;92:I-76.
587. Ramee SR, Kuntz RE, Schatz RA, et al. Preliminary experience with the POSSIS coronary AngioJet rheolytic thrombectomy catheter in the VEGAS-I Pilot study. J Am Coll Cardiol 1996;27:69A.

Intracoronary Thrombus

588. Ambrose JA, Winters SL, Stern A, et Al. Angiographic morphology and the pathogenesis of unstable angina pectoris. J Am Coll Cardiol 1985;5:609-616.
589. Fuster V, Badimon L, Badimon J, et al. The pathogenesis of coronary artery disease and the acute coronary syndromes. N Eng J Med 1992;326:242-250.
590. Cowley MJ, DiSciascio G, Vetrovec GW. Coronary thrombus in unstable angina: Angiographic observations and clinical relevance. In Hugenholtz PG and Goldman BG (eds): Unstable Angina: Current Concepatients and Management. Schattauer Press, Stuttgart, 1985;95-102.
591. Gotoh K, Minamino T, Katoh O, et al. The role of intracoronary thrombus in unstable angina: angiographic assessment and thrombolytic therapy during ongoing anginal attacks. Circulation 1988;77:526-534.
592. Mabin TA, Holmes DR, Smith HC. Intracoronary thrombus role in coronary occlusion complicating PTCA. J Am Coll Cardiol 1985;5:198-202.
593. Sugrue DR, Holmes DR, Smith HC. Coronary artery thrombus as a risk factor for acute vessel occlusion during PTCA: Improved Results. Br Heart J 1986;53:62-66.
594. Deligonul V, Gabliani GI, Caroles DG, et al. PTCA in patients with intracoronary thrombus. Am J Cardiol 1988;62:474-476.
595. Mooney MR, Fishman-Mooney J, Goldenberg I, et al. Percutaneous transluminal coronary angioplasty in the setting of large

intracoronary thrombus. Am J Cardiol 1990;65:427-431.
596. Schieman G, Cohen BM, Kozina J, et al. Intracoronary urokinase for intracoronary thrombus accumulation complicating percutaneous transluminal coronary angioplasty in acute ischemic syndromes. Circulation 1990;82:2052-2060.
597. Yanagida S, Mizuno K, Miyamolo A Comparison of findings between coronary angiography and angioscopy. Circulation 1989;80 (Supp II):376.
598. Ramee SR, White CJ, Collins TJ, et al. Percutaneous angioscopy during coronary angioplasty using a steerable microangioscope. J Am Coll Cardiol 1991;17:100-105.
599. Mizuno K, Satumora K, Miyamoto A, et al. Angioscopic evaluation of coronary-artery thrombi in acute coronary syndromes. New Engl J Med 1992;326:287-291.
600. Mizuno K, Miyamoto A, Satomura K, et al. Angioscopic coronary macromorphology in patients with acute coronary disorders. Lancet 1991,337:809-812.
601. Mizuno K, Hikita H, Miyamoto A, Satomura K, et al. The pathogenesis of an impending infarction and its treatment - an angioscopic analysis. Jpn Circ J 1992, 56:1160-5.
602. Hombach V, Hoher M, Kochs M, Eggeling T, et al. Pathophysiology of unstable angina pectoris-correlations with coronary angioscopic imaging. Eur Heart J 1988,;9:40-5.
603. Waxsman S, Sassower M, Zarich S, et al. Angioscopy can Identify lesion specific predictors of early adverse outcome following PTCA in patients with unstable angina. Circulation 1994;90:I-490.
604. Manzo K, Netso R, Sassower M, Leeman D, et al. Coronary lesion morphology by angioscopy vs angiography: the ability to detect thrombi. J Am Coll Cardiol 1994: 955-4023.
605. Annex BH, Ajluni SC, Larkin TJ, O'Neill WW, Safian RD. Angioscopic guided interventions in a saphenous vein bypass graft. Cathet Cardiovasc Diagn 1994;31:330-3.
606. den Heijer P, Foley D, Escaned J, Hillege HL, Serruys PW, Lie KI. Angioscopic versus angiographic detection of intimal dissection and intracoronary thrombus. J Am Coll Cardiol 1994;955-100.
607. White CJ, Ramee SR, Collins TJ, et al. Coronary thrombi increase PTCA risk: Angioscopy as a clinical tool. Circulation 1996:93:253-258.
608. Hillegass WB, Ohman EM, O'Hanesian MA, et al. The effect of preprocedural intracoronary thrombus on patient outcome after percutaneous coronary intervention. J Am Coll Cardiol 1995;21:94A.
609. Tan K, Sulke N, Taub N, Sowton E. Clinical and lesion morphologic determinants of coronary angioplasty success and complications: Current experience. J Am Coll Cardiol 1995;25:855-65.
610. Violaris AG, Herrman JP, Melkert R, et al. Does local thrombus formation increase long term luminal renarrowing following PTCA? A quantitative angiographic analysis. J Am Coll Cardiol 1994;February Special Issue:139A.
611. Tenaglia A, Fortin D, Califf R, Frid D, et al. Predicting the risk of abrupt vessel closure after angioplasty in an individual patient. J Am Coll Cardiol 1994;24:1004-11.
612. Myler R, Shaw R, Stertzer S, Hecht H, et al. Lesion morphology and coronary angioplasty: Current experience and analysis. J Am Coll Cardiol 1992;19:1641-52.
613. Sherman CT, Litvack F, Grundfest W, Lee M, et al. Coronary angioscopy in patients with unstable angina pectoris. N Engl J Med 1986, 315:913-9.
614. den Heijer P, van Dijk RB, Hillege HL, et al. Serial angioscopic and angiographic observations during the first hour after successful coronary angioplasty: A preamble to a multicenter trial addressing angioscopic markers for restenosis. Am Heart J 1994;128:656-63.
615. Siegel RJ, Fischbein MC, Chae JS, Helfant RH, Hickey A, Forrester JS. Comparative studies of angioscopy and ultrasound for the evaluation of arterial disease. Echocardiography 1990;7:495-502.
616. Chesebro J, Zoldhelyi P, Fuster V: Pathogenesis of Thrombosis in Unstable Angina. Am J Cardiol 1991;68:2B-10B.
617. Fuster V, Lewis A. Conner Memorial Lecture. Mechanisms leading to myocardial infarction: insights from studies of vascular biology. Circulation 1994;90:2126-2146.
618. Kawai C. Pathogenesis of acute myocardial infarction: novel regulatory system of bioactive substances in the vessel wall. Circulation 1994; 90:1033-1043.
619. Jang Y, Lincoff AM, Plow EF, Topol EJ. Cellular adhesion molecules in coronary artery disease. J Am Coll Cardiol 1994;24:1591-601.
620. Lefkovits J, Topol EJ. Direct thrombin inhibitors in cardiovascular medicine. Circulation 1994; 90:1522-1536.
621. Davies MJ, Thomas, AC. Plaque Fissuring--The Cause of Acute Myocardial Infarction, Sudden Ischemic Death, and Crescendo Angina. Br Heart J 1985;53:363-373.
622. Falk E. Plaque rupture with severe pre-existing stenosis precipitating coronary thrombosis. Characteristics of coronary atherosclerotic plaques underlying fatal occlusive thrombi. Br Heart 1983;50:127-134.
623. Davies MJ, Bland JM, Hangartner JRW, et al. Factors influencing the presence of absence of acute coronary artery thrombi in sudden ischemic death. Eur Heart J 1989;10:203-208.
624. Badimon L, Badimon JJ, Gahez A, et al. Influence of arterial damage and wall shear forces on platelet deposition. Ex vivo study u.a. swine model. Arteriosclerosis 1986;6:312-330.
625. Fernandez-Ortiz A, Badimon JJ, Falk E, et al. Characterization of the relative thrombogenicity of atherosclerotic plaque components: implications for consequences of plaque rupture. J Am Coll Cardiol 1994;23:1562-9.
626. Mehran R, Ambrose JA, Bongu M, et al. Angioplasty of complex lesions in ischemic rest angina: Results of the thrombolysis and angioplasty in unstable angina (TAUSA) trial. J Am Coll Cardiol 1995;26:961-966.
627. Pavlides GS, Schreiber TL, Gangadharan V, et al. Safety and efficacy of urokinase during elective coronary angioplasty. Am Heart J 1991;121:731-736.
628. Chapekis AT, George BS, Candela RJ. Rapid thrombus dissolution by continuous infusion of urokinase through an intracoronary

perfusion wire prior to and following PTCA: Results in native coronaries and patent saphenous vein grafts. Cathet Cardiovasc Diagn 1991;23:89-92.

629. Kiesz R, Hennecken J, Bailey S. Bolus administration of intracoronary urokinase during PTCA in the presence of intracoronary thrombus. Circulation 1991;84:II-346.
630. Laskey MAL, Deutsch E, Barnathan E, et al. Influence of heparin therapy on percutaneous transluminal coronary angioplasty outcome in unstable angina pectoris. Am J Cardiol 1990;65:1425-1429.
631. O'Neill WW, Sketch MH Jr, Steenkiste A, Detre K. New Device Intervention in the treatment of intracoronary thrombus: report of the NACI registry. Circulation 1993;88: I-595.
632. Sketch MH Jr, Davidson CJ, Popma J, et al. Morphologic and quantitative predictors of acute outcome with new devices in saphenous vein grafts. J Am Coll Cardiol 1994; 90:219A.
633. Holmes DR, Ellis SG, Garratt KN. Directional coronary atherectomy for thrombus containing lesions: Improved outcome. Circulation 1991;84:II-26.
634. Emmi R, Movsowitz H, Manginas A, Wells E, et al. Directional coronary atherectomy in lesions with co-existing thrombus. Circulation 1993;88:I-596.
635. Cowley MJ, Whitlow PL, Baim DS, et al. Directional coronary atherectomy of saphenous vein graft narrowings: multicenter investigational experience. Am J Cardiol 1993;72:30E-34E17.
636. Cowley MJ. DiSciascio G. Experience with directional atherectomy since pre-market approval. Am J Cardiol 1993;72:12E-20E.
637. Sabri MN, Johnson D, Warner M, Cowley MJ. Intracoronary thrombolysis followed by directional atherectomy. A combined approach for thrombotic vein graft lesions considered unsuitable for angioplasty. Cathet Cardiovasc Diagn 1992;26:15-18.
638. Saito S, Arai H, Kim K, Aoki N, et al. Primary directional atherectomy for acute myocardial infarction. Cathet Cardiovasc Diagn 1994;32:44-48.
639. Topol EJ, Leya F, Pinkerton CA, et al. A comparison of directional atherectomy with coronary angioplasty in patients with coronary artery disease. N Engl J Med 1993;329:221-7.
640. Adelman AG, Cohen EA, Kimball BP, et al. A comparison of directional atherectomy with balloon angioplasty for lesions of the left anterior descending coronary artery. N Engl J Med 1993;329:228-33.
641. Abdelmeguid AE, Ellis SG, Sapp SK, et al. Directional coronary atherectomy in unstable angina pectoris. J Am Coll Cardiol 1994;24:46-54.
642. Annex BH, Larkin TJ, O'Neill WW, Safian RD. Evaluation of thrombus removal by transluminal extraction atherectomy by percutaneous coronary angioscopy. Am J Cardiol 74:606-609.
643. Kaplan B, Safian RD, Goldstein JA, Grines CL, O'Neill WW. Efficacy of angioscopy in determining the effectiveness of intracoronary urokinase and TEC atherectomy thrombus removal from an occluded saphenous vein graft prior to stent implantation. Cathet Cardiovasc Diagn 1995;36:335-337.
644. Moses J, Yeh W, Popma J, Sketch M, NACI Investigators. Predictors of distal embolization with the TEC catheter: a NACI registry report. J Am Coll Cardiol 1995;27:179A.
645. Hong M, Wong S, Popma J, et al. Favorable results of debulking followed by immediate adjunct stent therapy for high risk saphenous vein graft lesions. J Am Coll Cardiol February Special Issue, 1996.
646. Al-Shaibi KF, Goods C, Jain S, Negus B, et al. Does transluminal extraction atherectomy reduce distal embolization in saphenous vein grafts? Circulation 1995;92:I-329.
647. Meany T, Leon M, Kramer B, Margolis J, et al. Transluminal extraction catheter for the treatment of diseased saphenous vein grafts: A multicenter experience. Cathet Cardiovasc Diagn 1995;34:112-120.
648. O'Neill WW, Kramer BL, Sketch MH et al. Mechanical extraction atherectomy. Report of the us transluminal extraction catheter investigation. Circulation 1992;86:I-79.
649. Annex BH, Larkin TJ, Safian RD. Evaluation of intracoronary thrombus by percutaneous coronary angioscopy before and after transluminal extraction atherectomy. Am J Cardiol 1994;74:606-609.
650. Dooris M, May M, Grines CL, Pavlides GS, et al. Comparative results of transluminal extraction atherectomy in saphenous vein graft lesions with and without thrombus. J Am Coll Cardiol 1995;25:1700-1705.
651. Safian RD, Grines CL, May MA, Lichtenberg A, et al. Clinical and angiographic results of transluminal extraction coronary atherectomy in saphenous vein bypass grafts. Circulation 1994;89:302-312.
652. Popma JJ, Leon MB, Mintz GS, Kent KH, et al. Results of coronary angioplasty using the transluminal extraction catheter. Am J Cardiol 1992;70:1526-32.
653. Hong MK, Popma JJ, Pichard AD, Kent et al. Clinical significance of distal embolization after Transluminal Extraction Atherectomy in diffusely diseased saphenous vein grafts. Am Heart J 1994;127:1496-503.
654. Moses JW, Tierstein PS, Sketch MH, et al. Angiographic determinants of risk and outcome of coronary embolus and myocardial infarction (MI) with the Transluminal Extraction Catheter (TEC): A report from the New Approaches for Coronary Intervention (NACI) Registry. J Am Coll Cardiol 1994;February Special Issue:219A.
655. Larkin TJ, O'Neill WW, Safian RD, et al. A prospective study of transluminal extraction atherectomy in high risk patients with acute myocardial infarction. J Am Coll Cardiol 1994;February Special Issue:226A.
656. Tomaru T, Nakamura F, Yanagisawa-Miwa A, et al. Reduced vasoreactivity and thrombogenicity with pulsed laser angioplasty: Comparison with balloon angioplasty. J Intervn Cardiol 1995;8:6:643-651.
657. Shefer A, Forrester JS, Litvack F. Recanalization of acute thrombus: Comparison of acute success and short-term patency after excimer laser coronary angioplasty, balloon angioplasty and intracoronary thrombolysis in pigs. J Am Coll Cardiol 1991;17:205A.
658. Estella P, Ryan TJ Jr, Landzberg JC, Bittl JA. Excimer laser assisted coronary angioplasty for lesions containing thrombus. J Am Coll Cardiol 1993;21:1550-6.
659. Baumbach A, Oswald H, Kvasnika J, Fleck E, et al. Clinical results of coronary excimer laser angioplasty: report from the European Coronary Excimer Laser Angioplasty Registry. Eur Heart J 1994;15:89-95.

660. Cook SI, Eigler NL, Shefer A, et al. Percutaneous excimer laser coronary angioplasty in lesions not ideal for balloon angioplasty. Circulation 1991;84:632-43.
661. Klein LW, Litvack F, Holmes D, et al. Prospective multicenter anlaysis of excimer laser coronary angioplasty (ELCA) in stenoses with complex morphology. J Am Coll Cardiol 1991:448A.
662. Chasteney EA, Ravichandran PS, Furnany AP, et al. Laser thrombolysis for bypass graft thrombosis. J Am Coll Cardiol 1994;February Special Issue:374A.
663. Grinstead WC, Kleiman NS, Marks GF, et al. Stenting of coronary arteries containing thrombus: Angiographic and clinical outcomes of 109 patients from the Gianturco-Roubin Flex-Stent™ Registry. J Am Coll Cardiol 1996 (in-press).
664. Agrawal SK, Ho DSW, Liu M, Iyer S, et al. Predictors of thrombotic complications after placement of the flexible coil stent. Am J Cardiology Vol. 73; 1216-1219.
665. Dooris M, Grines CL. Successful reversal of cardiogenic shock precipitated by saphenous vein graft distal embolization using aspiration thrombectomy. Cathet Cardiovasc Diagns 1994;33:267-71.
666. Fajadet J, Bar O, Jordan C, Robert G, et al. Human percutaneous thrombectomy using the new Hydrolyser catheter: preliminary results in saphenous vein grafts. J Am Coll Cardiol 1994;February Special Issue:220A.
667. Ramee S, Kuntz R, Schatz R, et al. Preliminary experience with the POSSIS coronary AngioJet Rheolytic Thrombectomy Catheter in the VeGAS I Pilot Study. J Am Coll Cardiol 1996;27:69A.
668. Hartnell GG, Saxton JM, Friedl SE, Abela GS, Rosenchein U. Ultrasound thrombus ablation: in vitro assessment of a novel device for intracoronary use. J Interven Cardiol 1993;6:69-76.
669. Siegel RJ, Gunn J, Ahsan A, Fiscbein MC, et al. Use of therapeutic ultrasound in percutaneous coronary angioplasty. Experimental in vitro and initial clinical experience. Circulation 1994;89:1587-92.
670. Gal D, Monteverde C, Hogan J, et al. In vivo assessment of ultrasound angioplasty of fibrotic total occlusions. Circulation 1991;84:II-422.
671. Nardone D, Bravette B, Shi Y, et al. Effect of microwave thermal angioplasty on intracoronary thrombus. Circualtion 1991;84:II-300.
672. Yamashita K, Satake S, Ohira H, Ohtomo K. Radiofrequency thermal balloon coronary angioplasty: a new device for successful percutaneous transluminal coronary angioplasty. J Am Coll Cardiol 1994;23:336-40.
673. Myler RK, Shaw NE, Stertzer SH, et al. Unstable angina and coronary angioplasty. Circulation 1990;82:88-95.
674. Hettleman BD, Aplin RA, Sullivan PR, et al. Three days of heparin pretreatment reduces major complications of coronary angioplasty in patients with unstable angina. J Am Coll Cardiol 1990;15:154A.
675. Pow TK, Varricchione TR, Jacobs AK, et al. Does pretreatment with heparin prevent abrupt closure following PTCA? J Am Coll Cardiol 1988;11:238A.
676. Lukas MA, Deutsch E, Hirshfeld JW Jr, et al. Influence of heparin therapy on percutaneous transluminal coronary angioplasty outcome in patients with coronary arterial thrombus. Am J Cardiol 1990;65:179-182.
677. Vaitkus PT, Laskey WK. Efficacy of adjunctive thrombolytic therapy in percutaneous transluminal coronary angioplasty. J Am Coll Cardiol 1994;24:1415-23.
678. Suryapranata H, DeFeyter PJ, Serruys PW. Coronary angioplasty in patients with unstable angina pectoris: is there a role for thrombolysis? J Am Coll Cardiol 1988;12:69A-77A.
679. Goudreau E, DiSciascio G, Vetrovec GW, et al. Intracoronary urokinase as an adjunct to percutaneous transluminal coronary angioplasty in patients with complex coronary narrowings or angioplasty - induced complications. Am J Cardiol 1992;69:57-62.
680. Ambrose J, Torre S, Sharma S, et al. Adjunctive urokinase for ptca in unstable angina. Circulation 1991;84:590.
681. Ambrose JA, Almeida OD, Sharma SK, et al. Adjunctive thrombolytic therapy during angioplasty for ischemic rest angina. Results of the TAUSA trial. Circulation 1994;90:69-77.
682. The TIMI IIIB Investigators. Effects of tissue plasminogen activator and a comparison of early invasive and conservative strategies in unstable angina and non Q wave myocardial infarction: Results of the TIMI IIIB trial. Circulation 1994;89:1545-1556.
683. The TIMI IIIA Investigators. Early effects of tissue-type plasminogen activator added to conventional therapy on the culprit coronary lesion in patients presenting with ischemic cardiac pain at rest. Results of the Thrombolysis in Myocardial Ischemia (TIMI IIIA) Trial. Circulation 1993;87:38-52.
684. Grines, C, Ajluni S, Savas V, Samyn J, Pavlides G, et al. Prolonged urokinase infusion for chronic total native coronary occlusions. J Am Coll Cardiol 1996;27
685. Hartmann JR, Mc Keever LS, Stamato NJ, et al. Recanalization of chronically occluded aortocoronary saphenous vein bypass grafts by extended infusion of urokinase: initial results and short term clinical follow-up. J Am Coll Cardiol 1991;18:1517-1523.
686. Taylor MA, Santoran EC, Aji J, Eldredge WJ, et al. Intracerebral hemorrhage complicating urokinase infusion into an occluded aortocoronary bypass graft. Cathet Cardiovasc Diagn 1994;31:206-210.
687. Brown DL, Topol EJ. Stroke complicating percutaneous coronary revascularization. Am J Cardiol 1993;72:1207-1209.
688. Gold GH, Gimple LW, Yasuda T, et al. Pharmacodynamic study of F (ab')2 fragments of murine monoclonal antibody 7E3 directed against human platelet glycoprotein IIb/IIIa in patients with unstable angina pectoris. J Clin Invest 1990;86:651-9.
689. Kleiman NS, Ohman EM, Ellis SG, et al. Profound inhibition of platelet aggregation with monoclonal antibody 7E3 Fab following thrombolytic therapy: results of the TAMI 8 Pilot study. Circulation 1993;86:I-260.
690. The EPIC Investigators. Use of a monoclonal antibody directed against the platelet glycoprotein IIb/IIIa receptor in high-risk coronary angioplasty. N Engl J Med 1994;330:956-61.
691. Topol EJ, Fuster V, Harrington RA, Califf RM, et al. Recombinant hirudin for unstable angina pectoris: a multicenter randomized trial. Circulation 1994;89:1557-1566.
692. Topol EJ, Bonan R, Jewitt D, Sigwart U, et al. Use of direct antithrombin, hirulog, in place of heparin during angioplasty. Circulation 1993;87:1622-1629.
693. van den Bos AA, Deckers JW, Heyndricks GR, et al. Safety and efficacy of recombinant hirudin (CGP 393) versus heparin in

patients with stable angina pectoris undergoing coronary angioplasty. Circulation 1993;88:2058-2066.

694. Antmann EM, for TIMI 9A Investigators. Hirudin in acute myocardial infarction. A safety report from the Thrombolysis in Myocardial Ischemia (TIMI) 9A Trial. Circulation 1994;90:1624-30.
695. Neuhaus KL, Essen RV, Tebbe U, Jessel A, et al. Safety observations from the pilot phase of the randomized r-hirudin for improvement of thrombolysis (HIT-III) study. A study of the Arbeitsgemeinschaft Leitender Kardiologischer Krankenhausarzte (ALKK). Circulation 1994;90:1638-42.
696. The Global Use of Strategies to Open Occluded Coronary Arteries (GUSTO) II Investigators. Randomized trial of intravenous heparin versus recombinant hirudin for acute coronary syndromes. Circulation 1994;90:1631-7.
697. Lincoff AM, Topol EJ, Ellis SG. Local drug delivery systems for the prevention of restenosis. Circulation 1994;90:2070-2084.
698. Nunes GL, Hanson SR, King SB 3rd, et al. Local delivery of a synthetic antithrombin with a hydrogel-coated angioplasty balloon catheter inhibits platelet-dependent thrombosis. J Am Coll Cardiol 1994;23:1578-83.
699. McKay R, Fram DB, Hirst JA, Kleman FJ, et al. Treatment of intracoronary thrombus with local urokinase using a new, site-specific drug delivery system: the Dispatch catheter. Cathet Cardiovasc Diagn 1994;33:181-88.
700. Muhlestein JB, Gomez MA, Karagounis L, Anderson G. "Rescue ReoPro": Acute utilization of Abciximab for the dissolution of coronary thrombus developing as a complication of coronary angioplasty. Circulation 1995;92:I-607.
701. Fram DB, Aretz T, Azrin MA, Mitchel JF,et al. Localized intramural drug delivery during balloon angioplasty using hydrogel-coated balloons and pressure augmented diffusion. J Am Coll Cardiol 1994;23:1570-7.
702. Plante S, Dupuis G, Mongeau CJ, Durand P. Porous balloon catheters for local delivery: Assessment of vascular damage in a rabbit iliac angioplasty model. J Am Coll Cardiol 1994;24:820-4.
703. Hong MK, Wong SC, Popma JJ, Kent KM, et al. A dual-purpose angioplasty-drug infusion catheter for treatment of intragraft thrombus. Cathet Cardiovasc Diagn 1994;32:193-5.
704. Gershony G, Glass PR. Coronary thrombosis: A novel catheter based approach to treatment. Cathet Cardiovasc Diagn 1994;31:147-149.
705. Grines C, Brodi B, Griffin J, Donohue B, et al. Which primary PTCA patients may benefit from new technologies? Circulation 1995;92:I-146.
706. Pavlides G, Schreiber TL, Gangadharan V, et al. Safety and efficacy of urokinase during elective coronary angioplasty. Am Heart J 121:731, 1991.
707. Lincoff AM, Popma JJ, Ellis SG, et al. Abrupt vessel closure complicating coronary angioplasty: Clinical, angiographic and therapeutic profile. J Am Coll Cardiol 19:926, 1992.
708. de Feyter PJ, van den Brand M, Jaarman G, et al. Acute coronary artery occlusion during and after percutaneous transluminal coronary angioplasty. Circulation 83:927, 1991.
709. Haft JI, Goldstein JE, Homoud MK, et al. PTCA following myocardial infarction: Use of bailout fibrinolysis to improve results. Am Heart J 120:243, 1990.
710. Gulba DC, Daniel WG, Simon R, et al. Role of thrombolysis and thrombin in patients with acute coronary occlusion during percutaneous transluminal coronary angioplasty. J Am Coll Cardiol 16:563, 1990.

Bifurcation Lesions

711. Pinkerton CA, Slack JD. Complex Coronary Angioplasty: A technique for dilatation of bifurcation stenosis. Angiology 1985:543-548.
712. Renkin J, Wijns W, Hanet C, et al. Angioplasty of coronary bifurcation stenoses. Cathet Cardiovasc Diagn 1991;22:167-173.
713. George BS, Myler RK, Stertzer SH, et al. Balloon angioplasty of coronary bifurcation lesions. Cathet Cardiovasc Diagn 1986;12:124-138.
714. Ciampricutti R, El-Gamol M, Van Golder B, et al. Coronary angioplasty of bifurcation lesions without protection of large sidebranches. Cathet Cardiovasc Diagn 1992;27:191-196.
715. Myler RK, Shaw RE, Stertzer SH, et al. Lesion morphology and coronary angioplasty: current experience and analysis. J Am Coll Cardiol 1992. In press.
716. Meier B, Gruentzig AR, King SB III, et al. Risk of side branch occlusion during coronary angioplasty. Am J Cardiol 1984;53:10-14.
717. Boxt LM, Meyeruvitz MF, Taus RH, et al. Sidebranch occlusion complicating percutanous transluminal coronary angioplasty. Radiology 1986;161:681-683.
718. Weinstein JS, Baim DS, Sipperly ME, et al. Salvage of branch vessels during bifurcation lesion angioplasty. Cathet Cardiovasc Diagn 1991;22:1-6.
719. Vetrovec GW, Cowley MJ, Wolfgang TC, et al. Effects of percutaneous transluminal coronary angioplasty in lesion associated branches. Am Heart J 1985;109:921-925.
720. Arora RR, Raymond RE, Dimas AP, et al. Side branch occlusion during coronary angioplasty: incidence, angiographic characteristics, and outcome. Cathet Cardiovasc Diagn 1989;18:210-212.
721. Thomas TS, Williams DO, Most AS. Efficacy of coronary angioplasty of bifurcation lesions: immediate and late outcome. Circulation 1988;78:II-632.
722. Shiu MF, Singh A. Spontaneous recanalization of sidebranches occluded during percutaneous transluminal coronary angioplasty. Brit Heart J 1985;54:215-217.
723. Eisenhauer AC, Clugston RA, Ruiz CE. Sequential directional atherectomy of coronary bifurcation lesions. Cathet Cardiovasc Diagn 1993;Suppl 1:54-60.
724. Hinohara T, Rowe MH, Robertson GC, et al. Effect of lesion characteristics on outcome of directional coronary atherectomy. J Am Coll Cardiol 1991;17:1112-20.

725. Grassman ED, Leya FS, Lewis BE, Johnson SA, et al. Examination of common PTCA guidewires used for sidebranch protection during directional coronary atherectomy of bifurcation lesions performed in vivo and in vitro. Cathet Cardiovasc Diagn 1993; Suppl 1:48-53.
726. Safian R, Schreiber T, Baim D. Specific indications for directional coronary atherectomy: Origin left anterior descending coronary artery and bifurcating lesions. Am J Cardiol 1993;72:35E-41E.
727. Mansour M, Fishman RF, Kuntz RE, Carrozza JP. Feasibility of directional atherectomy for the treatment of bifurcation lesions. Cor Art Dis 1992;3:761-765.
728. Lewis B, Leya F, Johnson S, et al. Acute procedural results in the treatment of 30 coronary artery bifurcation lesions with a double-wire atherectomy technique for side-branch protection. Am Heart J 1994;127:1600-1607.
729. Lewis B, Leya F, Johnson S, et al. Outcome of angioplasty (PTCA) and atherectomy (DCA) for bifurcation and non-bifurcation lesions in CAVEAT. Circulation 1993;88:I-601.
730. Campos-Esteve M, Laird J, Kufs W, Wortham CD. Side-branch occlusion with directional coronary atherectomy: Incidence and risk factors. Am Heart J 1994;128:686-690.
731. Kaufmann UP, Garratt KN, Vlietstra RE, Menke KK. Coronary atherectomy: First 50 patients at the Mayo Clinic. Mayo Clin Proc 1989;64:747-752.
732. Safian R, Gelbfish J, Erny R, Schnitt S, Schmidt D, Baim D. Coronary atherectomy. Clinical, angiographic, and histological findings and observations regarding potential mechanisms. Circulation 1990;82:69-79.
733. Rowe MH, Hinohara T, White NW, Robertson GC. Comparison of dissection rates and angiographic results following directional coronary atherectomy and coronary angioplasty. Am J Cardiol 1990;66:49-53.
734. Garratt K, Holmes D, Bell M, et al. Results of directional atherectomy of primary atheromatous and restenosis lesions in coronary arteries and saphenous vein grafts. Am J Cardiol 1992;70:449-454.
735. Fishman R, Kuntz R, Carrozza J, et al. Long-term results of directional coronary atherectomy: Predictors of restenosis. J Am Coll Cardiol 1992;20:1101-1110.
736. Baim D, Tomoaki H, Holmes D, et al. Results of directional coronary atherectomy during multicenter preapproval testing. Am J Cardiol 1993;72:6E-11E.
737. Cowley M, DiSciascio G. Experience with directional coronary atherectomy since pre-market approval. Am J Cardiol 1993;72:12E-20E.
738. Popma J, Mintz G, Satler L, et al. Clinical and angiographic outcome after directional coronary atherectomy: A qualitative and quantitative analysis using coronary arteriography and intravascular ultrasound. Am J Cardiol 1993;72:55E-64E.
739. Umans V, de Feyter P, Deckers J, et al. Acute and long-term outcome of directional coronary atherectomy for stable and unstable angina. Am J Cardiol 1993;74:641-646.
740. Guarneri E, Sklar M, Russo R, Claire D, Schatz R, Teirstein P. Escape from Stent Jail: An in vitro model. Circulation 1995;92:I-688.
741. Nakamura S, Hall P, Maiello L, Colombo A. Techniques of Palmaz-Schatz stent deployment in lesions with a large side branch. Cathet Cardiovas Diagn 1995;34:353-361.
742. Colombo A, Gaglione A, Nakamura S. "Kissing" stents for bifurcational coronary lesion. Cathet Cardiovas Diagn. 1993;30:327-330.
743. Iniguez A, Macaya C, Alfonso F, Goicolea J. Early angiographic changes of side branches arising from a Palmaz-Schatz Stented coronary segment: Results and clinical implications. J Am Coll Cardiol 1994;23:911-915.
744. Mazur W, Grinstead C, Hakim A, et al. Fate of side branches after intracoronary implantation of the Gianturco-Roubin flex-stent for acute or threatened closure after percutaneous transluminal coronary angioplasty. Am J Cardiol 1994;74:1207-1210.
745. Guarneri E, Sklar M, Russo R, Claire D, Schatz R, Teirstein P. Escape from Stent Jail: An in vitro model. Circulation 1995;92:I-688.
746. Bittl JA, Sanborn TA, Tcheng JE, et al. Clinical success, complications and restenosis rates with excimer laser coronary angioplasty: The PELCA Registry. Am J Cardiol 1992;70:1533-1539.
747. Holmes DR JR, Holubkov R, Vlietstra RE, et al. Comparison of complications during percutaneous transluminal coronary angioplasty from 1977 to 1981 and from 1985 to 1986. The National Heart, Lung, and Blood Institute Percutaneous Transluminal Coronary Angioplasty Registry. J Am Coll Cardiol 1988;12:1149-1155.
748. Fischman DL, Savage MP, Leon MB, et al. Fate of lesion-related sidebranches after coronary artery stenting. J Am Coll Cardiol 1993;22:1641-6.
749. Pan M, Medina A, de Lezo JS, et al. Follow-up patency of sidebranches covered by intracoronary Palmaz-Schatz stent. Am Heart J 1995;129:436-440.
750. Whitlow PL, Cowley M, Bass T, et al. Risk of high speed rotational atherectomy in bifurcation lesions. J Am Coll Cardiol 1993;21:445A.
751. Warth DC, Leon MB, O'Neill WW, et al. Rotational atherectomy multicenter registry: Acute results, complications and 6-month angiographic follow-up in 709 patients. J Am Coll Cardiol 1994;24:641-8.
752. Tan Kim, Sulke N, Taub N, Sowton E. Clinical and lesion morphologic determinants of coronary angioplasty success and complications: Current experience. J Am Coll Cardiol 1995;25:855-865.
753. Colombo A, Maiello L, Itoh A, et al. Coronary stenting of bifurcation lesions: Immediate and follow-up results. J Am Coll Cardiol 1996; 27:277A.
754. Mehta S, Popma J, Margolis JR, et al. Complications with new angioplasty devices. Are these device specific? J Am Coll Cardiol 1996;27:168A.
755. Caputo RP, Chafizedeh ER, Stoler RC, et al. "Stent Jail" — A minimum security prison. J Invas Cardiol 1996;8.

Proximal Tortuosity & Angulated Stenosis

756. Tan K, Sulke N, Taub N, Sowton E. Clinical and lesion morphologic determinants of coronary angioplasty success and complications: Current experience. J Am Coll Cardiol 1995;25:855-65.

757. Ellis SG, Vandormael MG, Cowley MJ, et al. Coronary morphologic and clinical determinants of procedural outcome with angioplasty for multivessel coronary disease. Implications for patient selection. Circulation 1990;82:1193-1202.
758. Gossman DE, Tuzcu EM, Simpfendorfer C, et al. Percutaneous transluminal angioplasty for Shepherd's Crook right coronary artery stenosis. Cathet Cardiovasc Diagn 1989;15:189-191.
759. Flood RD, Popma JJ, Chuang YC, Salter LF, et al. Incidence, angiographic predictors, and clinical significance of coronary perforation occurring after new device angioplasty. J Am Coll Cardiol 1994;23:301A.
760. Holmes DR, Berdan L, et al. Abrupt closure: The coronary angioplasty versus excisional atherectomy trial (CAVEAT) experience. J Am Coll Cardiol 1994;23:I-585A.
761. Ellis SG, Popma JJ, Buchbinder M, Franco I, et al. Relation of clinical presentation, stenosis morphology, and operator technique to the procedural results of rotational atherectomy and rotational atherectomy-facilitated angioplasty. Circulation 1994;89:882-892.
762. Hinohara T, Rowe MH, Robertson, GC, Selmon MR, et al. Effect of lesion characteristics on outcome of directional coronary atherectomy. J Am Coll Cardiol 1991;17:1112-20.
763. Ellis SG, De Cesare NB, Pinkerton CA, Whitlow P, et al. Relation of stenosis morphology and clinical presentation to the procedural results of directional coronary atherectomy. Circulation 1991;84:644-653.
764. Torre SR, Lai SM, Schatz RA. Relation of clinical presentation and lesion morphology to the procedural results of Palmaz-Schatz stent placement: A new approaches to coronary intervention (NACI) registry report. J Am Coll Cardiol 1994;23:135A.
765. Myler RK, Shaw RE, Stertzer SH, Hecht HS, et al. Lesion morphology and coronary angioplasty: Current experience and analysis. J Am Coll Cardiol 1992;19:1641-52.
766. Savas V, Puchrowicz S, Williams L, et al. Angioplasty outcome using long balloons in high-risk lesions. J Am Coll Cardiol 1992;19:34A.
767. Hermans WRM, Foley DP, Rensing BJ, Rutsch W, et al. Usefulness of quantitative and qualitative angiographic lesion morphology, and clinical characteristics in predicting major adverse cardiac events during and after native coronary balloon angioplasty. Am J Cardiol 1993;72:14-20.
768. Tenaglia AN, Zidar JP, Jackman JD, Fortin DF, et al. Treatment of long coronary artery narrowings with long angioplasty balloon catheters. Am J Cardiol 1993;71:1274-1277.
769. Ellis SG and Topol EJ. Results of percutaneous transluminal coronary angioplasty of high-risk angulated stenoses. Am J Cardiol 1990;66:932-937.
770. Barasch E, Conger JL, Janota T, Peters JJ, et al. PTCA of lesions on a bend: Effects of balloon material, balloon length, and inflation sequence. Circulation 1994;90:I-435.
771. Gray WA, Ghazzal ZMB, White HJ. The effects of balloon length and angle severity on the straightening force developed by polyethylene terephthalate (PET) angioplasty balloons. Circulation 1994;90:I-587.
772. Chevalier B, Commeau P, Favereau X, Gueri Y, et al. Limitations of rotational atherectomy in angulated coronary lesions. J Am Coll Cardiol 1994;23:285A.
773. Ghazzal ZMB, Hearn JA, Litvack F, Goldenberg T, et al. Morphological predictors of acute complications after percutaneous excimer laser coronary angioplasty. Results of a comprehensive angiographic analysis: Importance of the eccentricity index. Circulation 1992;86:820-827.
774. Bittl JA, Sanborn TA, Tcheng JE, Siegel RM, et al. Clinical success, complications, and restenosis rates with excimer laser coronary angioplasty. Am J Cardiol 1992;70:1533-1539.
775. Hong MK, Popma JJ, Wong SC, Kent KM, et al. Incidence of and factors associated with abrupt closure in patients undergoing elective, new device angioplasty in native coronary arteries. J Am Coll Cardiol 1995;25:122A.
776. Freed M, May M, Lichtenberg A, Strzelecki M, et al. Predictors of angiographic and clinical complications after new device coronary interventions. Circulation 1994;90:I-549.
777. Van Belle E, Bauters C, Lablanche JM, et al. Angiographic determinants of acute closure after coronary angioplasty: A prospective quantitative coronary angiographic study of 3679 procedures. J Am Coll Cardiol 1994;23:222A.
778. Meckel CR, Ahmed W, Ferguson JJ, Strony J, et al. Angiographic predictors of severe dissection during balloon angioplasty: A report from the Hirulog Angioplasty Study. Circulation 1994;90:I-64.

Calcified Stenosis

779. Mintz G, Popma J, et al. Patterns of calcification in coronary artery disease. A statistical analysis of intravascular ultrasound and coronary angiography in 1155 lesions. Circulation 1995;91:1959-1965.
780. Mintz GS, Pichard AD, Kovach JA, et al. Impact of preintervention intravascular ultrasound imaging on transcatheter treatment strategies in coronary artery disease. Am J Cardiol 1994;73:423-430.
781. Tan, K., N. Sulke, et al. Clinical and lesion morphologic determinants of coronary angioplasty success and complications: Current experience. J Am Coll Cardiol 195;25:855-65.
782. Braden GA, Herrington DM, Kerensky RA, Kutcher MA, Little WC. Angiography poorly predicts actual lesion eccentricity in severe coronary stenoses: Confirmation by intracoronary ultrasound imaging. J Am Coll Cardiol 1994;March Special Issue:413A.
783. Myler RK, Shaw RE, Stertzer SH, et al. Lesion Morphology and Coronary Angioplasty: Current Experience and Analysis. J Am Coll Cardiol 1992;19:1641-52.
784. Van Belle, E, Bauters C, Lablanche JM, McFadden EP, Quandalle P, Bertrand ME. Angiographic determinants of acute outcome after coronary angioplasty: A prospective quantitaitve coronary angiographic study of 3679 procedures. J Am Coll Cardiol 1994;March Special Issue:222A.
785. Danchin N, Buffet P, Dibon O, et al. Should specific angioplasty techniques be used to treat calcified coronary artery lesions? A retrospective study. Circulation 1994;90:I-436.
786. Hermans WR, Foley D, et al. Usefulness of quantitative and qualitative angiographic lesion morphology, and clinical characteristics

in predicting major adverse cardiac events during and after native coronary balloon angioplasty. Am J Cardiol 1993;72:14-20.
787. Ellis SG, Vandormael MG, Cowley MJ, et al. Coronary morphologic and clinical determinants of procedural outcome with angioplasty for multivessel coronary disease. Implications for patient selection. Circulation 1990;82:1193-1202.
788. Fitzgerald P, Ports T, Yock P. Contribution of localized calcium deposits to dissection after angioplasty: An observational study using IVUS. Circulation 1992;86:64-70.
789. Khurana S, Bakalyar D, Schreiber T, et al. Facilitated lumen enlargement by longitudinal force focused angioplasty. J Am Coll Cardiol 1995;March Special Issue:345A.
790. Solar RJ, Meaney DF, Miller RT, et al. Enhanced lumen enlargement with new focused force angioplasty device. Circulation 1995;92:I-147.
791. Mintz GS, Dusaillant GR, Wong SC, Pichard AD, et al. Rotational atherectomy followed by adjunct stents: The preferred therapy for calcified lesions in large vessels? Circulation 1995;92:I-329.
792. Warth D, Leon M, et al. Rotational atherectomy multicenter registry: Acute results, complications and 6-month angiographic follow-up in 709 patients. J Am Coll Cardiol 1994;24:641-648.
793. Ellis S, Popma J, et al. Relation of clinical presentation, stenosis morphology, and operator technique to the procedural results of rotational atherectomy-facilitated angioplasty. Circulation 1994;89:882-892.
794. MacIssac AI, Whitlow PL, Cowley MJ, Buchbinder M. Angiographic predictors of outcome of coronary rotational atherectomy from the completed multicenter registry. J Am Coll Cardiol 1994;March Special Issue:353A.
795. Altmann DB, Popma JJ, Kent KM, et al. Rotational atherectomy effectively treats calcified lesions. J Am Coll Cardiol 1993;21 (Part II):443A.
796. Reisman M, Devlin PG, Melikian J, Fenner J, Buchbinder M. Undilatable noncompliant lesions treated with the rotatblator: Outcome and angiographic follow-up. Circulation 1993;Speical Issue:2949.
797. Popma JJ, Mintz GS, Satler LF, et al. Clinical and angiographic outcome after directional coronary atherectomy. A qualitative and quantitative analysis using coronary arteriography and intravascular ultrasound. Am J Cardiol 1993;72:55E-64E.
798. Hinohara T, Rowe MH, Robertson GC, et al. Effect of lesion characteristics on outcome of directional coronary atherectomy. Circulation 1991;17:1112-1120.
799. Ellis SG, De Cesare NB, Pinkerton CA, et al. Relation of stenosis morphology and clinical presentation to the procedural results of directional coronary atherectomy. Circulation 1991;84:644-653.
800. IVT® Coronary TEC® Atherectomy Clinical Database Investigators Meeting. 1992.
801. Bittl JA, Sanborn TA, Tcheng JE, Watson LE. Excimer laser-facilitated angioplasty for undilatable coronary lesions: Results of a prospective, controlled study. Circulation 1993;88:I-24.
802. Bittl J, Sanborn T, et al. Clinical success, complications and restenosis rates with excimer laser coronary angioplasty. Am J Cardiol 1992;70:1533-1539.
803. Levine S, Mehta S, Krauthamer D, et al. Excimer laser coronary angioplasty of calcified lesions. J Am Coll Cardiol 1991;17(2):206A.
804. deMarchena EJ, Mallon SM, et al. Effectiveness of holmium laser-assisted coronary angioplasty. Am J Cardiol 1994;73:117-121.
805. Leon MB, Kent KM, Pichard AD, et al. Percutaneous transluminal coronary rotational angioplasty of calcified lesions. Circulation 1991;84(4):II-521.
806. Leguizamon JH, Chambre DF, Torresani EM, et al. High-speed coronary rotational atherectomy. Are angiographic factors predictive of failure, major complications or restenosis? A multivariate analysis. J Am Coll Cardiol 1995:Special Issue:95A.
807. Mintz G, Potkin B, et al. Intravascular ultrasound evaluation of the effect of rotational atherectomy in obstructive atherosclerotic coronary artery disease. Circulation 1992;86:1383-1393.
808. Kovach J, Mintz G, et al. Sequential intravascular ultrasound characterization of the mechanisms of rotational atherectomy and adjunct balloon angioplasty. J Am Coll Cardiol 1993;22 (4):1024-32.
809. Fitzgerald PJ, Stertzer SH, Hidalgo BO, Myler RK, et al. Plaque characteristics affect lesion and vessel response to coronary rotational atherectomy: An intravascular ultrasound Study. J Am Coll Cardiol 1994;March Special Issue:353A.
810. De Franco AC, Tuzcu EM, Moliterno DJ, et al. "Directional" coronary atherectomy removes atheroma more effectively from concentric than eccentric lesions: Intravascular ultrasound predictors of lesional success. J Am Coll Cardiol 1995;February Special Issue:137A.
811. Matar FA, Mintz GS, Kent KM, et al. Predictors of intravascular ultrasound endpoints after directional coronary atherectomy in 170 patients. J Am Coll Cardiol 1994;February Special Issue:302A.
812. DeLezo JS, Romero M, Medina A, et al. Intraocoronary ultrasound assessment of directional coronary atherectomy: Immediate and follow-up findings. J Am Coll Cardiol 1993;21:298-307.
813. Hong MK, Chuang YC, Prunka N, Satler LF. Predictors of early and late cardiac events in patients undergoing saphenous vein graft angioplasty with PTCA and new device modalities. Circulation 1993;88:I-601.
814. Henson KD, Flood R, Javier SP, et al. Transcatheter device synergy: Use of adjunct directional atherectomy after rotational atherectomy or excimer laser angioplasty. J Am Coll Cardiol 1994;February Special Issue:220A.
815. Ghazzal Z, Hearn J, et al. Morphological predictors of acute complications after percutaneous excimer laser coronary angioplasty. Results of a comprehensive angiographic analysis: Importance of the eccentricity index. Circulation 1992;86:820-827.
816. Baumbach A, Bittl J, Fleck E, et al. Acute complications of excimer laser coronary angioplasty: A detailed analysis of multicenter results. J Am Coll Cardiol 1994;23:1305-1313.
817. Mintz GS, Kovach JA, Javier SP, et al. Mechanisms of lumen enlargement after excimer laser angioplasty: An intravascular ultrasound study. Circulation 1995;92:3408-14.
818. Tamura T, Kimura T, Nosaka H, Nobuyoshi M. Predictors of restenosis after Palmaz-Schatz stent implantation. Circulation 1994;90:I-324.
819. Goldberg SL, Hall P, Almagor Y, Maiello L, et al. Intravascular ultrasound guided rotational atherectomy of fibro-calcific plaque

prior to intracoronary deployment of Palmaz-Schatz stents. J Am Coll Cardiol 1994;February Special Issue:290A.

820. Dussaillant GR, Mintz GS, Pichard AD, et al. The optimal strategy for treating calcified lesions in large vessels: Comparison of intravascular of intravascular ultrasound results of rotational atherectomy + adjunctive PTCA, DCA, or stents. J Am Coll Cardiol 1996;27:153A.

821. Dusaillant GR, Mintz GS, Pichard AD, et al. Mechanisms and immediate and long-term results of adjunct directional coronary atherectomy after rotational atherectomy. J Am Coll Cardiol 1996;27:1390-7.

Eccentric Lesions

822. Braden GA, Herrington DM, Kerensky RA, et al. Angiography poorly predicts actual lesion eccentricity in severe coronary stenoses: Confirmation by intracoronary ultrasound imaging. J Am Coll Cardiol 1994;Special Issue:413A.

823. Mintz GS, Popma JJ, Pichard AD, Kent KM, et al. Comparison of intravascular ultrasound and coronary angiography in the assessment of target lesion plaque distribution in coronary artery disease. TCT Meeting (Washington DC), February, 1995; Abstract.

824. Tan K, Sulke N, et al. Clinical and lesion morphologic determinants of coronary angioplasty success and complications: Current experience. J Am Coll Cardiol 1995;25:855-65.

825. Myler RK, Shaw RE, Stertzer SH, et al. Lesion morphology and coronary angioplasty: current experience and analysis. J Am Coll Cardiol 1992;19:1641-52.

826. Ellis SG, Vandormael MG, Cowley MJ, et al. Coronary morphologic and clinical determinants of procedural outcome with angioplasty for multivessel coronary disease. Implications for patient selection. Circulation 1990;82:1193-1202.

827. Kimball BP, Eric SB, Cohen EA, et al. Comparison of acute elastic recoil after directional coronary atherectomy versus standard balloon angioplasty. Am Heart J 1992;124:1459.

828. Baptista J, diMario C, Ozaki Y, de Feyter P, deJaegere P , Roelandt J, Serruys PW. Deterinants of lumen and plaque changes after balloon angioplasty: A quantitative ultrasound study. J Am Coll Cardiol 1994;March Special Issue:414A.

829. Fiscell TA, Bausback KN. Effects of luminal eccentricity on spontaneous coronary vasoconstriction after successful percutaneous transluminal coronary angioplasty. Am J Cardiol 1991;68:530.

830. Matar FA, Mintz GS, Kent KM, Pinnow E, et al. Predictors of intravascular ultrasound endpoints after directional coronary atherectomy in 170 patients. J Am Coll Cardiol 1994;March Special Issue:302A.

831. Ellis S, Popma J, et al. Relation of clinical presentation, stenosis morphology, and operator technique to the procedural results of rotational atherectomy-facilitated angioplasty. Circulation 1994;89:882-892.

832. Schiele TM, Marx R, Vogt M, Leschke M, et al. Eccentricity of coronary arteries is a predictor of chronic restenosis after directional coronary atherectomy. Circulation 1995;92:I-328.

833. Popma JJ, Mintz GS, Satler LF, et al. Clinical and angiographic outcome after directional coronary atherectomy. A qualitative and quantitative analysis using coronary arteriography and intravascular ultrasound. Am J Cardiol 1993;72:55E-64E.

834. Hinohara T, Vetter JW, Selmon MR, et al. Directional coronary atherectomy is effective treatment for extremely eccentric lesions. Circulation 1991;84:II-520.

835. Warth D, Leon M, et al. Rotational atherectomy multicenter registry: Acute results, complications and 6-month angiographic follow-up in 709 patients. J Am Coll Cardiol 1994;24:641-648.

836. IVT® Coronary TEC® Atherectomy Clinical Database Investigators Meeting. 1992.

837. Advanced Interventional Systems Coronary Excimer Laser Database. Goldenberg T. 1992.

838. Leon MB, Henson KD, Lavier SP, et al. Early results with directional laser angioplasty is unfavorable coronary lesions. Circulation 1993;88;I-23.

839. Ghazzal ZMB, Litvack F, Rothbaum DA, Shefer A, King SB. The directional laser catheter: Quantitative angiographic core lab analysis from the first five centers. Circulation 1993; 88:I-23.

840. Fitzgerald PJ. Lesion composition impacts size and symmetry of stent expansion: Initial report from the STRUT Registry. J Am Coll Cardiol 1995;February Special Issue;49A.

841. MacIssac AI, Whitlow PL, Cowley MJ, Buchbinder M. Angiographic predictors of outcome of coronary rotational atherectomy from the completed multicenter registry. J Am Coll Cardiol 1994;February Special Issue:353A.

842. Leguizamon JH, Chambre DF, Torresani EM, et al. High-speed coronary rotational atherectomy. Are angiographic factors predictive of failure, major complications or restenosis? A multivariate analysis. J Am Coll Cardiol 1995:February Special Issue:95A.

843. Hong MK, Chuang YC, Prunka N, Satler LF. Predictors of early and late cardiac events in patients undergoing saphenous vein graft angioplasty with PTCA and new device modalities. Circulation 1993;88:I-601.

844. Fitzgerald PJ, Stertzer SH, Hidalgo BO, Myler RK, Shaw RE, Yock PG. Plaque characteristics affect lesion and vessel response to coronary rotational atherectomy: An intravascular ultrasound study. J Am Coll Cardiol 1994;February Special Issue:353A.

845. Baumbach A, Bittl J, Fleck E, et al. Acute complications of excimer laser coronary angioplasty: A detailed analysis of multicenter results. J Am Coll Cardiol 1994;23:1305-1313.

846. Bittl J, Sanborn T, et al. Clinical success, complications and restenosis rates with excimer laser coronary angioplasty. Am J Cardiol 1992;70:1533-1539.

847. Ghazzal Z, Hearn J, et al. Morphological predictors of acute complications after percutaneous excimer laser coronary angioplasty. Results of a comprehensive angiographic analysis: Importance of the eccentricity index. Circulation 1992;86:820-827.

848. Rechavia E, Federman J, Shefer A, et al. Usefulness of a prototype directional excimer laser coronary angioplasty catheter in narrowings unfavorable for conventional excimer of balloon angioplasty. Am J Cardiol 1995;76:1144-46.

Ostial Lesions

849. Tan K, Sulke N, Taub N, Sowton E. Clinical and lesion morphologic determinants of coronary angioplasty success and complications: Current experience. J Am Coll Cardiol 1995;25: 855-65.
850. Tan K, Sulke N, Taub N, Karani S, Sowton E. Percutaneous transluminal coronary angioplasty of aorta ostial, non-aorta ostial, and branch ostial stenoses. J Am Coll Cardiol 1994;February Special Issue:351A.
851. Boehrer JD, Ellis SG, Pieper K, Holmes DR, Keeler GP, et al. Directional atherectomy versus balloon angioplasty for coronary ostial and nonostial left anterior descending coronary artery lesions: Results from a randomized multicenter trial. J Am Coll Cardiol 1995;25:1380-6.
852. Sawada Y, Kimura T, Shinoda E, Sato Y, Nosaka H, Nobuyoshi M. Poor outcome of balloon angioplasty (BA) for ostial left anterior descending and circumflex: Impact of new angioplasty devices. Circulation 1994;90:I-436.
853. Brown R, Kochar G, et al. Effects of coronary angioplasty using progressive dilation on ostial stenosis of left anterior descending artery. Am J Cardiol 1993;71:245-247.
854. Myler R, Shaw R, et al. Lesion morphology and coronary angioplasty: Current experience and analysis. J Am Coll Cardiol 1992;19:1641-1652.
855. Bedotto JB, McConahay DR, Rutherford BD. Balloon angioplasty of aorta coronary ostial stenoses revisited. Circulation 1991;84:II-251.
856. Mathias DW, Fishman-Mooney J, Lange HW, et al. Frequency of success and complications of coronary angioplasty of a stenosis at the ostium of a branch vessel. Am J Cardiol 1991;67:491-495.
857. Topol EJ, Ellis SG, Fishman J, et al. Multicenter study of percutaneous transluminal angioplasty for right coronary artery ostial stenosis. J Am Coll Cardiol 1987;9:1214-1218.
858. Waksman R, Ghazzal ZMB, Kennard ED, et al. Acute outcome and follow-up of ostial versus proximal lesions treated with new devices: Report of the NACI Registry. Circulation 1995;92:I-73.
859. Ellis S, Popma J, et al. Relation of clinical presentation, stenosis morphology, and operator technique to the procedural results of rotational atherectomy-facilitated angioplasty. Circulation 1994;89:882-892.
860. Cowley CA, Patterson PE, Kipperman RM, Chuang YC, Pacera JH, Popma JJ. Multicenter rotational coronary atherectomy registry experience in coronary artery ostial stenoses. TCT Course (Washington DC), February, 1995.
861. Commeau P, Zimarino M, Lancelin B, et al. Rotational coronary atherectomy for the treatment of aorto-ostial and branch-ostial lesions. Circulation 1994;90:I-213.
862. Koller P, Freed M, et al. Success, complications, and restenosis following rotational and transluminal extraction atherectomy of ostial stenoses. Cathet Cardiovasc Diagn. 1994;31:255-260.
863. Stephen WJ, Bates ER, Garratt KN, Hinohara T, Muller DWM. Directional atherectomy in coronary and saphenous vein graft ostial stenoses. Am J Cardiol 1995;75:1015-1018.
864. Popma J, Mintz G, et al. Clinical and angiographic outcome after directional coronary atherectomy: A qualitative and quantitative analysis using coronary arteriography and intravascular ultrasound. Am J Cardiol 1993;72:55E-64E.
865. Robertson GC, Simpson JB, Vetter JW. Directional coronary atherectomy for ostial lesions. Circulation 1991;84:II-251.
866. Litvack F, Eigler N, Margolis J, et al. Percutaneous excimer laser coronary angioplasty: results in the first consecutive 3,000 patients. J Am Coll Cardiol 1994;23:323-9.
867. deMarchena EJ, Mallon SM, et al. Effectiveness of holmium laser-assisted coronary angioplasty. Am J Cardiol 1994;73:117-121.
868. Sabri M, Cowley, et al. Immediate results of interventional devices for coronary ostial narrowing with angina pectoris. Amer J Cardiol 1994;73:122-125.
869. Brogan WC, Popma JJ, Pichard AD, et al. A lesion-specific approach to new device therapy in ostial lesions. J Am Coll Cardiol 1993;21:233A.
870. Rocha-Singh K, Morris N, et al. Coronary stenting for treatment of ostial stenoses of native coronary arteries or aortocoronary saphenous venous grafts. Am J Cardiol 1995;75: 26-29.
871. Zampieri PA, Colombo A, et al. Results of coronary stenting of ostial lesions. Am J Cardiol 1994;73:901-903.
872. Teirstein P, Stratienko AA, Schatz RA. Coronary stenting for ostial stenosis: Initial results and six month follow-up. Circulation 1991;84:II-250.
873. Wong SC, Pompa JJ, Chuang YC, et al. Angiographic and clinical outcomes in saphenous vein graft (SVG) versus native coronary aorto-ostial lesions. J Am Coll Cardiol 1994;March Special Issue:302A.
874. Colombo A, Itoh A, Maiello L, et al. Coronary stent implantation in aorto-ostial lesions: Immediate and follow-up results. J Am Coll Cardiol 1996;27:253A.
875. De Cesare NB, Galli S, Loaldi A, et al. Palmaz-Schatz stent for the treatment of left anterior descending ostial stenosis: Acute and long-term results. J Invas. Cardiol 1996;8.

Long Lesions

876. Tan K, Sulke N, Taub N, Sowton E. Clinical and lesion morphologic determinants of coronary angioplasty success and complications: Current experience. J Am Coll Cardiol 1995;25: 855-65.
877. Kaul U, Upasani PT, Agarwal R, Bahl VK, Wasir HS. In-hospital outcome of percutaneous transluminal coronary angioplasty for long lesions and diffuse coronary artery disease. Cathet Cardiol Diagn 1995;35:294-300.
878. Cates WU, Knopf WD, Lembo NJ, Bernstein C, et al. The 80 mm balloon: The first 95 vessel cumulative experience. J Am Coll Cardiol 1994;23:58A.
879. Mooney, M., J. Mooney-Fishman, et al. Directional atherectomy for long lesions: Improved results. Cathet Cardiovasc Diagn.

1993;1:26-30.
880. Myler R, Shaw R, et al. Lesion morphology and coronary angioplasty: Current experience and analysis. J Am Coll Cardiol 1992;19:1641-1652.
881. Zidar JP, Tenaglia AN, Jackman JD, et al. Improved acute results for PTCA of long coronary lesions using long angioplasty balloon catheters. J Am Coll Cardiol 1992;19:34A.
882. Savas V, Puchrowicz S, Williams L, et al. Angioplasty outcome using long balloons in high-risk lesions. J Am Coll Cardiol 1992;19:34A.
883. Goudreau E, DiSciascio G, Kelly K, et al. Coronary angioplasty of diffuse coronary artery disease. Am Heart J 1991;121:12-19.
884. Appleman YEA, Piek JJ, Strikwerda S, et al. Randomized trial of excimer laser angioplasty vs. balloon angioplasty for treatment of obstructive coronary artery disease. Lancet 1996;347:79-84.
885. Raymenants E, Bhandari S, Stammen F, De Scheerder ID, Desmet W, Piessens J. Effects of angioplasty balloon material and lesion characteristics on the incidence of coronary dissection in 2150 dilated lesions. J Am Coll Cardiol 1993;21:291A.
886. Raymenants E, Bhandari S, Stammen F, De Scheerder I, et al. Effects of angioplasty balloon material and lesion characteristics on the incidence of coronary dissection in 2150 dilated lesions. J Am Coll Cardiol 1993;21:291A.
887. Ellis SG, Roubin GS, King SB III, et al. Angiographic and clinical predictors of acute closure after native vessel coronary angioplasty. Circulation 1988;77:372-379.
888. Detre KM, Holmes DR Jr, Holubkov R, et al. Incidence and consequences of periprocedural occlusion. The 1985-1986 National Heart, Lung and Blood Institute Percutaneous Transluminal Coronary Angioplasty Registry. Circulation 1990;82:739-750.
889. Tenaglia AN, Fortin DF, Califf RM, et al. Predicting the risk of abrupt vessel closure after angioplasty in an individual patient. J Am Coll Cardiol 1994;23:1004-1011.
890. de Feyter PJ, van den Brand M, Jaarman G, et al. Acute coronary artery occlusion during and after percutaneous transluminal coronary angioplasty. Frequency, prediction, clinical course, management, and follow-up. Circulation 1991;83:927-936.
891. Hermans WR, Foley D, et al. Usefulness of quantitative and qualitative angiographic lesion morphology, and clinical characteristics in predicting major adverse cardiac events during and after native coronary balloon angioplasty. Am J Cardiol 1993;72:14-20.
892. Ellis SG, Vandormael MG, Cowley MJ, et al, and the Multivessel Angioplasty Prognosis Study Group. Coronary morphologic and clinical determinants of procedural outcome with angioplasty for multivessel coronary disease. Circulation 1990;82:1193-202.
893. Savage MP, Goldberg S, Hirshfeld JW, et al, for the M-Heart Investigators. Clinical and angiographic determinants of primary coronary angioplasty success. J Am Coll Cardiol 1991;17:22-8.
894. Hirshfeld JW Jr, Schwartz JS, Jugo R, et al. Restenosis after coronary angioplasty: A multivariate statistical model to relate lesion and procedure variables to restenosis. J Am Coll Cardiol 1991;18:647-656.
895. Ellis SG, Roubin GS, King SB III, et al. Importance of stenosis morphology in the estimation of restenosis risk after elective percutaneous transluminal coronary angioplasty. Am J Cardiol 1989;63:30-34.
896. Leimgruber PP, Roubin GS, Hollman J, et al. Restenosis after successful coronary angioplasty in patients with single-vessel disease. Circulation 1986;73:710-717.
897. Foley DP, Meilkert R, Umans VA, et al. Is the relationship between luminal increase and subsequent renarrowing linear or non-linear in patients undergoing coronary interventions? J Am Coll Cardiol 1994;Special Issue:302A.
898. Brymer JF, Khaja F, and Kraft L. Angioplasty of long or tandem coronary artery lesions using a new longer balloon dilatation catheter: A comparative study. Cathet and Cardiovasc Diagn 1991;23:84-88.
899. Banka V, et al. Effectiveness of decremental diameter balloon catheters (Tapered balloon). Am J Cardiol 1992;69:188.
900. Warth D, Leon MB, O'Neill W, Zacca N, Polissar NL, Buchbinder M. Rotational atherectomy multicenter registry: Acute results, complications and 6-month angiographic follow-up in 709 patients. J Am Coll Cardiol 1994;24: 641-648.
901. Ellis, S., J. Popma, et al. Relation of clinical presentation, stenosis morphology, and operator technique to the procedural results of rotational atherectomy-facilitated angioplasty. Circulation 1994;89:882-892.
902. Reisman M, Cohen B, Warth D, Fenner J, Gocka IT, Buchbinder M. Outcome of long lesions treated with high speed rotational ablation. J Am Coll Cardiol 1993;21:443A.
903. Teirstein PS, Warth DC, Haq N, et al. High speed rotational coronary atherectomy for patients with diffuse coronary artery disease. J Am Coll Cardiol 1991;18:1694-1701.
904. Robertson GC, Selmon MR, Hinohara T, et al. The effect of lesion length on outcome of directional coronary atherectomy. Circulation 1990;82:III-623.
905. IVT™ Coronary TEC™ Clinical Database. Investigators Meeting 1992.
906. Appelman YE, Piek J, Redekop WK, de Feyter PJ, et al. Excimer laser angioplasty versus balloon angioplasty in longer coronary lesions: A multivariate analysis. Circulation 1995;92:I-74.
907. Foley DP, Appleman YE, Piek JJ. Comparison of angiographic restenosis propensity of excimer laser coronary angioplasty and balloon angioplasty in the AMsterdam Rotterdam (AMRO) trial. Circulation 1995;92:I-477.
908. Litvack F, Eigler N, Margolis J, et al. Percutaneous excimer laser coronary angioplasty: Results in the first consecutive 3,000 patients. J Am Coll Cardiol 1994;23:323-9.
909. deMarchena EJ, Mallon SM, et al. Effectiveness of holmium laser-assisted coronary angioplasty. Am J Cardiol 1994;73:117-121.
910. Maiello L, Hall P, Nakamura S, et al. Results of stent implantation of diffuse coronary disease assisted by intravascular ultrasound. J Am Coll Cardiol 1995;February Special Issue:156A.
911. Akira I, Hall P, Maiello L, Blengino S, et al. Coronary stenting of long lesions greater than 20 mm) — a matched comparison of different stents. Circulation 1995;92:I-688.
912. Sutton JM, Ellis SG, Roubin GS, et al. Major clinical events after coronary stenting. The multicenter registry of acute and elective Gianturco-Roubin stent placement. Circulation 1994;89:1126-1137.
913. Hong MK, Popma JJ, Wong SC, Kent KM, et al. Incidence of and factors associated with abrupt closure in patients undergoing elective, new device angioplasty in native coronary arteries. J Am Coll Cardiol 1995;Feb Special Issue:122A.

914. Flood RD, Popma JJ, Chuang YC, et al. Incidence angiographic predictors, and clinical significance of coronary perforation occurring after new device angioplasty. J Am Coll Cardiol 1994;February Special Issue:301A.
915. Cohen BM, Weber VJ, Bass TA, et al. Coronary perforation during rotational ablation: Angiographic determinants and clinical outcome. J Am Coll Cardiol 1994;February Special Issue:354A.
916. Leguizamón JH, Chambre DF, Torresani EM, et al. High-speed coronary rotational atherectomy. Are angiographic factors predictive of failure, major complications or restenosis? A multivariate analysis. J Am Coll Cardiol 1995;February Special Issue:95A.
917. Popma J, Topol E, et al. Abrupt vessel closure after directional coronary atherectomy. J Am Coll Cardiol 1992;19:1372-1379.
918. Lincoff AM, Ellis SG, Leya F, Masden RR, et al. Are clinical and angiographic correlates of success the same during directional coronary atherectomy and balloon angioplasty? The CAVEAT Experience. Circulation 1993;88:I-601.
919. Baumbach A, Bittl J, Fleck E, et al. Acute complications of excimer laser coronary angioplasty: A detailed analysis of multicenter results. J Am Coll Cardiol 1994;23:1305-1313.
920. Ghazzal, Z., J. Hearn, et al. Morphological predictors of acute complications after percutaneous excimer laser coronary angioplasty. Results of a comprehensive angiographic analysis: Importance of the eccentricity index. Circulation 1992;86:820-827.
921. Appleman YE, Birnie E, Piek JJ, de Feyter PJ, et al. Excimer laser angioplasty versus balloon angioplasty in longer coronary lesions: A cost-effectiveness analysis. Circulation 1995;92:I-512.
922. Shaknovich A, Moses JW, Undemir C, Cohen NT, et al. Procedural and short-term clinical outcomes in multiple Palmaz-Schatz stents (PSSs) in very long lesions/dissections. Circulation 1995;92:I-535.
923. Hall P, Nakamura S, Maiello L, Blengino S, et al. Factors associated with late angiographic outcome after intravascular ultrasound guided Palmaz-Schatz coronary stent implantation: A multivariate analysis. J Am Coll Cardiol 1995;February Special Issue:36A.
924. Tamura T, Kimura T, Nosaka H, Nobuyoshi M. Predictors of restenosis after Palmaz-Schatz stent implantation. Circulation 1994;90:I-324.
925. Laird JR, Popma JJ, Knopf WD, et al. Angiographic and procedural outcome after coronary angioplasty in high-risk subsets using a decremental diameter (tapered) balloon catheter. Am J Cardiol 1996;77561-8.

Chronic Total Occlusion

926. Flameng W, Schwarz F, and Hehrlein FW. Intraoperative evaluation of the functional significance of coronary collateral vessels in patients with coronary artery disease. Am J Cardiol 1978;42:187-192.
927. Favereau X, Corcos T, Guerin Y, et al. Early reocclusion after successful coronary angioplasty of chronic total occlusions. J Am Coll Cardiol 1995;25:139A.
928. Tan K, Sulke N, Taub N, Sowton E. Clinical and lesion morphologic determinants of coronary angioplasty success and complications: Current experience. J Am Coll Cardiol 1995;25:855-65.
929. Ruocco NA Jr, Ring ME, Holubkov R, et al. Results of coronary angioplasty of chronic total occlusions (the National Heart, Lung, and Blood Institute 1985-1986 Percutaneous Transluminal Angioplasty Registry). Am J Cardiol 1992;69:69-76.
930. Myler R, Shaw R, Stertzer S, et al. Lesion morphology and coronary angioplasty: Current experience and analysis. J Am Coll Cardiol 1992;19:1641-1652.
931. Plante S. Laarman GJ, de Feyter PJ, et al. Acute complications of percutaneous transluminal coronary angioplasty for total occlusion. Am Heart J 1991;121:417.
932. Stone GW, Rutherford BD, McConahay DR, et al. Procedural outcome of angioplasty for total coronary artery occlusion: An analysis of 971 lesions in 905 patients. J Am Coll Cardiol 1990;15:849-856.
933. Safian RD, McCabe CH, Sipperly ME, et al. Initial success and long-term follow-up of percutaneous transluminal coronary angioplasty in chronic total occlusions versus conventional stenoses. Am J Cardiol 1988;61:23G-28G.
934. Kinoshitax I, Katoh O, Nariyama J, Otsuji S, et al. Coronary angioplasty of chronic total occlusions with bridging collateral vessels: Immediate and follow-up outcome from a large single-center experience. J Am Coll Cardiol 1995;26:409-15.
935. Ishizaka N, Issiki T, Saeki F, et al. Angiographic follow-up after successful percutaneous coronary angioplasty for chronic total coronary occlusion: Experience in 110 consecutive patients. Am Heart J 1994;127:8.
936. Tan KH, Sulke AN, Taub NA, Watts E, Sowton E. Coronary angioplasty of chronic total occlusions: Determinants of procedural success. J Am Coll Cardiol 1993;21:76A.
937. Shimizu M, Kato O, Otsuji S, et al. Progress in initial outcome of PTCA for complete occlusion. Circulation 1993;88:I-504.
938. Stewart J, Denne L, Bowker T, et al. Percutaneous transluminal coronary angioplasty in chronic coronary artery occlusion. J Am Coll Cardiol 1993;21:1371-1376.
939. Maiello L, Colombo A, Gianrossi R, et al. Coronary angioplasty of chronic occlusions: Factors predictive of procedural success. Am Heart J 1992;124:581-584.
940. Ivanhoe RJ, Weintraub WS, Douglas JS Jr, et al. Percutaneous transluminal coronary angioplasty of chronic total occlusions. Primary success, restenosis, and long-term clinical follow-up. Circulation 1992;85:106-115.
941. Bell MR, Berger PB, Reeder GS, et al. Successful PTCA of chronic total coronary occlusions reduces the need for coronary artery bypass surgery. Circulation 1991;84:II-250.
942. Shimizu M, Kato O, Otsuji S, et al. Progress in initial outcome of PTCA for complete occlusion. J Am Coll Cardiol 1993;88:I-504.
943. Bell MR, Berger PB, Reeder GS, et al. Initial and long-term outcome of 354 patients after coronary balloon angioplasty of total coronary artery occlusions. Circulation 1992;85:1003.
944. Melchior JP, Meier B, Urban P, et al. Percutaneous transluminal coronary angioplasty for chronic total coronary arterial occlusion. Am J Cardiol 1987;59:535-538.
945. Tenaglia A, Fortin D, Califf R. Predicting the risk of abrupt closure after angioplasty in an individual patient. J Am Coll Cardiol 1994;24:1004-1011.

946. Ruocco NA, Ring ME, Holubkov R, Jacobs AK. Results of coronary angioplasty of chronic total occlusions (the National Heart, Lung, and Blood Institute 1985-1986 Percutaneous Transluminal Angioplasty Registry). Am J Cardiol 1992;69:69-76.
947. Stone GW, Rutherford BD, McConahay DR, et al. Procedural outcome of angioplasty for total coronary artery occlusion: An analysis of 971 lesions in 905 patients. J Am Coll Cardiol 1990;15:849-856.
948. Burger W, Kadel C, Keul H, Vallbracht C, Kaltenbach M. A word of caution: Reopening chronic coronary occlusions. Cathet Cardiovasc Diagn 1992;27:35-39.
949. Bell MR, Berger PB, Bresnahan JF, Reeder GS. Initial and long-term outcome of 354 patients after coronary balloon angioplasty of total coronary artery occlusions. Circulation 1992;85:1003-1011.
950. Haerer W, Schmidt A, Eggeling T, et al. Angioplasty of chronic total coronary occlusions. Results of a controlled randomized trial. J Am Coll Cardiol 1991;17:113A.
951. Meier B. Total coronary occlusion: A different animal? J Am Coll Cardiol 1991;17:50B.
952. Anderson TJ, Knudtson ML, Roth DL, et al. Improvement in left ventricular function following PTCA of chronic totally occluded arteries. Circulation 1991;84:II-519.
953. Serruys PW, Umans V, Heyndrickx GR, et al. Elective PTCA of totally occluded coronary arteries not associated with acute myocardial infarction; short-term and long-term results. Eur Heart J 1985;6:2-12.
954. Danchin N, Angiol M, Beurrie D, et al. Late recanalization of chronic total coronary occlusion: Maintained vessel patency improves global and regional left ventricular function and avoids remodeling. J Am Coll Cardiol 195;25:345A.
955. Berger PB, Holmes DR, Ohman M, et al. Restenosis, reocclusion and adverse cardiovascular events after successful balloon angioplasty of occluded versus nonoccluded coronary arteries. Results from the Multicenter American Research Trial with Cilazapril after Angioplasty to Prevent Transluminal Coronary Obstruction and Restenosis (MARCATOR). J Am Coll Cardiol 1996;27:1-7.
956. Violaris A, Melkert R, Serruys P. Long-term luminal renarrowing after successful elective coronary angioplasty of total occlusions. A quantitative angiographic analysis. Circulation 1995;91:2140-2150.
957. Kadel C, Burger W, Hartmann A, et al. Long-term follow-up in 686 patients with attempted reopening of chronic coronary occlusions. Circulation 1993;88:I-505.
958. Finci L, Meier B, Fayre J et al. Long-term results of successful and failed angioplasty for chronic total coronary arterial occlusion. Am J Cardiol 1990;66:660.
959. Mintz G, Popma J, Pichard A, et al. Increased plaque burden affects procedural outcomes of total occlusions: An intravascular ultrasound study. J Am Coll Cardiol 1995;25:61A.
960. Sherman CT, Sheehan D and Simpson JB. Simultaneous cannulation: A technique for percutaneous transluminal coronary angioplasty of chronic total occlusions. Cathet Cardiovasc Diagn 1987;13:333-336.
961. Freed M, Boatman JE, Siegel N, Safian RD, Grines CL, O'Neill WW. Glidewire treatment of resistant coronary occlusions. Cathet Cardiovasc Diagn 1993;30:201-204.
962. Rees MR, Sivananthan MV, Verma SP. The use of hydrophilic terumo glidewires in the treatment of chronic coronary artery occlusions. Circulation 1991;84:II-519.
963. Hosny A, Lai D, Mancherje C, Lee G. Successful recanalization using a hydrophilic-coated guidewire in total coronary occlusions after unsuccessful PTCA attempts with standard steerable guidewires. J Interven Cardiol 1990;3:225-230.
964. Pande AK, Meier B, Urban P, de la Serna F. Magnum/magnarail versus conventional systems for recanalization of chronic total coronary occlusions: A randomized comparison. Am Heart J 1992;123:1182-1186.
965. Haerer W, Schmidt A, Eggeling T, et al. Angioplasty of chronic total coronary occlusions. Results of a controlled randomized trial. J Cardiol 1991;17:113A.
966. Serruys PW, Hamburger J, Fleck E, Koolen JJ, et al. Laser guidewire: A powerful tool in recanalization of chronic total coronary occlusion. Circulation 1995;92:I-76.
967. Rees M, Michalis L. Vibrational coronary angioplasty: Challenging chronic total occlusions. Preliminary clinical data. J Am Coll Cardiol 1995;25:368A.
968. Danchin N, Cassagnes J, Juilliere Y, Machescourt J. Balloon angioplasty versus rotational angioplasty in chronic coronary occlusions (the BAROCCO study). Am J Cardiol 1995;75:330-334.
969. Kaltenbach M, Vallbracht C, and Hartmann A. Recanalization of Chronic Coronary Occlusions by Low Speed Rotational Angioplasty (ROTACS). J Interven Cardiol 1991;4:155-165.
970. Appleman Y, Koolen J, deFeyter P, et al. Longterm outcome of excimer laser angioplasty versus balloon angioplasty in functional and total coronary occlusions. J Am Coll Cardiol 1995;25:330A.
971. Sato Y, Nosaka H, Kimura T, Nobuyoshi M. Randomized comparison of balloon angioplasty versus coronary stent implantation for total occlusion. J Am Coll Cardiol 1996;27:152A.
972. Zidar FJ, Kaplan BM, O'Neill WW, et al. Prosective, randomized trial of prolonged intracoronary urokinase infusion for chronic total occlusions in native coronary arteries. J Am Coll Cardiol 1996;27:1406-12.
973. Höpp HW, Franzen D, Deutsch HJ, et al. New option for balloon recanalization of total coronary occlusions. Cathet Cardiovasc Diagn 1991;24:226-230.
974. Little T, Rosenberg J, Seides S, et al. Probe ™ angioplasty of total coronary occlusion using the probing catheter ™ technique. Cathet Cardiovasc Diagn. 1990;21:124.
975. Hamm CW, Jupper W, Kuck K, et al. Recanalization of chronic total occluded coronary arteries by new angioplasty systems. Am J Cardiol 1990;66:1459.
976. Flood RD, Popma JJ, Chuang YC, Salter LF, et al. Incidence, angiographic predictors, and clinical significance of coronary perforation occurring after new device angioplasty. J Am Coll Cardiol 1994;23:301A.
977. Ajluni S, Jones D, Zidar F, Puchrowicz S, Margulis A. Prolonged urokinase infusion for chronic total native coronary occlusions: Clinical, angiographic, and treatment observations. Cath Cardiovas Diagn. 1995;34:106-110.

978. Cecena FA. Urokinase infusion after unsuccessful angioplasty in patients with chronic total occlusion of native coronary arteries. Cath Cardiovasc Diagn. 1993;28:214-218.
979. Vaska KJ, Whitlow PL. Selective tissue plasminogen activator infusion for chronic total occlusions of native coronary arteries failing angioplasty. Circulation 1991;84:II-250.
980. Dick R, Haudenschild C, Popma J, et al. Directional atherectomy for total coronary occlusions. Cor Art Dis 1991;2:189-199.
981. Hinohara T, Rowe M, Robertson G, et al. Effect of lesion characteristics on outcome of directional coronary atherectomy. J Am Coll Cardiol 1991;17:1112-1120.
982. Omoigui N, Reisman M, Franco I, Whitlow P. Rotational atherectomy in chronic total occlusions. J Am Coll Cardiol 1995;25:97A.
983. Stertzer SH, Rosenblum J, Shaw RE, et al. Coronary rotational ablation: Initial experience in 302 procedures. J Am Coll Cardiol 1993;21:287-95.
984. Klein L, Litvack F, Holmes D, et al. Prospective multicenter analysis of excimer laser coronary angioplasty (ELCA) in stenosis with complex morphology. J Am Coll Cardiol 1994:February Special Issue 448A.
985. Litvack F, Eigler N, Margolis J, et al. Percutaneous excimer laser coronary angioplasty: Results in the first consecutive 3,000 patients. J Am Coll Cardiol 1994;23:323-329.
986. Baumbach A, Bittl J, Fleck E, Geschwind H, Sanborn T. Acute complications of excimer laser coronary angioplasty: A detailed analysis of multicenter results. J Am Coll Cardiol 1994;23:1305-1313.
987. Holmes DR, Forrester JS, Litvack F, Reeder GS, et al. Chronic total obstruction and short-term outcome: The excimer laser coronary angioplasty registry experience. Mayo Clin Proc 1993;68:5-10.
988. Buchwald AB, Werner GS, Unterberg C, Voth E, Kreuzer H, Wiegand V. Restenosis after excimer laser angioplasty of coronary stenoses and chronic total occlusions. Am Heart J 1992;123:878-885.
989. deMarchena EJ, Mallon SM, Knopf WD, et al. Effectiveness of holmium laser-assisted coronary angioplasty. Am J Cardiol 1994;73:117-121.
990. Torre SR, Lai SM, Schatz RA. Relation of clinical presentation and lesion morphology to the procedural results of Palmaz-Schatz stent placement: A new approaches to coronary intervention (NACI) registry report. J Am Coll Cardiol 1994;23:135A.
991. Ooka M, Suzuki T, Yokoya K, Hayase M, et al. Stenting after revascularization of chronic total occlusion. Circulation 1995;92:I-94.
992. Hsu Y-S, Tamai H, Ueda K, et al. Clinical efficacy of coronary stenting in chronic total occlusions. Circulation 1994;90:I-613.
993. Almagor Y, Borrione M, Maiello L, Khalt B, Finci L, Colombo A. Coronary stenting after recanalization of chronic total coronary occlusions. Circulation 1993;88:I-504.
994. Bilodeau L, Iyer S, Cannon A, et al. Stenting as an adjunct to balloon angioplasty for recanalization of totally occluded coronary arteries: Clinical and angiographic follow-up. J Am Coll Cardiol 1993;21:292A.
995. Rothbaum DA, Linnemeier TJ, Krauthamer D, et al. Excimer laser angioplasty in total coronary occlusions: A registry report. Circulation 1991;84:II-744.
996. Ooka M, Suzuki T, Kosokawa H, et al. Stenting vs. non-stenting after revascularization of chronic total occlusion. Circulation 1994;90:I-613.
997. Saber RS, Edwards WD, Holmes DR Jr, et al. Balloon angioplasty of aortocoronary saphenous vein bypass grafts: A histopathologic study of six grafts from five patients, with emphasis on restenosis and embolic complications. J Am Coll Cardiol 1988;12:1501-1509.
998. Waller BF, Rothbaum DA, Gorfinkel HJ, et al. Morphologic observations after percutaneous transluminal balloon angioplasty of early and late aortocoronary saphenous vein bypass grafts. J Am Coll Cardiol 1984;4:784-792.
999. Kahn J, Rutherford B, McConahay D, et al. Initial and long-term outcome of 83 patients after balloon angioplasty of totally occluded bypass grafts. J Am Coll Cardiol 1994;23:1038-1042.
1000. Margolis JR, Mehta S, Kramer B, et al. Extraction atherectomy for the treatment of recent totally occluded saphenous vein grafts. J Am Coll Cardiol 1994;23:405A.
1001. Hartmann JR, McKeever LS, Stamato NJ, et al. Recanalization of chronically occluded aortocoronary saphenous vein bypass grafts by extended infusion of urokinase: Initial results and short-term clinical follow-up. J Am Coll Cardiol 1991;18:1517-1523.
1002. Hartmann JR, McKeever LS, O'Neill WW, White CJ, et al. Recanalization of chronically occluded aortocoronary saphenous vein bypass grafts with long-term, low dose direct infusion of urokinase (ROBUST): A serial trial. J Am Coll Cardiol 1996;27:60-6.
1003. Busch UW, Weingartner F, Renner U, Neumann FJ, et al. Balloon-occlusive-intravascular-lysis-enhanced-recanalization (B-O-I-L-E-R) of thrombotic saphenous vein graft occlusions: A new technique of selective intravascular thrombolysis. J Am Coll Cardiol 1993;21:451A.
1004. Katsuragawa M, Fujiwara H, Miyamae M, Sasayama S. Histologic studies in percutaneous transluminal coronary angioplasty for chronic total occlusion: comparison of tapering and abrupt types of occlusion and short and long occluded segments. J Am Coll Cardiol 1993;21:604-611.
1005. Jaup T, Allemann Y, Urban P, et al. The Magnum wire for percutaneous coronary balloon angioplasty in 723 patients. J Invas Cardiol 1995;7:259-64.
1006. Serruys PW, Leon M, Hamburger JN, et al. Recanalization of chronic total coronary occlusions using a laser guide wire: The Eu and US total experience. J Am Coll Cardiol 1996;27:152A.
1007. Moussa I, DiMario C, Blengino S, et al. Coronary stenting of chronic total occlusions without anticoagulation: Immediate and long-term outcome. J Invas. Cardiol 1996;8.
1008. Mehta S, Margolis JR, Bittl JA, Tcheng JE, et al. Finally, treatment of chronic total occlusions-ablation with excimer laser angiopalsty. J Invas. Cardiol 1996;8.
1009. Sharma SK, Duvvuri S, Cocke T, et al. Directional coronary atherectomy (DCA) of chronic total occlusions. J Invas. Cardiol 1996;8.

Saphenous Vein Graft & LIMA Intervention

1010. Campeau L, Enjalbert M, Lesperance J, et al. The relation of risk factors to the development of atherosclerosis in saphenous-vein bypass grafts and the progression of disease in the native circulation. N Engl J of Med 1984;311:1329-1332.
1011. Weintraub WS, Jones EL, Craver JM, Guyton RA. Frequency of repeat coronary bypass or coronary angioplasty after coronary artery bypass surgery using saphenous venous grafts. Am J Cardiol 1994;73:103-112.
1012. White C, Campeau L, Knatterud G, Probstfield J, Investigators atPCCT. Patency of saphaneous vein bypass grafts following elective angiography: Preliminary results from the POST CABG Clinical Trial. J Am Coll Cardiol 1993;21:18A.
1013. Reul GJ, Cooley DA, Ott DA, et al. Reoperation for recurrent coronary artery disease. Arch Surg 1979;114:1269-1275.
1014. Schaff HV, Orszulak TA, Gersh BJ, et al. The morbidity and mortality of reoperation for coronary artery disease and analysis of late results with use of actuarial estimate of event-free interval. J Thorac Cardiovasc Surg 1983;85:508-515.
1015. Foster ED, Fisher LD, Kaiser GC, et al. Comparison of operative mortality and morbidity for initial and repeat coronary artery bypass grafting: The coronary artery surgery study (CASS) registry experience. Ann of Thoracic Surg 1984;38:563-570.
1016. Pidgeon J, Brooks N, Magee P, et al. Reoperation for Angina After Previous Aortocoronary Bypass Surgery. Br Heart J 1985;53:269-75.
1017. Laird-Meeter K, VanDomBurg R, Vanden Brand MJBM, et al. Incidence, risk, and outcome of reintervention after aortocoronary bypass surgery. Br Heart J 1987;57:427-35.
1018. Lytle BW, Loop FD, Cosgrove DM, et al. Fifteen hundred coronary reoperations: results and determinants of early and late survival. J Thorac Cardiovasc Surg 1987;93:847-859.
1019. Verheul HA, Moulign AC, Hondema S, et al. Late results of 200 repeat coronary artery bypass operations. Am J of Cardiol 1991;67:24-30.
1020. Noyez L, van der Werf T, Janssen D, Klinkenberg T. Early results with bilateral internal mammary artery grafting in coronary reoperations. Am J Cardiol 1992;70:1113-1116.
1021. Verheul H, Moulijn A, Hondema S, Schouwink M. Late results of 200 repeat coronary artery bypass operations. Am J Cardiol 1991;67:24-30.
1022. Lytle B, Loop F, Cosgrove D, Taylor P. Fifteen hundred coronary reoperations. J Thorac Cardiovasc Surg. 1987;93:847-859.
1023. Loop F, Lytle B, Cosgrove D, et al. Reoperation for coronary atherosclerosis. Changing practice in 2509 consecutive patients. Ann Surg 1990;212:378-386.
1024. Lamas G, Mudge G, Collins J, et al. Clinical response to coronary artery operation. J Am Coll Cardiol 1986;8:274-279.
1025. Pidgeon J, Brook N, MaGee P, Pepper JR. Repoperation of angina after previous aortocoronary bypass surgery. Br Heart J 1985;53:269-275.
1026. Foster E, Fisher L, Kaiser G, Meyers W, CASS atPIo. Comparison of operative mortality and morbidity for initial and repeat coronary artery bypass grafting: The CASS Registry Experience. Ann Thorac Surg 1984;38:563-570.
1027. Schaff H, Orszulak T, Gersh B, Piehler J. The morbidity and mortality of reoperation for coronary artery disease and analysis of late results with use of actuarial estimate of event-free interval. J Thorac Cardiovasc Surg. 1983;85:508-515.
1028. Lytle BW, McElroy D, McCarthy P, Loop FD, et al. Influence of arterial coronary bypass grafts on the mortality in coronary reoperations. J Thorac Cardiovasc Surg 1994;107:675-82.
1029. Ivert TS, Ekestrom S, Petriffy A, Weiti R. Coronary artery reoperations. Early and late results in 101 patients. Scand J Thoracic Cardiovasc Surg 1988;22:111-8.
1030. Perrault L, Carrier M, Cartier R, Leclerc Y, Hebert Y, Diaz OS, Pelletier C. Morbidity and mortality of reoperation for coronary artery bypass grafting: signficance of atheromatous vein grafts. Can J Cardiol 1991;7:427-30.
1031. Gonzalez-Santos JM, Ennabli K, Grondin C. Repeat coronary artery bypass grafting in patients with patent atherosclerotic grafts: a special challenge. Thorac Cardiovasc Surg (West Germany) 1984;32:346-9.
1032. Tan K, Henderson R, Sulke N, Cooke R. Percutaneous transluminal coronary angioplasty in patients with prior coronary artery bypass grafting: ten years' experience. Cath Cardiovasc Diagn 1994;31:11-17.
1033. Morrison D, Crowley S, Veerakul G, Barbire C, Grover F, Sacks J. Percutaneous transluminal angioplasty of saphenous vein grafts for medically refractory unstable angina. J Am Coll Cardiol 1994;23:1066-1070.
1034. Unterberg C, Buchwald A, Wiegand V, Kreuzer H. Coronary angioplasty in patients with previous coronary artery bypass grafting. J Vasc Dis 1992:653-659.
1035. Miranda CP, Rutherford BD, McConahay DR, et al. Angioplasty of older saphenous vein grafts continues to be a sound therapeutic option. J Am Coll Cardiol 1992;19, 3:350A.
1036. Meester BJ, Samson M, Suryapranata H, et al. Long-term follow-up after attempted angioplasty of saphenous vein grafts: The Thoraxcenter Experience 1981-1988. Eur Heart J 1991;12:648-653.
1037. Plokker HWT, Meester BH, Serruys PW. The Dutch experience in percutaneous transluminal angioplasty of narrowed saphenous veins used for aortocoronary arterial bypass. Am J Cardiol 1991;67:361-366.
1038. Douglas JS, Weintraub WS, Liberman HA, et al. Update of saphenous graft (SVG) angioplasty: Restenosis and long-term outcome. Circulation 1991; 84: II-249.
1039. Jost S, Gulba D, Daniel WG, Amende I. Percutaneous transluminal angioplasty of aortocoronary venous bypass grafts and effect of the caliber of the grafted coronary artery on graft stenosis. Am J Cardiol 1991;68:27-30.
1040. Webb JG, Myler RK, Shaw RE, et al. Coronary angioplasty after coronary bypass surgery: Initial results and late outcome in 422 patients. J Am Coll Cardiol 1990;16:812-820.
1041. Dorros G, Lewin RF, Mathiak LM. Coronary angioplasty in patients with prior coronary artery bypass surgery: all prior coronary artery bypass surgery patients and patients more than 5 years after coronary bypass surgery. Cardiol Clin 1989;7:791-803.
1042. Platko WP, Hollman J, Whitlow PL, et al. Percutaneous transluminal angioplasty of saphenous vein graft stenosis: long-term follow-up. J Am Coll Cardiol 1989;14:1645-1650.

1043. Pinkerton CA, Slack JD, Orr CM, et al. Percutaneous transluminal angioplasty in patients with prior myocardial revascularization surgery. Am J Cardiol 1988;61:15G-22G.

1044. Cote GC, Myler RK, Stertzer SH, et al. Percutaneous transluminal angioplasty of stenotic coronary artery bypass grafts: 5 years' experience. J Am Coll Cardiol 1987;9:8-17.

1045. Ernst S, van der Feltz T, Ascoop C, et al. Percutaneous transluminal coronary angioplasty in patients with prior coronary artery bypass grafting. J Thorac Cardiovasc Surg 1987;93:268-275.

1046. Douglas J, Robinson K, Schlumpf M. Percutaneous transluminal angioplasty in aortocoronary venous graft stenoses: Immediate results and complications. Circulation 1986;74:II-363.

1047. Reeder G, Bresnahan J, Holmes DJ, et al. Angioplasty for aortocoronary bypass graft stenosis. Mayo Clin Proc 1986;61:14-19.

1048. Corbelli J, Franco I, Hollman J, et al. Percutaneous transluminal coronary angioplasty after previous coronary artery bypass surgery. Am J Cardiol 1985;56:398-403.

1049. Gamal M, Bonnier H, Michels R, Heijman J, Stassen E. Percutaneous transluminal angioplasty of stenosed aortocoronary bypass grafts. Br Heart J 1984;52:617-620.

1050. Block P, Cowley M, Kaltenbach M, Kent K, Simpson J. Percutaneous angioplasty of stenoses of bypass grafts or of bypass graft anastomotic sites. Am J Cardiol 1984;53:666-668.

1051. Douglas JS, Gruentzig AR, King SB, et al. Percutaneous transluminal coronary angioplasty in patients with prior coronary bypass surgery. J Am Colll Cardiol 1983;2:745-754.

1052. Douglas J, Weintraub W, King SI. Changing perspectives in vein graft angioplasty. J Am Coll Cardiol 1995;25:78A.

1053. Guzman LA, Villa AE, Whitlow P: New atherectomy devices in the treatment of old saphenous vein grafts: Are the initial results encouraging? Circulation 1992;86:I-780.

1054. Liu MW, Douglas JS, Lembo NJ, King SBI. Angiographic predictors of a rise in serum creatine kinase (distal embolization) after balloon angioplasty of saphenous vein coronary artery bypass grafts. Am J Cardiol 1993;72:514-517.

1055. Altmann D, Popma J, Hong M, et al. CPK-MB elevation after angioplasty of saphenous vein grafts. J Am Coll Cardiol 1993;21:232A.

1056. Tilli FV, Kaplan BM, Safian RD, Grines CL, O'Neill WW. Angioscopic plaque friability: a new risk factor for procedural complications following saphenous vein graft interventions. J Am Coll Cardiol 1996 (in-press).

1057. Challapalli RM, Eisenberg MJ, Sigmon K, Lemberger J. Platelet glycoprotein IIb/IIIa monocional antibody (c7E3) reduces distal embolization during percutaneous intervention of saphenous vein grafts. Circulation 1995;92:I-607.

1058. Abbo KM, Dooris M, Glazier S, O'Neill WW, et al. No-reflow after percutaneous coronary intervention: Clinical and angiographic characteristics, treatment, and outcome. Am J Cardiol 1995;75:778-782.

1059. de Feyter PJ, Serruys PW, van den Brand M, Meester H, Beatt K, Surypanyata H. Percutaneous transluminal angioplasty of totally occluded venous bypass grafts: a challenge that should be resisted. Am J Cardiol 1989;64:88-90.

1060. Weintraub WS, Cohen CL, Curling PE, et al. Results of coronary surgery after failed elective coronary angioplasty in patients with prior coronary surgery. J Am Coll Cardiol 1990;16:1341-1347.

1061. Kahn JK, Rutherford BD, McConahay DR, Johnson WL, Giorgi LV, Shimshak TM, Hartzler GO. Outcome following emergency coronary artery bypass grafting for failed elective balloon angioplasty in patients with prior coronary bypass. Am J Cardiol 1990;66:285-8.

1062. Lemmer JH, Ferguson DW, Rakel BA, Rossi NP. Clinical outcome of emergency repeat coronary artery bypass surgery. J Cardiovasc Surg (Torino) 1990;31:429-7.

1063. Ellis SG, Ajluni S, Arnold AZ, Popma JJ, Bittl JA, Eigler NL, Cowley MJ, Raymond RE, Safian RD, Whitlow PL. Increased coronary perforation in the new device era: incidence, classification, management and outcome. Circulation 1994;90:2725-2730.

1064. Ajluni SC, Glazier S, Blankenship L, O'Neill WW, Safian RD. Perforations after percutaneous coronary interventions: Clinical, angiographic, and theapeutic observations. Cathet Cardiovasc Diagn 1994;32:206-212.

1065. Douglas J, King SI. Ten year follow-up of patients undergoing vein graft angioplasty. Circulation 1994;90:I-333.

1066. Safian RD, Grines CL, May MA, Lichtenberg A, Juran N, Schreiber TL, Pavlides GS, Meany TB, Savas V, O'Neill WW. Clinical and angiographic results of transluminal extraction coronary atherectomy in saphenous vein bypass grafts. Circulation 1994;89:302-312.

1067. Popma JJ, Leon MB, MIntz GS, Kent KH, Satler LF, Garrand TJ, Pichard AJ. Results of coronary angioplasty using the Transluminal Extraction Catheter. Am J Cardiol 1992;70:1526-32.

1068. Meany T, Leon MB, Kramer B, et al. A multicenter experience of atherectomy of transluminal extraction in catheter for for the treatment of diseased of saphenous vein grafts. Cathet Cardiovasc Diagn 1995;34:112-120.

1069. Twidale N, Barth CW, Keperman RM, et al. Acute results and long-term outcome of transluminal extraction catheter atherectomy for saphenous vein graft stenoses. Cathet Cardiovasc Diagn 1994;31:187-191.

1070. Hong MK, Popma JJ, Pichard AD, Kent KH, Satler LF, Chuang YC, Mintz GS, Keller MB, Leon MB. Clinical significance of distal embolization after Transluminal Extraction Atherectomy in diffusely diseased saphenous vein grafts. Am Heart J 1994;127:1496-503.

1071. Kramer B. Optimal therapy for degenerated saphenous vein graft disease. J Invas Cardiol 1995;7:14D-20D.

1072. Annex B, Larkin T, O'Neill W, Safian R. Evaluation of thrombus removal by transluminal extraction coronary atherectomy by percutaenous coronary angioscopy. Am J Cardiol 1994;74:606-609.

1073. Kaplan BM, Safian RD, Grines CL, Goldstein JA, et al. Usefulness of adjunctive angioscopy and extraction atherectomy before stent implantation in high-risk aortocoronary saphenous vein grafts. Am J Cardiol 1995;76:822-826.

1074. Moses J, Lieberman S, Knopf W, et al. Mechanism of transluminal extraction catheter (TEC) atherectomy in degenerative saphenaous vein grafts (SVG). An angioscopic observational study. J Am Coll Cardiol 1993;21:442A.

1075. Moses J, Tierstein P, Sketch M, et al. Angiographic determinants of risk and outcome of coronary embolus and myocardial infarction (MI) with the transluminal extraction catheter (TEC): A report from the New Approaches to Coronary Intervention (NACI) Registry.

J Am Coll Cardiol 1994;23:220A.
1076. Dooris M, Hoffmann M, Glazier S, et al. Comparative results of transluminal extraction coronary atherectomy in saphenous vein graft lesions with and without thrombus. J Am Coll Cardiol 1995;25:1700-5.
1077. Al-Shaibi, KF, Goods CM, Jain SP, et al. Does transluminal extraction atherectomy reduce distal embolization in saphenous vein grafts? Circualtion 1995;92:I-329.
1078. Moses JW, Yeh W, Popma JJ, Sketch MH. Predictors of distal embolization with the TEC catheter: A NACI Registry Report. Circulation 1995;92:I-329.
1079. Hong M, Pichard A, Kent K, et al. Assessing a strategy of stand-alone extraction atherectomy followed by staged stnt placement in degenerated saphenous vein graft lesions. J Am Coll Cardiol 1995;25:394A.
1080. Parks JM. TEC before stent implantation. J Invas Cardiol 1995;7:10D-13D.
1081. Cowley MJ, Whitlow PL, Baim DS, Hinohara T, Hall K, Simpson JB. Directional coronary atherectomy of saphenous vein graft narrowings: mulitcenter investigational experience. Am J Cardiol 1993;72:30E-34E.
1082. Kaufmann UP, Garratt KN, Vliestra RE, Holmes DR. Transluminal atherectomy of saphenous vein aortocoronary bypass grafts. Am J Cardiol 1990:65:1430-1433.
1083. DiSciascio G, Cowley MJ, Vetrovec CW, et al. Directional coronary atherectomy of saphenou vein graft lesions unfavorable for balloon angioplasty: Results of a single-center experience. Cathet Cariovasc Diagn 1992;26:75.
1084. Pomerantz RM, Kuntz E, Carozza JP, Fishman RF, Mansour M, Schnitt SJ, Safian RD, Baim DS. Acute and long-term outcome of narrowed saphenous venous grafts treated by endoluminal stenting and directional atherectomy. Am J Cardiol 1992;70:161-167.
1085. Garratt KN, Holmes DR Jr, Bell MR, Berger PB, Kauffmann UP, Bresnahan JF, Vliestra RE. Results of directional atherectomy of primary atheromatous and restenosis lesions in coronary arteries and saphenous vein grafts. Am J Cardiol 1192;70:449-454.
1086. Selmon MR, Hinohara T, Robertson GC, Rowe MH, Vetter JW, Bartzokis TC, Braden IJ, Simpson JB. Directional coronary atherectomy for vein graft stenoses. J Am Coll Cardiol 1991;17:23A.
1087. Ghazzal ZMB, Douglas JS, Holmes DR, Ellis SG, Kereiakes DJ, Simpson JB, KIng SB, and the Directional Atherectomy Multicenter Investigational Group. Directional coronary atherectomy of saphenous vein grafts: recent multicenter experience. J An Coll Cardiol 1991;17:219A.
1088. Hinohara T, Robertson GC, Selmon MR, Vetter JW, Rowe MH, Braden LJ, McAuley BJ, Sheehan DJ, Simpson JB. Restenosis after directional coronary atherectomy. J Am Coll Cardiol 1992;20:623-632.
1089. Holmes D, Topol e, Califf R, et al. A multicenter, randomized trial of coronary angioplasty versus directional atherectomy for patients with saphenous vein bypass graft lesions. Circulation 1995;91:1966-1974.
1090. Strauss BH, Natarajan MK, Batchelor WB, Yardley DE, et al. Early and late quantitative angiographic results of vein graft lesions treated by excimer laser with adjunctive balloon angioplasty. Circulation 1995;92:348-356.
1091. Bittl JA, Sanborn TA, Yardley DE, Tcheng JE, Isner JM, Choksi SK, Strauss BH, Abela GS, Walter PD, Scmidhofer M, Power JA for the Percutaneous Excimer Laser Coronary Angioplasty Registry. Predictors of outcome of percutaneous excimer laser coronary angioplasty of saphenous vein bypass graft lesions. Am J Cardiol 1994;74:144-148.
1092. Litvack F, Eigler N, Margolis J, Rothbaum, D, et al. Percutaneous excimer laser coronary angioplasty: Results in the first consecutive 3,000 patients. J Am Coll Cardiol 1994;23:323-329.
1093. De Marchena EJ, Mallon SM, Knopf WD, et al. Effectiveness of Holmium laser-assisted coronary angioplasty. Am J Cardiol 1994;73:117-121.
1094. Serruys PW, de Jaegere P, Kiemeneij F, et al. A comparison of balloon-expandable stent implantation with balloon angioplasty in patients with coronary artery disease. N Engl J Med 1994;331: 489-95.
1095. Fischman DL, Leon MB, Baim DS et al. A randomized comparison of coronary -stent placement and balloon angioplasty in the treatment of coronary artery disease. N Engl J Med 1994;331:496-501.
1096. Savage M, Douglas J, Fischman D, et al. Coronary stents versus balloon angioplasty for aorto-coronary saphenous vein bypass graft disease: Interim results of a randomized trial. J Am Coll Cardiol 1995;25:79A.
1097. Wong SC, Baim D, Schatz R, et al. Immediate results and late outcomes after stent implantation in saphenous vein graft lesions: The multicenter US Palmaz-Schatz Stent experience. J Am Coll Cardiol 1995;26:704-712.
1098. Rechavia E, Litvack F, Macko G, Eigler N. Stent implantation of saphenous vein graft aorto-ostial lesions in patients with unstable ischemic syndromes: Immediate angiographic results and long-term clinical outcome. J Am Coll Cardiol 1995;25:866-870.
1099. Wong SC, Popma J, Pichard A, Kent K. Comparison of clinical and angiographic outcomes after saphenous vein grafts angioplasty using coronary versus "biliary" tubular slotted stents. Circulation 1995;91:339-350.
1100. Denardo SJ, Morris NB, Rocha-Singh, KJ, et al. Safety and efficacy of extended urokinase infusion plus stent deployment for treatment of o bstructed, older saphenous vein grafts. Am J Cardiol 1995;76:776-780.
1101. Piana RN, Moscucci M, Cohen DJ, Kugelmass AD, Senerchia C, Kuntz RE, Baim DS, Carozza JP Jr. Palmaz-Schatz stenting for treatment of focal vein graft stenosis: immediate results and long-term outcome. J Am Coll Cardiol 1994;23:1296-30.
1102. Eeckhout E, Goy JJ, Stauffer JC, Vogt P, Kappenberger L. Endoluminal stenting of narrowed saphenous vein grafts: long-term clinical and angiographic follow-up. Cathet Cardiovasc Diagn 1994;32:139-46.
1103. Keane D, Buis B, Reifart N, Plokker TH. Clinical and angiographic outcome following implantation of the new less shortening wallstent in aortocoronary vein grafts: Introduction of a second gemeration stent in the clinical arena. J Interven Cardiol 1994;7:557-564.
1104. Fenton S, Fischman D, Savage M, et al. Long-term angiographic and clinical outcome after implantation of balloon-expandable stents in aortocoronary saphenous vein grafts. Am J Cardiol 1994;74:1187-1191.
1105. Leon MB, Wong SC, Pichard A. Balloon expandable stent implantation in saphenous vein grafts. In Hermann HC, Hirschfeld JW (Eds). Clinical use of the Palmaz Schatz Intracoronary Stent. Futura Publishing Company Inc. 1993; 111-121.
1106. Fortuna R, Heuser R, Garratt K, Schwartz R, Buchbinder M. Wiktor intracoronary stent: Experience in the first 101 vein graft patients. Circulation 1993;88:I-309.

1107. Bilodeau L, Iyer S, Cannon A, et al. Flexible coil stent (Cook, Inc.) in saphenous vein grafts: clinical and angiographic follow-up. J Am Coll Cardiol 1992;19:264A.
1108. Strauss B, Serruys P, Bertrand M, Puel J. Quantitative angiographic follow-up of the coronary wallstent in native vessel and bypass grafts European experience-March 1986 to March 1990). Am J Cardiol 1992;69:475-481.
1109. deScheerder I, Strauss B, deFeyter P, Beatt K. Stenting of venous bypass grafts: a new treatment modality for patients who are poor candidates for reintervention. Am Heart J 1992;123:1046-1054.
1110. Urban P, Sigwart U, Golf S, Kaufmann U, Sadeghi H, Kappenberger L. Intravascular stenting for stenosis of aortocoronary venous bypass grafts. J Am Coll Cardiol 1989;13:1085-1091.
1111. Wong SC, Popma J, Hong M, et al. Procedural results and longterm clinical outcomes in aorto-osital saphenous vein graft lesions after new device angioplasty. J Am Coll Cardiol 1995;25:394A.
1112. Wong C, Popma J, Chuang Y, et al. Economic impact of reduced anticoagulation after saphenous vein graft stent placement. J Am Coll Cardiol 1995;25:80A.
1113. Sketch M, Wong C, Chuang Y, et al. Progressive deterioration in late (2-year) clinical outcomes after stent implantation in saphenous vein grafts: The Multicenter JJIS experience. J Am Coll Cardiol 1995;25:79A.
1114. Bass T, Gilmore P, Buchbinder M. Coronary rotational atherectomy (PTCRA) in patients with prior coronary revascularization: A registry report. Circulation 1992;86:I-653.
1115. Freed M, Niazi K, O'Neill W. Percutaneous coronary rotational atherectomy: The William Beaumont Hospital experience. p.297. In Restenosis After Intervention With New Mechanical Devices. ed. Dordrecht, The Netherlands: Kluwer Academic, 1992.
1116. van Ommen V, Veen Mat Daemen E, Habets J, Wellens H. In vivo evaluation of the safety to the vessel wall of the hydrolyser (a hydrodynamic thrombectomy catheter). J Am Coll Cardiol 1994;23:406A.
1117. Fajadet J, Bar O, Jordan C, Robert G, Laurent J, Callard J, Cassagneau B, Marco J. Human percutaneous thrombectomy using the new Hydrolyser catheter: preliminary results in saphenous vein grafts. J Am Coll Cardiol 1994;220A.
1118. Kahn J, Rutherfors B, McConahay D, et al. Initial and long-term outcome of 83 patients after balloon angioplasty of totally occluded bypass grafts. J Am Coll Cardiol 1994;23:1038-1042.
1119. Hartmann JR, McKeever LS, Stamato NJ, et al. Recanalization of Chronically Occluded aortocoronary Saphenous Vein Bypass Grafts by Extended Infusion of Urokinase: Initial Results and Short-term Clinical Follow-up. J Am Coll Cardiol 1991;18, 6:1517-1523.
1120. Hartmann J, McKeever L, Teran J. Prolonged infusion of urokinase for recanalization of chronically occluded aortocoronary bypass grafts. Am J Cardiol 1988;61:189-191.
1121. Sabri MN, Johnson D, Warner M, Cowley MJ. Intracoronary thrombolysis followed by directional coronary atherectomy: a combined approach for thrombotic vein graft lesions considered unsuitable for angioplasty. Cathet Cardiovasc Diagn 1992;26:15-18.
1122. Eagan J, Strumpf R, Heuser R. New treatment approach for chronic total occlusions of saphenous vein grafts: thrombolysis and intravascular stents. Cathet Cardiovasc Diagn 1993;29:62-69101.
1123. Blankenship JC, Modesto TA, Madigan NP. Acute myocardial infarction complicating urokinase infusion for total saphenous vein graft occlusion. Cath Cardiovasc Diagn 1993;28:39-43.
1124. Gurley JC, MacPhail BS. Acute myocardial infarction due to thrombolytic reperfusion of chronically occluded saphenous vein coronary bypass grafts. Am J Cardiol 1991;68:274-276.
1125. Taylor MA, Santoran EC, Aji J, Eldredge WJ, Cha SD, Dennis CA. Intracerebral hemorrhage complicating urokinase infusion into an occluded aortocoronary bypass graft. Cathet Cardiovasc Diagn 1994;31:206-210.
1126. Hartmann J, McKeever L, O'Neill W, White C, Whitlow P, Enger E. Recanalization of chronically occluded bypass grafts: The effect of angioplasty site following extended urokinase infusion on 6-month patency. J Am Coll Cardiol 1995;25:149A.
1127. Hartmann JR, McKeever LS, O'Neill WW, et al. Recanalization of chronically occluded aortocoronary saphenous vein bypass grafts with long-term, low dose direct infusion of urokinase (ROBUST): A Serial trial. J Am Coll Cardiol 1996; 27: 60-6.
1128. Torre S, Marotta C, Blum M, Banas J. "Pulse Spray" mini-urokinase infusion for recanalization of recently occluded saphenous vein grafts. J Am Coll Cardiol 1995;25:94A.
1129. de Feyter PJ, van Suylen RJ, de Jaegere PPT, Topol EJ, Serruys PW. Balloon angioplasty for the treatment of saphenous vein bypass grafts. J Am Coll Cardiol 1993;21:1539-49.
1130. Bredlau CE, Roubin GS, Leimgbruber PP, et Al. In-hospital morbidity and mortality in patients undergoing elective coronary angioplasty. Circulation 72;5:1044-1052.
1131. Dorogy ME, Highfill WT, Davis RC. Use of angioplasty in the management of complicated perioperative infarction following bypass surgery. Cathet Cardiovasc Diagn 1993;29:279-82.
1132. Kahn JK, Rutherford BD, McConahay DR, Giorgi LV, Johnson WL, Shimshak TM, Hartzler GO. Early postoperative balloon coronary angioplasty for failed coronary artery bypass grafting. Am J Cardiol 1990;66:943-6.
1133. Abdelmeguid A, Ellis S, Whitlow P, et al. Lack of graft age dependency for success of directional coronary atherectomy and Palmaz-Schatz stenting. J Am Coll Cardiol 1993;21:31A.
1134. Abdelmeguid A, Ellis S, Whitlow P, et al. Discordant results of extraction atherectomy in old and young saphenous vein grafts: The NACI Experience. J Am Coll Cardiol 1993;21:442A.
1135. Koller PT, Freed M, Grines CL, O'Neill WW. Success, complications and restenosis following rotational and transluminal extraction atherectomy of ostial stenoses. Cathet Cardiovasc Diagn 1994;31:255-260.
1136. Abdelmeguid AE, Whitlow PL, Simpfendorfer C, Sapp SK, et al. Percutaneous revascularization of ostial saphenous vein graft stenoses. J Am Coll Cardiol 1995;26:955-960.
1137. Stephan W, Bates E, Garratt K, Hinohara T, Muller D. Directional atherectomy of coronary and saphenous vein graft ostial stenoses. Am J Cardiol 1995;75:1015-1018.
1138. Hong M, Popma J, Chuang Y, et al. Predictive model of target-lesion revascularization after balloon and new device saphenous vein graft angioplasty. J Am Coll Cardiol 1994;23:139A.

1139. Glazier, Keiman FJ, Bauer JF, Mitchel DB, et al. Treatment of thrombotic saphenous vein graft stenoses/occlusions with local urokinase delivery with the dispatch catheter-initial results. Circulation 1995;92:I-671.
1140. Kaul U, Agarwal R, Mathur A, Wasir HS. Intracoronary stent placement in thrombus containing vein graft lesions. J Invas Cardiol 1995;7:248-250.
1141. Heuser R. Treatment alternatives for chronically occluded saphenous vein grafts. J Invas Cardiol 1995;7:94-96.
1142. Grines CL, Booth DC, Nissen SE, Gurley JC, Bennett KA, O,Connor WN, De Maria AN. Mechanisms of acute myocardial infarction in patients with prior coronary artery bypass grafting and therapeutic implications. Am J Cardiol 1990;66:1292-6.
1143. Santiago P, Vacek JL, Rosamond TL, Kramer KH, Crouse LJ, Beauchamp GD. Comparison of results of coronary angioplasty during acute myocardial infarction with and without prior coronary bypass surgery. Am J Cardiol 1993;72:1348-1351.
1144. Kahn JK, Rutherford BD, McConahay DR, Johnson W, Giorgi VL, Ligon R, Hartzler GO. Usefulness of angioplasty for acute myocardial infarction in patients with prior coronary artery bypass grafting. Am J Cardiol 1990;65: 698-702.
1145. Kaplan BM, Larkin T, Safian RD, O'Neill WW, et al. A propsective study of extraction atherectomy in patients with acute myocardial infarction. J Am Coll Cardiol 1996;27:365A.
1146. Spencer FC. The internal mammary artery: The ideal coronary bypass graft? N Engl J Med 1986;314:50-51.
1147. Loop FD, Lytle BW, Cosgrove DM, et al. Influence of internal mammary-artery graft on 10 year survival and other cardiac events. N Engl J Med 1986;314:1-6.
1148. Hearne S, Wilson J, Harrington J, et al. Angiographic and clinical follow-up after internal mammary artery graft angioplasty: A 9-year experience. J Am Coll Cardiol 1995;25:139A.
1149. Sketch MH Jr., Quigley PJ, Perez JA et al. Angiographic follow up after internal mammary artery angioplasty. Am J Cardiol 1992;70:401.
1150. Popma JJ, Cooke RH, Leon MB et al. Immediate procedural and long-term clinical results in internal mammary artery angioplasty. Am J Cardiol 1992;69:1237.
1151. Dimas AP, Arora RR, Whitlow PL, et al. Percutaneous transluminal angioplasty involving internal mammary artery grafts. Am Heart J 1991;122:423.
1152. Bell MR, Vliestra RE, et al. Percutaneous transluminal angioplasty of left internal mammary artery grafts: Two years experience with a femoral approach. Br Heart J 1989;61:417.
1153. Hill DM, McAuley BJ, Sheehan DJ et al. Percutaneous transluminal angioplasty of left internal mammary artery bypass grafts. J Am Coll Cardiol 1989;13:221A.
1154. Shimshak TM, Giorgi LV, Johnson WL et al. Application of percutaneous transluminal coronary angioplasty to the internal mammary artery graft. J Am Coll Cardiol 1988;12:1205.
1155. Pinkerton CA, Slack JD, Orr CM, Van Tassel JW. Percutaneous transluminal angioplasty involving internal mammary artery bypass grafts: a femoral approach. Cathet Cardiovasc Diagn 1987;13:414.
1156. Cote G, Myler RK, Stertzer SH et al. Percutaneous transluminal angioplasty of stenotic coronary artery bypass grafts. J Am Coll Cardiol 1987;9:8.
1157. Singh S,. Coronary angioplasty of internal mammary artery graft. Am J Med 1987,82:361.
1158. Steffenin OG, Meier B. Finci L, von Segesser L, Velebit V. Percutaneous transluminal angioplasty of right and left internal mammary artery grafts. Chest 1986;90:849-51.
1159. Brown RI, Galligan L, Penn IM, Weinstein L. Right internal mammary artery graft angioplasty through a right brachial approach using a new custom guide catheter: a case report. Cathet Cardiovasc Diagn 1992;25:42-5.
1160. Almagor Y, Thomas J, Colombo A. A balloon expandable stent ath the origin of the left internal mammary artery graft: a case report. Cathet Cardiovasc Diagn 1991;24:256-258.
1161. Bajaj RK, Roubin GS. Intravascular stenting of the right internal mammary artery. Cathet Cardiovasc Diagn 1991; 24:252-255.
1162. Hadjimiltiades S, Gourassas J, Louridas G, Tsifodimos D. Stenting the distal anastomotic site of the left internal mammary artery graft: a case report. Cathet Cardiovasc Diagn 1994;32:157-161.
1163. Dorros G, Lewin RF. The brachial artery method to transluminal internal mammary artery angioplasty. Cathet Cardiovasc Diagn 1986;12:341-346.
1164. Salinger M, Drummer B, Furey K, Bott-Silverman C, Franco I. Percutaneous angiplasty of internal mammary artery graft stenosis using the brachial approach: a case report. Cathet Cardiovasc Diagn 1986;12:261-5.
1165. Ishi K, Hirota Y, Kawamura K, Suma H, Takeuchi A. Coronary-subclavian steal corrected with percutaneous transluminal angioplasty. J Cardiovasc Surg (Torino) 1191;32:275-7.
1166. Laub GW, Muralidharan S, Naidech H, Fernandez H, Adkins M, McGrath LB. Percutaneous transluminal subclavian angioplasty in a patient with postoperative angina. Ann Thorac Surg 1991;52:850-1.
1167. Belz M, Marshall JJ, Cowley MJ, Vetrovec GW. Subclavian balloon angioplasty in the management of the coronary-subclavian steal syndrome. Cathet Cardiovasc Diagn 1992;25:161-3.
1168. Soulen MC, Sullivan KL. Subclavian artery angioplasty proximal to a left internal mammary coronary artery bypass graft: case report. Cardiovasc Intervent Radiol 1991;14:355-7.
1169. Feld H, Nathan P, Raninga D, Shani J. Symptomatic angina secondary to coronary-subclavian steal syndrome treated successfully by percutaneous transluminal angioplasty of the subclavian artery. Cathet Cardiovasc Diagn 1992;26:12-4.
1170. Holmes JR, Crane R. Coronary steal through a patent internal mammary artery graft: treatment by subclavian angioplasty. Am Heart J 1993;125:1166-7.
1171. Shapira S, Braun SD, Puram B, Patel G, Rotman H. Percutaneous transluminal angioplasty of proximal subclavian artery stenosis after left internal mammary to left anterior descending artery bypass surgery. J Am Coll Cardiol 1991;18:1120-3.
1172. Perrault LP, Carrier M, Hudon G, Lemarbre L, Hebert Y, Pelletier LC. Transluminal angioplasty of the subclavian artery in patients with internal mammary artery grafts. Ann Thorac Surg 1993,56:927-30.
1173. Motarjeme A, Gordon GI. Percutaneous transluminal angioplasty of the brachiocephalic vessels: guidelines for therapy. Int Angiol

1993;12:260-9.
1174. Rabah MM, Gangadharan V, Brodsky M, Safian RD. Unstable coronary ischemic syndromes due to coronary subclavian steal: Case reports and review of the literature. Am Heart J 1996;131:374-378.
1175. Ziomek S, Quinones-Baldrich WJ, Busuttil RW. The superiority of synthetic arterial grafts over autologous veins in carotid-subclavian bypass. J Vasc Surg 1986;3:140-5.
1176. McIvor ME, Williams GM, Brinker J. Subclavian coronary steal through a LIMIA-to LAD bypass graft. Cathet Cardiovasc Diagn 1988;14:100-104.
1177. Ishii K, Hirota Y, Kitz Y, Kawamura K, et al. Coronary-subclavian steal corrected with percutaneous transluminal angioplasty. J Cardiovasc Surg 1991;32:275-277.
1178. Benzuly K, Kaplan B, Bowers T, Safian RD. Coronary-subclavian steal due to fishulae from the left internal mammary artery to the pulmonary artery: Treatment by coil embolization. Cathet Cardiovasc Diagn (in-press).
1179. Laub GW, Muraldharan S, McGrath LB. Percutaneous transluminal subclavian angioplasty in a patient with postoperative angina. Ann Thorac Surg 1991;52:850-1.
1180. Perrault LP, Carrier M, Hudon G, Pelletier LC. Transluminal angioplasty of the subclavian artery in patients with internal mammary grafts. Ann Thorac Surg 1993;56:927-930.
1181. Dorros G, Lewin RF, Jamnadas P, Mathiak LM. Peripheral transluminal angioplasty of the subclavian and innominate arteries utilizing the brachial approach: acute outcome and follow-up. Cathet Cardiovasc Diagn 1990;19:71-76.
1182. Breall JA, Grossman W, Stillman IE, Gianturco LE, Kim D. Atherectomy of the subclavian artery for patients with symptomatic coronary-subclavian steal syndrome. J Am Coll Cadiol 1993;21:1564-1570.
1183. Breall JA, Kim D, Baim DS, Skillman JJ, Grossman W. Coronary-subclavian steal; and unusual cause of angina pectoris after successful internal mammary-coronary artery bypass grafting. Cathet Cardiovasc Diagn 1991;24:274-276.
1184. Sbarouni E, Corr L, Fenech A. Microcoil embolization of large intercostal branches of internal mammary artery grafts. Cathet Cardiovasc Diagn 1994;31:334-336.
1185. Mishkel GJ, Willinsky R. Combined PTCA and microcoil embolization of a left internal mammary artery graft. Cathet Cardiovasc Diagn 1192;27:141-6.
1186. Benzuly K, Kaplan B, Bowers T, Safian RD. Coronary-subclavian steal due to fishulae from the left internal mammary artery to the pulmonary artery: Treatment by coil embolization. Cathet Cardiovasc Diagn (in-press).
1187. Lytle BW, Cosgrove DM, Ratliff NB, Loop F. Coronary artery bypass grafting with the right gastroepiploic artery. J Thorac Cardiovasc Surg 1989;97:826-31.
1188. Verkkala K, Jarvinen A, Keto P, Virtanen K, Lehtola A, Pellinen T. Right gastroepiploic artery as a coronary bypass graft. Ann Thorac Surg 1989, 47:719-9.
1189. Grandjean JG, Boonstra PW, den Heyer P, Ebels T. Arterial revascularization with the right gastroepiploic artery and internal mammary arteries in 300 patients. J Thorac Surg 1994,107:1309-1315.
1190. Perrault LP, Carrier M, Hebert Y, Hudon G, Cartier R, Leclerc Y, Pelletier LC. Clinical experience with the right gastroepiploic artery in coronary bypass grafting. Ann Thorac Surg 1993;56:1082-4.
1191. Suma H, Wanibuchi Y, Terada Y, Fukuda S, Takayama T, Furuta S. The right gastroepiploic artery graft. Clinical and angiographic midterm results in 200 patients.
1192. Tanimoto Y, Matsuda Y, Fujii B, Kobayashi Y, Hatashi K, Takashiba K, Hamada Y, Hanazono S, Ando K, Hashimoto T. Angiography of the right gastroepiploic artery for coronary artery bypass graft. Cathet Cardiovasc Diagn 1989;16:35-8.
1193. Ishiki T, Yamaguchi T, Nakamura M, et al. Postoperative angiographic evaluation of gastroepiploic artery grafts: technical considerations and short-term patency. Cathet Cardiovasc Diagn 1991;21:233-8.
1194. Komiyama N, Nakanishi S, Yanagashita Y, Nishiyama S, Seki A, Watanabe Y, Konishi T, Fuse K. Percutaneous transluminal coronary angioplasty of gastroepiploic artery graft. Cathet Cardiovasc Diagn 1990;21:177-9.
1195. Watson LE, Schoolar EJ. PTCA of Gastroepiploic Bypass. Cathet Cardiovasc Diagn 1991;22:193-196.
1196. Ishiki T, Yamaguchi T, Tamura T, Saeki F, Furuta Y, Ikari Y, Chiku N, Suma H. Percutaneous angioplasty of stenosed gastroepiploic artery grafts. J Am Coll Cardiol 1993, 22:727-32.
1197. Bartlett JC, Tuzcu M, Simpfendorfer C, Dorosti K. Percutaneous transluminal coronary angioplasty of native coronary arteries via saphenous vein grafts. J Invas Cardiol 1991;3:62-65.
1198. Ramee S, Kuntz R, Schatz R, et al. Preliminary experience with the POSSIS coronary angiojet rheolytic thrombectomy catheter in the VeGAS 1 pilot study. J Am Coll Cardial 1996;27:69A.
1199. Hong M, Wong S, Popma J, et al. Favorable results of debulking followed by immediate adjunct stent therapy for high risk saphenous vein graft lesions. J Am Coll Cardial 1996;27:179A.
1200. Douglas J, Savage M, Bailey S, et al. Randomized trial of coronary stent and balloon angioplasty in the treatment of saphenous vein graft stenosis. J Am Coll Cardial 1996;27:178A.

PTCA Exotica

1201. Krucoff MW, Smith JE, Jackman JD Jr, et al. "Hugging balloons" through a single 8-french guide: salvage angioplasty with lytic therapy in the infarct vessel of a 40-year-old man. Cathet Cardiovasc Diagn 1991;24:45-50.
1202. Feld H, Valerio L and Shani J. Two hugging balloons at high pressures successfully dilate a lesion refractory to routine coronary angioplasty. Cathet Cardiovasc Diagn 1991;24:105-107.
1203. Arafah M, Aldridge HE and Schwartz L. Percutaneous transluminal angioplasty of stenotic saphenous vein right coronary bypass grafts utilizing a peripheral balloon dilatation catheter without a guiding catheter. Cathet Cardiovasc Diagn 1989;17:92-96.
1204. Villavicencio R, Urban P, Muller T., et al. Coronary balloon angioplasty through diagnostic 6 french catheters. Cathet Cardiovasc Diagn 1991;22:56-59.

1205. Feldman R, Glemser E, Kaizer J, et al. Coronary angioplasty using new 6 french guiding catheters. Cathet Cardiovasc Diagn 1991;23:93-99.

1206. Moles VP, Meier B, Urban P, et al. Percutaneous transluminal coronary angioplasty through 4 french diagnostic catheters. Cathet Cardiovasc Diagn 1992;25:98-100.

1207. Warren SG and Barnett JC. Guiding catheter exchange during coronary angioplasty. Cathet Cardiovasc Diagn 1990;20:212-215.

1208. Schreiber TL, Gangadharan V and O'Neill W. Guidewire facilitation of internal mammary artery cannulation. J Interven Cardiol 1990;3:23-26.

1209. Nakhjavan FK. Use of angioplasty guidewire for technically difficult angiography. Cathet Cardiovasc Diagn 1988;14:213.

1210. Das GS and Wysham DG. Double wire technique for additional guiding catheter support in anomalous left circumflex coronary artery angioplasty. Catheter Cardiovasc Diagn 1991;24:102-104.

1211. Hartzler GO. Three-wire technique. A unique approach to percutaneous transluminal coronary angioplasty of a trifurcation lesion. Cathet Cardiovasc Diagn 1987;13:174-177.

1212. Nakhjavan FK and Najmi M. Exit block: a new technique for difficult side branch angioplasty. Cathet Cardiovasc Diagn 1990;20:43-45.

1213. Lablanche JM, Fourrier JL, Gommeaux A, et al. Percutaneous aspiration of a coronary thrombus. Cathet Cardiovasc Diagn 1989;17:97-98.

1214. Brown SE, Segar DS, Weinberg BA, et al. Transcatheter Aspiration of Intracoronary Thrombus After Myocardial Infarction. Am Heart J 1990;120:688-690.

1215. Kahn JK and Hartzler GO. Thrombus Aspiration in Acute Myocardial Infarction. Cathet Cardiovasc Diagn 1990;20:54-57.

1216. Holmes, Lapeyre, Schuartz et al. Thrombectomy of occluded coronary arteries: an initial clinical experience. Circulation 1991;82:III-622.

1217. Kipperman RM, Feit AS, Einhorn AM, et al. Intracoronary thrombectomy: A new approach to total occlusion. Cathet Cardiovasc Diagn 1989;18:244-248.

1218. Haraphongse M and Rossall RE. Large air embolus complicating coronary angioplasty. Cathet Cardiovasc Diagn 1989;17:168-171.

1219. Burri C, Henkeneyer H, Passler HH. Katheterembolien. Schw Med Wschr 1971;101:1537.

1220. Hartzler G, Rutherford B, McConahay D. Retained percutaneous transluminal coronary angioplasty components and their management. Am J Cardiol 1987;60:1260-1264.

1221. Bogart DB, Earnest JB, and Miller JT. Foreign body retrieval using a simple snare device. Cathet Cardiovasc Diagn 1990;19:248-250.

1222. Mikolich JR and Hanson MW. Transcatheter retrieval of intracoronary detached angioplasty guidewire segment. Cathet Cardiovasc Diagn 1988:15:44-46.

1223. Savas V, Schreiber T and O'Neill W. Percutaneous extraction of fractured guidewire from distal right coronary artery. Cathet Cardiovasc Diagn 1991;22:124-126.

1224. Serota H, Deligonul U, Lew B, et al. Improved method for transcatheter retrieval of intracoronary detached angioplasty guidewire segments. Cathet Cardiovasc Diagn 1989;17:248-251.

1225. Gurley JC, Booth DC, Hixson C., et al. Removal of retained intracoronary percutaneous transluminal coronary angioplasty equipment by a percutaneous twin guidewire method. Cathet Cardiovasc Diagn 1990;19:251-256.

1226. Nyuyen K, Myler RK, Hieshima G, et al. Treatment of coronary artery stenosis and coronary arteriovenous fistula by interventional cardiology techniques. Cathet Cardiovasc Diagn 1989;18:240-243.

1227. Doorey AJ, Sullivan KL and Levin DC. Successful percutaneous closure of a complex coronary-to-pulmonary artery fistula using a detachable balloon: benefits of intra-procedural physiologic and angiographic assessment. Cathet Cardiovasc Diagn 1991;23:23-27.

1228. Jost S, Simon R, Amende I, et al. Transluminal balloon embolization of an inadvertent aorto-to-coronary venous bypass to the anterior cardiac vein. Cathet Cardiovasc Diagn 1989;17:28-30.

1229. Strunk BL, Hieshima GB and Shafton EP. Treatment of congenital coronary arteriovenous malformations with micro-particle embolization. Cathet Cardiovasc Diagn 1991;22:133-136.

1230. Jondeau G, Lacombe P, Rocha P, et al. Swan-ganz catheter-induced rupture of the pulmonary artery: successful early management by transcatheter embolization. Cathet Cardiovasc Diagn 1990;19:202-204.

1231. Watson LE. Snare loop technique for removal of broken steerable PTCA wire. Cathet Cardiovasc Diagn 1987;13:44-49.

1232. Interventional Radiology. Athanasoulis, Pfister, Greene, et al. 1982. W.B. Saunders, Co.

Coronary Artery Spasm

1233. Cowley M, Dorros G, Kelsey S, Van Raden M, Detre K. Acute coronary events associated with percutaneous transluminal coronary angioplasty. Am J Cardiol 1984;53:12C-16C.

1234. Holmes DJ, Holubkov R, Vlietstra R, et al. Comparison of complications during percutaneous transluminal coronary angioplasty from 1977 to 1981 and from 1985 to 1986: The National Heart, Lung, and Blood Institute Percutaneous Transluminal Coronary Angioplasty Registry. J Am Coll Cardiol 1988;12:1149-1155.

1235. Fitzgerald PJ, Stertzer SH, Hidalgo BO, et al. Plaque characteristics affect lesion and vessel response to coronary rotational atherectomy: An intravascular ultrasound study. J Am Coll Cardiol 1994:March Special Issue:353A.

1236. Fischell T, and Bausback K. Effects of luminal eccentricity on spontaneous coronary vasoconstriction after successful percutaneous transluminal coronary angioplasty. Am J Cardiol 1991;68:530-534.

1237. Corcos T, David PR, Bourassa MG, et al. Percutaneous transluminal coronary angioplasty for the treatment of variant angina. J Am Coll Cardiol 1985;5:1046-1054.

1238. David PR, Waters DD, Scholl M, et al. Percutaneous coronary angioplasty in patients with variant angina. Circulation 1982;66:695-702.
1239. Indolfi C, Piscione F, Esposito G, et al. Mechanisms of coronary vasoconstriction after successful single angioplasty of the left anterior descending artery. J Am Coll Cardiol 1993:February Special Issue:340A.
1240. Fischell T, Derby G, Tse T, Stadius M. Coronary artery vasoconstriction routinely occurs after percutaneous transluminal coronary angioplasty. A quantitative arteriographic analysis. Circulation 1988;78:1323-1334.
1241. Golino P, Piscione F, Benedict CF, et al. Local effect of serotonin released during coronary angioplasty. N Engl J Med 1994;330:523-8.
1242. Tousoulis D, Tentolouris C, Apostolopoulos T, Toutouzas P. Effects of intracoronary ketanserin in proximal and distal segments post angioplasty. J Am Coll Cardiol 1993:February Special Issue:341A.
1243. Hollman J, Austin GE, Gruentzig AR, et al. Coronary artery spasm at the site of angioplasty in the first two months after successful percutaneous transluminal coronary angioplasty. J Am Coll Cardiol 1983;2:1039-1045.
1244. Kirigaya H, Aizawa T, Ogasaware K, et al. Enhanced vasospastic activity to acetylcholine of the coronary arteries undergoing previous balloon angioplasty. J Am Coll Cardiol 1993:February Special Issue:341A.
1245. Cohen RA, Shepherd JT, and Vanhoutte PM. Inhibitory role of endothelium in the response of isolated coronary arteries to platelets. Science 1983;221:273-274.
1246. Lam JT, Chesebro JH, Steele PM, et al. Vasospasm related to platelet deposition? Relationship in a porcine preparation of arterial injury in vivo. Circulation 1987;75:243-248.
1247. Cohen RA, Zitany KM and Weisbrod RM. Accumulation of 5-hydroxy-tryptamine leads to dysfunction of adrenergic nerves in canine coronary artery following intimal damage in vivo. Circulation 1987;61:829-833.
1248. Gregorini L, Marco J, Fajadet J, Brunel, P, et al. Urapidil (α 1-sympathetic blocker) attenuates post-rotational ablation "elastic recoil". Circulation 1995;92:I-94.
1249. Ceravolo R, Piscoine F, Malone A, Stingone AM, et al. Reflex forearm vasoconstriction after successful angioplasty of the left anterior descending coronary artery. Circulation 1995;92:I-323.
1250. Ceravolo R, Indolfi C, Piscione F, et al. Coronary and limb vascular vasoconstriction after successful single angioplasty of the left anterior descending coronary artery. J Am Coll Cardiol 1995;February Special Issue:108A.
1251. Warth D, Leon M, et al. Rotational atherectomy multicenter registry: Acute results, complications and 6-month angiographic follow-up in 709 patients. J Am Coll Cardiol 1994;24:641-648.
1252. deMarchena EJ, Mallon SM, et al. Effectiveness of holmium laser-assisted coronary angioplasty. Am J Cardiol 1994;73:117-121.
1253. Bittl J, Sanborn T, et al. Clinical success, complications and restenosis rates with excimer laser coronary angioplasty. Am J Cardiol 1992;70:1533-1539.
1254. Ghazzal Z, Hearn J, et al. Morphological predictors of acute complications after percutaneous excimer laser coronary angioplasty. Results of a comprehensive angiographic analysis: Importance of the eccentricity index. Circulation 1992;86:820-827.
1255. Hinohara T, Rowe M, et al. Effect of lesion characteristics on outcome of directional coronary atherectomy. J Am Coll Cardiol 1991;17:1112-1120.
1256. Safian R, Niazi K, et al. Detailed Angiographic Analysis of High-Speed Mechanical Rotational Atherectomy in Human Coronary Arteries. Circulation 1993;88:961-968.
1257. Litvack F, Eigler N, et al. Percutaneous excimer laser coronary angioplasty: Results in the first consecutive 3,000 patients. J Am Coll Cardiol 1994;23:323-9.
1258. Baumback A, Bittl J, Fleck E, et al. Acute complications of excimer laser coronary angioplasty: A detailed analysis of multicenter results. J Am Coll Cardiol 1994;23:1305-1313.
1259. Mehta S, Popma JJ, Margolis JR, et al. Angiographic complications after new device angioplasty in native coronary arteries: A NACI Angiographic Core Laboratory Report. TCT Meeting (Washington DC),February, 1995.
1260. Bertrand M, Lablanche J, Leroy F, Bauters C. Percutaneous transluminal coronary rotary ablation with Rotablator (European experience). Am J Cardiol 1992;69:470-474.
1261. Teirstein PS, Warth DC, Haq N, et al. High-speed rotational coronary atherectomy for patients with diffuse coronary artery disease. J Am Coll Cardiol 1991;18:1694-1701.
1262. Initial results of the European Multicenter Registry on Coronary Excimer Laser Angioplasty. European Study Group. Circulation 1991;84:II-362.
1263. Babbitt DG, Perry JM, and Forman MB. Intracoronary verapamil for reversal of refractory coronary vasospasm during percutaneous transluminal coronary angioplasty. J Am Coll Cardiol 1988;12:1377-1381.
1264. McIvor ME, Undemir C, Lawson J, Reddinger J. Clinical effects and utility of intracoronary diltiazem. Cathet Cardiovasc Diagn. 1995;35:287-291.
1265. Ludmer PL. Selwyn AP, Shook TL, et al. Paradoxical vasoconstriction induced by acetylcholine in atherosclerotic coronary arteries. N Engl J Med 1988;315:1046-1051.
1266. Waters DD, Miller DD, Szlachcic J, et al. Factors influencing the long-term prognosis of treated patients with variant angina. Circulation 1983;63:258-265.
1267. Gaasch WH, Lufshanowski R, Leachment RD, et al. Surgical management of prinzmetal's variant angina. Chest 1974;66:614-621.
1268. Bertrand ME, LaBlanche JM, Thieuleux FA, et al. Comparative results of percutaneous transluminal coronary angioplasty in patients with dynamic versus fixed coronary stenosis. J Am Coll Cardiol 1986;8:504-508.
1269. Mehta S, Popma J, Margolis JR, et al. Complications with new angioplasty devices. Are these device specific? J Am Coll Cardiol 1996;27:168A.

Dissection & Acute Closure

1270. Ramee SR, White CJ, Jain A, et al. Percutaneous coronary angioscopy versus angiography in patients undergoing coronary angioplasty. J Am Coll Caridol 1991;17:125A.
1271. Tan K, Sulke N, Taub N, Sowton E. Clinical and lesion morphologic determinants of coronary angioplasty success and complications: Current experience. J Am Coll Cardiol 1995;25:855-65.
1272. Van Belle E, Bauters C, Lablanche J-M, McFadden E, Bertrand M. Angiographic determinants of acute outcome after coronary angioplasty: A prospective quantitative coronary angiographic study of 3679 procedures. J Am Coll Cardiol 1994:223A.
1273. Lincoff AM, Popma JJ, Ellis SG, Hacker J. Abrupt vessel closure complicating coronary angioplasty: Clinical, angiographic, and therapeutic profile. J Am Coll Cardiol 1992;19:926-935.
1274. Ellis S, Roubin G, King S, et al. In-hospital cardiac mortality after acute closure after coronary angioplasty: Analysis of risk factors from 8,207 procedures. J Am Coll Cardiol 1988;11:211-216.
1275. de Feyter PJ, van den Brand M, Jaarman G, van Domburg R. Acute coronary artery occlusion during and after percutaneous transluminal coronary angioplasty. Frequency, prediction, and clinical course, management, and follow-up. Circulation 1991;83:927-936.
1276. The Bypass Angioplasty Revascularization Investigation (BARI): Five year mortality and morbidity in a randomized study comparing CABG and PTCA in patients with multivessel coronary disease. The BARI Investigators. N Engl J Med (submitted).
1277. Simpfendorfer C, Belardi J, Bellamy G, Galan K. Frequency, management and follow-up of patients with acute coronary occlusions after percutaneous transluminal coronary angioplasty. Am J Cardiol 1987;59:267-269.
1278. Bansal A, Choksi NA, Levine AB, et al. Determinants of arterial dissection during PTCA: Lesion type versus inflation rate. J Am Coll Cardiol 1989;12:229A.
1279. Popma JJ, Topol EJ, Pinkerton CA, et al. Abrupt closure following directional coronary atherectomy: Clinical, angiographic and procedural outcome. J Am Coll Cardiol 1991;17:23A.
1280. Bertrand M, Lablanche J, Leroy F, Bauters C. Percutaneous transluminal coronary rotary ablation with Rotablator (European experience). Am J Cardiol 1992;69:470-474.
1281. Safian R, Lai S, Buchbinder M, Sanbron T, Sketch M. Incidence and management of abrupt closure after new device interventions. Report from the NACI Registry in 2988 lesions. Circulation 1993;88(Suppl.):I-585.
1282. Mehta S, Popma J, Margolis J, et al. Angiographic complications after new device angioplasty in native coronary arteries: A NACI Angiographic Core Laboratory Report. TCT Meeting (Washington DC), February, 1995.
1283. Popma J, Topol E, Hinohara T, et al. Abrupt vessel closure after directional coronary atherectomy. J Am Coll Cardiol 1992;19:1372-1379.
1284. Hinohara T, Rowe M, Robertson G, et al. Effect of lesion characteristics on outcome of directional coronary atherectomy. J Am Coll Cardiol 1991;17:1112-1120.
1285. Warth D, Leon M, O'Neill W, et al. Rotational atherectomy multicenter registry: Acute results, complications and 6-month angiographic follow-up in 709 patients. J Am Coll Cardiol 1994;24:641-648.
1286. Ellis S, Popma J, Buchbinder M, et al. Relation of clinical presentation, stenosis morphology, and operator technique to the procedural results of rotational atherectomy and rotational atherectomy--facilitated angioplasty. Circulation 1994;89:882-892.
1287. Safian R, Niazi K, et al. Detailed Angiographic Analysis of High-Speed Mechanical Rotational Atherectomy in Human Coronary Arteries. Circulation 1993;88: 961-968.
1288. Litvack F, Eigler N, Margolis J, et al. Percutaneous excimer laser coronary angioplasty: Results in the first consecutive 3,000 patients. J Am Coll Cardiol 1994;23:323-329.
1289. Painter J, Popma J, Pichard A, et al. A comparison of early and late clinical outcomes in patients undergoing concentric and directional laser coronary angioplasty. TCT Meeting (Washington DC), February, 1995.
1290. Chevalier B, Meyer P, Corcos T, et al. Delayed acute closure after rotational atherectomy: A multicenter registry. Circulation 1994;90:I-213.
1291. Huber M, Mooney J, Madison J, Mooney M. Use of a morphologic classification to predict clinical outcome after dissection from coronary angioplasty. Am J Cardiol 1991;68:467-471.
1292. Hermans WR, Foley DP, Rensing BJ, Rutsch W. Usefulness of quantitative and qualitative angiographic lesion morphology, and clinical characteristics in predicting major adverse cardiac events during and after native coronary balloon angioplasty. Am J Cardiol 1993;72:14-20.
1293. Bailey S, Ricci D, Kiesz S, et al. Incidence and clinical impact of dissections after PTCA and stent placement: Results from the Randomized STent REStenosis Study. TCT Meeting (Washington DC), February, 1995.
1294. Hermans WR, Rensing BJ, Foley DP, Deckers JW. Therapeutic dissection after successful coronary balloon angioplasty: No influence on restenosis or on clinical outcome in 693 patients. J Am Coll Cardiol 1992;20:767-780.
1295. Sharma SK, Israel DH, Kamean JL, Bodian CA. Clinical, angiographic, and procedural determinants of major and minor coronary dissection during angioplasty. Am Heart J 1993;126:39-47.
1296. Kovach J, Mintz G, Pichard A, et al. Sequential intravascular ultrasound characterization of the mechanisms of rotational atherectomy and adjunct balloon angioplasty. J Am Coll Cardiol 1993;22:1024-32.
1297. den Heijer P, Foley D, Escaned J, Hillege H. Angioscopic versus angiographic detection of intimal dissection and intracoronary thrombus. J Am Coll Cardiol 1994;24:649-654.
1298. Ghazzal Z, Hearn J, Litvack F, et al. Morphological predictors of acute complications after percutaneous excimer laser coronary angioplasty. Results of a comprehensive angiographic analysis: Importance of the eccentricity index. Circulation 1992;86:820-827.
1299. Baumbach A, Bittl J, Fleck E, Geschwind H, Sanborn T. Acute complications of excimer laser coronary angioplasty: A detailed analysis of multicenter results. J Am Coll Cardiol 1994;23:1305-1313.
1300. Dussaillant G, Popma J, Pichard A, et al. Rotational atherectomy vs. excimer laser angioplasty: A multivariable analysis of early and late procedural outcome. J Am Coll Cardiol 1995;25:330A.
1301. Brown D, Giordano F, Buchbinder M. Coronary dissection following rotational atherectomy: Clinical characteristics, angiographic

predictors and acute outcomes. J Am Coll Cardiol 1995;25:123A.

1302. Popma J, Knopf W, Davidson C, et al. Angiographic outcome after "cutting" balloon angioplasty. J Am Coll Cardiol 1995;25:268A.

1303. Knopf W, Yakubov S, Satler L, et al. Angiographic and procedural outcome after coronary angioplasty using a decremental diameter (tapered) balloon catheter. TCT Meeting (Washington DC), February, 1995.

1304. Fitzgerald PJ, Ports TA, Yock PG. Contribution of localized calcium deposits to dissection after angioplasty. An observational study using intravascular ultrasound. Circulation 1992;86:64-70.

1305. van Leeuwen T, Meertens J, Velema E, Post M, Borst C. Intraluminal vapor bubble induced by excimer laser pulse causes microsecond arterial dilation and invagination leading to extensive wall damage in the rabbit. Circulation 1993;87:1258.

1306. Tcheng J, Wells L, Phillips H, Deckelbaum L, Golobic R. Development of a new technique for reducing pressure pulse generation during 308-nm excimer laser coronary angioplasty. Cathet Cardiovas Diagn. 1995;34:15-22.

1307. Scott N, Weintraub W, Liberman H, Morris D, Douglas J, King S. Outcome after acute closure syndrome following coronary angioplasty. Circulation 1993;88:I-299.

1308. Popma J, Painter J, Pichard A, et al. Incidence, predictors, prognostic significance of coronary dissections after excimer laser coronary angioplasty (ELCA). TCT Meeting (Washington DC), February, 1995.

1309. Berry K, Drew T, McKendall G, et al. Balloon material as a risk factor for coronary angioplasty procedural complications. Circulation 1991;84:II-130.

1310. Mooney MR, Fishman-Mooney J, Longe TF, Brandenburg RO. Effect of balloon material on coronary angioplasty. Am J Cardiol 1992;69:1481-1482.

1311. Raymenants E, Bhandari S, Stammen F, De Scheerder I, Desmet W, Piessens J. Effects of angioplasty balloon material and lesion characteristics on the incidence of coronary dissection in 2150 dilated lesions. J Am Coll Cardiol 1993;21:291A.

1312. Talley JD, Blankenship S, Spokojny WA, Anderson HV, et al. Does the type of balloon material used in elective PTCA make a difference in clinical complications? Results from the CRAC study. Circulation 1995;92:I-74.

1313. Safian RD, Hoffmann MA, Almany S, et al. Comparison of coronary angioplasty with compliant and noncompliant balloons (The Angioplasty Compliance Trial). Am J Cardiol 1995;76:518-520.

1314. Cribier A, Elchaninoff H, Chan C, et al. Comparative effects of long (> 12 min) versus standard (<3 min) sequential balloon inflations in PTCA. Preliminary results of a prospective randomized study: Immediate results and restenosis rates. J Am Coll Cardiol 1994;23:58A.

1315. Remetz MS, Cabin HS, McConnell S, Cleman M. Gradual balloon inflation protocol reduces arterial damage following percutaneous transluminal coronary angioplasty. J Am Coll Cardiol 1988;11:131A.

1316. Ilia R, Cabin H, McConnell S. et al. Coronary angioplasty with gradual versus rapid balloon inflation. Cathet Cardiovasc Diagn 1993;29:199-202.

1317. Bansal A, Choksi N, Levein AB, et al. Determinants of arterial dissection after PTCA: lesion type versus inflation rate. J Am Coll Cardiol 1989;13:229A.

1318. Tenaglia AN, Quigley PJ, Kereiakes DJ, et al. Coronary angioplasty performed with a gradual and prolonged inflation using a perfusion balloon catheter: procedural success and restenosis rate. Am Heart J 1992;124:585-589.

1319. Farcot JC, Berland J, Stix A, et al. Gradual, low-pressure and prolonged (10 minutes) protected inflations decreased complications and improved results of proximal LAD angioplasty. Eur Heart J 1991;12:263.

1320. Shawl F, Dougherty K, Hoff S. Does inflation strategy influence acute outcome and long-term results. Circulation 1993;88:I-587.

1321. Blankenship J, Ford A, Henry S, Frey C. Coronary dissection resulting from angioplasty with slow oscillating vs. rapid inflation and slow vs. rapid deflation. Cath Cardiovasc Diagn. 1995;34:202-209.

1322. Foster C, Teskey R, Kells C, et al. Does the speed of balloon deflation affect the complication rate of coronary angioplasty. J Am Coll Cardiol 1993;21:290A.

1323. Banka V, Kochar G, Maniet A, Voci G. Progressive coronary dilation: An angioplasty technique that creates controlled arterial injury and reduces complications. Am Heart J 1993;125:61-71.

1324. McKeever LS, O'Donnell MJ, Stamato NJ, et al. The effect of predilatation on coronary angioplasty-induced vessel wall injury. Am Heart J 1991;122:1515-1518.

1325. Banka VS, Fail PS, Kochar GS, Maniet AR. Dual-balloon progressive coronary dilatation catheter: design and initial clinical experience. Am Heart J. 1994;127:430-435.

1326. Nobuyhshi M, Kimura T, Nosaka H, et al. Restenosis after successful percutaneous transluminal coronary angioplasty: Serial angiographic follow-up of 229 patients. J Am Coll Cardiol 1988;12:616-623.

1327. Cappelletti A, Margonato A, Berna G, Chierchia S. Spontaneous evolution of nonocclusive coronary dissection after PTCA: A 6-month angiographic follow-up study. J Am Coll Cardiol 1995;25:345A.

1328. Savage M, Dischman D, Bailey S, et al. Vascular remodeling of balloon-induced intimal dissection: Long-term angiographic assessment. J Am Coll Cardiol 1995;25:139A.

1329. Bell M, Berger PB, Reeder GS, et al. Coronary dissection following PTCA: Predictors of major ischemic complications. Circulation 1991;84:II-130.

1330. Bredlau CE, Roubin GS, Leimgruber PP, Douglas JS. In-hospital morbidity and mortality in patients undergoing elective coronary angioplasty. Circulation 1985;72:1044-1052. 71.

1331. Foley D, Hermans W, Rensing B, Serruys P. Predictability of major adverse cardiac events after balloon angioplasty from clinical data and quantitative and qualitative angiographic analysis. J Am Coll Cardiol 1993;21:339A.

1332. Ellis SG, Gallison L, Grines CL, et al. Incidence and predictors of early recurrent ischemia after successful percutaneous transluminal coronary angioplasty for acute myocardial infarction. Am J Cardiol 1989;63:263-268.

1333. Roubin GS, Lin S, Niederman A, et al. Clinical and anatomic descriptors for a major complication following PTCA. J Am Coll Cardiol 1987;9:20A.

1334. Ferguson J, Bittl J, Strony J, Adelman B. The relationship of dissection and thrombus after PTCA to in-hospital outcome: Results of a prospective multicenter study. Circulation 1993;88:I-217.

1335. Ellis S, Vandormael M, Cowley M, et al. Coronary morphologic and clinical determinants of procedural outcome with angioplasty for multivessel coronary disease. Circulation 1990;82:1193-1202.

1336. Detre KM, Holmes DR, Holubkow R, Cowley MJ. Incidence and consequences of periprocedural occlusion. The 1985-1986 National Heart, Lung, And Blood Institute Percutaneous Transluminal Coronary Angioplasty Registry. Circulation 1990;82:739-750.

1337. Ambrose J, Almeida O, Sharma S, Torre S. Adjunctive thrombolytic therapy during angioplasty for ischemic rest angina. Results of the TAUSA Trial. Circulation 1994;90:69-77.

1338. Ambrose J, Sharma S, Almeida O, et al. Delayed views post PTCA predict acute and in-hospital complications in patients with unstable angina. J Am Coll Cardiol 1995;25:392A.

1339. Tenaglia AN, Fortin DF, Frid DJ, Gardener LH. Long-term outcome following successful reopening of abrupt closure after coronary angioplasty. Am J Cardiol 1993;72:21-25.

1340. Barnathan E, Schwartz J, Taylor L, et al. Aspirin and dipyridamole in the prevention of acute coronary thrombosis complicating coronary angioplasty. Circulation 1987;76:125-134.

1341. Schwartz L, Bourassa MG, Lesperange J, Aldridge HE. Aspirin and dipyridamole in the prevention of restenosis after percutaneous transluminal coronary angioplasty. N Engl J Med 1988;318:1714-1719.

1342. Ellis S, Roubin G, King S, et al. Angiographic and clinical predictors of acute closure after native vessel coronary angioplasty. Circulation 1988;77:372-379.

1343. Tenaglia A, Fortin D, Califf R. Predicting the risk of abrupt closure after angioplasty in an individual patient. J Am Coll Cardiol 1994;24:1004-1011.

1344. Myler R, Shaw R, Stertzer S, et al. Lesion morphology and coronary angioplasty: Current experience and analysis. J Am Coll Cardiol 1992;19:1641-1652.

1345. Topol E, Bonan R, Jewitt D, et al. Use of a direct antithrombin, hirulog, in place of heparin during coronary angioplasty. Circulation 1993;87:1622.

1346. Ohman E, George B, White C, et al. Use of aortic counterpulsation to improve sustained coronary artery patency during acute myocardial infarction (Results of a randomized trial). Circulation 1994;90:792-799.

1347. Favereau X, Corcos T, Guerin Y, et al. Early reocclusion after successful coronary angioplasty of chronic total occlusions. J Am Coll Cardiol 1995;25:139A.

1348. Dougherty KG, Marsh KC, Edelman SK et al. Relationship between procedural activated clotting time and in-hospital post-PTCA outcome. Circulation 1990;82:111-189.

1349. Ellis SG, Myler RK, King SB, Douglas JS. Causes and correlates of death after unsupported coronary angioplasty: Implications for use of angioplasty and advanced support techniques in high-risk settings. Am J Cardiol 1991;68:1447-1451.

1350. Mufson L, Black A, Roubin G, et al. Randomized trial of aspirin in PTCA: Effect of high versus low dose aspirin on major complications and restenosis. J Am Coll Cardiol 1988;11:236A.

1351. Ogilby JD, Kopelman HA, Klein LW, et al. Adequate heparinization during PTCA: Assessment using activated clotting time. J Am Coll Cardiol 1988;11:237A.

1352. Gabliani G, Deligonul U, Kern M, Vandermael M. Acute coronary occlusion occurring after successful percutaneous transluminal coronary angioplasty: Temporal relationship to discontinuation of anticoagulation. Am Heart J 1988;116:696-700.

1353. Spielberg C, Schnitzer L, Linderer T, et al. Influence of catheter technology and adjunct medication on acute complications in percutaneous coronary angioplasty. Cathet Cardiovasc Diagn 1990;21:72-76.

1354. Ricci HR, Ray S, Buller CE, O'Neill B, et al. Six month follow-up of patients randomized to prolonged inflation of stent for abrupt occlusion during PTCA—Clinical and angiographic data: TASC II. Circulation 1995;92:I-475.

1355. de Muinck E, den Heijer P, van Dijk R. Autoperfusion balloon versus stent for acute or threatened closure during percutaneous transluminal coronary angioplasty. Am J Cardiol 1994;74:1002-1005.

1356. Barberis P, Marsico F, De Servi S, et al. Treatment of failed PTCA with perfusion balloon versus intracoronary stent: A short-term follow-up. J Am Coll Cardiol 1994:136A.

1357. Lincoff M, Topol E, Chapekis A, et al. Intracoronary stenting compared with conventional therapy for abrupt vessel closure complicating coronary angioplasty: A matched case-control study. J Am Coll Cardiol 1993;21:866-875.

1358. Bier J, Cannistra A, Mukherjee S, et al. Histopathologic findings following directional coronary atherectomy performed for failed balloon angioplasty. Circulation 1994;90:I-63.

1359. Berdan L, Holmes D, Davidson-Ray L, Lam L, Talley D, Mark D. Economic impact of abrupt closure following percutaneous intervention: The CAVEAT Experience. J Am Coll Cardiol 1994;23:434A.

1360. Movsowitz H, Emmi R, Manginas A, et al. Directional coronary atherectomy for failed balloon angioplasty: Outcome depends on the underlying pathology. Circulation 1993;88:I-601.

1361. Shaknovich A, Moses JW, Undemir C, Cohen NT, et al. Procedural and short-term clinical outcomes of multiple Palmaz-Schatz stents (PSSs) in very long lesions/dissections. Circulation 1995;92:I-535.

1362. Schieman G, Cohen BM, Kozina J, Erickson JS. Intracoronary urokinase for intracoronary thrombus accumulation complicating percutaneous transluminal coronary angioplasty in acute ischemic syndromes. Circulation 1990;82:2052-2060.

1363. Pavlides GS, Schreiber TL, Gangadharan V, et al. Safety and efficacy of urokinase during elective coronary angioplasty. Am Heart J 1991;121:731-737.

1364. Haft JL, Goldstein JE, Homoud MK, et al. PTCA following myocardial infarction: Use of bailout fibrinolysis to improve results. Am Heart J 1990;120:243-247.

1365. Hermann G, Zahorsky R, Meissner A, et al. Effects of acute rt-PA thrombolysis during PTA in patients with impending coronary occlusion. Eur Heart J 1990;11:23A.

1366. Gulba DC, Daniel WG, Simon R, Jost S. Role of thrombolysis and thrombin in patients with acute coronary occlusion during percutaneous transluminal coronary angioplasty. J Am Coll Cardiol 1990;16:563-568.

1367. Chapekis A, George B, Candela R. Rapid thrombus dissolution by continuous infusion of urokinase through an intracoronary perfusion wire prior to and following PTCA: Results in native coronaries and patent saphenous vein grafts. Cathet Cardiovasc Diagn 1991;23:89-92.
1368. Muhlestein JB, Gomez, MA, Karagounis LA, Anderson JL. "Rescue ReoPro": Acute utilization of abciximab for the dissolution of coronary thrombus developing as a complication of coronary angioplasty. Circulation 1995;92:I-607.
1369. Tenaglia AN, Fortin FD, Frid DJ, et al. Restenosis and long-term outcome following successful treatment of abrupt closure during and after angioplasty: Stabilization using a guidewire. Cathet Cardiovasc Diagn 1987;13:391-393.
1370. Piana RN, Ahmed WH, Ganz P, Dodge T Jr., et al. The legacy of uncomplicated abrupt vessel closure during coronary angioplasty: Increased ischemic events after hospital discharge. Circulation 1995;92:I-75.
1371. Abdelmeguid AE, Whitlow PL, Sapp SK, et al. Long-term outcome of transient, uncomplicated in-laboratory coronary artery closure. Circulation 1995;91:2733-2741.
1372. Deckelbaum LI, Natarajan MK, Bittl JA, et al. Effect of intracoronary saline infusion on dissection during excimer laser coronary angioplasty: A randomized trial. J Am Coll Cardiol 1995;26:1264-9.
1373. Holmes DR, Simpson JB, Berdan LG, et al. Abrupt closure: The CAVEAT I Experience. J Am Coll Cardiol 1995;26:1494-500.
1374. Zidar JP, Kruse KR, Thel MC, et al. Integrelin for emergency coronary artery stenting. J Am Coll Cardiol 1996;March Special Issue.
1375. Mehta S, Popma J, Margolis JR, et al. Complications with new angioplasty devices. Are these device specific? J Am Coll Cardiol 1996;March Special Issue.
1376. Popma JJ, Baim DS, Kuntz RE, et al. Early and late quantitative angiographic outcomes in the Optimal Atherectomy Restenosis Study (OARS). J Am Coll Cardiol 1996;March Special Issue.
1377. Ortiz-Fernandex A, Goicoles MJ, Perex-Vizcayno M, et al. Late clinical and angiographic outcome of bailout coronary stenting. A comparison study between Gianturco-Roubin and Palmaz-Schatz stents. J Am Coll Cardiol 1996;March Special Issue.
1378. Appleman YEA, Piek JJ, Strikwerda S, et al. Randomized trial of excimer laser angioplasty versus balloon angioplasty for treatment of obstructive coronary artery disease. Lancet 1996;347:79-84.
1379. Goy JJ, Eeckhout E, Stauffer J-C, Vogt P, Kappenberger L. Emergency endoluminal stenting for abrupt vessel closure following coronary angioplasty: A randomized comparison of the Wiktor and Palmaz-Schatz stents. Cathet Cardiovasc Diagn. 1995;34:128-132.
1380. Urban P, Chatelain P, Brzostek T, Jaup T, Verine V, Rutishauser W. Bailout coronary stenting with 6F guiding catheters for failed balloon angioplasty. Am Heart J 1995;129:1078-83.
1381. Metz D, Urban P, Camenzind E, Chatelain P, Hoang V, Meier B. Improving results of bailout coronary stenting after failed balloon angioplasty. Cathet Cardiovasc Diagn. 1994;32:117-124.
1382. Schomig A, Kastrati A, Mudra H, et al. Four-year experience with Palmaz-Schatz stenting in coronary angioplasty complicated by dissection with threatened or present vessel closure. Circulation 1994;90:2716-2724.
1383. Kiemeneij F, Laarman G, van der Wieken R, Suwarganda J. Emergency coronary stenting with the Palmaz-Schatz stent for failed transluminal coronary angioplasty: results of a learning phase. Am Heart J 1993;126:23-31.
1384. Reifart N, Haase J, Preusler W, Schwartz F, Storger H. Randomized trial comparing two devices: The Palmaz-Schatz stent and the Strecker stent in bail-out situations. J Interven Cardiol 1994;7:539-547.
1385. Chan C, Tan A, Koh T, Koh P. Intracoronary stenting in the treatment of acute or threatened closure in angiographically small coronary arteries (<3.0 mm) complicating percutaneous transluminal coronary angioplasty. Am J Cardiol 1995;75:23-25.
1386. Sutton J, Ellis S, Roubin G, et al. Major Clinical events after coronary stenting. The multicenter registry of acute and elective Gianturco-Roubin stent placement. Circulation 1994;89:1126-1137.
1387. Agrawal S, Ho D, Liu M, et al. Predictors of thrombotic complications after placement of the flexible coil stent. Am J Cardiol 1994;73:1216-1219.
1388. George B, Voorhees W, Roubin G, et al. Multicenter investigation of coronary stenting to treat acute or treated closure after percutaneous transluminal coronary angioplasty: Clinical and angiographic outcomes. J Am Coll Cardiol 1993;22:135-143.
1389. Roubin G, Cannon A, Agrawal S, et al. Intracoronary stenting for acute and threatened closure complicating percutaneous transluminal coronary angioplasty. Circulation 1992;85:916-927.
1390. Vrolix MC, Rutsch W, Piessens J, Kober G, Wiegand V. Bail-out stenting with Medtronic Wiktor: Results from the European stent study group. J Interven Cardiol 1994;7:549-555.
1391. Garratt K, White C, Buchbinder M, Whitlow P, Heuser R. Wiktor stent placement for unsuccessful coronary angioplasty. Circulation 1994;90:I-279.
1392. Ozaki Y, Keane D, Ruygrok P, de Feyter P, Stertzer S, Serruys P. Acute clinical and angiographic results with the new AVE micro coronary stent in bailout management. Am J Cardiol 1995;76:112-116.

No-Reflow

1393. Kloner RA, Ganote CE, Jennings RB. The "no-reflow" phenomenon after temporary coronary occlusion in the dog. J Clin Invest 1974;54:1496-1508.
1394. Kloner RA. No-reflow revisited. J Am Coll Cardiol 1989;14:1814-1815.
1395. Kitazume H, Iwama T, Kubo H, et al. No-reflow phenomenon during percutaneous transluminal coronary angioplasty. Am Heart J 1988;116:211-215.
1396. Wilson RF, Lesser JR, Laxson DD, et al. Intense microvascular constriction after angioplasty of acute thrombotic coronary arterial lesions. Lancet 1989:801-811.
1397. Piana RN, Paik GY, Moscucci M, et al. Incidence and treatment of no-reflow after percutaneous coronary intervention. Circulation 1994;89:2514-2518.

1398. Ellis SG, Popma JJ, Buchbinder M, et al. Relation of clinical presentation, stenosis morphology, and operator technique to the procedural results of rotational atherectomy and rotational atherectomy-facilitated angioplasty. Circulation 1994;89:882-892.

1399. Abbo KM, Dooris M, Glazier S, et al. No-reflow after percutaneous coronary intervention: Clinical and angiographic characteristics, treatment and outcome. Am J Cardiol 1995;75:778-782.

1400. Feld H, Schulhoff N, Lichstein E, et al. Direct angioplasty as primary treatment for acute myocardial infarction resulting in the no-reflow phenomenon predicts a high mortality rate. Circulation 1992;86 (suppl);I-135.

1401. Pomerantz RM, Kuntz RE, Diver DJ, et al. Intracoronary verapamil for the treatment of distal microvascular spasm following PTCA. Cath and Cardiovasc Diagn 1991;24:283-288.

1402. Ritchie JL, Hansen D, Johnson C, et al. Combined mechanical and chemical thrombolysis in an experimental animal model: Evaluation by angiography and angioscopy. Am Heart J 1990;119-164.

1403. Wyrens FJ, Mooney J, Lesser J, Mooney MR. Intracoronary diltiazem for microvascular spasm after interventional therapy. Am J Cardiol 1995;75:849-850.

1404. Shani J, Feld H, Frankel R, Hollander G. Clinical cardiology: percutaneous transluminal coronary angioplasty in ischemic syndromes. Circulation 1992;86:I-852.

1405. Safian RD, Niazi KA, Strzelecki M, et al. Detailed angiographic analysis of high-speed mechanical rotational atherectomy in human coronary arteries. Circulation 1993;88:961-968.

1406. Ellis SG, Popma JJ, Buchbinder M, et al. Relation of clinical presentation, stenosis morphology, and operator technique to the procedural results of rotational atherectomy and rotational atherectomy-facilitated angioplasty. Circulation 1994;89:882-892.

1407. Warth DC, Leon MB, O'Neill W, et al. Rotational atherectomy multicenter registry: Acute results, complications and 6-month angiographic follow-up in 709 patients. J Am Coll Cardiol 1994;24:641-8.

1408. Ramee SR, White CJ, Jain A, et al. Percutaneous coronary angioscopy versus intravascular ultrasound in patients undergoing coronary angioplasty. J Am Coll Cardiol 1991;17:125A.

1409. Kloner RA, Alker KJ. The effect of streptokinase on intramyocardial hemorrhage, infarct size, and the "no-reflow" phenomenon during coronary reperfusion. Circulation 1984;70:513-521.

1410. Kloner RA, Alker K, Campbell C, et al. Does tissue-type plasminogen activator have direct beneficial effects on the myocardium independent of its ability to lyse intracoronary thrombi? Circulation 1989;79:1125-1136.

Perforation

1411. 1410.Ajuni SC, Glazier S, Blankenship L, et al. Perforations after percutaneous coronary interventions: clinical, angiographic, and therapeutic observations. Cath Cardiovasc Diagn. 1994;32:206-212.

1412. Ellis SG, Ajluni S, Arnold AZ, et al. Increased coronary perforation in the new device era. Incidence, classification, management, and outcome. Circulation 1994;90:2725-2730.

1413. Flood RD, Popma JJ, Chuang, Ya Chien, et al. Incidence, angiographic predictors, and clinical significance of coronary perforation occurring after new device angioplasty. J Am Coll Cardiol 1994;23:301A.

1414. Lansky A, Popma JJ, Baim DS, et al. Angiographic outcome after new devices saphenous vein graft Angioplasty. Abstract from Transcatheter Cardiovascular Therapeutics, 1995.

1415. Bittl JA, Ryan TJ, Keaney JF, et al. Coronary artery perforation during excimer laser coronary angioplasty. J Am Coll Cardiol 1993;21:1158-1165.

1416. Holmes DR, Reeder GS, Ghazzai ZM, et al. Coronary perforation after excimer laser coronary angioplasty: the excimer laser coronary angioplasty registry experience. J Am Coll Cardiol 1994;23:330-335.

1417. Cowley MJ, Dorros G, and Kelsey SF. Acute coronary events associated with percutaneous transluminal coronary angioplasty. Am J Cardiol 1984;53:12C-16C.

1418. Saffitz JE, Rose TE, Oaks JB, et al. Coronary arterial rupture during coronary angioplasty. Am J Cardiol 1983;51:902-904.

1419. Kimbiris DM, Iskandrian AS, Goel I, et al. Transluminal coronary angioplasty complicated by coronary artery perforation. Cathet Cardiovasc Diagn 1982;8:481-487.

1420. Iannone LA and Iannone DP. Iatrogenic left coronary artery fistula-to-left ventricle following PTCA: A previously unreported complication with nonsurgical treatment. Am Heart J 1990;120:1215-1217.

1421. Cherry S and Vandormael M. Rupture of a coronary artery and hemorrhage into the ventricular cavity during coronary angioplasty. Am Heart J 1990;113:386-388.

1422. Teirstein PS and Hartzler GO. Nonoperative management of aortocoronary saphenous vein graft rupture during percutaneous transluminal coronary angioplasty. Am J Cardiol 1987;60:377-378.

1423. Meier B. Benign coronary perforation during percutaneous transluminal coronary angioplasty. Br Heart J 1985;54:33-35.

1424. Grollier G, Bories H, Commeau P, et al. Coronary artery perforation during coronary angioplasty. Clin Cardiol 1986;9:27-29.

1425. Benzuly K, Safian RD. Coronary artery perforation: an unreported complication after stenting. Cathet Cardiovasc Diagn (in-press).

1426. Cohen BM, Weber VJ, Bass TA, et al. Coronary perforation during rotational ablation: Angiographic determinants and clinical outcome. J Am Coll Cardiol 1994;23:354A.

1427. Mehta S, Popma J, Margolis JR, Moore L, et al. Complications with new angioplasty devices. Are these device specific? J Am Coll Cardiol 1996;27 (supplement A):168A.

1428. Dorros G, Jain A, Kumar K. Management of coronary artery rupture: Covered stent or microcoild embolization. Cathet Cardiovasc Diagn. 1995;36:148-154.

1429. Kaplan BM, Stewart RE, Sakwa MP, et al. Repair of a coronary pseudoaneurysm with percutaneous placement of a saphenous vein allograft attached to a biliary stent. Cathet Cardiovasc Diagn. 1996;37:208-212.

Emergent CABG for Failed PTCA

1430. Craver JM, Weintraub WS, Jones EL, et. al. Emergency coronary artery bypass surgery for failed percutaneous coronary angioplasty. An Surg 1992; 215:425-433.
1431. Vogel JH. Changing trends for surgical standby in patients undergoing percutaneous transluminal coronary angioplasty. Am J Cardiol. 1992; 69:25F-35F.
1432. Cameron DE, Stinson DC, Greene PS, et al. Surgical standby for percutaneous coronary angioplasty: "A survey of patterns of practice." An Thoracic Surg 1990;50:35-39.
1433. Iniguez A, Macaya C, Hernandez R, et al. Comparison of results of percutaneous Transluminal coronary angioplasty with and without selective requirement of surgical standby. Am J of Cardiology; 1992; 69:1161-1165.
1434. Klinke WP and Hui W. Percutaneous transluminal angioplasty without on-site surgical facilities. Am J Cardiology 1992;70:1520-1525.
1435. Richardson SG, Morton P, Murtagh JG, et al. Management of acute coronary occlusion during percutaneous coronary angioplasty: "Experience of complications in a hospital without on-site facilities for cardiac surgery." British Med J 1990;300:355-358.
1436. Meier B. Surgical standby for PTCA. In: Textbook of Interventional Cardiology, E. Topol (Ed) WB Sanders 1994; p. 565-575.
1437. Feyter PJ, Jaegere PP, Murphy ES, et al. Abrupt coronary artery occlusion during percutaneous transluminal coronary angioplasty. Am Heart J 1992;123:1633-1642.
1438. Scott NA, Weintraub WS, Carlin SF, et al. Recent changes in the management and outcome of acute closure after percutaneous transluminal coronary angioplasty. Am J of Cardiology 1993;71:1159-1163.
1439. Lazar HL, Faxon DP, Paone G, et al. Changing profiles of failed coronary angioplasty patients: Impact on surgical results. Ann Thorac Surg 1992;53:269-273.
1440. Greene MA, Gary LA, Slater D, et al. Emergency aortocoronary bypass after failed angioplasty. Ann Thorac Surg 1991;51:194-199.
1441. Taylor PC, Boylan MJ, Lytle BW, et al. Emergent coronary bypass for failed PTCA: A 10-year experience with 253 patients. J Invasive Cardiol 1994;6:97-98.
1442. Carey JA, Davres SW, Balcon R, et al. Emergency surgical revascularization for coronary angioplasty complications. Br. Heart J 1994; 72:428-435.
1443. Glick DB, Liddicoat JR, Karp RB. Alternative conduits for coronary artery bypass grafting. Advances in Cardiac Surgery. RB Karp (Ed) Mosby Year Book 1990 p. 191-201.
1444. Piana RN, Paik GY, Moscucci M, et al. Incidence and treatment of no-reflow after percutaneous coronary intervention. Civc 1994;89:2514-2518.
1445. Denny TL, Magovern JA, Kao RL, et al. Resuscitation of injured myocardium with adenosine and biventricular assist. Ann Thorac Surg 1993;105:864-884.
1446. Allen BS, Buckberg GD, Fontain RM, et al. Superiority of controlled surgical reprfusion versus percutaneous transluminal coronary angioplasty in acute coronary occlusion. J Thorac Cardiovasc Surg; 1993;105:864-884.
1447. Lazar HL, Haan CK. Determinants of myocardial infarction following emergency coronary artery bypass for failed percutaneous coronary angioplasty. Ann Thorac Surg 1987;44:646-650.
1448. Pelletier LC, Pardini A, Renkin J, et al. Myocardial revascularization after failure of percutaneous transluminal coronary angioplasty. J Thorac Cardiovasc Surg 1985;90:265-271.
1449. Brediau CE, Roubin GS, Leimgruber PP, et al. In-hospital morbidity and mortality in patients undergoing elective coronary angioplasty. Circulation 1985;72:1044-1052.
1450. Acinapura AJ, Cummingham JN Jr, Jacobowitz IJ, et al. Efficacy of percutaneous transluminal coronary angioplasty compared with single-vessel bypass. J Thorac Cardiovasc Surg 1985;89:35-41.
1451. Killen DA, Hamaker WR, Reed WA. Coronary artery bypass following percutaneous transluminal coronary angioplasty. Ann Thorac Surg 1985;40:133-138.
1452. Golding LA, Loop FD, Hollman JL, et al. Early results of emergency surgery after coronary angioplasty. Circulation 1986;74:, III-26.
1453. Parsonnet V, Fisch D, Gielchinsky I, et al. Emergency operation after failed angioplasty. J Thorac Cardiovasc Surg 1988; 96:198-203.
1454. Naunheim KS, Fiore AC, Fagan D et al. Emergency coronary artery bypass grafting for failed angioplasty: Risk factors and outcome. Ann Thorac Surg 1989;47:816-823.
1455. Stark KS, Satler LF, Krucoff MW, et al. myocardial salvage after failed coronary angioplasty. J Am Coll Cardiol 1990;15:78-82.
1456. Kahn JK, Rutherford BD, McConahy DR, et al. Outcome following emergency coronary artery bypass grafting for failed elective balloon coronary angioplasty in patients with prior coronary bypass. Am J Cardiol 1990; 66: 285-288.
1457. Barner HB, LEA IV JW, Naunheim KS, et al. Emergency coronary bypass not associated with pre-operative cardiogenic shock in failed angioplasty, after thrombolysis and for acute myocardial infarction. Civc Suppl. I 1989;79:I152-I159.
1458. Clark RE, Acinapura J, Anderson RD, et al. Data analysis of the Society of Thoracic Surgeons. National Cardiac Surgery Database. 1994, p78.
1459. Boerher JD, Kereiakes DJ, Maveita FL, et al. Effects of profound platelet inhibition with c 7E3 before coronary angioplasty an complications of coronary bypass surgery. Am J Cardiol. 1994;74: 1166-1170.

Restenosis

1460. Gruentzig AR. Transluminal dilatation of coronary artery stenoses. Lancet 1978;1:263.
1461. Baim DS (ed): A symposium: Interventional Cardiology-1987. Am J Cardiol 1988;61:1g-117g.

1462. Detre K, Holubkov R, Kelsey S, et al. Percutaneous transluminal coronary angioplasty in 1985-1986 and 1977-1981. The National Heart, Lung and Blood Institute Registry. N Engl J Med 1988;318:265-270.

1463. Gruentzig AR, King SB III, Schlumpf M., et al. Long-term follow-up after percutaneous transluminal coronary angioplasty. The early Zurich experience. N Engl J Med. 1987;316:1127-1132.

1464. Parisi AF, Folland ED, Hartigan P. A comparison of angioplasty with medical therapy in the treatment of single vessel coronary disease. Veterans Affairs ACME Investigators. N Engl J Med 1992;326:10-16.

1465. Goy JJ, Eeckhout E, Burnand B et al. Coronary angioplasty versus left internal mammary artery grafting for isolated proximal left anterior descending artery stenosis. Lancet 1994;343:1449-1453.

1466. Coronary angioplasty versus coronary artery bypass surgery: the Randomized Intervention Treatment of Angina (RITA) trial. Lancet 1993;341:573-380.

1467. Roubin G, King SI, Douglas J, JR. Restenosis after percutaneous transluminal coronary angioplasty: The Emory University Hospital experience. Am J Cardiol 1987;60:39B-43B.

1468. Gould K, Lipscomb K, Hamilton G. Physiological basis for assessing critical coronary stenosis: instantaneous flow response and regional distribution during coronary hyperemia as measures of coronary flow reserve. Am J Cardiol 1974;33:87-97.

1469. Beatt KJ, Serruys PW, Renseing BJ, Hugenoltz PG. Restenosis after coronary angioplasty: New standards for clinical studies. J Am Coll Cardiol 1990;15:491-498.

1470. Beatt KJ, Luijten H, de Feyter P, van den Brand M, Reiber J, Serruys P. Change in diameter of coronary artery segments adjacent to stenosis after percutaneous transluminal coronary angioplasty: Failure of percent diameter stenosis measurement to reflect morphologic changes induced by balloon dilation. J Am Coll Cardiol 1988;12:315-323.

1471. Rensing BJ, Hermans WM, Deckers JW, deFeyter PJ. Lumen narrowing after percutaneous transluminal coronary balloon angioplasty follows a near gaussian distribution: A quantitative angiographic study in 1,445 successfully dilated lesions. J Am Coll Cardiol 1992;19:939-945.

1472. Kuntz R, Safian R, Levine M, Reis G, Diver D, Baim D. Novel approach to the analysis of restenosis after the use of three new coronary devices. J Am Coll Cardiol 1992;19:1493-1499.

1473. Gordon PC, Gibson M, Cohen DJ, Carrozza J, Kuntz R, Baim D. Mechanisms of restenosis and redilation within coronary stents-quantitative angiographic assessment. J Am Coll Cardiol 1993;21:1166-1174.

1474. Kuntz RE, Gibson CM, Nobuyoshi M, Baim DS. Generalized model of restenosis after conventional balloon angioplasty, stenting and directional atherectomy. J Am Coll Cardiol 1993;21:15-25.

1475. Schwartz R, Huber K, Murphy J, et al. Restenosis and the proportional neointimal response to coronary artery injury: Results in a porcine model. J Am Coll Cardiol 1992;19:267-274.

1476. Beatt KJ, Serruys PW, Luijten HE, et al. Restenosis after coronary angioplasty: The paradox of increased lumen diameter and restenosis. J Am Coll Cardiol 1992;19:258-266.

1477. Holmes D, Vlietstra R, Smith H, et al. Restenosis after percutaneous transluminal coronary angioplasty (PTCA): a report from the PTCA Registry of the NHLBI. Am J Cardiol 1984;53:77C-81C.

1478. Gruentzig AR, King SB III, Schlumpf M, et al. Long term follow-up after percutaneous transluminal coronary angioplasty. The early Zurich experience. N Engl J Med 1987;316:1127-1132.

1479. Fishman D, Leon M, Baim D. A randomized comparison of coronary stent placement and balloon angioplasty in the treatment of coronary artery disease. N Engl J Med 1994;331:496-501.

1480. Serruys P, deJegere P, Kiemeneij F, et al. A comparison of balloon expandable stent implantation with balloon angioplasty in patients with coronary artery disease. N Engl J Med 1994;331(8):489-495.

1481. Rodriguez A, Santaera O, Larribau M, et al. Coronary stenting decreases restenosis in lesions with early loss in luminal diameter 24 hours after successful PTCA. Circulation 1995;91:1397-1402.

1482. Rensing BJ, Hermans WRM, Beatt KJ, et al. Quantitative angiographic assessment of elastic recoil after percutaneous transluminal coronary angiography. Am J Cardiol 1990;66:1039-1044.

1483. Rodriguez A, Lassileau M, Santaera O, et al. Early decreases in minimal luminal diameter after PTCA are associated with higher incidence of late restenosis. J Am Coll Cardiol 1993;21:34A.

1484. LaBlanche JM on behalf of the FACT Investigators. Recoil twenty-four hours after coronary angioplasty: A computerized angiographic study. J Am Coll Cardiol 1993;21:34A.

1485. Johnson DE, Hinohara T, Selmon MR, Braden LJ. Primary peripheral arterial stenoses and restenoses excised by transluminal atherectomy: A histopathologic study. J Am Coll Cardiol 1990;15:419-425.

1486. Garratt K, Edwards W, Kaufmann U, Vlietstra R, Holmes D. Differential histopathology of primary atherosclerotic and restenotic lesions in coronary arteries and saphenous vein bypass grafts: Analysis of tissue obtained from 73 patients by directional atherectomy. J Am Coll Cardiol 1991;17:442-448.

1487. Post M, Borst C, Kuntz R. The relative importance of arterial remodeling compared with intimal hyperplasia in lumen renarrowing after balloon angioplasty (A study in the normal rabbit and the hypercholesterolemic Yucatan micropig). Circulation 1994;89:2816-2821.

1488. Lafont A, Guzman L, PLW. Restenosis after experimental angioplasty. Intimal, medial and adventitial changes associated with constrictive remodeling. Circ Res 1995;76:996-1002.

1489. Mintz G, Kovach J, Javier S, Ditrano C, Leon M. Geometric remodeling is the predominant mechanism of late lumen loss after coronary angioplasty. Circulation 1993;88:I-654.

1490. Serruys PW, Luijten HE, Beatt KJ, et al. Incidence of restenosis after successful coronary angioplasty: a time-related phenomenon. A quantitative angiographic study in 342 consecutive patients at 1, 2, 3, and 4 months. Circulation 1988;77:361-371.

1491. Nobuyoshi M, Kimura T, Nosaka H, Mioka S. Restenosis after successful percutaneous transluminal coronary angioplasty: Serial angiographic follow-up of 229 patients. J Am Coll Cardiol 1988;12:616-623.

1492. Guidance for the Submission of Research and Marketing Applications for Interventional Cardiology Devices: PTCA Catheters,

Atherectomy Catheters, Lasers, Intravascular Stents. Interventional Cardiology Devices Branch, Division of Cardiovascular, Respiratory and Neurology Devices, Office of Device Evaluation, US Food and Drug Administration, May 1993:29.

1493. Kimura T, Yokoi H, Tamura T, Nakagawa Y, Nosaka H, Nobuyoshi M. Three years clinical and quantitative angiographic follow-up after the Palmaz-Schatz coronary stent implantation. J Am Coll Cardiol 1995;25:375A.

1494. Hermiller J, Fry E, Peters T, et al. Late lesion regression within the Gianturco-Roubin Flex stent. J Am Coll Cardiol 1995;25`:375A.

1495. Kimura T, Nosaka H, Yokoi H, Iwabuchi M. Serial angiographic follow-up after Palmaz-Schatz stent implantation: Comparison with conventional balloon angioplasty. J Am Coll Cardiol 1993;21:1557-1563.

1496. Kuntz R, Safian R, Carrozza J, Fishman R, Mansour M, Baim D. The importance of acute luminal diameter in determining restenosis after coronary atherectomy or stenting. Circulation 1992;86:1827-1835.

1497. Topol E, Leya F, Pinkerton C, et al. A comparison of directional atherectomy with coronary angioplasty in patients with coronary artery disease. N Engl J Med 1993;329:221-227.

1498. Vandormael M, Reifart N, Preusler W, et al. Comparison of excimer laser angioplasty and rotational atherectomy with balloon angioplasty for complex lesions: ERBAC study final results. J Am Coll Cardiol 1994;57A.

1499. Spears JR, Reyes VP, Wynne J, et al. Percutaneous coronary laser balloon angioplasty: Initial results of a multicenter experience. J Am Coll Cardiol 1990;16:293-303.

1500. Umans VAWM, Keane D, Foley D, et al. Optimal use of directional coronary atherectomy is required to ensure long-term angiographic benefit: A study with matched procedural outcome after atherectomy and angioplasty. J Am Coll Cardiol 1994;24:1652-1659.

1501. Garratt KN, Holmes DR, Bell MR, et al. Restenosis after directional coronary atherectomy: differences between primary atheromatous and restenosis lesions and influence of subintimal tissue resection. J Am Coll Cardiol 1990;16:1665-1671.

1502. Kuntz RE, Hinohara T, Safian RD, et al. Restenosis after directional coronary atherectomy: Effects of luminal diameter and deep wall excision. Circulation 1992;86:1394-1399.

1503. Carrozza JR, Kuntz RE, Fishman RF, Baim DS. Restenosis after arterial injury caused by coronary stenting in patients with diabetes mellitus. Ann Intern Med. 1993;118(5):344-349.

1504. Simons M, Leclerc G, Safian RD, Isner JM. Relation between activated smooth-muscle cells in coronary artery lesions and restenosis after atherectomy. N Engl J Med 1993;328:608-613.

1505. Kuntz RE, Hinohara T, Robertson GC, et al. Influence of vessel selection on the observed restenosis rate after endoluminal stenting or directional coronary atherectomy. Am J Cardiol 1992;70:1101-1108.

1506. Hirshfeld JW, Schwartz JS, Jugo R, et al. Restenosis after coronary angioplasty: A multivariate statistical model to relate lesion and procedure variables to restenosis. J Am Coll Cardiol 1991;18:647-656.

1507. Hermans WR, Rensing BJ, Kelder JC, et al. Postangioplasty restenosis rate between segments of the major coronary arteries. Am J Cardiol 1992;194-200.

1508. Violaris A, Melkert R, Serruys P. Influence of serum cholesterol and cholesterol subfractions on restenosis after successful coronary angioplasty. A quantitative angiographic analysis of 3336 lesions. Circulation 1994;90:2267-2279.

1509. Fishman RF, Kuntz RE, Carrozza JP, Miller MJ, et al. Long-term results of directional coronary atherectomy: Predictors of restenosis. J Am Coll Cardiol 1992;20:1101-1110.

1510. Williams DO, Gruentzig A, Kent K, Detre K, Kelsey S, To T. Efficacy of repeat percutaneous transluminal coronary angioplasty for coronary restenosis. Am J Cardiol 1984;53:32C-35C.

1511. Dimas AP, Grigera F, Arora RR, et al. Repeat coronary angioplasty as treatment for restenosis. J Am Coll Cardiol 1992;19:1310-1314.

1512. Meier B, King SBI, Gruentzig AR. Repeat coronary angioplasty. J Am Coll Cardiol 1984;4:463-466.

1513. Moscucci M, Piana R, Kuntz R, Kugelmass A, et al. The effect of prior coronary restenosis on the risk of subsequent restenosis after stent placement or directional atherectomy. Am J Cardiol 1994;73:1147-1153.

1514. Glazier J, Varricchione T, Ryan T. Factors predicting recurrent restenosis after percutaneous transluminal coronary balloon angioplasty. Am J Cardiol 1989;63:902-905.

1515. Quigley P, Hlatky M, Hinohara T. Repeat percutaneous transluminal coronary angioplasty and predictors of recurrent restenosis. Am J Cardiol 1989;63:409-413.

1516. Hinohara T, Robertson G, Selmon M, et al. Restenosis after directional coronary atherectomy. J Am Coll Cardiol 1992;20:623-632.

1517. Teirstein P, Hoover C, Ligon R. Repeat coronary angioplasty: Efficacy of a third angioplasty for a second restenosis. J Am Coll Cardiol 1989;13:291-296.

1518. Hillegass WB, Ohman ME and Califf RM. Restenosis: the clinical issues. In Topol EJ (ed). Textbook of Interventional Cardiology, 2nd Edition, Philadelphia, WB Saunders Company, 1993; 415-435.

1519. Topol E, Califf R, Weisman H, et al. Randomized trial of coronary intervention with antibody against platelet IIb/IIIa integrin for reduction of clinical restenosis: results at six months. Lancet 1994;343:881-86.

1520. Emanuelsson H, Beatt K, Bagger J. Long-term effects of angiopeptine treatment in coronary angioplasty. Reduction of clinical events but not of angiographic restenosis. European Angiopeptin Study Group. Circulation 1995;91:1689-1696.

1521. Safian RD, Hoffmann MA, Almany S, et al. Comparison of coronary angioplasty with compliant and noncompliant balloons (The Angioplasty Compliance Trial). Am J Cardiol 1995;76:518-520.

1522. DiSciascio G, Vetrovec GW, Lewis SA, et al. Clinical and angiographic recurrence following PTCA for nonacute total occlusions: comparisons of one versus five minute inflations. Am Heart J 1990;120:529-532.

1523. Ohman EM, Marquis JF, Ricci DR, et al. A randomized comparison of the effects of gradual prolonged versus standard primary balloon inflation on early and late outcome. Results of a multicenter clinical trial. Perfusion Balloon Catheter Study Group. Circulation 1994;89:1118-1125.

1524. Roubin GS, Douglas JS, King SB, et al. Influence of balloon size on initial success rate, acute complications, and restenosis after PTCA. Circulation 1988;78:557-565.

1525. Piana R, Moscucci M, Cohen D, et al. Palmaz-Schatz stenting for treatment of focal vein graft stenosis: Immediate results and long-term outcome. J Am Coll Cardiol 1994;23:1296-304.
1526. Wong SC, Baim DS, Schatz RA, et al. Immediate results and late outcomes after stent implantation in saphenous vein graft lesions: the multicenter U.S. Palmaz-Schatz stent experience. J Am Coll Cardiol 1995;26:704-712.
1527. Simonton CA, Leon MB, Kuntz RE, et al. Acute and late clinical and angiographic results of directional atherectomy in the optimal atherectomy restenosis study (OARS). Circulation 1995;92:I-545.
1528. Baim DS, Kuntz RE, Sharma SK, et al. Acute and late results of the Balloon versus Optimal Atherectomy Trial (BOAT). Circulation 1995;92:I-544.
1529. Colombo A, Hall P, Nakamura S, et al. Intracoronary stenting without anticoagluation accomplished with intravascular ultrasound guidance. Circulation 1995;91:1676-1688.
1530. Russo RJ, Teirstin PS for the AVID investigators. Angiography versus intravascular ultrasound-directed stent placement. Circulation 1995;92:I-546.
1531. Bengston J, Mark D, Honan M. Detection of restenosis after elective percutaneous transluminal angioplasty using the exercise treadmill test. Am J Cardiol 1990;65:28-34.
1532. Hecht H, DeBord L, Shaw R. Usefulness of supine bicycle stress echocardiography for the detection of restenosis after percutaneous transluminal coronary angioplasty. Am J Cardiol 1993;71:293-296.
1533. Pfisterer M, Rickenbacher P, Klowski W, Muller-Brand J. Silent ischemia after percutaneous transluminal coronary angioplasty: Incidence and prognostic significance. J Am Coll Cardiol 1993;22:1446-1454.
1534. Manyari D, Knudtson M, Kloiber R. Sequential thallium-201 myocardial perfusion studies after successful percutaneous transluminal coronary angioplasty: delayed resolution of exercise-induced scintigraphic abnormalities. Circulation 1988;77:86-95.
1535. Miller D, Verani M. Current status of myocardial perfusion imaging after percutaneous transluminal coronary angioplasty. J Am Coll Cardiol 1994;24:260-266.
1536. Baim D, Levine M, Leon M, Levine S, Ellis S, Schatz R. Management of restenosis within the Palmaz-Schatz coronary stent (the U.S. multicenter experience). Am J Cardiol 1993;71:364-366.
1537. Ellis SG, Savage M, Fishman D, et al. Restenosis after placement of Palmaz-Schatz stents in native coronary arteries. Initial results of a multicenter experience. Circulation 1992;86:1836-1844.
1538. Colombo A, Almagor Y, Maiello L, et al. Results of coronary stenting for restenosis. J Am Coll Cardiol 1994;23:118A.
1539. Penn I, Ricci D, Almond DG, et al. Stenting results in increased early complications and fewer late reinterventions: Final clinical data from the trial of Angioplasty and Stents in Canada (TASC) I. Circulation 1995;92:I-475.
1540. Waksman R, Weintraub WS, Ziyad MB, Douglas JS, Shen Y, King SB. Balloon angioplasty, Palmaz-Schatz stent, and directional coronary atherectomy for restenotic lesions: Retrospective comparison in a single center. J Am Coll Cardiol 1995;25;330A.
1541. Muller DWM. Restenosis: site-specific therapy. In Topol EJ (ed). Textbook of Interventional Cardiology, 2nd Edition, Philadelphia, WB Saunders Company, 1993; 436-448.
1542. Muller DWM. Gene therapy for cardiovascular disease. Br Heart J 1994;71:309-311.
1543. Mitchell JR, Arzin MA, Fram DB, et al. Inhibition of platelet deposition and lysis of intracoronary thrombus during balloon angioplasty using urokinase-coated hydrogel balloons. Circulation 1994;90:1979-1988.
1544. Ohno T, Gordon D, San H, et al. Gene therapy for vascular smooth muscle cell proliferation after arterial injury. Science 1994;265:781-784.
1545. von der Leyen HE, Gibbons GH, Morishita R, et al. Gene therapy inhibiting neointimal vascular lesion: in vivo transfer of endothelial cell nitric oxide synthase gene. Proc Natl Acad Sci USA 1995;92:1137-1141.
1546. Change MW, Barr E, Seltzer J, et al. Cytostatic gene therapy for vascular proliferative disorders with a constitutively active form of the retinoblastoma gene product. Science 1995;267:518-522.
1547. Asahara T, Bauters C, Pastroe C, et al. Local delivery of vascular endothelial growth factor accelerates reendothelialization and attenuates intimal hyperplasia in balloon-injured rat carotid artery. Circulation 1995;91:2793-2801.
1548. Simons M, Edelman ER, Dekeyser JL, et al. Antisense c-myb oligonucleotides inhibit intimal arterial smooth muscle cell accumulation in vivo. Nature 1992;359:67-70.
1549. Morhisita R, Gibbons GH, Ellison KE, et al. Initimal hyperplasia after vascular injury is inhibited by antisense cdk2kinase oligonucleotides. J Clin Invest 1994;93:1458-1464.
1550. O'Keefe JH, Lapeyre AC, Holmes DR, et al. Usefulness of early radionuclide angiography for identifying low-risk patients for late restenosis after percutaneous transluminal coronary angioplasty. Am J Cardiol 1988;61:51-54.
1551. El-Tamimi H, Davies GJ, Hackett D, et al. Very early prediction of restenosis after successful coronary angioplasty: Anatomic and functional assessment. J Am Coll Cardiol 1990;15:259-264.
1552. Wijns W, Serruys P, Reiber J, et al. Early detection of restenosis after successful percutaneous transluminal coronary angioplasty by exercise-redistribution thallium scintigraphy. Am J Cardiol 1985;55:357-361.
1553. Wijns W, Serruys PW, Simoons ML, van den Brand M, de Feyter PJ, Reiber JH, Hugenholtz PG. Predictive value of early maximal exercise test and thallium scintigraphy after successful percutaneous transluminal coronary angioplasty. Br Heart J 1985;53:194-200.
1554. Scholl JM, Chaitman BR, David PR, et al. Exercise electrocardiography and myocardial scintigraphy in the serial evaluation of the results of percutaneous transluminal coronary angioplasty. Circulation 1982;66:380-390.
1555. Ernst SMPG, Hillebrand FA, Kelin B, et al. The value of exercise tests in the follow-up of patients who underwent transluminal coronary angioplasty. Int J Cardiol 1985;7:267-279.
1556. Rosing DR, Van Raden MJ, Mincemoyer RM, et al. Exercise, electrocardiographic and functional responses after percutaneous transluminal coronary angioplasty. Am J Cardiol 1984;53:36C-41C.
1557. Honan MB, Bengtson JR, Pryor DB, et al. Exercise treadmill testing is a poor predictor of anatomic restenosis after angioplasty for acute myocardial infarction. Circulation 1989;80:1585-94.

1558. Hillegass WB, Ancukiewicz M, Bengtson JR, et al. Does follow-up exercise testing predict restenosis after successful balloon angioplasty? Circulation 1992;I-137.
1559. Hardoff R, Shefer A, Gips S, et al. Predicting late restenosis after coronary angioplasty by very early (12 to 24 h) thallium-201 scintigraphy: implications with regard to mechanisms of late coronary restenosis. J Am Coll Cardiol 1990;15:1486-1492.
1560. Jain A, Mahmarian JJ, Borges-Neto S, et al. Clinical significance of perfusion defects by thallium-201 single photon emission tomography following oral dipyridamole early after coronary angioplasty. J Am Coll Cardiol 1988;11:970-976.
1561. Lam JYT, Chaitman BR, Byers S, et al. Can dipyridamole thallium imaging predict restenosis after coronary angioplasty? Circulation 1987;76:373.
1562. DePuey EF, Leatherman RD, Dear WE, et al. Restenosis after transluminal coronary angioplasty detected with exercise-gated radionuclide ventriculography. J Am Coll Cardiol 1984;4:1103-1113.
1563. DePuey EG, Boskovic D, Krajcer Z, et al. Exercise radionuclide ventriculography in evaluating successful transluminal coronary angioplasty. Cathet Cardiovasc Diagn 1983;9:153-166.

Medical & Peripheral Complications

1564. Porter GA. Experimental contrast-associated nephropathy and its clinical implications. Am J Cardiol 1990;66:18F-22F.
1565. Cronin RE. Renal failure following radiologic procedures. Am J Med Sci 1989;298:342-356.
1566. Porter GA. Contrast-associated nephropathy. Am J Cardiol 1989;64:22E-26E.
1567. Manske CL, Sprafka JM, Strong JT, et al. Contrast nephropathy in azotemic diabetic patients undergoing coronary angiography. Am J Med 1990;89(5):615-620.
1568. Davidson CJ, Hiatky M, Morris KG, et al. Cardiovascular and renal toxicity of a nonionic radiographic contrast agent after cardiac catheterization. A prospective trial. Ann Intern Med 1989;110:119-124.
1569. Jeunikar AM, Finnie KJ, Dennis B, et al. Nephrotoxicity of high-and-low-osmolality contrast media. Nephron 1988;48:300-305.
1570. Weinstein JM, Heyman S, Brezis M. Potential deleterious effect of furosemide in radiocontrast nephropathy. Nephron 1992;62:413-5.
1571. Weisberg LS, Kurnid PB, Kurnid BRC. Risk of radiocontrast nephropathy in patients with and without diabetes mellitus. Kidney Int 1994;45:259-65.
1572. Opie LH. Drugs for the heart.
1573. Ansell G, Tweedie MCK, West CR, et al. The current status of reactions to intravenous contrast media. Invest Radiol 1980;15:532-539.
1574. Bilazarian SD, Mittal S, Mills RM. Recognizing the extrarenal hazards of intravascular contrast agents. J Crit Illness 1991;6:859-869.
1575. Lasser EC, et al. Pre-Treatment with corticosteroids to alleviate reactions to intravenous contrast material. N Engl J Med 1987;317:845-849.
1576. Lang DM, Alpern MB, Visintainer PF, et al. Increased risk for Anaphylactoid reaction from contrast media in Patients on β-adrenergic blockers or with asthma. Ann Intern Med 1991;115:270-276.
1577. Zuckerman LS, Friehling TD, Wolf NM, et al. Effect of calcium-binding additives on ventricular fibrillation and repolarization changes during coronary angiography. J Am Coll Cardiol 1987;10:1249-1253.
1578. Lembo NJ, King SB III, Roubin GS, et al. Effects of nonionic versus ionic contrast media on complications of percutaneous transluminal coronary angioplasty. Am J Cardiol 1991;67:1046-1050.
1579. Katayama H, Yamaguchi K, Kozuka T, et al. Adverse reactions to ionic and nonionic contrast media. Radiology 1990;175:621-628.
1580. Fischer HW, Spataro RF. Use of low-osmolality contrast media in patients with previous reactions. Radiol 1988;23:I186-I188.
1581. Piessens, et al. Effects of an ionic versus a nonionic low osmolar contrast agent on the thrombotic complications of coronary angioplasty. Cathet Cardiovasc Diagn 1993;28:99-105.
1582. Grines CL, Zidar F, Jones D, et al. A randomized trial of ionic vs. nonionic contrast in myocardial infarction or unstable angina patients undergoing coronary angioplasty. Circulation 1993;88:1886.
1583. Aguirre FV, Topol EJ, Donohue TJ, et al. Impact on ionic and non-ionic contrast media on post-PTCA ischemic complications: results from the EPIC trial. J Am Coll Cardiol 1995;March, Special Issue:8A.
1584. Bonan R, Lesperance J, Gosselin G, et al. Recoil 15 minutes post-coronary angioplasty and contrast media: A randomized double-blind comparative study. Circulation 1994;90:I488.
1585. Lembo NJ, King SB III, Roubin GS, et al. Effects of nonionic versus ionic contrast media on complications of percutaneous transluminal coronary angioplasty Am J Cardiol 1991;67:1046-50.
1586. Schwab SJ, Hlatky MA, Pieper KS, et al. Contrast nephrotoxicity: A randomized controlled trial of a nonionic and an ionic radiographic contrast agent. N Engl J Med 1989;320:149-153.
1587. Taliercio CP, Vlietstra RE, Ilstrup DM, et al. A randomized comparison of the nephrotoxicity of Iopamidol and diatrizoate in high risk patients undergoing cardiac angiography. J Am Coll Cardiol 1991;17:384-390.
1588. Shehadi WH. Adverse reactions to intravascularly administered contrast media: a comprehensive study based on prospective survey. Am J Radiol 1975;124:145-52.
1589. Shehadi WH, Toniolo G. Adverse reactions to contrast media. Radiology 1980;137:299-302.
1590. Palmer FJ, The RACR survey of intravenous contrast media reactions: a preliminary report. Australas Radiol 1988;32:8-11.
1591. Katayama H. Report of the Japanese committee on the safety of contrast media. Presented at the Radiological Society of North America Meeting, November, 1988.
1592. Lasser EC, Berry CC, Talner LB, et al. Pretreatment with corticosteroids to alleviate reactions to intravenous contrast material. N Engl J Med 1987;317:845-9.
1593. Greenberg MA, Levine B, Menegus MA, et al. Single dose pre-treatment prevents adverse events associated with the use of ionic

contrast agents. J Am Coll Cardiol 1995;March, Speical Issue:319A.
1594. Wyman RM, et al. Current complications of diagnostic and therapeutic cardiac catheterization. J Am Coll Cardiol 1988;12:1400.
1595. Muller DWM, Shamir KJ, Ellis SG, et al. Peripheral vascular complications after conventional and complex percutaneous coronary interventional procedures. Am J Cardiol 1992;69:63-68.
1596. Schaub F, Theiss W. Heinz M, et al. New Aspects in ultrasound-guided compression repair of post catheterization femoral artery injuries. Circulation 1994;90:1861-5.
1597. Hessel SJ, Adams DF, Abrams HL. Complications of angiography. Radiology 1981;138:273-281.
1598. Rappaport S, Sniderman KW, Morse SS. Pseudoaneurysm: A complication of faulty technique in femoral artery puncture. Radiology 1985;529-530.
1599. Moote JJ, Hilborn MD, Harris KA, et al. Postarteriographic femoral pseudoaneurysms: treatment with ultrasound-guided compression. Annals of Vascular Surgery 1994;8:325-31.
1600. Cox GS, Young JR, Gray BR, et al. Ultrasound-guided compression repair of postcatheterization pseudoaneurysms: results of treatment in one hundred cases. J Vascular Surg 1994;19:683-6.
1601. Humphries AW, et al. Evaluation of the natural history and result of treatment involving the lower extremities: Fundamentals of vascular grafting. McGraw-Hill, New York 1973.
1602. Raithel D. Surgical Treatment of acute embolization and acute arterial thrombosis. J Cardiovas Surgery. Barcelona, 1973.
1603. Johnson LW, Lozner EC, Johnson S, et al. Coronary arteriography 1984-1987: A report of the registry of the society for cardiac angiography and interventions. Cathet Cardiovasc Diagn 1989;17:5-10.
1604. Rooke TW. Vascular complications of interventional procedures. Radiology 1981;138;273-281.
1605. Lauk EK. A survey of complications of percutaneous retrograde arteriography. Radiology 1963;81:257-263.
1606. Bourassa MA, Noble J. Complication rate of coronary arteriography. Circulation. 1976;53:106-114.
1607. Guss SB, Zin LM, Garrison HB, et al. Coronary occlusion during coronary angiography. Circulation 1975;52:1063-1068.
1608. Feit A, Kahn R, Chowdry I, et al. Coronary artery dissection secondary to coronary arteriography: Case report and review. Cathet Cardiovas Diagn 1984;10:177-181.
1609. Morise AP, Hardin NJ, Bovili EG, et al. Coronary artery dissection secondary to coronary arteriography: Presentation of three cases. Cathet Cardiovasc Diagn 1981;7:283-296.
1610. Connors JP, Thanavaro S, Shaw RC, et al. Urgent myocardial revascularization for dissection of the left main coronary artery. J Thorac Cardiovasc Surgery 1982;84:349-352.
1611. Shires TG. Principles of surgery. Fourth Edition. McGraw-Hill, New York, 1984:240-241.
1612. Boylis SM, Lausing EH, Gilas NW. Traumatic retroperitoneal hematoma. Am J Surgery 1962;103:477.
1613. Caravajial JA. A thrombolism. Arch Intern Med 1967;119:539.
1614. Gore J, Collins WDP. Review of the literature and a report of 16 additional cases. Am J Clin Pathol 1960;33:416.
1615. Haimovici H. Vascular emergencies. Appleton Century Crafts. 1982.
1616. Colt HG, Begg RJ, Saporito JJ, et al. Cholesterol emboli after cardiac catheterization. Medicine 1988;57:389-400.
1617. Gaines DA. Cholesterol embolization: A lethal complication of vascular catheterization. Lancet 1988;1:168.
1618. Grines CL, Glazier S, Bakalyar D, et al. Predictors of bleeding complications following coronary angioplasty. Circulation 1991;(Suppl II);84:II-591.
1619. Brown KJ, Morcher JH, Whitman GR, et al. The incidence and analysis of bleeding and vascular complications following percutaneous coronary interventional procedures. Circulation 1994;88:I-196.
1620. Hillgrass WB, Brott BC, Narins CR, et al. Predictors of blood loss and bleeding complications after angioplasty. J Am Coll Cardiol 1994;March, Special Issue:69A.
1621. Mansour KA, Moscucce M, Kent C, et al. Vascular complications following directional coronary atherectomy or Palmaz-Schatz stenting. J Am Coll Cardiol 1994;23:136A.
1622. Oweida SW, Roubin GS, Smith RB, et al. Postcatheterization vascular complication associated with percutaneous transluminal coronary angioplasty. J Vasc Surgery 1990;12:310-315.
1623. Muller D, Shamir KJ, Ellis SG, et al. Peripheral vascular complications after conventional and complex percutaneous coronary interventional procedures. Am J Caridol 1992;69:63-68.
1624. Popma JJ, Satler LF, Pichard AD, et al. Vascular complications after balloon and new device angioplasty. Circulation 1993;88:1569-1578.
1625. Schweiger MJ, Wiseman A, Wolfe MW, et al. Bleeding complications of coronary angioplasty: A prospective multicenter study. Circulation 1994;90:I-621.
1626. Friedman HZ, Cragg DR, Glazier SM, et al. Randomized prospective evaluation of prolonged versus abbreviated intravenous heparin therapy after coronary angioplasty. J Am Coll Cardiol 1994;24:1214-1219.
1627. Carere RG, Webb JG, Dodek A. Collagen plug closure of femoral arterial punctures. Are complications excessive? Circulation 1994;90:I-621.
1628. Webb JG, Carere RA, Dodek AA. Collagen plug hemostatic closure of femoral arterial puncture sites following implantation of intracoronary stents. Cathet Cardiovasc Diag 1993;30:314-6.
1629. Silber S, Bjorvik A, Rosch A. Advantages of sealing arterial puncture sites after PTCA with a single collagen plug: a randomized prospective trial. J Am Coll Cardiol 1995;February, Special Issue:262A.
1630. Camenzind E, Grossholz M, Urban P, et al. Mechanical compression (Femostop) alone versus combined collagen application (Vasoseal) and Femostop for arterial puncture site closure after coronary stent implantation: A randomized trial. J Am Coll Cardiol 1994;Sprecial Issue:355A.
1631. Vetter JW, Hinohara T, Ribeiro EE, et al. Percutaneous vascular surgery: suture mediated percutaneous closure of femoral artery access site following coronary intervention. J Am Coll Cardio 1995;March, Special Issue:901-21.
1632. Clark C, Popma JJ, Bucher TA, et al, A randomized study of the Femostop compression device to prevent vascular complications

after coronary angioplasty. J Am Coll Cardiol 1994;March, Special Issue:106A.
1633. Sridhar K, Porter K, Gupta B, et al. Reduction in peripheral vascular complications after coronary stenting by the use of a pneumatic vascular compression device. Circulation 1994;90:I-621.
1634. Simon AW. Use of mechanical pressure device for hemostasis following cardiac catheterization. Am J Crit Care 1994;3:62-4.

Coronary Stents

1635. Dotter CT, Judkins MR. Transluminal treatment of arteriosclerotic obstructions. Circulation 1964;30:654.
1636. Eeckhout E, Kappenberger L, Goy JJ. Stents for intracoronary placement: Current status and future directions. J Am Coll Cardiol 1996;27:757-65.
1637. Sigwart U, Puel J, Mirkovitch V, et al. Intravascualr stents to prevent occlusion and restenosis after transluminal angioplasty. N Engl J Med 1987;316:701.
1638. Serruys PW, Strauss BH, Beatt KJ, et al. Angiographic follow-up after placement of a self-expanding coronary-artery stent. N Engl J Med 1991 324:13.
1639. Macander PJ, Agrawal SK, Roubin GS. The Gianturco-Roubin balloon-expandable intracoronary flexible coil stent. J Interven Cardiol 1991;3:85.
1640. Schatz RA. A view of vascular stents. Circulation 1989;79:445.
1641. Medina A, Hernandez E, de Lezo J, Pan M. Divided Palmaz-Schatz stent for discrete coronary stenosis. J Inv Cardiol 1992;4:389-392.
1642. Nordrehaug JE, Priestly K, Chronos N, Buller N, Sigwart U. Implantation of half Palmaz-Schatz stents in short aorto-ostial lesions of saphenous vein grafts. Cathet Cardiovasc Diagn 1993;30:141-143.
1643. Mehan V, Kaufmann U, Salzmann C, Meier B. Use of half (disarticulated) Palmaz-Schatz stents for thrombus-containing coronary lesions. Cathet Cardiovasc Diagn. 1994;33:370-372.
1644. Mehan V, Kaufmann U, Urban P, Chatelain P, Meier B. Stenting with the half (disarticulated) Palmaz-Schatz Stent. Cathet Cardiovas Diagn. 1995;34:122-127.
1645. Wong P, Wong CM, Ko P. Clinical application of a new Palmaz-Schatz coronary stent delivery system with a short (8mm) nonarticulated stent. Cathet Cardiovasc Diagn. 1995;34:82-87.
1646. Koh, Tai-Hai. Method of preparing, mounting, and implanting a Palmaz-Schatz coronary half-stent from the stent delivery system. Cathet Cardiovasc Diagn 1995;36:164-170.
1647. Satler, Lowell F. Editorial Comment. Cathet Cardiovasc Diagn 1995;35:171-172.
1648. Buchwald A, Unterberg C, Werner G, et al. Initial clinical results with the Wiktor stent: A new balloon-expandable coronary stent. Clin Cardiol 1991;14:374.
1649. Cragg A, Lund G, Rysavy J, et al. Nonsurgical placement of arterial endoprostheses: A new technique using nitinol wire. Radiol 1983;147:261.
1650. den Heijer P, van Dijk R, Twisk SP, Lie K. Early stent occlusion is not always caused by thrombosis. Cathet Cardiovasc Diagn. 1993;29:136-140.
1651. Ozaki Y, Keane D, Ruygrok P, vd Giessen W, de Feyter P. Six-month clinical and angiographic follow-up of the new less shortening Wallstent in native coronary arteries. Circulation 1995;92:I-79.
1652. Colombo A, Hall P, Martini G. Ultrasound-guided coronary stenting without anticoagulation. In: Current Review of Interventional Cardiology, Second Edition. Topol EJ, Serruys PW (eds). Current Medicine, Philadelphia, PA. 1995, pg. 115.
1653. Kiemeneij F, Laarman G, Slagboom T. Mode of deployment of coronary Palmaz-Schatz stents after implantation with the stent delivery system: An intravascular ultrasound study. Am Heart J 1995;129:638-644.
1654. Mudra H, Regar E, Wener F, Rothman MftMI. A focal high pressure dilatation of Palmaz-Schatz stents can safely achieve maximal stent expansion using a single balloon catheter approach. First results from the MUSCAT Trial. Circulation 1995;92:I-280.
1655. Kiemeneij F, Laarman GJ, Slagboom T, Stella P. Transradial Palmaz-Schatz coronary stenting on an outpatient basis: Results of a prospective pilot study. J Inv Cardiol 1995;7:5A-11A.
1656. Kiemeneij F, Laarman GJ. Transradial artery Palmaz-Schatz coronary stent implantation: Results of a single center feasibility study. Am Heart J 1995;130:14-21.
1657. Kiemeneij F, Laarman GJ, Slagboom T. Percutaneous tranradial coronary Palmaz-Schatz stent implantation, guided by intravascular ultrasound. Cathet Cardiovasc Diagn. 1995;34:133-136.
1658. Kiemeneij F, Laarman G, Slagboom T, van der Wieken R. Transradial coronary stenting in outpatients. Circulation 1995;92:I-535.
1659. Holmes D, Berger P, Garratt K, Bell M, Bresnahan J. Stenting in cardiac interventional practice, off label versus approved indication. Circulation 1995;92:I-85.
1660. Penn I, Ricci D, Brown R, et al. Randomized study of stenting versus prolonged balloon dilatation in failed angioplasty (PTCA): Preliminary data from the trial of Angioplasty and Stents in Canada (T.A.S.C. II). Circulation 1993;88:I-601.
1661. Ricci D, Buller C, O'Neill B, et al. Coronary stent vs. prolonged perfusion balloon for failed coronary angioplasty. A randomized trial. Circulation 1994;90:I-651.
1662. Ray S, Penn I, Ricci D, et al. Mechanism of benefit of stenting in failed PTCA. Final results from the trial of Angioplasty and Stents in Canada (TASC II). J Am Coll Cardiol 1995;25:156A.
1663. Ricci D, Ray S, Buller C, et al. Six month followup of patients randomized to prolonged inflation or stent for abrupt occlusion during PTCA-clinical and angiographic data: TASC II. Circulation 1995;92:I-475.
1664. Hui N, Brass N, Klinke P. Effect of coronary stents on PTCA practice in a hospital without cardiac surgery. Circulation 1995;92:I-409.
1665. Goy JJ, Eeckhout E, Stauffer J-C, Vogt P, Kappenberger L. Emergency endoluminal stenting for abrupt vessel closure following coronary angioplasty: A randomized comparison of the Wiktor and Palmaz-Schatz stents. Cathet Cardiovasc Diagn. 1995;34:128-

132.
1666. Urban P, Chatelain P, Brzostek T, Jaup T, Verine V, Rutishauser W. Bailout coronary stenting with 6F guiding catheters for failed balloon angioplasty. Am Heart J 1995;129:1078-83.
1667. Metz D, Urban P, Camenzind E, Chatelain P, Hoang V, Meier B. Improving results of bailout coronary stenting after failed balloon angioplasty. Cathet Cardiovasc Diagn. 1994;32:117-124.
1668. Schomig A, Kastrati A, Mudra H, et al. Four-year experience with Palmaz-Schatz stenting in coronary angioplasty complicated by dissection with threatened or present vessel closure. Circulation 1994;90:2716-2724.
1669. Kiemeneij F, Laarman G, van der Wieken R, Suwarganda J. Emergency coronary stenting with the Palmaz-Schatz stent for failed transluminal coronary angioplasty: results of a learning phase. Am Heart J 1993;126:23-31.
1670. Reifart N, Haase J, Preusler W, Schwartz F, Storger H. Randomized trial comparing two devices: The Palmaz-Schatz stent and the Strecker stent in bail-out situations. J Interven Cardiol 1994;7:539-547.
1671. Hermann H, Buchbinder M, Cleman M, et al. Emergent use of balloon-expandable coronary artery stenting for failed percutaneous coronary angioplasty. Circulation 1992;86:812-819.
1672. Chan C, Tan A, Koh T, Koh P. Intracoronary stenting in the treatment of acute or threatened closure in angiographically small coronary arteries (<3.0 mm) complicating percutaneous transluminal coronary angioplasty. Am J Cardiol 1995;75:23-25.
1673. Sutton J, Ellis S, Roubin G, et al. Major Clinical events after coronary stenting. The multicenter registry of acute and elective Gianturco-Roubin stent placement. Circulation 1994;89:1126-1137.
1674. Agrawal S, Ho D, Liu M, et al. Predictors of thrombotic complications after placement of the flexible coil stent. Am J Cardiol 1994;73:1216-1219.
1675. George B, Voorhees W, Roubin G, et al. Multicenter investigation of coronary stenting to treat acute or treated closure after percutaneous transluminal coronary angioplasty: Clinical and angiographic outcomes. J Am Coll Cardiol 1993;22:135-143.
1676. Roubin G, Cannon A, Agrawal S, et al. Intracoronary stenting for acute and threatened closure complicating percutaneous transluminal coronary angioplasty. Circulation 1992;85:916-927.
1677. Vrolix MC, Rutsch W, Piessens J, Kober G, Wiegand V. Bail-out stenting with Medtronic Wiktor: Results from the European stent study group. J Interven Cardiol 1994;7:549-555.
1678. Garratt K, White C, Buchbinder M, Whitlow P, Heuser R. Wiktor stent placement for unsuccessful coronary angioplasty. Circulation 1994;90:I-279.
1679. Ozaki Y, Keane D, Ruygrok P, de Feyter P, Stertzer S, Serruys P. Acute clinical and angiographic results with the new AVE micro coronary stent in bailout management. Am J Cardiol 1995;76:112-116.
1680. Metz D, Urban P, Hoang V, Camenzind E, Chatelain P, Meier B. Predicting ischemic complications after bailout stenting following failed coronary angioplasty. Am J Cardiol 1994;74:271-274.
1681. Carrozza J, George C, Curry C. Palmaz-Schatz stenting for non-elective indications: Report from the new approaches to coronary intervention (NACI) Registry. Circulation 1995;92:I-86.
1682. Gordon P, Gibson M, Cohen D, Carrozza J, Kuntz R, Baim D. Mechanisms of restenosis and redilation within coronary stents-quantitative angiographic assessment. J Am Coll Cardiol 1993;21:1166-1174.
1683. Hermiller J, Fry E, Peters T, Orr C, Van Tassel J, Pinkerton C. Multiple Gianturco-Roubin stent for long dissections causing acute and threatened coronary artery closure. J Am Coll Cardiol 1994;23:73A.
1684. Sankardas M, Garrahy J, McEniery PT. Sequential implantation of dissimilar tandem stents for long dissections complicating percutaneous transluminal coronary angioplasty. Cathet Cardiovasc Diagn. 1995;34:155-158.
1685. Meckel C, Kjelsberg M, Ahmed W, et al. Bailout stenting for abrupt closure during coronary angioplasty. Circulation 1995;92:I-688.
1686. Agrawal S, Liu M, Hearn J, et al. Can preemptive stenting improve the outcome of acute closure? J Am Coll Cardiol 1993;21:291A.
1687. Lincoff M, Topol E, Chapekis A, et al. Intracoronary stenting compared with conventional therapy for abrupt vessel closure complicating coronary angioplasty: A matched case-control study. J Am Coll Cardiol 1993;21:866-875.
1688. Stauffer JC, Eeckhout E, Goy JJ, et al. Major dissection during coronary angioplasty: Outcome using prolonged balloon inflation versus coronary stenting. J Invas Cardiol 1995;7:221-227.
1689. Garratt K, Voorhees W, Bell M, et al. Complications related to intracoronary stents placed for moderate and severe dissections: Cook FlexStent Registry report. J Am Coll Cardiol 1994;23:102A.
1690. Pilon C, Foley JB, Penn I, Brown R. A costing study of coronary stenting in failed angioplasty. J Am Coll Cardiol 1994;23:73A.
1691. Gaspard P, Didier B, Lienhart Y, et al. Emergency temporary stenting should be preferred to permanent stenting for abrupt closure during coronary angioplasty. J Am Coll Cardiol 1994;23:103A.
1692. Mahrer J, Eigler N, Khorsandi M, et al. Development of the Heat Activated Recoverable Temporary Stent (HARTS) with a slotted-tube design for coronary application. J Am Coll Cardiol 1994;23:103A.
1693. Hall P, Nakamura S, Maiello L, et al. Clinical and angiographic outcome after Palmaz-Schatz stent implantation guided by intravascular ultrasound. J Inv Cardiol 1995;7:12A-22A.
1694. Morice M-C. Advances in post stenting medication protocol. J Inv Cardiol 1995;7:32A-35A.
1695. Colombo A, Maiello L, Nakamura S, et al. Preliminary experience of coronary stenting with the MicroStent. J Am Coll Cardiol 1995;25:239A.
1696. Hamasaki N, Nosaka H, Nobuyoshi M. Initial experience of Cordis stent implantation. J Am Coll Cardiol 1995;25:239A.
1697. Karouny E, Khalife K, Monassier J-P, et al. Clinical experience with Medtronic Wiktor stent implantation: A report from the French Multicenter Registry. J Am Coll Cardiol 1995;25:239A.
1698. Savage M, Fischman D, Schatz R, et al. Long-term angiographic and clinical outcome after implantation of a balloon-expandable stent in the native coronary circulation. J Am Coll Cardiol 1994;24:1207-1212.
1699. Popma J, Colombo A, Chuang YC, et al. Late angiographic outcome after ultrasound-guided stent deployment in native coronary arteries using adjunct high pressure balloon dilatation. Circulation 1994;90:I-612.
1700. Webb J, Abel J, Allard M, Carere R, Evans E, Dodek A. AVE Microstent: Initial human experience. Circulation 1994;90:I-612.

1701. de Jaegere P, Serruys P, Bertrand M, et al. Angiographic predictors of recurrence of restenosis after Wiktor stent implantation in native coronary arteries. Am J Cardiol 1993;72:165-.
1702. Carrozza J, Kuntz R, Levine M, et al. Angiographic and clinical outcome of intracoronary stenting: Immediate and long-term results from a large single-center experience. J Am Coll Cardiol1992;20:328-337.
1703. Strauss B, Serruys P, Bertrand M, et al. Quantitative angiographic follow-up of the coronary Wallstent in native vessels and bypass grafts (European experience--March 1986 to March 1990). Am J Cardiol 1992;69:475-481.
1704. Dawkins K, Emanuelson H, wine VdG, et al. Preliminary results of a European multicenter feasability and safety registry of an innovative stent: The West Study. Circulation 1995;92:I-280.
1705. Chevalier B, Royer T, Glatt B, Diab N, Rosenblatt E. Preliminary experience of coronary stenting with the MicroStent. Circulation 1995;92:I-409.
1706. Goy J, Eeckhout G, Stauffer J-C, Vogt P. Stenting of the right coronary artery for de novo stenoses. A comparison of the Wiktor and the Palmaz-Schatz stents. Circulation 1995;92:I-536.
1707. Levine M, Leonard B, Burke J, et al. Clinical and angiographic results of balloon-expandable intracoronary stents in right coronary artery stenoses. J Am Coll Cardiol 1990;16:332-339.
1708. Fischman D, Savage M, Zalewski A. Overview of the Palmaz-Schatz stent. J Interven Cardiol 1991;3:75.
1709. Wong SC, Baim D, Schatz R, et al. Immediate results and late outcomes after stent implantation in saphenous vein graft lesions: The multicenter U.S. Palmaz-Schatz Stent Experience. J Am Coll Cardiol 1995;26:704-712.
1710. Fischman DL, Leon MB, Baim DS, Schatz RA, et al. A randomized comparison of coronary stent placement and balloon angioplasty in the treatment of coronary artery disease. N Engl J Med 1994;331:496-501.
1711. Serruys P, de Jaegere P, Kiemeneij F, et al. A comparison of balloon expandable stent implantation with balloon angioplasty in patients with coronary artery disease. N Engl J Med 1994;331:489-495.
1712. Mashman W, Gatlin S, King S, Klein L. Medtronic Wiktor TM stent implantation and follow-up: results from the core laboratory. J Am Coll Cardiol 1994;23:117A.
1713. Kuntz RE, Safian RD, Levine MJ, Reis GJ, Diver D, Baim D. Novel approach to the analysis of restenosis after the use of three new coronary devices. J Am Coll Cardiol 1992;19:1493-1499.
1714. de Jaegere P, Serruys P, van Es G, et al. Recoil following Wiktor stent implantation for restenotic lesions of coronary arteries. Cathet Cardiovasc Diagn 1994;32:147-156.
1715. Rodriguez A, Santaera O, Larribau M, et al. Coronary stenting decreases restenosis in lesions with early loss in luminal diameter 24 hours after successful PTCA. Circulation 1995;91:1397-1402.
1716. Penn I, Ricci D, Almond D, et al. Coronary artery stenting reduces restenosis: Final results from the Trial of Angioplasty and Stents in Canada (TASC) I. Circulation 1995;92:I-279.
1717. Mintz G, Pichard A, Kent K, et al. Endovascular stents reduce restenosis by eliminating geometric arterial remodeling: A serial intravascular ultrasound study. J Am Coll Cardiol 1995;25:36A.
1718. Fernandez-Ortiz A, Goicolea J, Perez-Vizcaynio M, et al. Is coronary stent recoil different for Gianturco-Roubin and Palmaz-Schatz stent? Circulation 1995;92:I-94.
1719. Kastrati A, Schomig A, Dietz R, Neumann F-J. Time course of restenosis during the first year after emergency coronary stenting. Circulation 1993;87:1498-1505.
1720. Kimura T, Nosaka H, Yokoi H, Iwabuchi M, Nobuyoshi M. Serial angiographic follow-up after Palmaz-Schatz stent implantation: Comparison with conventional balloon angioplasty. J Am Coll Cardiol 1993;21:1557-1163.
1721. Kimura T, Yokoi H, Tamura T, Nakagawa Y, Nosaka H, Nobuyoshi M. Three years clinical and quantitative angiographic follow-up after the Palmaz-Schatz coronary stent implantation. J Am Coll Cardiol 1995;25:375A.
1722. Hermiller J, Fry E, Peters T, et al. Late lesion regression within the Gianturco-Roubin Flex stent. J Am Coll Cardiol 1995;25:375A.
1723. Macaya C, Serruys P, Suryapranata H, et al. One year clinical follow-up of the Benestent trial. J Am Coll Cardiol 1995;25:374A.
1724. Hermiller J, Fry E, Berkompas D, et al. Five-year clinical follow-up of the Gianturco-Roubin stent: No late stent restenosis. Circulation 1995;92:I-280.
1725. Painter J, Mintz G, Wong C, Popma J. Serial intravascular ultrasound studies fail to show evidence of chronic palmaz-schatz stent recoil. Am J Cardiol 1995;75:398-400.
1726. Laham R, Carrozza J, Berger C, Cohen D, Baim D. Long-term (4-6 year) outcome of Palmaz-Schatz coronary stenting. Circulation 1995;92:I-281.
1727. Debbas N, Sigwart U, Eeckhout E, Stauffer J-C, Vogt P, Goy J-J. Late clinical follow-up 9 years after intracoronary stenting with the Wallstent. Circulation 1995;92`:I-280.
1728. Kern M, Rupprecht H, Wolf T, Meyer J. Five year follow-up after Palmaz-Schatz coronary stent implantation. Circulation 1995;92:I-686.
1729. Ali N, Lowry R, Tawa C, et al. Predictors of restenosis after Gianturco-Roubin coronary stent deployment. Analysis of 135 consecutive patients from a single center. J Am Coll Cardiol 1994;23:71A.
1730. Ellis S, Savage M, Dischman D, Baim D, Leon M, Goldberg S. Restenosis after placement of palmaz-schatz stents in native coronary arteries. Initial results of a multicenter experience. Circulation 1992;86:1836-1844.
1731. Baim D, Levine M, Leon M, Levine S, Ellis S, Schatz R. Management of restenosis within the palmaz-schatz coronary stent (the U.S. multicenter experience). Am J Cardiol 1993;71:364-366.
1732. Wong SC, Zidar J, Chuang YC, et al. Stents improve late clinical outcomes: Results from the combined (I + II) STent REStenosis Study. Circulation 1995;92:I-281.
1733. Hall P, Nakamura S, Maiello L, et al. Factors associated with late angiographic outcome after intravascular ultrasound guided Palmaz-Schatz coronary stent implantation: A multivariate analysis. J Am Coll Cardiol 1995;25:36A.
1734. Wong SC, Chuang Y, Schatz R, et al. Predictors for adverse clinical events are different in stents and PTCA: Results from the Stent Restenosis Study. J Am Coll Cardiol 1995;25:125A.

1735. Segal J, Reiner J, Thompson M, et al. Residual stenosis and MLD following coronary stenting do not predict restenosis in the Strecker stent. J Am Coll Cardiol 1994;23:134A.

1736. Yokol H, Kimura T, Nobuyoshi M. Palmaz-Schatz coronary stent restenosis: Pattern and management. J Am Coll Cardiol 1994;23:117A.

1737. Ikari Y, Hara K, Tamura T, Saeki F, Tamaguchi T. Luminal lost and site of restenosis after palmaz-schatz coronary stent implantation. Am J Cardiol 1995;76:117-120.

1738. Macander P, Roubin G, Agrawal S, Cannon A, Dean L, Baxley W. Balloon angioplasty for treatment of in-stent restenosis: Feasibility, safety, and efficacy. Cathet Cardiovasc Diagn. 1994;32:125-131.

1739. Ribichini F, Steffenino G, Dellavalle A, et al. Restenosis after coronary stenting is associated with high plasma angiotensin-converting enzyme levels. Circulation 1995;92:I-86.

1740. Markovitz J, Roubin G, Parks JM. Platelet activation and restenosis following intracoronary stenting. Circulation 1995;92:I-87.

1741. Haude M, Erbel R, Issa H, et al. Subacute thrombotic complication after intracoronary implantation of palmaz-schatz stents. Am Heart J 1993;126:15-22.

1742. Liu MW, Voohees W, Agrawal S, Dean L, Roubin G. Stratification of the risk of thrombosis after intracoronary stenting for threatened or acute closure complicating coronary balloon angioplasty: A Cook registry study. Am Heart J 1995;130:8-13.

1743. Rechavia E, Litvack F, Macko G, Eigler N. Stent implantation of saphenous vein graft aorto-ostial lesions in patients with unstable ischemic syndromes: Immediate angiographic results and long-term clinical outcome. J Am Coll Cardiol 1995;25:866-870.

1744. Wong SC, Popma J, Pichard A, Kent K. Comparison of clinical and angiographic outcomes after saphenous vein grafts angioplasty using coronary versus "biliary" tubular slotted stents. Circulation 1995;91:339-350.

1745. Piana R, Moscucci M, Cohen D, et al. Palmaz-Schatz stenting for treatment of focal vein graft stenosis: Immediate results and long-term outcome. J Am Coll Cardiol 1994;23:1296-304.

1746. Eeckhout E, Goy J, Stauffer J, Vogt P, Kappenberger L. Endoluminal stenting of narrowed saphenous vein grafts: Long-term clinical and angiographic follow-up. Cathet Cardiovasc Diagn 1994;32:139-146.

1747. Keane D, Buis B, Reifart N, Plokker TH. Clinical and angiographic outcome following implantation of the new less shortening Wallstent in aortocoronary vein grafts: Introduction of a second generation stent in the clinical arena. J Interven Cardiol 1994;7:557-564.

1748. Fenton S, Fischman D, Savage M, et al. Long-term angiographic and clinical outcome after implantation of balloon-expandable stents in aortocoronary saphenous vein grafts. Am J Cardiol 1994;74:1187-1191.

1749. Leon MB, Wong SC, Pichard A. Balloon expandable stent implantation in saphenous vein grafts. In Hermann HC, Hisrschfeld JW (Eds). Clinical use of the Palmaz-Schatz Intracoronary Stent. Futura Publishing Company Inc. 1993; 111-121.

1750. Fortuna R, Heuser R, Garratt K, Schwartz R, M B. Intracoronary stent: experience in the first 101 vein graft patients. J Am Coll Cardiol 1993;26:I-308.

1751. Pomerantz R, Kuntz R, Carrozza J, et al. Acute and long-term outcome of narrowed saphenous venous grafts treated by endoluminal stenting and directional atherectomy. Am J Cardiol 1992;70:161-167.

1752. Bilodeau L, Iyer S, Cannon A, et al. Flexible coil stent (Cook, Inc) in saphenous vein grafts: Clinical and angiographic follow-up. J Am Coll Cardiol 1992;19:264A.

1753. de Scheerder I, Strauss B, de Feyter P, et al. Stenting of venous bypass grafts: A new treatment modality for patients who are poor candidates for reintervention. Am Heart J 1992;123:1046-1054.

1754. Urban P, Sigwart U, Golf S, Kaufmann U. Intravascular stenting for stenosis of aortocoronary venous bypass grafts. J Am Coll Cardiol 1989;13:1085-1091.

1755. Wong SC, Kent K, Chuang YC, et al. Is bigger really better for stent placement in large saphenous vein grafts? Circulation 1994;90:I-279.

1756. Savage M, Douglas J, Fischman D, et al. Coronary stents versus balloon angioplasty for aorto-coronary saphenous vein bypass graft disease: Interim results of a randomized trial. J Am Coll Cardiol 1995;25:79A.

1757. Wong SC, Chuang Y, Hong M, et al. Stent placement is safe and effective in the treatment of older (>4 years) saphenous vein graft lesions. J Am Coll Cardiol 1995;25:79A.

1758. Sketch M, Wong C, Chuang Y, et al. Progressive deterioration in late (2-year) clinical outcomes after stent implantation in saphenous vein grafts: The Multicenter JJIS experience. J Am Coll Cardiol 1995;25:79A.

1759. Wong SC, Chuang Y, Popma J, et al. Comparative analysis of long term clinical outcomes after native coronary versus saphaneous vein graft stent implantation. J Am Coll Cardiol 1995;25:198A.

1760. Hadjimiltiades S, Gourassas J, Louridas G, Tsifodimos D. Stenting the distal anastomotic site of the left internal mammary artery graft: A case report. Cathet Cardiovasc Diagn. 1994;32:157-161.

1761. Kaplan BM, Safian RD, Grines CL, Goldstein JA, et al. Usefulness of adjunctive angioscopy and extraction atherectomy before stent implantation in high-risk aortocoronary saphenous vein grafts. Am J Cardiol 1995;76:822-824.

1762. Hong M, Pichard A, Kent K, et al. Assessing a strategy of stand-alone extraction atherectomy followed by staged stent placement in degenerated saphenous vein graft lesions. J Am Coll Cardiol 1995;25:394A.

1763. Denardo SJ, Morris NB, Rocha-Singh KJ, Curtis GP, et al. Safety and efficacy of extended urokinase infusion plus stent deployment for treatment of obstructed, older saphenous vein grafts. Am J Cardiol 1995;76:776-780.

1764. Guarneri E, Sklar M, Russo R, Claire D, Schatz R, Teirstein P. Escape from StentJail: An in vitro model. Circulation 1995;92:I-688.

1765. Nakamura S, Hall P, Maiello L, Colombo A. Techniques of Palmaz-Schatz stent deployment in lesions with a large side branch. Cathet Cardiovas Diagnos 1995;34:353-361.

1766. Colombo A, Gaglione A, Nakamura S. "Kissing" stents for bifurcational coronary lesion. Cathet Cardiovas Diag. 1993;30:327-330.

1767. Zampieri P, Colombo A, Almagor Y, Mairello L, Finci L. Results of coronary stenting of ostial lesions. Am J Cardiol 1994;73:901-903.

1768. Rocha-Singh K, Morris N, Wong C, Schatz R, Teirstein P. Coronary stenting for treatment of ostial stenoses of native coronary

arteries or aortocoronary saphenous venous grafts. Am J Cardiol 1995;75:26-29.
1769. Maiello L, Hall P, Nakamura S, et al. Results of stent implantation for diffuse coronary disease assisted by intravascular ultrasound. J Am Coll Cardiol 1995;25:156A.
1770. Wong SC, Hong M, Popma J, et al. Stent placement for the treatment of aorto-ostial saphenous vein graft lesions. J Am Coll Cardiol 1994;23:118A.
1771. Fenton S, Fischman D, Savage M, et al. Does stent implantation in ostial saphenous vein graft lesions reduce restenosis? J Am Coll Cardiol 1994;23:118A.
1772. Wong SC, Popma J, Hong M, et al. Procedural results and long term clinical outcomes in aorto-ostial saphenous vein graft lesions after new device angioplasty. J Am Coll Cardiol 1995;25:394A.
1773. Eeckhout E, Stauffer J-C, Vogt P, Debbas N, Kappenberger L, Goy J-J. A comparison of intracoronary stenting with conventional balloon angioplasty for the treatment of new onset stenoses of the right coronary artery. J Am Coll Cardiol 1995;25:196A.
1774. Colombo A, Almagor Y, Maiello L, et al. Results of coronary stenting for restenosis. J Am Coll Cardiol 1994;23:118A.
1775. Penn I, Ricci D, Almond DG, et al. Stenting results in increased early complications and fewer late reinterventions: Final clinical data from the trial of Angioplasty and Stents in Canada (TASC) I. Circulation 1995;92:I-475.
1776. Teirstein P, Schatz R, Russo R, Guarneri E, Stevens M. Coronary stenting of small diameter vessels: Is it safe? Circulation 1995;92:I-281.
1777. Hall P, Colombo A, Itoh A, et al. Gianturco-Roubin stent implantation in small vessels without anticoagulation. Circulation 1995;92:I-795.
1778. Wong SC, Hirshfeld J, Teirstein P, Schatz R, Shaknovich A, Nobuyoshi M. Differential impact of stent versus PTCA on restenosis in large (> or less 3 mm) vessels in the Stent Restenosis Trial. J Am Coll Cardiol 1995;25:375A.
1779. Azar AJ, Detre K, Goldberg S, Kiemeneij F, et al. A meta-analysis on the clinical and angiographic outcomes of stents vs PTCA in the different coronary vessel sizes in the Benestent-I and Stress ½ trials. Circulation 1995;92:I-475.
1780. Rechavia E, Litvack F, Macko G, Eigler NL. Influence of expanded balloon diameter on Palmaz-Schatz stent recoil. Cathet Cardiovasc Diagn 1995;36:11-16.
1781. Medina A, Melian F, deLezo J, et al. Effectiveness of coronary stenting for the treatment of chronic total occlusion in angina pectoris. Am J Cardiol 1994;73:1222-1224.
1782. Hsu Y-S, Tamai H, Ueda K, et al. Clinical efficacy of coronary stenting in chronic total occlusions. Circulation 1994;90:I-613.
1783. Ooka M, Suzuki T, Kosokawa H, Kukkutomi T, Yamashita K, Hayase M. Stenting vs. non-stenting after revascularization of chronic total occlusion. Circulation 1994;90:I-613.
1784. Maiello, Luigi, Hall, Patrick, Nakamura, Shigeru Blengino, Simonetta, et al. Results of stent implantation for diffuse coronary disease assisted by ultravascular ultrasound. J Am Coll Cardiol 1995;25:156A.
1785. Reimers B, Di Mario C, Nierop P, Pasquetto G, Camenzind E, Ruygrok P. Long-term restenosis after multiple stent implantation. A quantitative angiographic study. Circulation 1995;92:I-327.
1786. Shaknovich A, Moses J, Undemir C, et al. Procedural and short-term clinical outcomes of multiple Palmaz-Schatz stents (PSS) in very long lesions/dissections. Circulation 1995;92:I-535.
1787. Akira I, Hall P, Maielli L, et al. Coronary stenting of long lesions (greater than 20 mm)-A matched comparison of different stents. Circulation 1995;92:I-688.
1788. Sato Y, Kimura T, Nosaka H, Nobuyoshi M. Randomized comparison of balloon angioplasty (BA) versus coronary stent implantation (CS) for total occlusion (TO): Preliminary result. Circulation 1995;92:I-475.
1789. Kaul U, Agarwal R, Mathur A, Wasir HS. Intracoronary stent placement in thrombus containing vein graft lesions. J Inv Cardiol 1995;7:248-250.
1790. Annex BH, Ajluni SC, Larkin TJ, et al. Angioscopic guided interventions in a saphenous vein bypass graft. Cathet Cardiovasc Diagn 1994;31:330-333.
1791. Hong MK, Pichard A, Kent KM, et al. Assessing a strategy of stand-alone extraction atherectomy followed by staged stent placement in degenerated saphenous vein graft lesions. J Am Coll Cardiol 1995;25:394A.
1792. Glazier J, Kiernan F, Bauer H, et al. Treatment of thrombotic saphenous vein graft stenoses/occlusions with local urokinase delivery with the dispatch catheter-initial results. Circulation 1995;92:I-671.
1793. Walton AS, Oesterle SN, Yeung AC. Coronary artery stenting for acute closure complicating primary angioplasty for acute myocardial infarction. Cathet Cardiovasc Diagn. 1995;34:142-146.
1794. Ahmad T, Webb JG, Carere RR, Dodek A. Coronary stenting for acute myocardial infarction. Am J Cardiol 1995;76:77-80.
1795. Wong PH, Wong CM. Intracoronary stenting in acute myocardial infarction. Cathet Cardiovasc Diagn. 1994;33:39-45.
1796. Benzuly KH, Goldstein JA, Almany SL, et al. Feasibility of stenting in acute myocardial infarction. Circulation 1995;92:I-616.
1797. Iyer S, Bilodeau L, Cannon A, et al. Stenting the infarct related artery within 15 days of the acute event: Immediate and long term outcome using the Flexible Metallic Coil stent. J Am Coll Cardiol 1993;21:291A.
1798. Capers Q, Thomas C, Weintraub W, King S, Douglas J, Scott N. Emergent stent placement: Worse out come in the patients with a recent myocardial infarction. J Am Coll Cardiol 1994;23:71A.
1799. Levy G, De Boisgelin X, Volpiliere R, Gallay P, Bouvagnet P. Intracoronary stenting in direct angioplasty: Is it dangerous? Circulation 1995;92:I-139.
1800. Saito S, Kim K, Hosokawa G, Hatano K, Tanaka S. Primary Palmaz-Schatz implantation without coumadine in acute myocardial infarction. Circulation 1995;92:I-796.
1801. Malosky S, Hirshfeld J, Herrmann H. Comparison of results of intracoronary stenting in patients with unstable vs. stable angina. Cathet Cardiovasc Diagn 1994;31:95-101.
1802. Guameri EM, Schatz RA, Sklar MA, Norman SL, et al. Acute coronary syndromes: Is it safe to stent? Circulation 1995;92:I-616.
1803. Fajadet J, Brunel P, Jordan C, Cassagneau B, Marco J. Is stenting of left main coronary artery a reasonable procedure? Circulation 1995;92:I-74.

1804. Stefanadis C, Vlachopoulos C, Kallikazaros I, et al. Autologous vein graft coating applied to vascular stents: the ideal coated stent? J Am Coll Cardiol 1994;23:135A.
1805. Dorros G, Jain A, Kumar K. Management of coronary artery rupture: Covered stent or microcoil embolization. Cathet Cardiovasc Diagn. 1995;36:148-154.
1806. Kaplan BM, Stewart RE, Sakwa MP, et al. Repair of a coronary pseudoaneurysm with percutaneous placement of a saphenous vein allograft attached to a biliary stent. Cathet Cardiovasc Diagn 1996 (in-press).
1807. Stefanadis C, Tsiamis E, Toutouzas K, et al. Autologous vein graft-coated stent in coronary artery disease: The first implantation in de novo lesions in humans. Circulation 1995;92`:I-544.
1808. Fenton S, Fischman D, Savage M, Rake R, Goldberg S. Influence of gender on outcome after elective coronary stent implantation. Circulation 1995;92:I-86.
1809. Ooka M, Suzuki T, Yokoya K, et al. Stenting after revascularization of chronic total occlusion. Circulation 1995;92:I-94.
1810. Goldberg SL, Colombo A, Maiello L, Borrione M, et al. Intracoronary stent insertion after balloon angioplasty of chronic total occlusion. J Am Coll Cardiol 1995;26:713-719.
1811. Mintz G, Dussaillant G, Wong SC, et al. Rotational atherectomy followed by adjunct stents: The preferred therapy for calcified lesions in large vessels? Circulation 1995;92:I-329.
1812. Kruse, Tanguay J-F, Armstrong B, Phillips h. Coumadin versus Ticlopidine in an animal model of stent thrombosis: A comparative study. Circulation 1995;92:I-485.
1813. Brunel P, Jordon C, Fajadet J, Cassagneau B, Marco J. Successive steps in the management of coronary stenting. Circulation 1995;92:I-87.
1814. Heyndrickx G. Benestent-II Pilot Study: In-hospital results of phase I,2,3, and 4. Circulation 1995;92:I-279.
1815. Serruys P. Benestent-II Pilot Study: 6 months follow-up of phase I,II. Circulation 1995;92:I-542.
1816. Suryapranata H, Group ObotBS. Evolving changes in technique of stent deployment during the course of the BENESTENT-II Pilot Study. Circulation 1995;92:I-687.
1817. Morice M-C, Bourdonnec C, Lefevre T, et al. Coronary stenting without coumadin. Phase III. Circulation 1994;90:I-125.
1818. Morice M, Zemour G, Benveniste E, et al. Intracoronary stenting without coumadin: One month results of a french multicenter study. Cathet Cardiovasc Diagn. 1995;35:1-7.
1819. Lablanche J-M, Grollier G, Danchin N, et al. Full antiplatelet therapy without anticoagulation after coronary stenting. J Am Coll Cardiol 1995;25:181A.
1820. Barragan P, Silverstri M, Sainsous J, et al. Prevention of subacute occlusion after coronary stenting with ticlopidine regimen without intravascular ultrasound guided stenting. J Am Coll Cardiol 1995;25:182A.
1821. Colombo A, Nakamura S, Hall P, Maiello L, Ferraro M, Martini G. A prospective study of Gianturco-Roubin coronary stent implantation without anticoagulation. J Am Coll Cardiol 1995;25:50A.
1822. Wong C, Popma J, Chuang Y, et al. Economic impact of reduced anticoagulation after saphenous vein graft stent placement. J Am Coll Cardiol 1995;25:80A.
1823. Buszman P, Clague J, Gibbs S, et al. Improved post stent management: High gain at low risk. J Am Coll Cardiol 1995;25:182A.
1824. Fajadet J, Jordon C, Carvalho H, et al. Percutaneous transradial coronary stenting without coumadin can reduce vascular access complications and hospital stay. J Am Coll Cardiol 1995;25:182A.
1825. Blasini R, Mudra H, Schuhlen H, et al. Intravascular ultrasound guided optimized emergency coronary Palmaz-Schatz stent placement without post procedural systemic anticoagulation. J Am Coll Cardiol 1995;25:197A.
1826. Colombo A, Nakamura S, Hall P, Maiello L, Finci L, Martini G. A prospective study of Wiktor coronary stent implantation without anticoagulation. J Am Coll Cardiol 1995;25:239A.
1827. Colombo A, Hall P, Nakamura S, et al. Intracoronary stenting without anticoagulation accomplished with intravascular ultrasound guidance. Circulation 1995;91:1676-1688.
1828. Mehan V, Saizmann C, Kaufmann U, Meier B. Coronary stenting without anticoagulation. Cathet Cardiovasc Diagn. 1995;34:137-140.
1829. Reifart N, Haase J, Vandormael M, et al. Gianturco-Roubin Stent Acute Closure Evaluation (GRACE): Thirty-day outcomes compared to drug regimen. Circulation 1995;92:I-409.
1830. Lablanche J-M, Grollier G, Bonnet J-L, et al. Ticlopidine Aspirin Stent Evaluation (TASTE); A French multicenter study. Circulation 1995;92:I-476.
1831. Russo R, Schatz R, Morris N, Stevens M, Teirstein P. Ultrasound-guided coronary stent placement without warfarin anticoagulation: Six-month clinical follow-up. Circulation 1995;92:I-543.
1832. Haase H, Reifart N, Baier T, et al. Bail-out stenting (Palmaz-Schatz) without anticoagulation. Circulation 1995;92:I-795.
1833. Goods C, Al-Shaibi K, Iyer S, et al. Flexible coil coronary stenting without anticoagulation or intravascular ultrasound: A prospective observational study. Circulation 1995;92:I-795.
1834. Belli G, Whitlow P, Gross L, et al. Intracoronary stenting without oral anticoagulation: The Cleveland Clinic Registry. Circulation 1995;92:I-796.
1835. Morice M, Breton C, Bunouf P, et al. Coronary stenting without anticoagulant, without intravascular ultrasound. Results of the French Registry. Circulation 1995;92:I-796.
1836. Carvalho H, Fajadet J, Jordan C, Cassagneau B, Robert C, Marco J. A lower rate of complications after Gianturco-Roubin coronary stenting using a new antiplatelet and anticoagulant protocol . Circulation 1994;90:I-125.
1837. Barragan P, Sainsous J, Silestri M, et al. Ticlopidine and subcutaneous heparin as an alternative regimen following coronary stenting. Cathet Cardiovasc Diagn. 1994;32:133-138.
1838. Jordan C, Carvalho H, Fajadet J, Cassagneau B, Robert G, Marco J. Reduction of acute thrombosis rate after coronary stenting using a new anticoagulant protocol. Circulation 1994;90:I-125.
1839. Wong SC, Popma J, Mintz G, et al. Preliminary results from the Reduced Anticoagulation in Saphenous Vein Graft Stent (RAVES)

Trial. Circulation 1994;90:I-125.
1840. Colombo A, Nakamura S, Hall P, Maiello L, Blengino S, Martini G. A prospective study of Wiktor Coronary stent implantation treated only with antiplatelet therapy. Circulation 1994;90:I-124.
1841. Elias J, Monassier JP, Puel J, et al. Medtronic Wiktor stent implantation without coumadin: Hospital outcome. Circulation 1994;90:I-124.
1842. Hall P, Colombo A, Nakamura S, Maiello L, Blengino S. A prospective study of Gianturco-Roubin coronary stent implantation without subsequent anticoagulation. Circulation 1994;90:I-124.
1843. Aubry P, Royer T, Spaulding C, et al. Coronary stenting without coumadin: Phase II and III, the bail-out group. Circulation 1994;90:I-124.
1844. Blengino S, Maiello L, Hall P, Nakamura S, Martini G, Colombo A. Randomized trial of coronary stent implantation without anticoagulation: aspirin vs. ticlopidine. Circulation 1994;90:I-124.
1845. Gaglion A, Tiecco F, Hall P, et al. High pressure assisted intracoronary stent implantation without subsequent anticoagulation. Circulation 1994;90:I-622.
1846. Painter J, Mintz G, Wong C, et al. Intravascular ultrasound assessment of biliary stent implantation in saphenous vein graft. Am J Cardiol 1995;75:731-734.
1847. Fajadet J. New coronary stenting management. J Inv Cardiol 1995;7:30A-31A.
1848. May A, Neumann F-J, Gawaz M, Ott I. Monocyte function after coronary stent implantation. Effect of two different antithrombotic regimens. Circulation 1995;92:I-86.
1849. Ho Jeong M, Owen W, Staab M, et al. Does ticlopidine affect platelet deposition and acute stent thrombosis? Circulation 1995;92:I-489.
1850. Colombo A, Hall P, Nakamura S, et al. Preliminary experience using protamine to reverse heparin immediately following a successful coronary stent implantation. J Am Coll Cardiol 1995;25:182A.
1851. Russo R, Schatz R, Sklar M, Johnson A, Tobis J, Teirstein P. Ultrasound-guided coronary stent placement without prolonged systemic anticoagulation. J Am Coll Cardiol 1995;25:50A.
1852. Schuhlen H, Blasini R, Mudra H, Klauss V, Kastrati A, Zitzmann E. Stenting for progressive dissection during PTCA: Clinical, angiographic and intravascular ultrasound criteria to define a low-risk group not requiring subsequent anticoagulation. J Am Coll Cardiol 1995;25:125A.
1853. Schomig A, Schuhlen H, Blasini R, et al. Anticoagulation versus antiplatetet therapy after intracoronary Palmaz-Schatz placement-A prospective randomized trial. Circulation 1995;92:I-280.
1854. Bruining N, di Mario C, Prati F, et al. Dynamic three-dimensional reconstruction of implanted intracoronary stent structures using IVUS images based on an ECG gated pull-back device. Circulation 1995;92:I-17.
1855. Nakamura S, Colombo A, Gaglione A, et al. Intracoronary ultrasound observations during stent implantation. Circulation 1994;89:2026-2034.
1856. Mudra H, Klauss V, Blasini R, Kroetz M. Ultrasound guidance of Palmaz-Schatz intracoronary stenting with a combined intravascular ultrasound balloon catheter. Circulation 1994;90:1252-1261.
1857. Caputo R, Lopez J, Ho K, et al. Intravascular ultrasound analysis of routine high pressure balloon post-dilatation after Palmaz-Schatz stent deployment. J Am Coll Cardiol 1995;25:49A.
1858. Gorge G, Haude M, Ge J, et al. Intravascular ultrasound after low and high inflation pressure coronary artery stent implantation. J Am Coll Cardiol 1995;26:725-730.
1859. Gil R, Prati F, Ligthart J, von Birgelen C, van Camp G, Serruys P. Is quantitative angiography a substitute for intracoronary ultrasound in guidance of stent deployment? Circulation 1995;92:I-327.
1860. Fitzgerald P. Lesion composition impacts size and symmetry of stent expansion: Initial report from the STRUT registry. J Am Coll Cardiol 1995;25:49A.
1861. Metz J, Mooney M, Walter P, et al. Significance of edge tears in coronary stenting: Initial observations from the STRUT Registry. Circulation 1995;92:I-546.
1862. Popma J, Colombo A, Mintz G, Wong SC, Pichard A. The impact of intravascular (IVUS) on post-stent deployment balloon dilatation. J Am Coll Cardiol 1995;25:49A.
1863. Jain S, Liu M, Iyer S, Parks M, Babu R, Yadav S. Do high-pressure balloon inflations improve acute gain within flexible metallic coil stents? An intravascular ultrasound assessment. J Am Coll Cardiol 1995;25:49A.
1864. Mudra H, Klauss V, Blasini R, et al. Intracoronary ultrasound guidance of stent deployment leads to an increase of luminal gain not discernible by angiography. J Am Coll Cardiol 1994;23:71A.
1865. Nunez B, Foster-Smith K, Berger P, Melby S, Garratt K, Higano S. Benefit of intravascular ultrasound guided high pressure inflations in patients with a "perfect" angiographic result: The Mayo Clinic Experience. Circulation 1995;92:I-545.
1866. Blasini R, Schuhlen H, Mudra H, et al. Angiographic overestimation of lumen size after coronary stent placement impact of high pressure dilatation. Circulation 1995;92:I-223.
1867. Caputo R, Ho K, Lopez J, Stoler R, Cohen D, Carrozza J. Quantitative angiographic comparison of Palmaz-Schatz stent implantation with and without intravascular ultrasound. Circulation 1995;92:I-545.
1868. Russo R, Teirstein P. Angiography versus intravascular ultrasound-directed stent placement. Circulation 1995;92:I-546.
1869. Goldberg S, Colombo A, Almagor Y, et al. Has the introduction of intravascular ultrasound guidance led to different clinical results in the deployment of intracoronary stents? Circulation 1994;90:I-612.
1870. Hall P, Nakamura S, Maiello L, Blengino S, Martini G, Colombo A. Factors associated with procedural complications during high pressure optimized Palmaz-Schatz intracoronary stent implantation. Circulation 1994;90:I-612.
1871. Hall P, Maiello L, Colombo A, et al. In vivo evidence that Palmaz-Schatz stents do not recoil immediately following deployment. Circulation 1995;92:I-327.
1872. Prati F, Di Mario C, Gil R, et al. Usefulness of on-line three-dimensional reconstruction of intracoronary ultrasound for guidance

of stent deployment. Circulation 1995;92:I-546.
1873. Teirstein P, Schatz R, Wong C, Rocha-Singh K. Coronary stenting with angioscopic guidance. Am J Cardiol 1995;75:344-347.
1874. Shaknovich A, Lieberman S, Kreps E, et al. Qualitative comparison of intravascular ultrasound and angioscopy with angiographic assessment of Palmaz-Schatz (PS) coronary stents. J Am Coll Cardiol 1994;23:72A.
1875. Kern M, Aguirre F, Thomas D, Bach R, Caracciolo E. Impact of lumen narrowing of coronary flow after angioplasty and stent: Intravascular ultrasound Doppler and imaging data in support of physiological-guided coronary angioplasty. Circulation 1995;92:I-263.
1876. Verna E, Gil R, Di Mario C, Sunamura M, Gurne O, Porenta GobotDSG. Does coronary stenting following balloon angioplasty improve distal coronary flow reserve? Circulation 1995;92:I-536.
1877. Haude M, Baumgart D, Caspari G, Erbel R. Does adjunct coronary stenting in comparison to balloon angioplasty has an impact of Doppler flow velocity parameters? Circulation 1995;92:I-547.
1878. Mintz G, Pichard A, Dussalilant G, et al. Acute results of adjunct stents following directional coronary atherectomy. Circulation 1995;92:I-328.
1879. Holmes D, Garratt K, Schwartz R. Timing of stent occlusion/thrombosis after stent placement. J Am Coll Cardiol 1994;23:70A.
1880. Mitchel J, McKay R. Treatment of acute stent thrombosis with local urokinase therapy using catheter-based, drug delivery systems: A case report. Cathet Cardiovasc Diagn. 1995;34:149-154.
1881. Metz D, Urban P, Hoang V, Camenzin E, Chatelain P. Predicting the risk of ischemic complications after bail-out stenting for failed angioplasty. J Am Coll Cardiol 1994;23:72A.
1882. Moscucci M, Mansour K, Kuntz R, et al. Vascular complications of Palmaz-Schatz stenting: Predictors, management and outcome. J Am Coll Cardiol 1994;23:134A.
1883. Bartorelli A, Sganzerla P, Fabbiocchi F, et al. Prompt and safe femoral hemostasis with a collagen device after intracoronary implantation of Palmaz-Schatz stents. Am Heart J 1995;130(1):26-32.
1884. Mansour K, Moscucci M, Kent C, et al. Vascular complications following directional coronary atherectomy or Palmaz-Schatz stenting. J Am Coll Cardiol 1994;23:136A.
1885. Dean L, Voorhees W, Sutor C, Roubin G. Female gender: A risk factor for complications following intracoronary stenting? A Cook multicenter registry report. Circulation 1994;90:I-620.
1886. Cishek MB, Laslett L, Gershony G. Balloon catheter retrieval of dislodged coronary artery stents: A novel technique. Cathet Cardiovasc Diagn 1995;34:350-352.
1887. Rozenman Y, Burstein M, Hasin Y, Gotsman M. Retrieval of occluding unexpanded palamaz-Schatz stent from a saphenous aorto-coronary vein graft. Cathet Cardiovasc Diagn. 1995;34:159-161.
1888. Iniguez A, Macaya C, Alfonso F, Goicolea J. Early angiographic changes of side branches arising from a Palmaz-Schatz stented coronary segment: Results and clinical implications. J Am Coll Cardiol 1994;23:911-915.
1889. Mazur W, Grinstead C, Hakim A, et al. Fate of side branches after intracoronary implantation of the Gianturco-Roubin flex-stent for acute or threatened closure after percutaneous transluminal coronary angioplasty. Am J Cardiol 1994;74:1207-1210.
1890. Cohen D, Krumhotz H, Sukin C, et al. Economic outcomes in the randomized stent restenosis study (STRESS): In-hospital and one-year follow-up costs. Circulation 1994;90:I-620.
1891. Cohen D, Breall J, Ho K, et al. Evaluating the potential cost-effectiveness of stenting as a treatment for symptomatic single-vessel coronary disease. Use of a decision-analytic model. Circulation 1994;89:1859-1874.
1892. Cohen D, Baim D. Coronary stenting: Costly or cost-effective? J Inv Cardiol 1995;7:36A-42A.
1893. Weintraub W, Bernard J, Hicks F, Canup D, Mauldin P, Becker E. How coronary stents impact costs in interventional cardiology. Circulation 1995;92:I-436.
1894. Eccleston D, Eisenberg M. Ticlopidine without intravascular ultrasound or coumadin reduces high marginal costs of elective coronary stent deployment. Circulation 1995;92:I-796.
1895. Goods C, Liu M, Iyer S. A cost analysis of coronary stenting without anticoagulation versus stenting with anticoagulation using warfarin. Circulation 1995;92:I-796.
1896. Wong SC, Popma JJ, Chuang YC, et al. Economic impact of reduced anticoagulation after saphenous vein graft stent placement. J Am Coll Cardiol 1995;25:80A.
1897. Blengino S, Nakamura S, Hall P, et al. A cost analysis of intravascular ultrasound guided coronary stenting without anticoagulation vs. the traditional method of stenting with anticoagulation. J Am Coll Cardiol 1995;25:197A.
1898. Aggarwal R, Ireland D, Azrin M, Ezekowitz M, de Bono D, Gershlick A. Antithrombotic properties of stents eluting platelet glycoprotein IIb/IIIa antibody. Circulation 1995;92:I-488.
1899. Chronos N, Robinson K, Kelly A, et al. Thrombogenicity of tantalum stenosis decreased by surface heparin bonding: Scintigraphy of 111 in-plaletet deposition in baboon carotid arteries. Circulation 1995;92:I-490.
1900. De Scheerder I, Wang K, Wilczek K, Meuleman D, Piessens J. Heparin coating of metallic coronary stents decrease their thrombogenicity but does not decreases neointimal hyperplasia. Circulation 1995;92:I-537.
1901. Chronos N, Robinson K, Kelly A, et al. Thromboresistant phosphorylcholine coating for coronary stents. Circulation 1995;92:I-685.
1902. Laird J, Carter A, Kufs W, et al. Inhibition of neointimal proliferation with a beta particle emitting stent. J Am Coll Cardiol 1995;25:287A.
1903. Wiedermann J, Marboe C, Amois H, Schwartz A, Weinberger J. Intracoronary irradiation fails to reduce neointimal proliferation after oversized stenting in a porcine model. Circulation 1995;92:I-146.
1904. Hehrlein C, Kaiser S, Kollum M, Kinscherf R, Fehsenfeld P. Effects of very low dose endovascular irradiation via an activated guidewire on neointima formation after stent implantation. Circulation 1995;92:I-146.
1905. Hehrlein C, Gollan C, Donges K, Metz J, et al. Low-dose radioactive endovascular stents prevent smooth muscle cell proliferation and neointimal hyperplasia in rabbits. Circulation 1995;92:1570-1575.
1906. Slepian M, Massia S, Weselcouch E, Khosravi F, Roth L. Photopolymerization of hydrogel barriers on endoluminal surfaces of

porcine stented arteries reduces stent and adjacent arterial wall thrombogenicity. Circulation 1995;92:I-687.
1907. Waksman R, Robinson KA, Crocker IR, Gravanis MB, et al. Intracoronary radiation before stent implantation inhibits neointima formation in stented porcine coronary arteries. Circulation 1995;92:1383-1386.
1908. Teirstein P, Massullo V, Jani S, et al. Catheter-based radiation therapy to inhibit restenosis following coronary stenting. Circulation 1995;92:I-543.
1909. Sawa H, Vinogradsky B, Guala A, Fujii S. Genetically engineered endothelial cells: Increased surface fibrinolysis and potential adaptation to endovascular stenting. Circulation 1995;92:I-537.
1910. Murphy JG, Schwartz R, Edwards W, Camrud A. Percutaneous polymeric stents in porcine coronary arteries. Initial experience with polethylene terephthalate stents. Circulation 1992;86:1596-1604.
1911. Morice MC, Valelx B, Marco J, et al. Preliminary results of the MUST trial, major clinical events during the first month. J Am Coll Cardiology 1996;27:137A.
1912. Goods CM, Al-Shaibi KF, Dean LS, et al. Is ticlopidine a necessary component of antiplatelet regimens following coronary artery stenting. J Am Coll Cardiology 1996;27:137A.
1913. Marco J, Fajadt J, Brunel P, et al. First use of the second-generation Gianturco-Roubin stent without coumadin. Am J Cardiol 1996 (in-press).
1914. Elias J, Monassier JP, Carrie D, et al. Final results of phases II, III, IV and V of Medtronic Wiktor stent implantation without coumadin. J Am Coll Cardiology 1996;27:15A.
1915. Monassier JP, Ellias J, Meyer P, et al. STENTIM I: The French Registry of stenting of acute myocardial infarction. J Am Coll Cardiology 1996;27:68A.
1916. Hong MK, Wong SC, Popma JJ, et al. Favorable results of debulking followed by immediate adjunct stent therapy for high risk saphenous vein graft lesions. J Am Coll Cardiology 1996;27:179A.
1917. Douglas JS, Savage MP, Bailey S, Bailey R, et al. Randomized trial of coronary stent and balloon angioplasty in the treatment of saphaneous vein graft stenosis. J Am Coll Cardiology 1996;27:178A.
1918. Erbel R, Hande M, Hopp HW, et al. REstenosis STent (REST) study: Randomized trial comparing stenting and balloon angioplasty for treatment of restenosis after balloon angioplasty. J Am Coll Cardiology 1996;27:139A.
1919. Zidar JP, Kruse KR, Thel MC, et al. Integrelin for emergency coronary artery stenting. J Am Coll Cardiology 1996;27:138A.
1920. Sato Y, Nosaka H, Kimura AT, et al. Randomized comparison of balloon angioplasty versus coronary stent implantation for total occlusion. J Am Coll Cardiology 1996;27:152A.
1921. Fernandez-Ortiz A, Goicoles J, Perez-Vizcayno MJ, et al. Late clinical and angiographic outcome of bailout coronary stenting. A comparison between Gianturco-Roubin and Palmaz-Schatz stents. J Am Coll Cardiology 1996;27:111A.
1922. Caputo RP, Chafizedeh ER, Stoler RC, et al. "Stent Jail"— A minimum security prison. Am J Cardiol 1996 (in-press).
1923. Colombo A, Maiello L, Itoh A, Hall P, et al. Coronary stenting of bifurcation lesions immediate and follow-up results. J Am Coll Cardiology 1996;27:277A.
1924. Golderberg SL, Hall P, Nakamura S, et al. Is there a benefit from intravascular ultrasound when high-pressure stent expansion is routinely performed prior to ultrasound imaging? J Am Coll Cardiology 1996;27:306A.
1925. Serruys PQW, Azar AJ, Sigwart U, et al. Long-term follow-up of "stent-like" (≤ 30% diameter stenosis post) angioplasty: A case for provisional stenting. J Am Coll Cardiology 1996;27:15A.
1926. Colombo A, Itoh A, Maiello L, et al. Coronary stent implantation in aorto-ostial lesions: Immediate and follow-up results. J Am Coll Cardiology 1996;27:253A.
1927. Russo RJ, Teirstein PS, et al. Angiography versus intravascular ultrasound-directed stent placement. J Am Coll Cardiology 1996;27:306A.
1928. Teirstein P, Massullo V, Shirish J, et al. A Randomized, Clinical Trial of Radiation Therapy to Reduce Restenosis Following Coronary Stenting-Early Results. J Am Coll Cardiology 1996;27:15A.
1929. Lefevre T, Morice M, Labrunie B, et al. Coronary stenting in elderly patients. Results from the Stent Without Coumadin French Registry. J Am Coll Cardiology 1996;27:252A.
1930. Serruys P, Emanuelsson H, van der Giessen W, et al. Heparin-coated Palmaz-Schatz Stents in human coronary arteries. Early outcome of the Benestent-II pilot study. Circulation 1996;93:412-422.
1931. Schomig A, Neumann FJ, Kastrati A, et al. A randomized comparison of antiplatelet and anticoagulant therapy after the placement of coronary artery stents. N Engl J Med 1996;334:1084-9.
1932. Klugherz BD, DeAngelo DL, Kim BK, et al. Three-year clinical follow-up after Palmaz-Schatz stenting. J Am Coll Cardiol 1996;27:1185-91.
1933. Macaya C, Serruys PW, Ruygrok P, et al. Continued benefit of coronary stenting vs. balloon angioplasty: One-year clinical follow-up of Benestent trial. J Am Coll Cardiol 1996;27:255-61.
1934. Mak KH, Belli G, Ellis SG, Moliterno DJ. Subacute stent thrombosis: Evolving issues and current concepts. J Am Coll Cardiol 1996;27:494-503.
1935. Hall P, Nakamura S, Maiello L, et al. A randomized comparison ofr combined ticlopidine and aspirin therapy versus aspirin therapy alone after successful intravascular ultrasound-guided stent implantation. Circulation 1996;93:215-22.
1936. Lindsay J, Hong MK, Pinnow EE, Pichard AD. Effects of endoliminal coronary stents on the frequency of coronary artery bypass grafting after unsuccessful percutaneous transluminal coronary revascularization. Am J Cardiol 1996;77:647-9.
1937. Hermiller JB, Fry ET, Peters TF, et al. Late coronary artery stenosis regression within the Gianturco-Roubin intracoronary stent. Am J Cardiol 1996;77:247-51.
1938. Kaul U, Agarwal R, Jain P, Wasir H. Safety and efficacy of intracoronary stenting for thrombus-containing lesions. Am J Cardiol 1996;77:425-7.
1939. Garcia-Cantu E, Spaulding C, Corcos T, et al. Stent implantation in acute myocardial infation. Am J Cardiol 1996;77:451-4.
1940. Sankardas MA, McEniery PT, Aroney CN, Bett JHN. Elective implantation of intracoronary stents without intravascular ultrasound

guidance or subsequent warfarin. Cathet Cardiovasc Diagn 1996;37:355-9.

Rotablator Atherectomy

1941. Fourrier JL, Stankowiak C, Lablanche JM, et al. Histopathology after rotational angioplasty of peripheral arteries in human beings. J Am Coll Cardiol 1988;11:109A.
1942. Kovach J, Mintz G, Pichard A, Kent K, et al. Sequential intravascular ultrasound characterization of the mechanisms of rotational atherectomy and adjunct balloon angioplasty. J Am Coll Cardiol 1993;22:1024-32.
1943. Mintz G, Potkin B, Keren G, Satler L, et al. Intravascular ultrasound evaluation of the effect of rotational atherectomy in obstructive atherosclerotic coronary artery disease. Circulation 1992; 86:1383-1393.
1944. Cowley M, Buchbinder M, Warth D, Dorros G, et al. Effect of coronary rotational atherectomy abrasion on vessel segments adjacent to treated lesions . J Am Coll Cardiol 1992;19:333A.
1945. Prevosti LG, Cook JA, Unger EF, Sheffield CD, et al. Particulate debris from rotational atherectomy: size distribution and physiologic effect. Circulation 1988;78:II-83.
1946. Friedman HZ, Elliott MA, Gottlieb GJ, O'Neill WW. Mechanical rotary atherectomy: The effects of microparticle embolization on myocardial blood flow and function. J Interv Cardiol 1989;2:77-83.
1947. Hansen DD, Auth DC, Hall M, Ritchie JL. Rotational endarterectomy in normal canine coronary arteries: preliminary report. J Am Coll Cardiol 1988; 11:1073-77.
1948. Sherman C, Brunken R, Chan A, et al. Myocardial perfusion and segmental wall motion after coronary rotational atherectomy. Circulation 1992;86:I-652.
1949. Pavlides G, Hauser A, Grines C, et al. Clinical, hemodynamic, electrocardiographic, and mechanical events during nonocclusive coronary atherectomy and comparison to balloon angioplasty. Am J Cardiol 1992;70:841-845.
1950. Williams MJA, Dow CJ, Weyman AE, et al. Myocardial dysfunction after rotational coronary atherectomy: Serial evaluation by echocardiography. Circulation 1994;90:I-395.
1951. Huggins GS, Williams MJA, Yang J, et al. Transient wall motion abnormalities following rotational atherectomy are reflective of myocardial stunning more than myocardial infarction. J Am Coll Cardiol 1995;25:96A.
1952. Nunez BD, Keelan ET, Lerman A, et al. Coronary hemodynamics after rotational atherectomy. J Am Coll Cardiol 1995;25:95A.
1953. Safian R, Freed M, Lichtenberg A, et al. Are residual stenoses after excimer laser angioplasty and coronary atherectomy due to inefficient or small devices? Comparison with balloon angioplasty. J Am Coll Cardiol 1993;22:628-1634.
1954. Reisman M, Buchbinder M, Bass T, et al. Improvement in coronary dimensions at early 24-hour follow-up after coronary rotational ablation: Implications for restenosis. Circulation 1992;86:I-332.
1955. Kovach JA, Mintz GS, et al. Sequential intravascular ultrasound characterization of the mechanisms of rotational atherectomy and adjunct balloon angioplasty. J Am Coll Cardiol 1993;22:1024-32.
1956. Mintz GS, Douek P, et al. Target lesion calcification in coronary artery disease: An intravascular ultrasound study. J Am Coll Cardiol 1992;20:1149-55.
1957. Nino C, Free M, Blankenship L, et al. Procedural cost and benefits of new interventional devices. Am J Cardiol 1994;74:1165-1166.
1958. Vandormael M, Reifart N, Preusler W, et al. In-hospital costs comparison of excimer laser angioplasty, rotational atherectomy (Rotablator) and balloon angioplasty for complex coronary lesions: A randomized trial (ERBAC). J Am Coll Cardiol 1994;89:223A.
1959. Cohen B, et al. Intracoronary cocktail infusion during rotational ablation: Safety and Efficacy. Cathet Cardiovasc Diagn (in press).
1960. Reisman M, Harms V. Guidewire bias: A potential source of complications with rotational atherectomy. Cathet Cardiovasc Diagn (in press).
1961. Mintz GS, Pichard AD, et al. Transcatheter device synergy: preliminary experience with adjunct directional coronary atherectomy following high-speed rotational atherectomy or excimer laser angioplasty in the treatment of coronary artery disease. Cathet Cardiovasc Diagn 1993;28:37-44.
1962. Mintz GS, Dussaillsnt GR, Wong SC, et al. Rotational atherectomy followed by adjunct stents: The preferred therapy for calcified large vessels? Circulation 1995;92:I-329.
1963. Mintz GS, Pichard AD, et al. Impact of preintervention intravascular ultrasound imaging on transcatheter treatment strategies in coronary artery disease. Am J Cardiol 1994;73:423-430.
1964. MacIsaac A, Whitlow P, Cowley M, Buchbinder M. Angiographic predictors of outcome of coronary rotational atherectomy from the completed multicenter registry. J Am Coll Cardiol 1994;23:353A.
1965. Redwood SR, Popma JJ, Kent KM, Pichard AD, et al. "Minor" CPK-MB elevations are associated with increased mortality following new-device angioplasty in native coronary arteries. Circulation 1995;92:I-544.
1966. Safian RD, Niazi KA, et al. Detailed angiographic analysis of high-speed mechanical rotational atherectomy in human coronary arteries. Circulation 1993;88:961-8.
1967. Vandormael M, Reifart N, Preusler W, et al. Comparison of excimer laser, rotablator and balloon angioplasty for the treatment of complex lesions: ERBAC study final results. J Am Coll Cardiol, 1994;23:57A.
1968. Dietz UR, Erbel R, et al. Angiographic and histologic findings in high frequency rotational ablation in coronary arteries in vitro. Zeitschrift fur Kardiologie 1991;80:222-9.
1969. Borrions M, Hall P, et al. Treatment of simple and complex coronary stenosis using rotational ablation followed by low pressure balloon angioplasty. Cath Cardiovasc Diagn 1993;30:131-7.
1970. Guerin Y, Rahal S, et al. Coronary angioplasty combining rotational atherectomy and balloon dilatation. Results in 67 complex stenoses. Arch Mal du Coeur 1993;86:1535-41.
1971. Gilmore PS, Bass TA, et al. Single site experience with high-speed coronary rotational atherectomy. Clin Cardiol 1993;16:311-6.

1972. Warth DC, Leon MB, et al. Rotational atherectomy multicenter registry: Acute results, complications and 6-month angiographic follow-up in 709 patients. J Am Coll Cardiol 1994;24:641-8.
1973. Stertzer SH, Rosenblum J, et al. Coronary rotational ablation: initial experience in 302 procedures. J Am Coll Cardiol 1993;21:287-95.
1974. Ellis SG, Popma JJ, et al. Relation of clinical presentation, stenosis morphology, and operator technique to the procedural results of rotational atherectomy and rotational atherectomy facilitated angioplasty. Circulation 1994;89:882-92.
1975. MacIsaac AI, Bass TA, Buchbinder M, et al. High speed rotational atherectomy: Outcome in calcified and noncalcified coronary artery lesions. J Am Coll Cardiol 1995;26:531-6.
1976. Leguizamon JH, Chambre DF, Torresani EM, et al. High speed coronary rotational atherectomy: Are angiographic factors predictive of failure, major complications or restenosis? J Am Coll Cardiol 1995;25:95A.
1977. Altmann D, Popma J, Kent K, et al. Rotational atherectomy effectively treats calcified lesions. J Am Coll Cardiol 1993;21:443A.
1978. Dussaillant GR, Mintz GS, Walsh CL, et al. Volumetric intravascular ultrasound analysis shows that rotational atherectomy effectively ablates soft atherosclerotic plaque. Circulation 1995;92:I-17.
1979. Reisman M, Cohen B, Warth D, Fenner J, et al. Outcome of long lesions treated with high speed rotational ablation. J Am Coll Cardiol 1993;21:443A.
1980. Favereaux X, Chevalier B, Commeau P, et al. Is rotational atherectomy more effective than balloon angioplasty for the treatment of long coronary lesions? SCA & I Meeting Abstracts, 92.
1981. Koller PT, Freed M, Grines CL, O'Neill WW. Success, complications, and restenosis following rotational and transluminal extraction atherectomy of ostial stenoses. Cathet and Cardiovas Diagn 1994;31:255-260.
1982. Popma J, Brogan W, Pichard A, et al. Rotational coronary atherectomy of ostial stenoses. Am J Cardiol 1993;71:436-438.
1983. Zimarino M, Corcos T, Favereau X, et al. Rotational coronary atherectomy with adjunctive balloon angioplasty for the treatment of ostial lesions. Cathet Cardiovas Diagn 1994;33:22-27.
1984. Sabri MN, Cowley MJ, DiSciascio G, DeBottis D, et al. Immediate results of interventional devices for coronary ostial narrowing with angina pectoris. Am J Cardiol 1994;73:122-125.
1985. Omoigui N, Booth J, Reisman M, et al. Rotational atherectomy in chronic total occlusions. J Am Coll Cardiol 1995;25:97A.
1986. Reisman M, Devlin P, Melikian J, et al. Undilatable noncompliant lesions treated with the Rotablator: outcome and angiographic follow-up. Circulation 1993;88: I-547.
1987. Brogan W, Popma J, Pichard A, Satler L, et al. Rotational coronary atherectomy after unsuccessful coronary balloon angioplasty. Am J Cardiol 1993;71:794-798.
1988. Rosenblum J, Stertzer S, Shaw R, et al. Rotational ablation of balloon angioplasty failures. J Inva Cardiol 1992;4:312-317.
1989. Sievert H, Tonndorf S, Utech A, Schulze R. [High frequency rotational angioplasty (rotablation) after unsuccessful balloon dilatation] Z Cardiol 1993;82:411- 414.
1990. Bass T, Gilmore P, Buchbinder M, et al. Coronary rotational atherectomy (PTCA) in patients with prior coronary revascularization: a registry report. Circulation 1992;86:I-653.
1991. Chevalier B, Commeau P, Favereau X, et al. Limitations of rotational atherectomy in angulated coronary lesions. J Am Coll Cardiol 1994;23:285A.
1992. Dussaillant GR, Mintz GS, Pichard AD, et al. The optimal strategy for treating calcified lesions in large vessels: Comparison of intravascular ultrasound results of rotational atherectomy + adjunctive PTCA, DCA, or stents. J Am Coll Cardiol 1996;27:153A.
1993. O'Murchu B, Foreman RD, Shaw RE, et al. Role of intraaortic balloon pump counterpulsation in high risk coronary rotational atherectomy. J Am Coll Cardiol 1995;26:1270-5.
1994. Reisman M, DeVore LJ, ferguson M, et al. Analysis of heat generation during high-speed rotational ablation: Technical implications. J Am Coll Cardiol 1996;27:292A.
1995. Coletti RH, Haik BJ, Wiedermann JG, et al. Marked reduction in slow-reflow after rotational atherectomy through the use of a novel flushing solution. TCT Meeting 1996;Washington DC
1996. Stertzer SH, Pomerantsev EV, Fitzgerald PJ, et al. Effects of technique modification on immediate results of high speed rotational atherectomy in 710 procedures on 656 patients. Cathet Cardiovasc Diagn 1995;304-310.
1997. Dusaillant GR, Mintz GS, Pichard AD, et al. Mechanisms and immediate and long-term results of adjunct directional coronary atherectomy after rotational atherectomy. J Am Coll Cardiol 1996;27:1390-1397.
1998. Walton AS, Pomerantsev EV, Oesterle SN, et al. Outcome of narrowing related sidebranches after high-speed rotational atherectomy. Am J Cardiol 1996;77:370-3.
1999. Stertzer SH, Pomerantsev EV, Fitzgerald PS, et al. Effects of technique modification on immediate results of high-speed rotation atherectomy in 710 procedures in 656 patients. Cathet Cardiovasc Diagn 1995;36:304-10.

Directional Coronary Atherectomy

2000. Topol E, Califf R, Weisman H, et al. Randomized trial of coronary intervention with antibody against platelet IIb/IIIa integ reduction of clinical restenosis: results at six months. Lancet 1994;343:881-886.
2001. Mintz GS, Pichard AD, Kent KM, Kovach JA, Popma JJ, Satler LF, Leon MB. Transcatheter device synergy: Pr experience with adjunct directional coronary atherectomy following high-speed rotational atherectomy or excimer laser a in the treatment of coronary artery disease. Cathet Cardiovasc Diagn 1993;Suppl 1:37-44.
2002. Dussaillant GR, Griffin J, Weaver TK, Deible RA, Pichard AD. Transcatheter device synergy: Intravascular ultrasoun of rotational atherectomy followed by adjunct directional coronary atherectomy in the treatment of calcified coronary a Circulation 1995;92:I-329.
2003. Leon M, Kuntz R, Popma J, et al. Acute angiographic, intravascular ultrasound and clinical results of directional the optimal atherectomy restenosis study. J Am Coll Cardiol 1995;25:137A.

2004. Simonton CA, Leon MB, Kuntz RE, et al. Acute and late clinical and angiographic results of directional atherectomy in the optimal atherectomy restenosis study (OARS). Circulation 1995;92:I-545.
2005. Doi T, Tamai H, Ueda K, Hsu YS, Ono S, et al. Impact of intracoronary ultrasound-guided directional atherectomy on restenosis. Circulation 1995;92:I-545.
2006. Bauman RP, Yock PG, Fitzgerald PJ, Annex BH, et al. "Reference Cut" method of intracoronary ultrasound guided directional coronary atherectomy: Initial and six month results. Circulation 1995;92:I-546.
2007. Baim D, Kuntz R, Popma J, Leon M. Results of directional atherectomy in the "Pilot" phase of BOAT. Circulation 1994;90:I-214.
2008. Baim DS, Kuntz RE, Sharma SK, Fortuna R, Feldman R, et al. Acute results of the randomized phase of the balloon versus optimal atherectomy trial (BOAT). Circulation 1995;92:I-544.
2009. Mintz GS, Pichard AD, Dussaillant GR, Satler LF, Wong SC, Walsh CL, et al. Acute results of adjunct stents following directional coronary atherectomy. Circulation 1995;92:I-326.
2010. Waksman R, Weintraub WS, Ghazzal ZMB, Douglas JS, et al. Directional coronary atherectomy (DCA): Is much bigger much better? Circulation 1995;92:I-329.
2011. Safian R, Gelbfish J, Erny R, Schnitt S, Schmidt D, Baim D. Coronary atherectomy. Clinical, angiographic, and histological findings and observations regarding potential mechanisms. Circulation 1990;82:69-79.
2012. Baim D, Kuntz R. Directional coronary atherectomy: How much lumen enlargement is optional? Am J Cardiol 1993;72:65E-70E.
2013. Penny W, Schmidt D, Safian R, Erny R, Baim D. Insights into the Mechanism of Luminal Improvement After Directional Coronary Atherectomy. Am J Cardiol 1991;67:435-437.
2014. Matar F, Mintz G, Farb A, Douek P. The contribution of tissue removal to lumen improvement after directional coronary atherectomy. Am J Cardiol 1994;74:647-650.
2015. Tenaglia AN, Buller CE, Kisslo KB, Stack RS. Mechanisms of balloon angioplasty and directional coronary atherectomy as assessed by intracoronary ultrasound. J Am Coll Cardiol 1992;20:685-691.
2016. Braden G, Herrington D, Downes T, et al. Qualitative and quantitative contrasts in the mechanisms of lumen enlargement by coronary balloon angioplasty and directional coronary atherectomy. J Am Coll Cardiol 1994;23:40-48.
2017. Umans V, Baptisla J, di Mario C, et al. Angiographic, ultrasound, and angioscopic assessment of the coronary artery wall and lumen area configuration after directional atherectomy: The mechanism revisited. Am Heart J 1995;130:217-227.
2018. Fortuna R, Walston D, Hansell H, Schulz G. Directional coronary atherectomy: Experience in 310 patients. J Invas Cardiol 1995;7:57-64.
2019. Umans V, de Feyter P, Deckers J, et al. Acute and long-term outcome of directional coronary atherectomy for stable and unstable angina. Am J Cardiol 1993;74:641-646.
2020. Popma J, Mintz G, Satler L, et al. Clinical and angiographic outcome after directional coronary atherectomy: A qualitative and quantitative analysis using coronary arteriography and intravascular ultrasound. Am J Cardiol 1993;72:55E-64E.
2021. Cowley M, DiSciascio G. Experience with directional coronary atherectomy since pre-market approval. Am J Cardiol 1993;72:12E-20E.
2022. Baim D, Tomoaki H, Holmes D, et al. Results of directional coronary atherectomy during multicenter preapproval testing. Am J Cardiol 1993;72:6E-11E.
2023. Feld H, Schulhoff N, Lichstein E, et al. Coronary atherectomy versus angioplasty: The CAVA study. Am Heart J 1993;126:31-38.
2024. Popma J, Topol E, Hinohara T, et al. Abrupt vessel closure after directional coronary atherectomy. J Am Coll Cardiol 1992;19:1372-1379.
2025. Garratt K, Holmes D, Bell M, et al. Results of directional atherectomy of primary atheromatous and restenosis lesions in coronary arteries and saphenous vein grafts. Am J Cardiol 1992;70:449-454.
2026. Ellis S, DeCesare N, Pinkerton C, Whitlow P. Relation of stenosis morphology and clinical presentation to the procedural results of directional coronary atherectomy. Circulation 1991;84:644-653.
2027. Hinohara T, Rowe MH, Robertson GC, et al. Effect of lesion characteristics on outcome of directional coronary atherectomy. J Am Coll Cardiol 1991;17:1112-20.
2028. Rowe MH, Hinohara T, White NW, Robertson GC. Comparison of dissection rates and angiographic results following directional coronary atherectomy and coronary angioplasty. Am J Cardiol 1990;66:49-53.
2029. Kaufmann UP, Garratt KN, Vlietstra RE, Menke KK. Coronary atherectomy: First 50 patients at the Mayo Clinic. Mayo Clin Proc 1989;64:747-752.
2030. Cowley M, Whitlow P, Baim D, Hinohara T, et al. Directional coronary atherectomy of saphenous vein graft narrowings: Multicenter investigational experience. Am J Cardiol 1993;72:30E-34E.
2031. Pomerantz R, Kuntz R, Carrozza J, et al. Acute and long-term outcome of narrowed saphenous venous grafts treated by endoluminal stenting and directional atherectomy. Am J Cardiol 1992;70:161-167.
2032. DiScasio G, Cowley MJ, Vetrovec GW, Goudreau E, et al. Directional coronary atherectomy of saphenous vein graft lesions unfavorable for balloon angioplasty: Results of a single center experience. Cathet Cardiovasc Diagn 1992;26:75.
2033. Ghazzal ZMB, Douglas JS, Holmes DR, et al. Directional atherectomy of saphenous vein grafts: Recent multicenter experience. J Am Coll Cardiol 1991;17:219A.
2034. Selmon MR, Hinohara T, Robertson GC, Rowe MH, et al. Directional coronary atherectomy for saphenous vein graft stenoses. J Am Coll Cardiol 1991;17:23A.
2035. Kaufmann U, Garratt K, Vlietstra R, Holmes D. Transluminal atherectomy of saphenous vein aortocoronary bypass grafts. Am J Cardiol 1990;65:1430-1433.
2036. Stephan W, Bates E, Garratt K, Hinohara T, Muller D. Directional atherectomy of coronary and saphenous vein graft ostial stenoses. Am J Cardiol 1995;75:1015-1018.
2037. Fishman R, Kuntz R, Carrozza J, et al. Long-term results of directional coronary atherectomy: Predictors of restenosis. J Am Coll Cardiol 1992;20:1101-1110.

2038. Bergelson B, Fishman R, Tomaso C, et al. Acute and long-term outcome of failed percutaneous transluminal coronary angioplasty treated by directional coronary atherectomy. Am J Cardiol 1994;73:1224-1226.
2039. Harris W, Berger P, Holmes D, Garratt K. "Rescue" directional coronary atherectomy after unsuccessful percutaneous transluminal coronary angioplasty. Mayo Clin Proc 1994;69:717-722.
2040. McCluskey E, Cowley M, Whitlow P. Multicenter clinical experience with rescue atherectomy for failed angioplasty. Am J Cardiol 1993;72:42E-46E.
2041. Movsowitz H, Emmi R, Manginas A, et al. Directional coronary atherectomy for failed balloon angioplasty: Outcome depends on the Underlying pathology. Circulation 1993;88:I-601.
2042. Hofling B, Gonschior P, Simpson L, Bauriedel G. Efficacy of directional coronary atherectomy in cases unsuitable for percutaneous transluminal coronary angioplasty (PTCA) and after unsuccessful PTCA. Am Heart J 1992;124:341-348.
2043. Mansour M, Fishman RF, Kuntz RE, Carrozza JP. Feasibility of directional atherectomy for the treatment of bifurcation lesions. Cor Art Dis 1992;3:761-765.
2044. Eisenhauer AC, Clugston RA, Ruiz CE. Sequential directional atherectomy of coronary bifurcation lesions. Cathet Cardiovasc Diagn 1993;Suppl 1:54-60.
2045. Groassman ED, Leya FS, Lewis BE, Johnson SA, et al. Examination of common PTCA guide wires used for side branch protection during directional coronary atherectomy of bifurcation lesions performed in vivo and in vitro. Cathet Cardiovasc Diagn 1993;1:48-53.
2046. Popma JJ, Dick RJL, Haudenschild CC, Topol EJ, Ellis S. Atherectomy of right coronary ostial stenoses: Initial and long-term results, technical features and histologic findings. Am J Cardiol 1991;67:431-433.
2047. Lewis B, Leya F, Johnson S, et al. Acute procedural results in the treatment of 30 coronary artery bifurcation lesions with a double-wire atherectomy technique for side-branch protection. Am Heart J 1994;127:1600-1607.
2048. Mooney M, Mooney-Fishman J, Madison J, Nahhan A, Van Tassel R. Directional atherectomy for long lesions: Improved results. Cathet Cardiovasc Diagn 1993;1:26-30.
2049. Laster S, Rutherford B, McConahay D, Giorgi L, Johnson W. Directional atherectomy of left main stenoses. Cathet Cardiovasc Diagn 1994;33:317-322.
2050. Dick RJL, Haudenschild CC, Popma JJ, Ellis SG. Directional atherectomy for total coronary occlusions. Cor Art Dis 1991;2:189-199.
2051. Baldwin TF, Lash RE, Whitfeld SS, Toalson WB. Directional coronary atherectomy in acute myocardial infarction. J Inv Cardiol 1993;5:288-294.
2052. Emmi R, Movsoqitz H, Manginas A, et al. Directional coronary atherectomy in lesions with coexisting thrombus. Circulation 1993;88:3204.
2053. Topol E, Leya F, Pinkerton C, et al. A comparison of directional atherectomy with coronary angioplasty in patients with coronary artery disease. N Engl J Med 1993;329:221-227.
2054. Adelman A, Cohen E, Kimball B, et al. A comparison of directional atherectomy with balloon angioplasty for lesions of the left anterior descending coronary artery. N Engl J Med 1993;329:228-233.
2055. Holmes D, Topol E, Califf R, et al. A multicenter, randomized trial of coronary angioplasty versus directional atherectomy for patients with saphenous vein bypass graft lesions. Circulation 1995;91:1966-1974.
2056. Gordon P, Kugelmass A, Cohen D, et al. Balloon postdilation can safety improve the results of successful (but suboptimal) directional coronary atherectomy. Am J Cardiol 1993;72:71E-79E.
2057. Carrozza J, Baim J. Complications of directional coronary atherectomy: Incidence, causes, and management. Am J Cardiol 1993;72:47E-54E.
2058. Carrozza JP, Baim DS, Safian RD, et al. Risks and complications of coronary atherectomy. In: Atherectomy, eds. Holmes DR, Garratt KN; Blackwell Scientific Publication, 1992, p.132-148.
2059. Van Suylen RJ, Serruys PW, Simpson JB, et al. Delayed rupture of right coronary artery after directional coronary atherectomy for bail-out. Am Heart J 1991;121:914-917.
2060. Selmon MR, Robertson GC, Simpson JB, et al. Retrieval of media and adventitia by directional coronary atherectomy and angiographic correlation. Circulation 1990;82:III-624.
2061. Safian R, Schreiber T, Baim D. Specific indications for directional coronary atherectomy: Origin left anterior descending coronary artery and bifurcating lesions. Am J Cardiol 1993;72:35E-41E.
2062. Campos-Esteve M, Laird J, Kufs W, Wortham CD. Side-branch occlusion with directional coronary atherectomy: Incidence and risk factors. Am Heart J 1994;128:686-690.
2063. Tauke JT, Kong TW, Meyers SN, et al. Prognostic value of creatinine kinase elevation following elective coronary artery interventions. J Am Coll Cardiol 1995;25:269A.
2064. Hinohara T, Vetter JW, Robertson GC, Selmon MR, et al. CK MB elevation following directional coronary atherectomy. Circulation 1995;92:I-544.
2065. Kugelmass AD, Cohen DJ, Moscucci M, et al. Elevation of the creatine kinase myocardial isoform following otherwise successful directional coronary atherectomy and stenting. Am J Cardiol 1994;74:748-754.
2066. Lefkovits J, Anderson K, Weisman H, Topol E. Increased risk of non-Q MI following DCA: Evidence for a platelet dependant mechanism from the EPIC Trial. Circulation 1994;90:I-214.
2067. Cutlip DE, Ho KKL, Senerchia C, Baim DS, et al. Classification of myocardial infarction after directional coronary atherectomy and relation to clinical outcome: Results of the OARS trial. Circulation 1995;92:I-616.
2068. Omoigui N, Califf R, Pieper K, et al. Peripheral vascular complications in the coronary angioplasty versus excisional atherectomy trial (CAVEAT-I). J Am Coll Cardiol 1995;26:922-930.
2069. Elliott J, Berdan L, Holmes D, et al. One-year follow-up in the coronary angioplasty versus excisional atherectomy trial (CAVEAT I). Circulation 1995;91:2158-2166.

2070. Umans V, Keane D, Foley D, Boersma E, et al. Optimal use of directional coronary atherectomy is required to ensure long-term angiographic benefit: A study with matched procedural outcome after atherectomy and angioplasty. J Am Coll Cardiol 1994;24:1652-1659.

2071. Morris D, Weintraub W, Liberman H, Douglas J, King S. A case matched comparison of directional atherectomy to balloon angioplasty. Circulation 1993;88:3232.

2072. Mintz GS, Fitzgerald PJ, Kuntz RE, Simonton CA, et al. Lesion site and reference segment remodeling after directional coronary atherectomy: An analysis from the optimal atherectomy restenosis study. Circulation 1995;92:I-93.

2073. Mintz GS, Kent KM, Satler LF, Wong SC, Hong MK, Griffin J, Pichard AD. Dimorphic mechanisms of restenosis after DCA and stents: A serial intravascular ultrasound study. Circulation 1995;92:I-546.

2074. Mitsuo K, Degawa T, Nakamura S, Ui K, et al. Serial intravascular ultrasound evaluation of the mechanism of restenosis after directional coronary atherectomy. Circulation 1995;92:I-149.

2075. Kosuga K, Tamai H, Ueda K, Hsu YS, et al. Efficacy of tranilast on restenosis after directional coronary atherectomy (DCA). Circulation 1995;92:I-346.

2076. Popma JJ, DeCesare NB, Ellis SG, Holmes DR. Clinical, angiographic and procedural correlates of quantitative coronary dimensions after directional coronary atherectomy. J Am Coll Cardiol 1991;18:1183-1189.

2077. Umans V, Robert A, Foley D, et al. Clinical, histological and quantitative angiographic predictors pf restenosis after directional coronary atherectomy: A multivariate analysis of the renarrowing process and late outcome. J Am Coll Cardiol 1994;23:49-58.

2078. Hinohara T, Robertson G, Selmon M, et al. Restenosis after directional coronary atherectomy. J Am Coll Cardiol 1992;20:623-632.

2079. Garratt KN, Kaufmann UP, Edwards WD, Vlietsra RE. Safety of percutaneous coronary atherectomy with deep arterial resection. Am J Cardiol 1989;64:538-542.

2080. Kuntz RE, Gibson MC, Nobuyoshi M, Baim DS. Generalized Model of Restenosis After Conventional Balloon Angioplasty, Stenting and Directional Atherectomy. J Am Coll Cardiol 1993;21:15-25.

2081. Garratt K, Holmes D, Bell M, et al. Restenosis after directional coronary atherectomy: Differences between primary atheromatous and restenosis lesions and the influence of subintimal resection. J Am Coll Cardiol 1990;16:1665-1671.

2082. Kuntz R, Hinohara T, Safian R, Selmon M, Simpson J, Baim D. Restenosis after directional coronary atherectomy. Effects of luminal diameter and deep wall excision. Circulation 1992;86:1394-1399.

2083. Bell M, Garratt K, Bresnahan J, Edwards W, Holmes D. Relation of deep arterial resection and coronary artery aneurysms after directional coronary atherectomy. J Am Coll Cardiol 1992;20:1474-1481.

2084. Abdelmeguid A, Ellis S, Sapp S, Simpfendrofer C. Directional coronary atherectomy in unstable angina. J Am Coll Cardiol 1994;24:46-54.

2085. Ghazzal Z, Hinohara T, Scott N, et al. Directional coronary atherectomy in patients with recent myocardial infarction. A NACI Registry Report. J Am Coll Cardiol 1993;21:32A.

2086. Robertson G, Hinohara T, Vetter J, et al. Directional coronary atherectomy for patients with recent myocardial infarction. J Am Coll Cardiol 1994;23:219A.

2087. Poelnitz AV, Backa D, Bauriedel G, Nerlich A. Coronary directional atherectomy: Rescue for failed balloon angioplasty and treatment of complicated lesions. J Interven Cardiol 1991;4:5-11.

2088. Movsowitz H, Manginas A, Emmi R, et al. Directional coronary atherectomy can be successfully performed in the elderly. Am J Cardiol 1994;31:261-263.

2089. Strauss B, Umans V, van Suylen R-J, et al. Directional atherectomy for treatment of restenosis within coronary stents: Clinical, angiographic and histologic results. J Am Coll Cardiol 1992;20:1465-1473.

2090. Lewis B, Leya F, Johnson S, et al. Outcome of angioplasty (PTCA) and atherectomy (DCA) for bifurcation and non-bifurcation lesions in CAVEAT. Circulation 1993;88:I-601.

2091. Waksman R, Weintraub WS, Ziyad MB, Douglas JS, Shen Y, King SB. Balloon angioplasty, Palmaz-Schatz stent, and directional coronary atherectomy for restenotic lesions: Retrospective comparison in a single center. J Am Coll Cardiol 1995;25;330A.

2092. Escaned J, van Suylen R, MacLeod D, et al. Histologic characteristics of tissue excised during directional coronary atherectomy in stable and unstable angina pectoris. Am J Cardiol 1993;71:1442-1447.

2093. Rosenschein U, Ellis S, Haudenschild C, et al. Comparison of histopathologic coronary lesions obtained from directional atherectomy in stable angina versus acute coronary syndromes. Am J Cardiol 1994;73:508-510.

2094. Miller M, Kuntz R, Friedrich S, et al. Frequency and consequences of intimal hyperplasia in specimens retrieved by directional atherectomy of native primary coronary artery stenoses and subsequent restenoses. Am J Cardiol 1993;71:652-657.

2095. DiSciascio G, Cowley M, Goudreau E, Vetrovec G, Johnson D. Histopathologic correlates of unstable ischemic syndromes in patients undergoing directional coronary atherectomy: In vivo evidence of thrombosis, ulceration, and inflammation. Am Heart J 1994;128:419-26.

2096. Arbustini E, De Servi S, Bramucci E, et al. Comparison of coronary lesions obtained by directional coronary atherectomy in unstable angina, stable angina, and restenosis after either atherectomy or angioplasty. Am J Cardiol 1995;75:675-682.

2097. Annex B, Denning S, Channon K, et al. Differential expression of tissue factor protein in directional atherectomy specimens from patients with stable and unstable coronary syndromes. Circulation 1995;91:619-622.

2098. Holmes DR, Simpson JB, Berdan LG, et al. Abrupt closure: The CAVEAT I Experience. J Am Coll Cardiol 1995;26:1494-500.

2099. Mehta S, Popma J, Margolis JR, et al. Complications with new angioplasty devices. Are these device specific? J Am Coll Cardiol 1996;27:168A.

2100. Popma JJ, Baim DS, Kuntz RE, Mintz GS, et al. Early and late quantitative angiographic outcomes in the Optimal Atherectomy Restenosis Study (OARS). J Am Coll Cardiol 1996;27:91A.

2101. Dusaillant GR, Mintz GS, Pichard AD, et al. Mechanisms and immediate and long-term results of adjunct directional coronary atherectomy after rotational atherectomy. J Am Coll Cardiol 1996;27:1390-1397.

TEC Atherectomy

2102. Annex BH, Larkin TJ, O'Neill WW, Safian RS. Evaluation of thrombus removal by transluminal extraction coronary atherectomy by percutaneous coronary angioscopy. Amer J Cardiol 1994;74:606-9.
2103. Kaplan BM, Safian RS, Grines CL, Goldstein JA, et al. Usefulness of adjunctive angioscopy and extraction atherectomy before stent implantation in high risk narrowings in aorto-coronary artery saphenous vein grafts. Amer J Cardiol 1995;76:822-824.
2104. Moses JW, Lieberman SM, Knopf WD, et al. Mechanism of transluminal extraction catheter (TEC) atherectomy in degenerative saphenous vein grafts (SVG): An Angioscopic Observational Study. J Am Coll Cardiol 1993;21:442A.
2105. Popma JJ, Leon MB, Mintz GS, et al. Results of coronary angioplasty using the transluminal extraction catheter. Am J Cardiol 1992;70:1526-1532.
2106. Pizzulli L, Kohler U, Manz M, Luderitz B. Mechanical dilatation rather than plaque removal as major mechanism of transluminal extraction atherectomy. J Intervent Cardiol 1993;6:31-39.
2107. IVT Coronary TEC Atherectomy Clinical Database. 1995.
2108. Safian RS, May MA, Lichtenberg A, et al. Detailed clinical and angiographic analysis of complex lesions in native coronary arteries. J Am Coll Cardiol 1995;25:848-854.
2109. Safian RD, Freed M, Reddy V, et al. Do excimer laser and rotational atherectomy facilitate balloon angioplasty? Implications for lesion-specific coronary intervention. J Am Coll Cardiol (in-press)
2110. Ishizaka N, Ikari Y, Hara K, Saeki F, et al. Angiographic follow-up of patients after transluminal extraction atherectomy. Am Heart J 1994; 128(4): 691-696.
2111. Safian RS, Grines CL, May MA, et al. Clinical and angiographic results of transluminal extraction coronary atherectomy in saphenous vein bypass grafts. Circulation 1994; 89(1): 302-312.
2112. Meany TB, Leon MB, Kramer BL, et al. Transluminal extraction catheter for the treatment of diseased saphenous vein grafts: A multicenter experience. Cathet Cardio Diagn 1995; 34: 112-120.
2113. Twidale N, Barth III, CW, Kipperman RM, et al. Acute results and long-term outcome of transluminal catheter atherectomy for saphenous vein graft stenoses. Cath and Cardio Diagn 1994; 31: 187-91.
2114. Kaplan BM, Benzuly KH, Bowers TR, et al. Prospective study of intracoronary verapamil and nitroglycerin for the treatment of no-reflow after interventions on degenerated saphenous vein grafts. Circ 1995; 92:I-330.
2115. Piana RN, Paik GY, Moscucci M, Cohen DJ, et al. Incidence and treatment of "no-reflow" after percutaneous coronary intervention. Circulation 1994; 89(6): 2514-2518.
2116. Pomerantz RM, Kuntz RE, Diver DJ, Safian RD, Baim DS. Intracoronary verapamil for the treatment of distal microvascular coronary artery spasm following PTCA. Cathet Cardio Diagn 1991; 24: 283-285.
2117. Hong MK, Popma JJ, Pichard AD, Kent KM, et al. Clinical significance of distal embolization after transluminal extraction atherectomy in diffusely diseased saphenous vein grafts. Am Heart J 1994; 127(6): 1496-1503.
2118. Moses JW, Yeh W, Popma JJ, Sketch Jr. MH, NACI Investigators. Predictors of distal embolization with the TEC catheter: A NACI Registry Report. Circ 1995; 92:I-329.
2119. Hong MH, Pichard AD, Kent KM, et al. Assessing a strategy of stand-alone extraction atherectomy followed by staged stent placement in degenerated saphenous vein graft lesions. J Amer Coll Cardiol 1995;27:394A.
2120. Al-Shaibi KF, Goods CM, Jain SP, et al. Does transluminal extraction atherectomy reduce distal embolization in saphenous vein grafts? Circ 1995; 92:I-329.
2121. Kaplan BM, Larkin TJ, Safian RS, O'Neill WW, et al. A Prospective pilot trial of direct and rescue extraction atherectomy for acute myocardial infarction. 1995 (to be submitted for publication).
2122. Dooris M, Hoffman M, Glazier S, et al. Comparative results of transluminal extraction coronary atherectomy in saphenous vein graft lesions with and without thrombus. J Am Coll Cardiol 1995; 25: 1700-1705.
2123. Kaplan BM, O'Neill WW, Grines CL, et al. Rescue extraction atherectomy after failed primary angioplasty in right coronary artery infarction. Am J Cardiol (in-press).
2124. Tilli FV, Kaplan BM, Safian RD, Grines CL, O'Neill WW. Angioscopic plaque friability: a new risk factor for procedural complications following saphenous vein graft interventions. J Am Coll Cardiol (in-press).

Laser Angioplasty

2125. Grundfest WS, Segalowitz J, Laudenslager J, et al. The physical and biological basis for laser angioplasty: In coronary laser angioplasty. Litvack F (ed), Blackwell Scientific Publications, 1992.
2126. Mintz GS, Kovach JA, Javier SP, et al. Mechanisms of lumen enlargement after excimer laser coronary angioplasty: An intravascular ultrasound study. Circulation. 1995;92:3408-3414.
2127. Honye J, Mahon DJ, Nakamura S, Wallis J, et al. Intravascular ultrasound imaging after excimer laser angioplasty. Cathet Cardiovasc Diagn 1994;32:213-222.
2128. van Leeuwen TG, Meertens JH, Velema E, et al. Intraluminal vapor bubble induced by excimer laser pulse causes microsecond arterial dilation and invagination leading to extensive wall damage in the rabbit. Circulation 1993;87:1258-1263.
2129. Serruys PW, Leon MB, Hamburger JN, et al. Recanalization of chronic total coronary occlusions using a laser guide wire: The European and US total experience. J Am Coll Cardiol 1996;March Special Issue.
2130. Bittl JA, Sanborn TA. Excimer laser-facilitated coronary angioplasty. Circulation 1992;86:71-80.
2131. Margolis JR, Mehta S. Excimer laser coronary angioplasty. Am J Cardiol 92;69:3F-11F.
2132. Litvack F. Excimer Laser Coronary Angioplasty. In Textbook of Interventional Cardiology. Topol (ed) Second Edition, 1990, pp. 840-858.

2133. Litvack F, Eigler N, Margolis J, et al. Percutaneous excimer laser coronary angioplasty: Results in the first consecutive 3,000 patients. J Am Coll Cardiol 1994;23:323-329.
2134. Bittl JA, Sanborn RA, Tcheng JE, et al. Clinical success complications and restenosis rates with excimer laser coronary angioplasty. Am J Cardiol 1992;70:1553-1539.
2135. Bittl JA, Sanborn TA, Siegel RM, et al. Which complex lesions are suitable for excimer laser coronary angioplasty: Multivariate analysis in 701 patients. J Am Coll Cardiol 1992;263A.
2136. Dussaillant GR, Popma JJ, Picard AD, et al. Rotational atherectomy vs. excimer laser angioplasty: A multivariable analysis of early and late procedural outcome. Abstract presented at TCT, 1995.
2137. Strikwerda S, vanSwijndregt EM, Foley DP, et al. Immediate and late outcome of excimer laser and balloon coronary angioplasty: A quantitative angiographic comparison based on matched lesions. J Am Coll Cardiol 1995;26:939-46.
2138. Foley DP, Appelman YE, Piek JJ on behalf of the AMRO group. Comparison of angiographic restenosis propensity of excimer laser coronary angioplasty (ELCA) and balloon angioplasty (BA) in the Amsterdam Rotterdam (AMRO) Trial. Circulation 1995;92: I-477.
2139. Koolen J, Appelman Y, Strikwerda S, et al. Initial and long-term results of excimer laser coronary angioplasty versus balloon angioplasty in functional and total coronary occlusions. Eur Heart Journal 1994:832.
2140. Appelman YEA, Piek JJ, Strikwerda S, et al. Randomized trial of excimer laser angioplasty versus balloon angioplasty for treatment of obstructive coronary artery disease. Lancet 1996;347:79-84.
2141. Vandormael M, Reifart N, Preusler W, et al. Six months follow-up results following excimer laser angioplasty, rotational atherectomy and balloon angioplasty for complex lesions: ERBAC Study. Circulation 1994:90:I-213.
2142. Ghazzal ZM, Hearn JA, Litvack F, et al. Morphological predictors of acute complications after percutaneous excimer laser coronary angioplasty. Circulation 1992;86:820-827.
2143. Baumbach A, Bittl JA, Fleck E, et al. Acute complications of coronary excimer laser angioplasty: Analysis of 2 multicenter registries. Circulation 1992;86:4 510.
2144. Baumbach A, Bittl JA, Fleck E, et al. Coinvestigators of the U.S. and European percutaneous excimer laser coronary angioplasty (PELCA) registries. J Am Coll Cardiol 1994;23:1305-13.
2145. Bittl JA, Kuntz RE, Estella P, et al. Analysis of late lumen narrowing after excimer laser-facilitated coronary angioplasty. J Am Coll Cardiol 1994;23:1314.
2146. Ghazzal ZMB, Burton E, Wintraub, WS, et al. Predictors of restenosis after excimer laser coronary angioplasty. Am J Cardiol 1995;75:1012-1014.
2147. Deckelbaum LI, Natarajan MK, Bittl JA, et al. For the percutaneous excimer laser coronary angioplasty (PELCA) investigators: Effect of intracoronary saline infusion on dissection during excimer laser coronary angioplasty: A randomized trial. J Am Coll Cardiol 1995;26:1264-9.
2148. Tcheng JE, Wells LD, Phillips HR, et al. Development of a new technique for reducing pressure pulse generation during 308-nm excimer laser coronary angioplasty. Cathet Cardiovasc Diagn 1995;34:15-22.
2149. Rechavia E, Federman J, Shefer A, et al. Usefulness of a prototype directional catheter for excimer laser coronary angioplasty in narrowings unfavorable for conventional excimer or balloon angioplasty. Am J Cardiol 1995;76:1144-1146.
2150. Bittl JA, Brinker JA, Sanborn TA, et al. The changing profile of patient selection, procedural techniques, and outcomes in excimer laser coronary angioplasty. J Interven Cardiol 1995;8:653-660.

Intravascular Ultrasound

2151. Zir LM, Miller SW, Dinsmore RE, Gilber JP, Harthorne JW. Interobserver variability in coronary angiography. Circulation 1976;53:627-632.
2152. Vlodaver Z, Frech R, van Tassel RA, Edwards JE. Correlation of the antemortem coronary angiogram and the postmortem specimen. Circulation 1973;47:162-168.
2153. White CW, Wright CB, Doty DB, Hirtza LF, et al. Does visual interpretation of the coronary arteriogram predict the physiologic importance of a coronary stenosis? N Engl J Med 1984;310:819-24.
2154. Waller BF: "Crackers, breakers, stretchers, drillers, scrapers, shavers, burners, welders, and melters": The future treatment of atherosclerotic coronary artery disease? A clinical-morphologic assessment. J Am Coll Cardiol 1989;13:969-87.
2155. Nissen SE, Gurley JC, Grines CL, Booth DC, et al. Intravascular ultrasound assessment of lumen size and wall morphology in normal subjects and coronary artery disease patients Circulation 1991;84:1087-1099.
2156. St. Goar FG, Pinto FJ, Alderman EL, Fitzgerald PJ, et al. Detection of coronary atherosclerosis in young adult hearts using intravascular ultrasound, Circulation 1992;86:756-763.
2157. Fitzgerald PJ, St. Goar FG, Connolly AJ, Pinto JF, et al. Intravascular ultrasound imaging of coronary arteries. Is three layers the norm? Circulation 1992;86:154-158.
2158. Tobis JM, Mallery J, Mahon D, Lehmann K, et al. Intravascular ultrasound imaging of human coronary arteries in vivo. Analysis of tissue characterizations with comparison to in vitro histological specimens. Circulation 1991;83:913-926.
2159. Nissen SE, Tuzcu EM, De Franco AC. Coronary intravascular ultrasound: Diagnostic and interventional applications. In: Topol EJ ed. Update to Textbook of Interventional Cardiology, W B Saunders, Philadelphia, PA, pages 207-222, 1994.
2160. Nissen SE, De Franco AC, Raymond RE, Franco I, et al. Angiographically unrecognized disease at "normal" reference sites: a risk factor for sub-optimal results after coronary interventions. Circulation 1993;88:I-412A.
2161. Glagov S, Weisenberg E,Zarins CK et al. Compensatory enlargement of human coronary arteries. N Engl J of Med 1987;316:1371-1375.
2162. White CJ, Ramee SR, Collin TJ, Jain A, Mesa JE. Ambiguous coronary angiography: clinical utility of intravascular ultrasound. Cathet Cardiovasc Diagn 1992;26:200-203.

2163. Tuzcu EM, Hobbs H, Rincon G , Bott-Silverman C , et al. Occult and frequent transmission of atherosclerosis coronary disease with cardia transplantation. Circulation 1995; 91:1706-1713.
2164. Nissen SE, Grines CL, Gurley JC, Sublett K, et al. Application of a new phased-array ultrasound imaging catheter in the assessment of vascular dimensions: In vivo comparison to cineangiography. Circulation 1990;81:660-666.
2165. DeFranco AC, Tuzcu E, Abdelmeguid A, Lincoff AM, et al. Intravascular ultrasound assessment of PTCA results: Insights into the mechanisms of balloon angioplasty. J Am Coll Cardiol 1993,21:485A.
2166. Tuzcu EM, Berkalp B, De Franco AC, Ellis SG, et al. Dilemma of Diagnosing Coronary Calcification: Angiography vs. Intravascular Ultrasound. J Am Coll Cardiol 1995, (in press).
2167. Popma JJ, Mintz GS et al. Clinical and angiographic outcome after directional coronary atherectomy. A qualitative and quantitative analysis using angiography and intravascular ultrasound. Am J Cardiol 1994;72:55E-64E.
2168. DeFranco AC, Tuzcu EM, Moliterno DJ, et al. "Directional" coronary atherectomy removes atheroma more effectively from concentric than eccentric lesions: intravascular ultrasound predictors of lesional success. J Am Coll of Cardiol 1995;25:137A.
2169. Kovach JA, Mintz GS, Pichard AD, Kent KM, et al. Sequential intravascular ultrasound characterization of the mechanism of rotational atherectomy and adjunct balloon angioplasty. J Am Coll Cardiol 1993;22:1024-1032.
2170. Donohue TJ, Kern MJ, Aguirre FV, Bach RG, et al. Assessing the hemodynamic significance of coronary artery stenoses: analysis of translesional pressure velocity relations in patients. J Am Coll Cardiol 1993;22:449-458.
2171. Kern MJ, Bach RG, Donohue TJ, Caracciolo EA, Aguirre FV. Coronary Stenoses with Low Translesional Gradient and Abnormal Flow Reserve. Cathet Cardiovas Diagn 1994;32:354-58.
2172. Kern MJ, Donohue TJ, Aguirre FV, Bach RG, et al. Clinical Outcome of Deferring Angioplasty in Patients with a Normal Translesional Flow-Velocity Measurements. J Am Coll Cardiol 1995;25:178-187.
2173. Patrick W. Serruys. Personal communication, Results of the Doppler Endpoints Balloon Angioplasty Trial Europe (DEBATE trial).
2174. Russo RJ, Teirstein PS. Angiography versus intravascular ultrasound-directed stent placement. J Am Coll Cardiol 1996;27:306A.
2175. Goldberg SL, Hall P, Nakamura S, et al. Is there a benefit from intravascular ultrasound when high-pressure stent expansion is routinely performed prior to ultrasound imaging? J Am Coll Cardiol 1996;27:306A.

Angioscopy

2176. Sherman TC, Litvack F, Grundfest W, et al. Coronary angioscopy in patients with unstable angina pectoris. N Eng J Med 1986;315:913-919.
2177. Litvack F, Grundfest WS, Lee ME, et al. Angioscopic visualization of blood vessel interior in animals and humans. Clin Cardiol 1985;8:65-70.
2178. Grundfest WS, Litvack F, Sherman T, et al. Delineation of peripheral and coronary detail by intraoperative angioscopy. Ann Surg 1985;202:394-400.
2179. Sanborn TA, Rygaard JA, Westbrook BM, et al. Intraoperative angioscopy of saphenous vein and coronary arteries. J Thorac Cardiovasc Surg 1986;91:339-343.
2180. King SB III. Role on new technologies in balloon angioplasty. Circulation 1991;84:2574-2579.
2181. Forrester JS, Eigler N, Litvack F: interventional Cardiology: The decade ahead. Circulation 1991;84:942-944.
2182. Schweiger MJ, Roccario E, Weil T. Treatment of patients following bypass surgery: a dilemma for the 1990s. Am Heart J 1992;123:268-272.
2183. White CJ, Ramee SR, Collins TJ, et al. Percutaneous angioscopy of saphenous vein coronary bypass grafts. J Am Coll Cardiol 1993;21:1181-1185.
2184. Annex, BH, Larkin TJ, O'Neill WW, et al. Evaluation of thrombus removal by transluminal extraction coronary atherectomy by percutaneous coronary angioscopy. Am J Cardiol 1994;74:606-609.
2185. Annex BH, Ajluni SC, Larkin TJ, et al. Angioscopic guided interventions in a saphenous vein bypass graft. Cathet Cardiovasc Diagn 1994;31:330-333.
2186. Nath FC, Muller DWM, Ellis SG, et al. Thrombosis of a flexible coil coronary stent: frequency, predictors and clinical outcome. J Am Coll Cardiol 1993;21:622-627.
2187. Hermann HC, Buchbinder M, Clemen MW, et al. Emergent use of balloon-expandable coronary artery stenting for failed percutaneous transluminal coronary angioplasty. Circulation 1992;86:812-819.
2188. Kaplan BM, Safian RD, Grines CL, et al. Usefulness of adjunctive angioscopy and extraction atherectomy before stent implantation in high-risk aorto-coronary saphenous vein grafts. Am J Cardiol 1995;76:822-824.
2189. Tilli FV, Kaplan BM, Safian RD, Grines CL, O'Neill WW. Angioscopic plaque friability: A new risk factor for procedural complications following saphenous vein graft interventions. J Am Coll Cardiol (in-press).
2190. White CJ, Ramee SR, Collins TJ, et al. Percutaneous coronary angioscopy: Applications in interventional cardiology. J Interven Cardiol 1993;6:61-67.
2191. Sassower MA, Abela GS, Koch JM, et al. Angioscopic evaluation of periprocedural and postprocedural abrupt closure after percutaneous coronary angioplasty. Am Heart J 1993;126:444-450.
2192. Teirstein PS, Schatz RA, Rocha-Singh KJ, et al. Coronary stenting with angioscopic guidance. J Am Coll Cardiol 1992;19:223A.
2193. Nakamura F, Kvasnicka J, Uchida Y, et al. Percutaneous angioscopic evaluation of luminal changes induced by excimer laser angioplasty. Am Heart J 1992;124:1467-1472.
2194. Eltchaninoff H, Cribier A, Koning R, et al. Comparative angioscopic findings after rotational atherectomy and balloon angioplasty. J Am Coll Cardiol 1995;25:95A.
2195. Waxman S, Mittleman MA, Manxo K, Saaower M, et al. Culprit lesion morphology in subtypes of unstable angina as assessed by angioscopy. Circulation 1995;92:I-79.
2196. Waxman S, Saaower M, Mittleman MA, Nesto RW, et al. Characterization of the culprit lesion underlying thrombus: Insights from

angioscopy. Circulation 1995;92:I-353.

2197. Uchida Y, Nakamura F, Tomaru T, Mortia T, et al. Prediction of acute coronary syndromes by percutaneous coronary angioscopy in patients with stable angina. Am Heart J 1995;130:195-203.

2198. Silva JA, Escobar A, Collins TJ, Ramee SR, White CJ. Unstable angina. A comparison of angioscopic findings between diabetic and nondiabetic patients. Circulation 1995;92:1731-1736.

2199. Bauters C, Lablanche JM, McFadden E, Hamon M, Bertrand ME. Angioscopic thrombus is associated with a high risk of angiographic restenosis. Circulation 1995;92:I-401.

2200. Waxman S, Mittleman MA, Saaower M, Kowalker W, Nesto RW. Can angioscopy predict initial procedural success of PTCA in acute coronary syndromes? Circulation 1995;92:I-785.

2201. Feld S, Ganim M, Vaughn WK, Kelly R, et al. Utility of angioscopy and intravascular ultrasound in predicting outcome following coronary intervention. Circulation 1995;92:I-18.

2202. Uretsky BF, Denys BG, Counihan P, et al. Accuracy of angioscopy in diagnosing endoluminal lesions. J Am Coll Cardiol;1994:23:407A.

2203. Lablanche, JM, Geschwind H, Cribier A, et al. Coronary angioscopy safety survey: European multicenter experience. J Am Coll Cardiol 1995;25:154A.

2204. Wolff, MR, Resar JR, Stuart RS, et al. Coronary artery rupture and pseudoaneurysm formation resulting from percutaneous coronary angioscopy. Cathet Cardiovasc Diagn 1993;28:47-50.

2205. Alfonso F, Hernandez R, Goicolea J, et al. Angiographic deterioration of the previously dilated coronary segment induced by angioscopic examination. Am J Cardiol 1994;74:604-606.

2206. White CJ, Ramee SR, Collins TJ, et al. Coronary thrombi increase PTCA risk: Angioscopy as a clinical tool. Circulation 1996;93:253-8.

Doppler FloWire

2207. Benchimol A, Stegall HF, Gartlan JL. New method to measure phasic coronary blood velocity in man. Am Heart J 1971;81:93-101.

2208. Doucette JW, Corl PD, Payne HM, et al. Validation of a Doppler guidewire for intravascular measurement of coronary artery flow velocity. Circulation 1992;85:1899-1911.

2209. Segal J, Kern MJ, Scott NA, King III SB, et al. Alterations of phasic coronary artery flow velocity in humans during percutaneous coronary angioplasty. J Am Coll Cardiol 1992;20:276-286.

2210. Ofili EO, Kern MJ, Labovitz AJ, St. Vrain JA, et al. Analysis of coronary blood flow velocity dynamics in angiographically normal and stenosed arteries before and after endoluminal enlargement by angioplasty. J Am Coll Cardiol 1993;21:308-316.

2211. Marcus ML, Chilian WM, Kanatuka H, Dellsperger KC, et al. Understanding the coronary circulation through studies at the microvascular level. Circulation 1990;82:1-7.

2212. Bone RM, Rubio R. Coronary circulation, in Berne R, Sperelakis N, (eds): Handbook of Physiology, Section 2: The Cardiovascular System, Volume 1, The Heart. Baltimore, Williams & Wilkins CO, 1979, pp 873-952.

2213. Wilson RF, Laxson DD. Caveat Emptor: A clinician's guide to assessing the physiologic significance of arterial stenoses. Cathet Cardiovasc Diagn 1993;29:93-98.

2214. Gould KL, Lipscomb K, Hamilton GW. Physiologic basis for assessing critical coronary stenosis. Am J Cardiol 1974;33:87-94.

2215. Gould KL, Lipscomb K, Calvert J. Compensatory changes of the distal coronary vascular bed during progressive coronary constriction. Circulation 1975;51:1085-1094.

2216. Kirkeeide R, Gould KL, Parsel L. Assessment of coronary stenoses by myocardial imaging during coronary vasodilation. VII. Validation of coronary flow reserve as a single integrated measure to stenosis severity accounting for all its geometric dimensions. J Am Coll Cardiol 1986;7:103-113.

2217. Gould KL, Kirkeeide R, Buchi M. Coronary flow reserve as a physiologic measure of stenosis severity. Part I. Relative and absolute coronary flow reserve during changing aortic pressure. Part II. Determination from arterographic stenosis dimensions under standardized conditions. J Am Coll Cardiol 1990;15:459-474.

2218. Demer L, Gould KL, Kirkeide RL. Assessing stenosis severity: Coronary flow reserve, collateral function, quantitative coronary arteriography, position imaging, and digital subtraction angiography: a review and analysis. Prog Cardiovasc Dis 1988;30:307-322.

2219. Gould KL. Identifying and measuring severity of coronary artery stenosis: quantitative coronary arteriography and position emission tomography. Circulation 1988;78:237-245.

2220. Wilson RF, Marcus ML, White CW. Prediction of the physiologic significance of coronary arterial lesions by quantitative lesion geometry in patients with limited coronary artery disease. Circulation 1987;75:723-732.

2221. Shammas NW, Thondapu V, Gerasimou EM, Antonio J, et al. Effect of pretreatment with nitroglycerin on coronary flow reserve measured using bolus intracoronary adenosine. Circulation 1995;92:I-264.

2222. Ofili EO, Lasovitz AJ, Kern MJ. Coronary flow velocity dynamics in normal and diseased arteries. Am J Cardiol 1993;71:3D-9D.

2223. Kajiya F, Ogasawara Y, Tsujioka K, et al. Analysis of flow characteristics in post-stenotic regions of the human coronary artery during bypass graft surgery. Circulation 1987;76:1092-1100.

2224. Donohue TJ, Kern MJ, Aguirre FV, Bach RG, et al. Assessing the hemodynamic significance of coronary artery stenosis. Analysis of translesional pressure-flow velocity relations in patients. J Am Coll Cardiol 1993;22:449-458.

2225. Kern MJ, Aguirre FV, Bach RG, Caracole EA, Donohue TJ. Translesional pressure-flow velocity assessment in patients: Part I. Cathet Cardiovasc Diagn 1994;313:49-60.

2226. Kern MJ, Deligonul, Tatineni S, Serota H, et al. IV adenosine continuous infusion and low dose bolus administration for determination of coronary vascular reserve in patients with and without coronary artery disease. J Am Coll Cardiol 1991;18:718-729.

2227. Miller DD, Donohue TJ, Younis LT, Bach RG, et al. Correlation of pharmacologic Technesium 99m-Sestamibi myocardial perfusion imaging with post-stenotic coronary flow reserve in patients with angiographically intermediate coronary artery stenoses.

Circulation 1994;89:2150-2160.

2228. Joye JD, Schulman DS, Lesorde D, Farah T, et al. Intracoronary Doppler guide wire versus stress single-photon emission computer tomographic thallium 201 imaging in assessment of intermediate coronary stenoses. J Am Coll Cardiol 1994;24:940-947.

2229. Gadallah S, Thaker KB, Kawanishi D, Rashtian M, et al. Comparison of the hyperemic response to intracoronary and intravenous adenosine by intracoronary Doppler flow recording. Circulation 1995;92:I-326.

2230. White CW, Wilson RF, Intracoronary Doppler Ultrasound in Nanda P (ed): Doppler Ultrasound. Philadelphia, Lea & Febiger, 1994, pp 403-412.

2231. McGinn AL, White CW, Wilson RF. Interstudy variability of coronary flow reserve. Influence of heart rate, arterial pressure and ventricular preload. Circulation 1990;81:1319-1330.

2232. De Bruyne B, Bartunek J, Stanislas US, et al. Feasibility and hemodynamic dependency of invasive indexes of coronary stenosis. Circulation 1995;92:I-324.

2233. Claeys MJ, Vrints CJ, Bosmans JM, Cools F, et al. Coronary flow reserve measurement during coronary angioplasty in the infarct related vessel. Circulation 1995;92:I-326.

2234. Kern MJ, Donohue TJ, Aguirre FV, Bach RG, et al. Clinical outcome of deferring angioplasty in patients with normal translesional pressure-flow velocity measurements. J Am Coll Cardiol 1995;25:178-187.

2235. Lesser JT, Wilson RF, White CW. Physiologic assessment of coronary stenosis of intermediate severity can facilitate patient selection for coronary angioplasty. Coronary Art Dis 1990;1:697-705.

2236. Cannon RO III, Camici PG, Epstein SE. Pathophysiological dilemma of Syndrome X. Circulation 1992;85:883-892.

2237. Marcus ML, Doty DB, Hirratzka LF, Wright CB, Enpthan CE. Decreased coronary reserved a mechanism of angina pectoris in patients with aortic stenosis and normal coronary arteries. N Eng J Med 1982;37:1362-1366.

2238. Houghton JL, Prisant LM, Carr AA, van Dohlen TW, Frank MJ. Relationship of left ventricular mass to impairment of coronary vasodilator reserve in hypertensive heart disease. Am Heart J 1991;21:1107.

2239. Cannon RO, Bonow RO, Bacharach SL, et al. Left ventricular dysfunction in patients with angina pectoris, normal epicardial coronary arteries, and abnormal vasodilator reserve. Circulation 1985;71:218-226.

2240. McGinn AL, Wilson RF, Olisan MT et al. Coronary vasodilator reserve following human orthotopic cardiac transplantation. Circulation 1988;78:1200-1209.

2241. Wilson RE, Wilson ML, White CW. Effects of coronary bypass surgery and angioplasty on coronary blood flow and flow reserve. Prog Cardiovasc Dis 1988;31:95-114.

2242. Wilson RE, White CW. Does coronary bypass graft surgery restore normal CFR. The effect of diffuse atherosclerosis and focal obstruction lesions. Circulation 1987;76:563-571.

2243. Stewart RE, Bowers TR, Ponto R, Miller DD, et al. Coronary Doppler flow velocity and PET myocardial blood flow are highly correlated and predict post-infarction perfusion in patients with TIMI-3 flow. J Am Coll Cardiol 1995;25:427A.

2244. Aguirre FV, Donohue TJ, Bach RG, Caracole EA, et al. Coronary flow velocity of infarct-related arteries: Physiologic differences between complete (TIMI III) and incomplete (TIMI 0,I,II) angiographic coronary perfusion. J Am Coll Cardiol 1995;25:401A.

2245. Ishihara M, Sato H, Tateishi H, Kawagoe T, Shimatani Y, et al. Time course of impaired coronary vasodilatory reserve after reperfusion in acute myocardial infarction. J Am Coll Cardiol 1995;25:2008A.

2246. Wakatsuk T, Nakamura M, Tsundoa T, Ui K, Degawa T, Yamaguchi T. Coronary angioplasty predicts recovery of regional wall motion in acute myocardial infarction. J Am Coll Cardiol 1995;25:161A.

2247. Kim HS, Tahk SJ, Shin JH, Kim W, Cho YK, et al. Coronary flow reserve in infarct related artery and myocardial viability in patients with recent myocardial infarction. Circulation 1995;92:I-600.

2248. Segal J. Applications of coronary flow velocity during angioplasty and other coronary interventional procedures. Am J Cardiol 1993;71:17D-25D.

2249. Bowers TR, Stewart RE, O'Neill WW, Reddy VM, et al. Plaque pulvariation during Rotablator atherectomy: does it impair coronary flow dynamics? J Am Coll Cardiol 1995;25:96A.

2250. Bach R, Kern MJ, Bell C, et al. Clinical application of coronary flow velocity for stent placement during coronary angioplasty. Am J Heart 1993;125:873-880.

2251. Bowers TR, Safian RD, Stewart RE, Benzuly KH, et al. Normalization of CFR after stenting, but not after PTCA. J Am Coll Cardiol 1996 (in-press).

2252. Larman DJ, Serruys PW, Suryapranata H, et al. Inability of coronary blood flow reserve measurements to assess the efficacy of coronary angioplasty in the first 24-hours in unselected patients. Am Heart J 1991;122:631-639.

2253. Wilson RF, Johnson MR, Marcus ML, Aylward PEG, et al. The effect of coronary angioplasty on coronary flow reserve. Circulation 1988;77:873-885.

2254. Kern MJ, Deligonul U, Vandormael M, Labovitz A, et al. Impaired coronary vasodilator reserve in the immediate post coronary angioplasty period: Analysis of coronary artery flow velocity indexes and regional cardiac venous efflux. J Am Coll Cardiol 1989;13:860-872.

2255. Kern MJ, Aguirre FV, Donohue TJ, Bach RG, et al. Impact of residual lumen narrowing on coronary flow after angioplasty and stent: Intravascular ultrasound Doppler and imaging data in support of physiologically-guided coronary angioplasty. Circulation 1995;92:I-263.

2256. Verna E, Gil R, Di Mario C, Sunamura M, Gurne O, Porenta G. Does coronary stenting following balloon angioplasty improve distal coronary flow reserve? Circulation 1995;92:I-536.

2257. Haude M, Baumgart D, Caspari G, Erbel R. Does adjunct coronary stenting in comparison to balloon angioplasty has an impact on Doppler flow velocity parameters? Circulation 1995;92:I-547.

2258. The D.E.B.A.TE. Study Group. Are flow velocity measurements after PTCA predictive of recurrence of angina or of a positive exercise stress test early after balloon angioplasty? Circulation 1995;92:I-264.

2259. The D.E.B.A.T.E. Study Group. Doppler guide wire as a primary guide wire for PTCA. Feasibility, safety, and continuous

monitoring of the results. Circulation 1995;92:I-263.
2260. Eichhorn E, Grayburn PA, Willard JE, Anderson HV, et al. Spontaneous alterations in coronary blood flow velocity before and after coronary angioplasty in patients with severe angina. J Am Coll Cardiol 1991;17:43-52.
2261. Anderson HV, Kirkeeide RL, Stuart Y, Smalling RW, et al. Coronary artery flow monitoring following coronary interventions. Am J Cardiol 1993;71:62D-69D.
2262. Kern MJ, Donohue TJ, Bach RG, Aguirre FV, Bell C. Monitoring cyclical coronary blood flow alterations following coronary angioplasty for stent restenosis using a Doppler guidewire. Am Heart J 1993;125:1159-1160.
2263. Kern MJ, Aguirre FV, Donohue TJ, Bach RG, et al. Continuous coronary flow velocity monitoring during coronary interventions: Velocity trend patterns associated with adverse events. Am Heart J 1994;128:426-34.
2264. The D.E.B.A.T.E. Study Group. Cyclic flow variations after PTCA are predictive of immediate complications. Circulation 1995;92:I-725.
2265. Anderson HV, Revana M, Rosales O, Brannigan L, et al. Intravenous administration of monoclonal antibody to the platelet GP IIb/IIIa receptor to treat abrupt closure during coronary angioplasty. Am J Cardiol 1992;69:1373-1376.
2266. Yaniyama Y, Iwakure K, Ito H, Takiuchi S, et al. Coronary flow velocity pattern in patients with TIMI flow grade 2: Its relation to residual coronary stenosis and microvascular dysfunction. Circulation 1995;92:I-149.
2267. Nemoto T, Kimure K, Shimizu T, Mochida Y, et al. Coronary artery flow velocity waveform in acute myocardial infarction with angiographic no-reflow. Circulation 1995;92:I-325.
2268. Geschwind HJ, Melnik L, Kvasnicka J, Dupouy P. Dynamic detection of coronary stenosis by Doppler-tipped guidewire. J Am Coll Cardiol 1995;25:336A.
2269. Ferrari M, Werner GS, Nargang L, Figulla HR. Turbulent flow as a cause for underestimating the coronary flow reserve. Circulation 1995;92:I-77.
2270. Wilson RF, Laughlin DE, Ackell PH, Chilian WM. Transluminal subselective measurement of coronary blood flow velocity and vasodilator reserve in man. Circulation 1985;72:82-92.
2271. White CW, Marcus ML, Wilson RF. Methods of measuring coronary flow in humans. Prog Cardiovasc Dis 1988;31:79-94.
2272. Sibley DH, Millar HD, Hartley CJ, Whitlow PL. Subselective measurement of coronary blood flow velocity using a steerable Doppler catheter. J Am Coll Cardiol 1986;8:1332-1340.
2273. Vanyi J, Bowers TR, Jarvis G, White CW. Can an intracoronary Doppler wire accurately measure changes in coronary blood flow velocity? Cathet Cardiovasc Diagn 1993;29:240-246.
2274. Zijlstra F, Juilliere Y, Serruys PW, Roelandt JRTC. Value and limitations of intracoronary adenosine for the assessment of coronary flow reserve. Cathet Cardiovasc Diagn 1988;15:76-80.
2275. Wilson RF, Wych K, Christensen BV, Zimmer S, Laxson DD. Effects of adenosine on human coronary arterial circulation. Circulation 1990;82:1595-1606.
2276. Wilson RF, White CW. Intracoronary papaverine: An ideal vasodilator for studies of the coronary circulation in conscious humans. Circulation 1986;73:444-452.
2277. Ranhosty A, Kempthorne-Rawson J. Intravenous Dipyridamole Thallium Imaging Study Group. The safety of intravenous dipyridamole thallium myocardial perfusion imaging. Circulation 1990;81:1205-1209.

Adjunctive Pharmacotherapy

2278. Davidson JAH, Boom SJ. Warming lignocaine to reduce pain associated with injection. BMJ 1992;305:617-8.
2279. Mader TJ, Playe SJ, Garb JL. Reducing the pain of local anesthetic infiltration: warming and buffering have a synergistic effect. Annals of Emergency Medicine 1994;23:550-4.
2280. Lasser EC, et al. Pre-Treatment with Corticosteroids to alleviate reactions to intravenous contrast material. N Engl J Med 1987;317:845-849.
2281. Lang DM, Alpern MB, Visintainer PF, et al. Increased risk for anaphylactoid reaction from contrast media in patients on β-adrenergic blockers or with asthma. Ann Intern Med 1991;115:270-276.
2282. Schwartz L, Bourassa MG, Lespérance J, et al. Aspirin and Dipyridamole in the prevention of restenosis after percutaneous transluminal coronary angioplasty. N Engl J Med 1988;318:1714-1719.
2283. Mufson L, Black A, Roubin G, et al. A randomized trial of aspirin in PTCA: Effect of high vs. low dose aspirin on major complications and restenosis. J Am Coll Cardiol 1988;11:236A.
2284. Levine MN, Hirsh J, Landefeld S, Raskob G. Hemorrhagic complications of long-term anticoagulant therapy. Chest 1992;102:352S-363S.
2285. Ridker PM, Manson JE, Gaziano JM, Buring JE, et al. Low-dose aspirin therapy for chronic stable angina: A randomized, placebo-controlled clinical trial. Ann Intern Med 1991;114:835-839.
2286. Chesebro JH, Webster MWI, Smith HC, Frye RI, Holmes DR, et al. Antiplatelet therapy in coronary disease progression: Reduced infarction and new lesion formation. Circulation 1989:80:II-266.
2287. Lewis HD Jr, Davis JW, Archibald DG, Steinke WE, Smitherman TC, et al. Protective effects of aspirin against acute myocardial infarction and death in men with unstable angina: Results of a Veterans Administration Cooperative Study. N Engl J Med 1983;309:396-403.
2288. Cairns JA, Gent M, Singer J, Finnie KJ, Froggatt GM, Holder DA, Jablonsky G,et al. Aspirin, sulfinpyrazone, or both in unstable angina. N Engl J Med 1985:313:1369-1375.
2289. Theroux P, Quimet H, McCans J, Latour JG, Joly P, et al. Aspirin, heparin, or both to treat acute unstable angina. N Engl J Med 1988;319:1105-1111.
2290. ISIS-2 Collaborative Group: Randomized trial of intravenous streptokinase, oral aspirin, both or neither among 17,187 cases of suspected acute myocardial infarction: ISIS-2. Lancet 1988;318:349-360.

2291. Henderson W, Goldman S, Copeland J, Moritz TE, Harker L. Antiplatelet or anticoagulant therapy after coronary artery bypass surgery: A meta-analysis of clinical trials. Ann Intern Med 1989;743-750.

2292. White CW, Chaitman B, Knudtson ML, et al. Antiplatelet agents are effective in reducing the acute ischemic complications of angioplasty but do not prevent restenosis: results from the ticlopidine trial. Coronary Artery Dis 1991;2:757.

2293. Chronos NA, Patel D, Sigwart U, et al. Intracoronary activation of human platelets following balloon angioplasty despite aspirin and heparin: a flow cytometric study. Circulation 1994;90:I-181.

2294. Di Minno G, Cerbone AM, Mattioli PL. Turco S, et al. Functionally thrombasthenic state in normal platelets following the administration of ticlopidine. J Clin Intest 1985;75:328-338.

2295. Cattaneo M, Lombardi R, Bettega D et al. Shear-induced platelet aggregation is potentiated by desmopressin and inhibited by Ticlopidine. Arteriosclerosis and Thrombosis 1993;13:393-397.

2296. Dembinska-Kiec A, Virgolini I, Rauscha F, et al. Ticlopidine and platelet function in healthy volunteer, Thrombosis Research 1992;65:559-570.

2297. Cattaneo M, Akkawat B, Kinlough-Rathbone RL, et al. Ticlopidine facilitates the deaggregation of human platelets aggravated by thrombin. Thrombosis and Hemostasis 1994,71:91-94.

2298. Heptinstall S, May JA, Glenn JR, Sanderson HM, et al. Effects of Ticlopidine administered to healthy volunteers on platelet function in whole blood. Thrombosis and Haemostasis 1995;74:1310-5.

2299. Khurana S, Westley S, Mattson J, Safian RD. Is it possible to expedite the antiplatelet effect of Ticlopidine? 1996 Transcatheter Therapeutics (TCT-VIII) meeting Washington Hospital, Washington D.C. J Inv. Card. 1996;8:65.

2300. Balsano F, Rizzon P, Violi F, et al. Antiplatelet treatment with ticlopidine in unstable angina: A controlled multicenter clinical trial. Circulation 1990;82:17.

2301. Hass WK, Easton JD, Adams HP et al. A randomized trial comparing ticlopidine hydrochloride with aspirin for the prevention of stroke in high-risk patients. Ticlopidine Aspirin Stroke Study Group. N Engl J Med 1989;321:501.

2302. de Caterina R, Sicari R, Bornane W et al. Benefit/risk profile of combined antiplatelet therapy with Ticlopidine and Aspirin Thrombosis and Haemostasis 1991;65:504-510.

2303. Lembo NJ, Black AJR, Roubin GS et al. Effect of pretreatment with aspirin versus aspirin plus dipyridamole on frequency and type of acute complications of percutaneous transluminal coronary angioplasty. Am J Cardiol 1990;65:422-426.

2304. Danchin N, Juilliere Y, Kettani C, Buffet P, et al. Effect of early acute occlusion rate of adjunctive antithrombotic treatment with intravenously administered dipyridamole during percutaneous transluminal coronary angioplasty. American Heart Journal 1994;127:494-8.

2305. The EPIC Investigators. Use of a monoclonal antibody directed against the platelet glycoprotein IIb/IIIa receptor in high-risk coronary angioplasty. N Engl J Med 1994;330:956-61.

2306. Ferguson JJ. All ACTs are not created equal. Texas Heart Inst J. 1992;19:1-3.

2307. Rath B, Bennett DH. Monitoring the effect of heparin by measurement of activated clotting time during and after percutaneous transluminal coronary angioplasty. Br Heart J. 1990;63:18-21.

2308. Hattersly PG. Activated coagulation time of whole blood. JAMA 1966;196:436-440.

2309. Bull BS, Huse WM, Bauer FS, Korpman RA: Heparin therapy during extracorporeal Circulation. The use of a dose-response curve to individualize heparin and protamine dosage. J Thorac Cardiovascular Surg 1975;69:685-689.

2310. Ferguson JJ, Dougherty KG, Gaos CM et al. Relation between procedural ACT and outcome after PTCA. J Am Cardiol Coll 1994;23:1061-5.

2311. Neuenschwander C, Attenhofer C, Kiowski W, et al. Activated clotting times and heparin need during coronary angioplasty in acute myocardial infarction and angina pectoris. Circulation 1993;88:I-1107.

2312. Freidman HZ, Cragg DR, Glazier SM et al. Randomized prospective evaluation of prolonged versus abbreviated intravenous heparin therapy after coronary angioplasty. J Am Coll Cardiol 1994, 24:1214-9.

2313. Dougherty KG, Gaos CM, Bush HS, Leachman R, Ferguson JJ. Activated clotting times and activated partial thromboplastin times in patients undergoing coronary angioplasty who receive bolus doses of heparin. Catheterization and Cardiovascular Diagnosis 1992;26:260-263.

2314. Granger CB, Miller JM, Bovill EG, GA, et al. Rebound increase in thrombin generation and activity after cessation of intravenous heparin in patients with acute coronary syndromes. Circulation 1995;91:1929-1935.

2315. Gabliani G, Deligonul U, Kern MJ, et al. Acute closure occlusion occurring after successful percutaneous transluminal coronary angioplasty: Temporal relationship to discontinuation of anticoagulation. Am Heart J 1988;116:696.

2316. Chesebro JH, Badimon L, Fuster V. Importance of antithrombin therapy during coronary angioplasty. J Am Coll Cardiol 1991;17:96B-100B.

2317. Schachinger V, Allert M, Kasper W et al. Adjuvant intracoronary infusion of antithrombin III during PTCA: Results of a prospective, randomized trial. Circulation 1994;90:2258-2266.

2318. Mabin TA, Holmes DR Jr., Smith HC et al. Intracoronary thrombus: Role in coronary occlusion complicating PTCA. J Am Coll Cardiol 1985;3:198-202.

2319. Becker PS, Miller VT. Heparin-induced thrombocytopenia. Stroke 1989;20:1449-1459.

2320. Kappa J, Fisher C, Todd B, Stenach N, Bell P, Campbell F, Ellison N, Addonizio VP. Intraoperative management of patients with heparin-induced thrombocytopenia. Ann Thorac Surg 1990;49:714-23.

2321. Warkentin TE, Levine MN, Hirsh J, Horsewood P, et al. Heparin-induced thrombocytopenia in patients treated with low-molecular-weight heparin or unfractionated heparin. N Engl J Med 1995;332:1330-5.

2322. Aster RH. Heparin-induced thrombocytopenia and thrombosis. New Engl J Med 332:1374.

2323. Eichinger S, Kyrle PA, Brenner B, et al. Thrombocytopenia associated with low-molecular-weight heparin. Lancet 1991;1:1425-6.

2324. Warkentin TE, Hayward CPM, Boshkov LK, Santos AV, et al. Sera from patients with heparin-induced thrombocytopenia generate platelet-derived microparticles with procoagulant activity: An explanation for the thrombotic complications of heparin-induced thrombocytopenia. Blood 1994;84:3691-3699.

2325. Amiral J, Bridey F, Wolf M, et al. Antibodies to macromolecular platelet factor 4-heparin complexes in heparin-induced thrombocytopenia: a study of 44 cases. Thromb Haemost 1995;73:21-8.

2326. Fareed J, Hoppensteadt DA, Walenger JM. Current perspectives on low molecular weight heparins. Seminars in Thromb Heamostasis 1993;19:I-11.

2327. Faxon DP, Spiro TE, Minor S, Coté G, Douglas J, Gottlieb R, Califf R, et al. Low molecular weight heparin in prevention of restenosis after angioplasty. Circulation 1994;90:908-914.

2328. Lefkovits J, Topol E. Direct thrombin inhibitors in cardiovascular medicine. Circulation 1994;90:1522-1536.

2329. Heras M, Cheseboro JH, Webster MWI et al. Hirudin, heparin, and placebo during deep arterial injury in the pig: the in vivo role of thrombin in platelet-mediated thrombosis. Circulation 1990;82:1476-1484.

2330. Van den Bos AA, Deckers JW, Heyndrckx GR, et al. Safety and efficacy of recombinant hirudin (CGP 39 393) versus heparin in patients with stable angina undergoing coronary angioplasty. Circulation 1993;88:2058-2066.

2331. Bittl JA, Strony J, Brinker JA, Ahmed WH, et al. Treatment with bivalirudin (Hirulog) as compared with heparin during coronary angioplasty for unstable or post-infarction angina. N Engl J Med 1995;333:764-9.

2332. Serruys PW, Herrman JPR, Simon R, Rutsch W, Bode C, et al. A Comparison of Hirudin with heparin in the prevention of restenosis after coronary angioplasty. N Engl J Med 1995;333:757-63.

2333. Topol EJ, Bonan R, Jewitt D, Sigwart U, Kakkar VV, et al. Use of a direct antithrombin, Hirulog, in place of heparin during coronary angioplasty. Circulation 1993;87:1622-1629.

2334. The Global Use of Strategies to Open Occluded Coronary Arteries (GUSTO) IIa Investigators. Randomized trial of intravenous heparin versus recominant hirudin for acute coronary syndromes. Circulation 1994;90:1631-1637.

2335. Antman EM, for the TIMI 9A Investigators. Hirudin in acute myocardial infarction, Safety report from the thrombolysis and thrombin inhibition in myocardial infarction (TIMI) 9A trial. Circulation 1994;90:1624-1630.

2336. Neuhaus KL, Essen R.v, Tebbe U, Jessel A, Heinrichs H, Mäurer W, et al. Safety Observations from the pilot phase of the randomized r-Hirudin for improvement of thrombolysis (HIT-III) study. Circulation 1994;90:1638-1642.

2337. Fuchs J, Cannon CP, TIMI 7 Investigators. Hirulog in the treatment of unstable angina, results of the Thrombin Inhibition in Myocardial Ischemia (TIMI) 7 Trial. Circulation 1995;92:727-733.

2338. The TIMI IIIA Investigators. Early effects of tissue-type plasminogen activator added to conventional therapy on the culprit coronary lesion in patients presenting with ischemic cardiac pain at rest, results of the Thrombolysis in Myocardial Ischemia (TIMI IIIA) Trial. Circulation 1993;87:38-52.

2339. The TIMI IIIB Investigators. Effects of tissue plasminogen activator and a comparison of early invasive and conservative strategies in unstable angina and non-Q-wave myocardial infarction. Results of the TIMI IIIB Trial. Circulation 1994;89:1545-1556.

2340. Ambrose JA, Almeida OD, Sharma SK, Torre SR, Marmur JD, Israel DH, et al. Adjunctive thrombolytic therapy during angioplasty for ischemic rest angina, results of the TAUSA Trial. Circulation 1994;90:69-77.

2341. Goudreau E, DiSciascio G, Vetrovec GW, et al. The role of intracoronary urokinase in combination with coronary angioplasty in patients with complex lesion morphology. J Am Coll Cardiol 1990;15:154A.

2342. Cohen BM, Buchbinder M, Kozina J, et al. Rethrombosis during angioplasty in myocardial infarction and unstable syndromes: Efficacy of intracoronary urokinase and redilation. Circulation 1988;78:II-8.

2343. Schieman G, Cohen BM, Kozina J, et al. Intracoronary urokinase for intracoronary thrombus accumulation complicating percutaneous transluminal coronary angioplasty in acute ischemic syndromes. Circulation 1990;82:2052-2060.

2344. Intracoronary t-PA Registry Investigators. Clinical experience with intracoronary tissue plasminogen activator: Results of a multicenter registry. Catheterization and Cardiovascular Diagnosis 1995;34:196-201.

2345. Ambrose JA. Thrombolysis as an adjunct to angioplasty. Am J Cardiol 1993;72:34G-39G.

2346. Spielberg C, Schnitzer L, Linderer T, et al. Influence of catheter technology and adjunct medication on acute complications in percutaneous coronary angioplasty. Cathet and Cardiovasc Diagn 1990;21:72-76.

2347. Swanson KT, Dogs, Dextran, and Dilitation: A story of empiricism run wild. Cath and Cardiovasc Diag 1994;32:203-205.

2348. Taylor MA, DiBlasi SL, Bender RM, Santoian EC, Cha SD, Dennis CA. Adult respiratory distress syndrome complicating intravenous infusion of low-molecular weight dextran. Catheterization and Cardiovascular Diagnosis 1994;32:249-253.

2349. Brown KJ, Prcela L, Kerrick et al. Analysis of hypotension in percutaneous coronary intervention patients. Circulation 1994;90(Part 2)I-205.

2350. Johansson SR, Lamm C, Bondjers G, et al. Role of beta-adrenergic blockers after percutaneous transluminal coronary angioplasty. Am J Cardiol 1990;66:915-920.

2351. Kern MJ, Walsh RA, Barr WK, et al. Improved myocardial oxygen utilization by diltiazem in patients. Am Heart J 1985;110:986-990.

2352. Kern MJ, Deligonul U, Labovitz A, et al. Effects of nitroglycerin and nifedipine on coronary and systemic hemodynamics during transient coronary artery occlusion. Am Heart J 1988;115:1164.

2353. Serruys PW, van den Brand M, Brower RW. Hugenholtz PG. Regional cardioplegia and cardioprotection during transluminal angioplasty. Which role for nifedipine? Eur Heart J 1984;4:115.

2354. Kern MJ, Pearson A, Woodruff R, et al. Hemodynamic and echocardiographic assessment of the effects of diltiazem during transient occlusion of the left anterior descending coronary artery during percutaneous transluminal coronary angioplasty. Am J Cardiol 1989;64:849-855.

2355. Hanet C, Rousseau MF, Vincent MF, et al. Myocardial protection by intracoronary nicardipine administration during percutaneous transluminal coronary angioplasty. Am J Cardiol 1987;59:1035-1040.

2356. Mager A, Strasberg B, Rechavia E, et al. Clinical significance and predisposing factors to symptomatic bradycardia and hypotension after PTCA. Am J Cardiol 1994;74:1085-1088.

2357. Maffrand JP, Herbert JM. Effect of clopidogrel and ticlopidine on the binding of [^{3}H]-2 Methyl-Thio-ADP to RAT platelets.

Thromb Haemost 1993;69:637.
2358. Tcheng JE. Effects of Integrelin™, A competitive platelet integrin glycoprotein IIb/IIIa inhibitor, in preventing ischemic complications of percutaneous coronary intervention. (Manuscript submitted for publication).

Local Drug Delivery

2359. Riessen R, Isner JM. Prospects for site-specific delivery of pharmacologic and molecular therapies. J Am Coll Cardiol 1994;23:1234-44.
2360. Lincoff AM, Topol EJ, Ellis SG. Local drug delivery for the prevention of restenosis: Fact, Fancy and Future. Circulation 1994;90:2070-2083.
2361. Wilensky RL, March KL, Gradus-Pizlo I, et al. Methods and devices for local drug delivery in coronary and peripheral arteries. Trends Cardiovasc Med 1993;3:163-170.
2362. Goldman B, Blanke H, Wolinsky H. Influence of pressure on permeability of normal and diseased muscular arteries to horseradish peroxidase. Atherosclerosis 1987;65:215-225.
2363. Lopez-Sendon J, Sobrino N, Gamallo C, Lorenzo A, et al. Locally delivered heparin reduces intimal hyperplasia and lumen stenosis following arterial balloon injury in swine. European Heart Journal 1993;14(supplement):191 (abstract).
2364. Meyer BJ, Fernandez-Ortiz A, Mailhac A, Falk E, et al. Local delivery of r-hirudin by a double-balloon perfusion catheter prevents mural thrombosis and minimizes platelet deposition after angioplasty. Circulation 1994;90:2474-2480.
2365. Jorgensen B, Tonnesen KH, Bulow L, et al. Femoral artery recanalisation with percutaneous angioplasty and segmentally enclosed plasminogen activator. Lancet 1989;1:1106-8.
2366. Nabel EG, Plautz G, Nabel GJ. Site-specific gene expression in vivo by direct gene transfer into the arterial wall. Science 1990;249:1285-8.
2367. Nabel EG, Yang Z, Liptay S, et al. Recombinant platelet-derived growth factor B gene expression in porcine arteries reduces intimal hyperplasia in vivo. J Clin Invest 1993;91:1822-9.
2368. Wolinsky H, Thung SN. Use of a perforated catheter to deliver concentrated heparin into the wall of the normal canine artery. J Am Coll Cardiol 1990;15:475-81.
2369. Wolinsky H, Lin CS. Use of the perforated balloon catheter to infuse marker substances into diseased coronary artery walls after experimental postmortem angioplasty. J Am Coll Cardiol 1991;17:174B-178B.
2370. Gimple LW, Gertz SD, Haber HL, Ragosta M, et al. Effect of chronic subcutaneous or intramural administration of heparin on femoral artery restenosis after balloon angioplasty in hypercholesterolemic rabbits. A quantitative angiographic and histopathological study. Circulation 1992;86:1536-46.
2371. Gellman J, Enger CD, Sigal SL, True LD, et al. The successful application of a local infusion angioplasty catheter in a rabbit model of focal femoral atherosclerosis. J Am Coll Cardiol 1990;15:164A (abstract).
2372. Muller DWM, Topol EJ, Abrams GD, Gallagher K, Ellis SG. Intramural methotrexate therapy for prevention of neointimal thickening after balloon angioplasty. J Am Coll Cardiol 1992;20:460-466.
2373. Franklin SM, Kalan JM, Currier JW, Mejias Y, Cody C, Haudenschild CC, Faxon DP. Effects of local delivery of doxorubicin or saline on restenosis following angioplasty in atherosclerotic rabbits. Circulation 1992;86:I-52 (abstract).
2374. Wilensky RL, Gradus-Pizlo I, Marck KL, Sandusky GE, Hathaway DR. Efficacy of local intramural injection of colchicine in reducing restenosis following angioplasty in the atherosclerotic rabbitt model. Circulation 1992;86:I-52 (abstract).
2375. Wilensky RL, March KL, Hathaway DR. Restenosis in an atherosclerotic rabbit model is reduced by thiol protease inhibitor. J Am Coll Cardiol 1991;17:286A (abstract).
2376. Hong MK, Bhatti T, Mathews BJ, Stark KS, et al. Locally delivered angiopeptin reduces intimal hyperplasia following balloon injury in rabbits. Circulation 1991;84:II-72 (abstract).
2377. Shi Y, Fard A, Galeo A, Hutchinson HG, et al. Transcatheter delivery of c-myc antisense oligomers reduces neointimal formation in a porcine model of coronary artery balloon injury. Circulation 1994;90:944-951.
2378. Flugelman MY, Jaklitsch MT, Newman KD, Casscell W, et al. Low level in vivo gene transfer into the arterial wall through a perforated balloon catheter. Circulation 1992;85:1110-7.
2379. Chapman GD, Lim CS, Gammon RS, et al. Gene transfer into coronary arteries of intact animals with a percutaneous balloon catheter. Circ Res 1992;71:27-33.
2380. Stadius ML, Collins C, Kernoff R. Local infusion balloon angioplasty to obviate restenosis compared with conventional balloon angioplasty in an experimental model of atherosclerosis. Am Heart J 1993;126:47-56.
2381. Lambert CR, Leone JE, Rowland SM. Local drug delivery catheters: functional comparison of porous and microporous designs. Cor Art Dis 1993;4:469-475.
2382. Herdeg C, Oberhoff M, Baumbach A, Kamenz J, et al. Application of porous balloon catheter with two different injection pressures: differences in outcome. European Heat Journal 1994:15 (Supplement):561 (abstract).
2383. French BA, Mazur W, Finnigan JP, Carter Grinstead W, et al. Gene transfer into intact porcine coronary arteries via infusion balloon catheter: influences of delivery volume and pressure. Circulation 1992;86:I-799 (abstract).
2384. Lambert CR, LeoneJ, Rowland S. The microporous balloon: A minimal trauma local drug delivery catheter. Circulation 1992;86:I-381 (abstract).
2385. Thomas CN, Robinson KA, Cipolla GD, Jones M, King SB. In-vivo local delivery of heparin to coronary arteries with a microporous infusion balloon. J Am Coll Cardiol 1994;23:187A (abstract).
2386. Lincoff AM, Furst JG, Penn MS, Lee P, MacIssac AI, Chisolm GM, Topol EJ, Ellis SG. Efficiency of solute transfer by a microporous balloon catheter in the porcine coronary model of arterial injury. J Am Coll Cardiol 1994;23:18A (abstract).
2387. Cumberland DC, Gunn J, Tsikaderis D, Arafa S, Ahsan A. Initial clinical experience of local drug delivery via a porous balloon during percutaneous coronary angioplasty. J Am Coll Cardiol 1994;23:186A (abstract).

2388. Fram DB, Aretz TA, Azrin MA, Mitchel JF, et al. Localized intramural drug delivery during balloon angioplasty using hydrogel-coated balloons and pressure-augmented diffusion. J Am Coll Cardiol 1994;23:1570-7.

2389. Azrin MA, Mitchel JF, Fram DB, Pedersen CA, et al. Decreased platelet deposition and smooth muscle cell proliferation following intramural heparin delivery with hydrogel-coated balloons. Circulation 1994:90:433-441.

2390. Mitchel JF, Azrin MA, Fram DB, Hong MK, et al. Inhibition of platelet deposition and lysis of intracoronary thrombus during balloon angioplasty with urokinase-coated hydrogel balloons. Circulation 1994:90:1979-88.

2391. Nunes GL, Hanson SR, King SB, Sahatjian RA, Scott NE. Local delivery of a synthetic antithrombin with a hydrogel-coated angioplasty balloon inhibits platelet-dependent thrombosis. J Am Coll Cardiol 1994;23:1578-83.

2392. Azrin MA, Mitchel JF, Pedersen C, Curley TM, et al. Inhibition of smooth muscle cell proliferation in-vivo following local delivery of antisense oligonucleotides during angioplasty. J Am Coll Cardiol 1994;23:396A (abstract).

2393. Riessen R, Rahimizadeh H, Blessing E, Takeshita S, et al. Arterial gene transfer using pure DNA applied directly to a hydrogel-coated angioplasty balloon. Hum Gene Ther 1993;4:749-58.

2394. Mitchel JF, Hirst JA, Kiernan FJ, Fram DB, et al. Local, intracoronary thrombolysis using urokinase-coated hydrogel balloons. Circulation 1994;90(4):I-493 (abstract).

2395. Fram DB, Mitchel JF, Azrin MA, Schwedick MW, et al. Local heparin delivery in porcine coronary arteries with the Dispatch catheter: delivery, washout and effect on platelet deposition following balloon angioplasty. Circulation 1994;90(4):I-493 (abstract).

2396. Mitchel JF, Fram DB, Palme DF, Foster R, et al. Enhanced local thrombolysis with urokinase using the Dispatch catheter. Circulation 1995;91:785-793.

2397. Camenzind E, di Mario C, de Jaegere P, de Feyter P, et al. Left ventricular and coronary hemodynamics during local drug delivery with a new infusion catheter: First experience in humans. European Heat Journal 1994;15 (Supplement):561 (abstract).

2398. McKay RG, Fram DB, Kiernan FJ, Hirst JA, et al. Localized thrombolysis of intracoronary thrombus using a new drug delivery system - The Dispatch catheter. Cathet Cardiovasc Diagn 1994;33:181-188.

2399. Mitchel JF, McKay RG. Treatment of acute stent thrombosis with local drug delivery systems. Cathet Cardiovasc Diagn 1995;34:149-154.

2400. Mitchel JF, Fram DB, Palme DF, Foster R, et al. Enhanced intracoronary thrombolysis using the Dispatch catheter. Circulation 1994;90(4):I-493 (abstract).

2401. Mitchel JF, Fram DB, Hirst JA, Kiernan FJ, et al. Local dissolution of intracoronary thrombus with urokinase using the Dispatch catheter: clinical studies. J Am Coll Cardiol 1995;25:347A (abstract).

2402. Hong MK, Wong SC, Farb A, Mehlman MD, et al. Feasibility and drug delivery efficiency of a new balloon angioplasty catheter capable of performing simultaneous local drug delivery. Cor Art Dis 1993;4:1023-1027.

2403. Hong MK, Wong SC, Haudenschild CC, Mehlman MD, et al. Local delivery with low molecular weight heparin by the Channelled balloon during simultaneous angioplasty in atherosclerotic rabbit iliac arteries. Circulation 1994;90(4):I-157 (abstract).

2404. Mitchel JF, Fram DB, Azrin MA, Bow L, et al. Localized intracoronary delivery of urokinase with the Channelled balloon: pharmacokinetics of drug delivery and washout. J Am Coll Cardiol 1995;25:347A (abstract).

2405. Feldman LJ, Steg PG, Zheng LP, Barry JJ, et al. Efficient percutaneous adenovirus-mediated arterial gene transfer using a channelled angioplasty balloon. Circulation 1994;90(4):I-20 (abstract).

2406. Thomas CN, Barry JJ, King SB, Scott NA. Local delivery with heparin with a PTCA infusion balloon inhibits platelet-dependent thrombosis. J Am Coll Cardiol 1994;23:4A (abstract).

2407. Kaplan AV, Kermode J, Grant G, Klein E, et al. Intramural delivery of marker agent in ex vivo and in vivo models using a novel drug delivery sleeve. J Am Coll Cardiol 1994;23:187A (abstract).

2408. Moura A, Lam JYT, Hebert D, Letchacovski G, et al. Local heparin delivery decreases the thrombogenicity of the balloon-injured artery. Circulation 1994;90(4):I-449 (abstract).

2409. Azrin MA, Mitchel JF, Bow LM, Alberghini TV, et al. Local delivery of urokinase to porcine coronary arteries using the Localmed infusion sleeve. J Am Coll Cardiol 1995;25:347A (abstract).

2410. Kaplan AV, Vandormael M, Bartorelli A, Hofman M, et al. Local delivery at the site of angioplasty with a novel drug delivery sleeve: Initial clinical series. J Am Coll Cardiol 1995;25:286A (abstract).

2411. Chien YW, Banga AK: Iontophoretic delivery of drugs: Overview of historical development. J Pharm Sci 1989;78:353-354.

2412. Fernandez-Ortiz A, Meyer BJ, Mailhac A, Falk E, et al. A new approach for local intravascular drug delivery. The iontophoretic balloon. Circulation 1994;89:1518-1522.

2413. Mitchel JF, Azrin MA, Schwedick MW, Bow LM, et al. Local delivery of heparin with a novel iontophoretic catheter - quantitative heparin delivery and effect on platelet deposition following balloon angioplasty. Circulation 1994;90(4):I-492 (abstract).

2414. Mitchel JF, Azrin MA, Fram DB, Feroze H, et al. Localized intracoronary delivery of heparin with iontophoresis. J Am Coll Cardiol 1995;25:285A (abstract).

— INDEX —

PHYSICIANS' PRESS

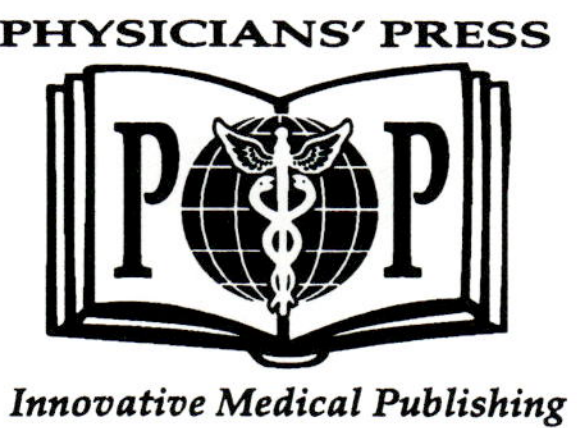

Innovative Medical Publishing

Other Services & Interventional Cardiology Publications from Physicians' Press

(see p. 723 for table of contents)

(see page 725 for order form)

(see page 725 for order form)

Detailed Step-by-Step Instruction:

9. **Deploy the Stent by Inflating the Delivery Balloon (Figure 8)**
    - Gradually apply positive pressure (3.0 mm stent: 8 ATM; 3.5 mm stent: 7 ATM; 4.0 mm stent: 6 ATM) to the delivery balloon while monitoring balloon expansion under fluoroscopy; the deployment inflation can be limited to 15 seconds if the balloon is fully inflated.

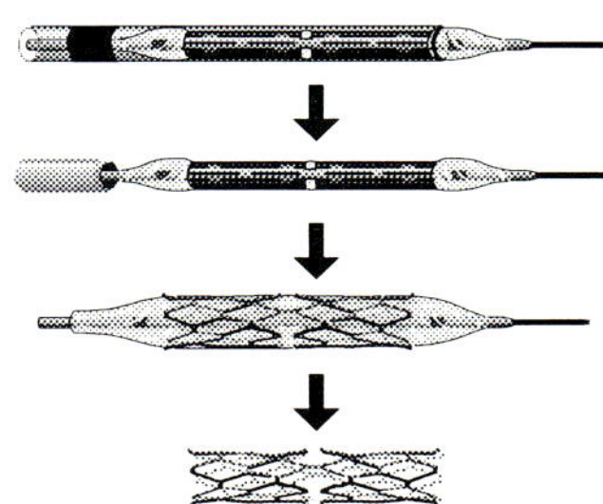

Figure 8. Stent Deployment Sequence

- Film the delivery balloon at maximal expansion.
- Apply negative pressure to the indeflator and ensure full deflation of the delivery balloon prior to its withdrawal.
- Remove the deflated balloon and delivery sheath while main-

2. **Test the Burr Outside the Patient**
    - Activate the burr and set the speed **outside** the body to 10,000-20,000 RPM higher than desired platform speed (Table 3); this compensates for additional friction encountered as the device passes through the guiding catheter and coronary artery.
    - **A 5-point checklist is crucial at this time:**
        1. *Verify the target burr speed is achieved (i.e., 10,000-20,000 RPM higher than desired platform speed).*
        2. *Confirm the advancer knob has full excursion (advancement and retraction).*
        3. *Ensure a continuous spray of flush at the tip of the sheath while the burr is activated.*
        4. *Confirm the guidewire is "locked" & immobile during burr rotation.*
        5. *Pre-advance the advancer by 2 cm, and "lock-in" this position before inserting the burr into the guiding catheter.*

Table 3. Recommended Rotablator Speeds

Burr Size (mm)	Platform Speed (RPM)	Ablation Speed (RPM)
1.25	180,000	150-180,000
1.50	180,000	150-180,000
1.75	180,000	150-180,000
2.00	180,000	150-180,000
2.15	160,000	140-180,000

Lesion-Specific Techniques & more...

Angulation < 45°

Stenting is readily accomplished in lesions with mild-to-moderate angulation. Useful tips include strong guiding catheter position and the use of extra-support guidewires. Use of overlapping disarticulated half-stents (Figure 9) may avoid placing the articulation site at the angle vertex.

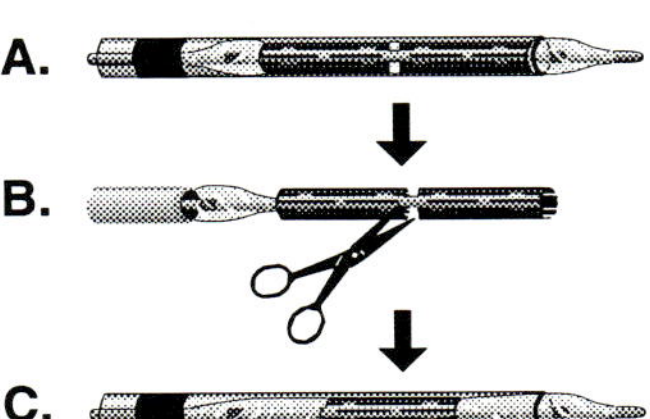

Figure 9. Technique for Disarticulating the Palmaz-Schatz Stent

A. *Remove the Palmaz-Schatz stent delivery system from its package.*
B. *Retract the stent delivery sheath, and slide the stent forward on the delivery balloon until the articulation is freely exposed. Cut the stent at the articulation using sterile scissors. Save the half-*

Angulated Lesions

Severely angulated lesions (>60°) should not be routinely considered for the Rotablator. For angulated lesions that are highly calcified, initial debulking may be considered, using a burr-to-artery ratio of 0.5-0.6. All angulated lesions need to be assessed for guidewire bias (Figure 5, p. 65), which may result in tangential ablation. As shown in Figure 7, lesions on the outer curve may be better suited for the Rotablator than lesions on the inner curve.

NOTE: To minimize guidewire bias and the risk of perforation, select a final burr-to-artery ratio ≤ 0.6 and employ a stepped-burr approach. Gentle forward advancement using a "pecking" motion is required to decrease tangential cutting. Burr deceleration may be due to the lesion itself, vessel angulation, or both.

WARNING: Continuous forward pressure ("leaning" on the lesion) increases the risk of vessel perforation and should be avoided.

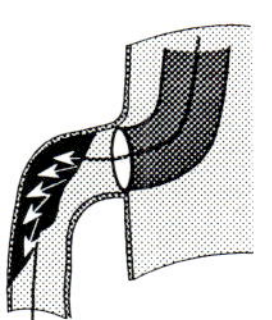

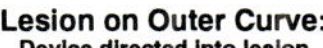

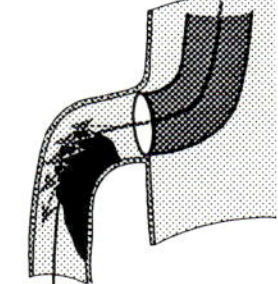

Lesion on Outer Curve: Device directed into lesion

Lesion on Inner Curve: Device deflected into disease-free wall

(See order form on page 725 for information)

Special Emphasis on Stents

STENT DESIGN

Balloon-Expandable Stents

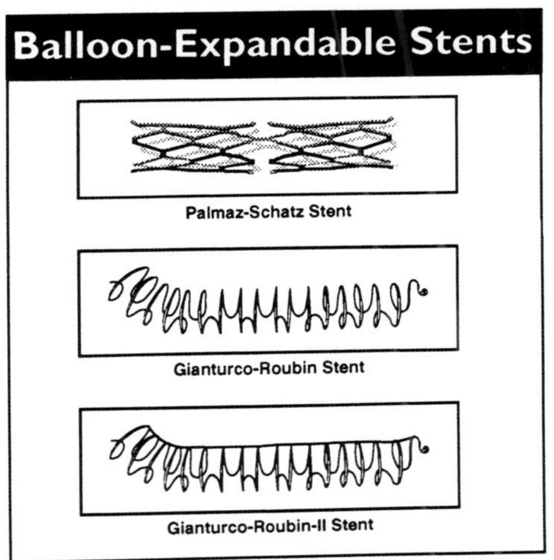

TRIAL RESULTS

Benestent-I Trial: I Year Follow-up

516 patients with stable angina & a de novo coronary lesion randomized to Palmaz-Schatz stent or PTCA.

	Stent (%)	PTCA (%)	*P*
Death	1.2	0.8	NS
MI	5.0	4.2	NS
CABG	6.9	5.1	NS
Repeat PTCA	10	21	0.001
Combined Endpoint	23	32	0.004

CCL: Benefit of elective stenting of native coronaries is maintained at 1 year.

JACC 1996: 255: 2-7

SEE NEXT PAGE FOR MORE DETAILS!

LESION-SPECIFIC TECHNIQUES

Stenting of Aorto-Ostial Lesions

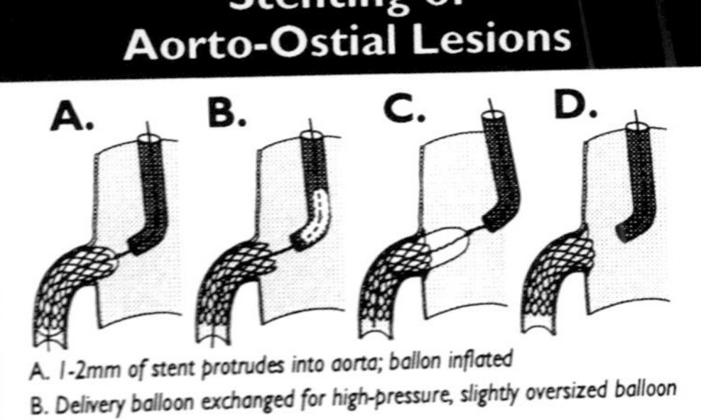

A. 1-2mm of stent protrudes into aorta; ballon inflated
B. Delivery balloon exchanged for high-pressure, slightly oversized balloon
C. Proximal stent flared
D. Final result

Also Includes

- **Figures of equipment and technique**

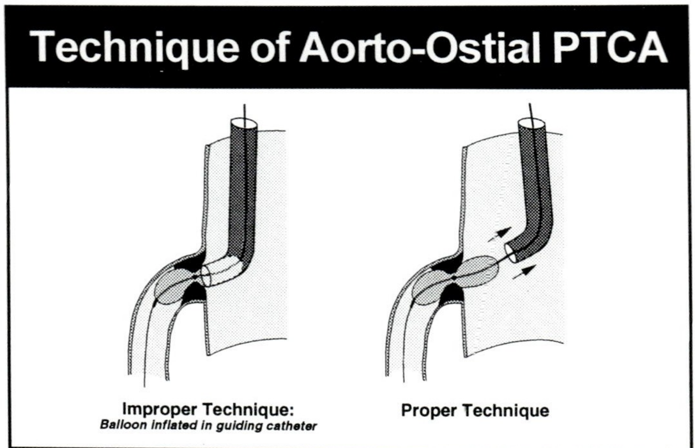

PTCA *vs* CABG for Multivessel Disease: *The BARI Trial*

5 year outcome	All patients PTCA	All patients CABG	Diabetics PTCA	Diabetics CABG
Death	14	11	35	19*
Repeat revasc.	54	8*	62	8*

*$p < 0.05$

Conclusion: CABG may be preferred over PTCA in diabetics. However, data do not reflect improving PTCA results and use of stents.

- **1996 Trial results**
- **Triage and management algorithms**

- **Angiograms, photos, and photomicro-graphs**

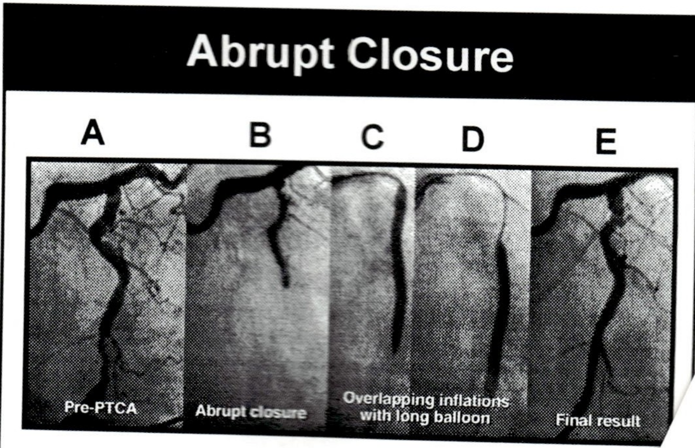

TABLE OF CONTENTS – *Manual of Interventional Cardiology*
LIST OF LECTURES – *Slide Series*

I. **Simple & Complex Angioplasty:** PTCA Equipment & Technique • Brachial & Radial Approach • Single & Multivessel Angioplasty • High-Risk Intervention • PTCA for Unstable Ischemic Syndromes • LV Dysfunction • Patient Characteristics

II. **Coronary Intervention by Lesion Morphology & Location:** Overview of Interventional Devices • Intracoronary Thrombus • Bifurcation Lesions • Tortuosity & Angulation • Calcified Lesions • Eccentric Lesions • Ostial Lesions • Long Lesions • Chronic Total Occlusions • Coronary Artery Bypass Grafts • PTCA Exotica

III. **Complications:** Coronary Artery Spasm • Dissection & Acute Closure • No-reflow • Perforation • Emergency Bypass Surgery • Restenosis • Medical & Peripheral Complications

IV. **New Interventional Devices:** Coronary Stents • Rotablator Atherectomy • Directional Coronary Atherectomy • TEC Atherectomy • Excimer Laser Coronary Angioplasty • Intravascular Ultrasound • Coronary Angioscopy • Doppler Blood Flow

V. **Miscellaneous Topics:** Adjunctive Pharmacotherapy • Local Drug Delivery • Peripheral & Visceral Intervention • Balloon Valvuloplasty • Special Considerations for Cath Lab Personnel

(see page 725 for order form)

Fax / Mail Order Form

Fax: (810) 642-4949

ITEM	DESCRIPTION	PRICE	ITEM	DESCRIPTION	PRICE
1A	Manual of Interventional Cardiology: *Soft Cover*	84.95	4B	Slide Series: PTCA Miniset (175 slides) *See I, p. 723 for list of lectures*	299.00
1B	Manual of Interventional Cardiology: *Hard Cover*	99.95	4C	Slide Series: New Devices Miniset (175 slides) *See IV, p. 723 for lectures*	299.00
2	The Device Guide	39.95	5	Interventional Library: *Manual + Device Guide + "Tough Calls!"*	229.95* (save $25)
3	"Tough Calls!" in Interventional Cardiology	129.95	6	Interventional Library + Slide Series (entire set of 650 slides)	899.95* (save $105)
4A	Slide Series (Entire set; 650 slides)	750.00	* Price includes Soft Cover Manual; add $15 for Hard Cover Manual		

***Sales Tax*:** Michigan residents add 6%; Canadians add 7% GST

***Shipping & Handling*:** Charges based on weight of shipment & destination

- *USA:* Orders sent out within 24 hours by UPS: 1 book - $7; add $4 for each addtl book; Slide Series - $10. Overnight delivery - extra charge.
- *Outside USA*: **Express air carrier (FEDEX, UPS, DHL)** — usually arrives 3-5 days after order is placed: 1 book - $60; add $30 for each additional book; Slide Series - $80. **US Postal Service** — arrives in 2-4 weeks: 1 book - $30; add $20 for each addtl. book; Slide Series not available by this route.

ITEM	QUANTITY	TOTAL
Sales Tax; see above		
Shipping: see above		
TOTAL (U.S. Dollars)		

METHOD OF PAYMENT

☐ Check enclosed (U.S. dollars from U.S. bank)

☐ Credit Card: ☐ Visa ☐ MasterCard ☐ American Express

Credit Card #:

Expiration date:

Signature:

Name & Address *(Please print) (We cannot deliver to PO Box):*

Phone number:
(important)

Fax number:
(if available)

3 Ways To Order:

Mail To:
Physicians' Press
555 So. Woodward Ave, # 1409
Birmingham, MI, USA 48009

To Order by Phone:
USA: (800) 642-5494
Outside USA: (810) 645-6443

To Order by Fax:
(810) 642-4949

Fax / Mail Order Form

Fax: (810) 642-4949

ITEM	DESCRIPTION	PRICE	ITEM	DESCRIPTION	PRICE
1A	Manual of Interventional Cardiology: *Soft Cover*	84.95	4B	Slide Series: PTCA Miniset (175 slides) *See I, p. 723 for list of lectures*	299.00
1B	Manual of Interventional Cardiology: *Hard Cover*	99.95	4C	Slide Series: New Devices Miniset (175 slides) *See IV, p. 723 for lectures*	299.00
2	The Device Guide	39.95	5	Interventional Library: *Manual + Device Guide + "Tough Calls!"*	229.95* (save $25)
3	"Tough Calls!" in Interventional Cardiology	129.95	6	Interventional Library + Slide Series (entire set of 650 slides)	899.95* (save $105)
4A	Slide Series (Entire set; 650 slides)	750.00	* Price includes Soft Cover Manual; add $15 for Hard Cover Manual		

***Sales Tax*:** Michigan residents add 6%; Canadians add 7% GST

***Shipping & Handling*:** Charges based on weight of shipment & destination

- *USA:* Orders sent out within 24 hours by UPS: 1 book - $7; add $4 for each addtl book; Slide Series - $10. Overnight delivery - extra charge.
- *Outside USA*: **Express air carrier (FEDEX, UPS, DHL)** — usually arrives 3-5 days after order is placed: 1 book - $60; add $30 for each additional book; Slide Series - $80. **US Postal Service** — arrives in 2-4 weeks: 1 book - $30; add $20 for each addtl. book; Slide Series not available by this route.

ITEM	QUANTITY	TOTAL	METHOD OF PAYMENT
			☐ Check enclosed (U.S. dollars from U.S. bank)
			☐ Credit Card: ☐ Visa ☐ MasterCard ☐ American Express
			Credit Card #:
Sales Tax; see above			Expiration date:
Shipping: see above			Signature:
TOTAL (U.S. Dollars)			

Name & Address *(Please print) (We cannot deliver to PO Box):*

Phone number:
(important)

Fax number:
(if available)

3 Ways To Order:

Mail To:
Physicians' Press
555 So. Woodward Ave, # 1409
Birmingham, MI, USA 48009

To Order by Phone:
USA: (800) 642-5494
Outside USA: (810) 645-6443

To Order by Fax:
(810) 642-4949

Fax / Mail Order Form

Fax: (810) 642-4949

ITEM	DESCRIPTION	PRICE	ITEM	DESCRIPTION	PRICE
1A	Manual of Interventional Cardiology: *Soft Cover*	84.95	4B	Slide Series: PTCA Miniset (175 slides) *See I, p. 723 for list of lectures*	299.00
1B	Manual of Interventional Cardiology: *Hard Cover*	99.95	4C	Slide Series: New Devices Miniset (175 slides) *See IV, p. 723 for lectures*	299.00
2	The Device Guide	39.95	5	Interventional Library: *Manual + Device Guide + "Tough Calls!"*	229.95* (save $25)
3	"Tough Calls!" in Interventional Cardiology	129.95	6	Interventional Library + Slide Series (entire set of 650 slides)	899.95* (save $105)
4A	Slide Series (Entire set; 650 slides)	750.00	* Price includes Soft Cover Manual; add $15 for Hard Cover Manual		

Sales Tax: Michigan residents add 6%; Canadians add 7% GST
Shipping & Handling: Charges based on weight of shipment & destination

- *USA:* Orders sent out within 24 hours by UPS: 1 book - $7; add $4 for each addtl book; Slide Series - $10. Overnight delivery - extra charge.
- *Outside USA*: **Express air carrier (FEDEX, UPS, DHL)** — usually arrives 3-5 days after order is placed: 1 book - $60; add $30 for each additional book; Slide Series - $80. **US Postal Service** — arrives in 2-4 weeks: 1 book - $30; add $20 for each addtl. book; Slide Series not available by this route.

ITEM	QUANTITY	TOTAL
Sales Tax; see above		
Shipping: see above		
TOTAL (U.S. Dollars)		

METHOD OF PAYMENT

☐ Check enclosed (U.S. dollars from U.S. bank)

☐ Credit Card: ☐ Visa ☐ MasterCard ☐ American Express

Credit Card #:

Expiration date:

Signature:

Name & Address *(Please print) (We cannot deliver to PO Box):*

Phone number:
(important)

Fax number:
(if available)

3 Ways To Order:

Mail To:
Physicians' Press
555 So. Woodward Ave, # 1409
Birmingham, MI, USA 48009

To Order by Phone:
USA: (800) 642-5494
Outside USA: (810) 645-6443

To Order by Fax:
(810) 642-4949

GWUMC
P176H5